NEONATAL INTENSIVE CARE NURSING

This new edition of *Neonatal Intensive Care Nursing* is comprehensive, up to date and evidence based. With more pedagogical features and a practice-focused approach, this is an essential text for nurses and allied health professionals caring for sick newborn infants.

Neonatal Intensive Care Nursing focuses on the common problems and related care occurring within the neonatal specialty. It is thoroughly updated throughout, with three entirely new chapters on antenatal and perinatal care, continuing care beyond the neonatal unit, and specific diagnostic neonatal practice. There is new content on psychologically informed care of the family, community-based care, perinatal optimisation, health inequalities, diagnostic procedures, drug mechanisms, and more. The accessible and interactive approach used in the book enables readers to recognise, rationalise, and understand clinical problems using an evidence-based approach. Divided into four parts, the book provides an overview of neonatal care and a detailed look at the physical and emotional wellbeing of the neonate and family, a range of clinical aspects of neonatal care, and key practices and procedures. The book's web-based companion includes online resources, case studies with answer guides, and learning activities, and can be found at www.routledge.com/cw/petty

Neonatal Intensive Care Nursing will be essential reading for both new and experienced nurses, allied health professionals, and students learning about neonatal care, including those undertaking qualifications in the neonatal specialism and pre-registration students taking relevant modules or placements.

Julia Petty is an adult, paediatric, and neonatal nurse who trained and worked as a practice educator at Great Ormond Street hospital before becoming a senior lecturer at City University, London, UK. There, she co-led the neonatal nursing education portfolio for 12 years before moving to the University of Hertfordshire in 2013. Her current role is Associate Professor (learning and teaching) and Senior Lecturer in Children's Nursing.

Lisa Kaiser has been a neonatal nurse in the UK since 2008, having gained her paediatric nursing diploma in Vienna in 2007. During this time, Lisa has developed extensive clinical expertise across Level 1, 2, and 3 neonatal units, including specialist surgical neonatal care. She qualified as an advanced neonatal nurse practitioner in 2014 and gained her MSc in 2019.

Glenys Boxwell (Connelly) was an advanced neonatal nurse practitioner for Plymouth Hospitals NHS Trust. She was previously a senior lecturer at Homerton College, Cambridge, and has now retired from clinical practice. Glenys was the editor of *Neonatal Intensive Care Nursing* for the 1st and 2nd editions in 2000 and 2010, respectively, continuing as part of the editing team for the 3rd edition, published in 2020. We are very grateful to Glenys for the original development of this key, widely reputed neonatal nursing care textbook that has formed the basis of this revised 4th edition.

NEONATAL INTENSIVE CARE NURSING FOURTH EDITION

Edited by Julia Petty, Lisa Kaiser
and Glenys Boxwell

Routledge
Taylor & Francis Group
LONDON AND NEW YORK

Designed cover image: Getty Images

Fourth edition published 2027
by Routledge
4 Park Square, Milton Park, Abingdon, Oxon, OX14 4RN

and by Routledge
605 Third Avenue, New York, NY 10158

Routledge is an imprint of the Taylor & Francis Group, an informa business

First edition published by Routledge 2000
Third edition published by Routledge 2020

British Library Cataloguing-in-Publication Data
A catalogue record for this book is available from the British Library

ISBN: 978-1-032-96951-0 (hbk)
ISBN: 978-1-032-96935-0 (pbk)
ISBN: 978-1-003-59140-5 (ebk)

DOI: 10.4324/9781003591405

Typeset in Akziden Grotesk
by Apex CoVantage, LLC

Access the companion website: www.routledge.com/cw/petty

In memory of Dr Oliver Rackham.

His unwavering dedication to babies and their families, his commitment to supporting and inspiring colleagues, and his enduring passion for excellence in neonatal care left a lasting impact on all who knew him. His legacy continues to guide us and shape the care we provide.

CONTENTS

FIGURES

TABLES

ABOUT THE EDITORS

Dr Julia Petty Julia is an adult, paediatric, and neonatal nurse who trained and worked as a practice educator at Great Ormond Street hospital before becoming a senior lecturer at City University, London, UK. There, she co-led the neonatal nursing education portfolio for 12 years before moving to University of Hertfordshire in 2013. Her current role is Associate Professor (learning and teaching) and Senior Lecturer in Children's Nursing. Julia leads a range of pre-registration children's nursing modules, including curricula relating to nursing research, communication, and neonatal care. She is a principal fellow of the Higher Education Academy and holds a National Teaching Fellowship (NTF). Julia is a newborn life support instructor for the UK Resuscitation Council and a Trustee of the UK Neonatal Nurses Association and is on the board of the Council of International Neonatal Nurses. Julia combines research with her education role and has a wide range of book, chapter, and peer-reviewed journal publications as both author and editor.

Lisa Kaiser Having gained her paediatric nursing diploma in Vienna in 2007, Lisa has been a neonatal nurse in the UK since 2008. During this time, Lisa has developed extensive clinical expertise across Level 1, 2, and 3 neonatal units, including specialist surgical neonatal care. She qualified as an advanced neonatal nurse practitioner in 2014 and gained her MSc in 2019. Based in North Wales, Lisa's role combines advanced clinical practice with a strong commitment to multiprofessional education at both local and national levels. She is an experienced instructor for Neonatal Life Support (NLS), Advanced Resuscitation of the Newborn Infant (ARNI), and Multiprofessional Neonatal Emergency Training (MoNET) and contributes to wider service development and workforce training. Lisa is actively engaged in neonatal research and has held key leadership roles within major studies. She served as Principal Investigator for the SurfON trial and is currently Co-Principal Investigator for the PALOH-UK study.

Glenys Boxwell (Connelly) was an advanced neonatal nurse practitioner for Plymouth Hospitals NHS Trust. She was previously a senior lecturer at Homerton

College, Cambridge and has now retired from clinical practice. Glenys was the editor of *Neonatal Intensive Care Nursing* for the 1st and 2nd editions in 2000 and 2010, respectively, continuing as part of the editing team for the 3rd edition, published in 2020. We are very grateful to Glenys for the original development of this key, widely reputed neonatal nursing care textbook that has formed the basis of this revised 4th edition.

CONTRIBUTORS

Natalie Anders qualified with a BSc in children's nursing before specialising in neonatal care, gaining the 'qualified-in-speciality' (QIS) and Enhancing Neonatal Nursing qualifications, as well as a master's in advanced neonatal nursing. She has extensive experience from Band 5 nurse to advanced neonatal nurse practitioner (ANNP), including roles in a neonatal surgical intensive care unit and transport team. Since 2023, she has worked for the North West Neonatal Operational Delivery Network (ODN), initially leading a project to develop a sustainable screening model for retinopathy of prematurity and now serving as Senior Network Educator for 22 units across the region. She has served as nurse representative on the BAPM executive committee, championing the neonatal nursing voice nationally.

Jo Bennett has been a neonatal nurse for 35 years. For the majority of this time, she worked on a tertiary NICU. Always having an interest in family support both on the neonatal unit and after discharge home, she became a senior sister for transitional care, neonatal outreach, palliative care, and bereavement care. She initiated and led a 7-day/week neonatal outreach service and collaborated in developing a bereavement support service for families experiencing a loss on the neonatal unit. Jo now works for the South West Neonatal ODN as Lead Nurse for Transition. She is also a professional nurse advocate. In 2022 Jo was honoured to be named the Neonatal Nurses Association Neonatal Nurse of the Year.

Rebecca Chilvers is a consultant clinical psychologist with extensive experience in working with neonatal families and staff teams in the NHS and independent practice. She is currently the Lead Psychologist for the East of England Neonatal ODN and the author of a new book to support neonatal parents: *Not Alone in NICU: A Compassionate Companion for Parents of a Baby in Neonatal Care.*

Alexandra Connolly is a clinical lead neonatal speech and language therapist at University College London Hospital. She is also one of the SLT leads for London's Neonatal ODN and is training to be a lactation consultant. Alex is passionate about quality improvement and cultural change in neonatal feeding practice. She champions cue-based, psychologically informed feeding approaches for babies and families.

Jo Cookson is a senior neonatal lecturer at Keele University with a clinical background in midwifery and neonatal intensive care. She holds a BSc in women's health and an MA in medical ethics and law. Jo leads a well-established portfolio of pre- and post-registration education programmes and contributes to national neonatal education workstreams. Her professional interests include perinatal bereavement and neonatal ethics. She is currently leading initiatives to support student midwives in managing the emotional demands of clinical practice.

Julia Cooper: With over 30 years in neonatal nursing, Julia specialises in familycentred and integrated care, leading regional initiatives that strengthen support for parents of sick and preterm babies. As Lead Care Coordinator for the East of England Neonatal ODN, she works across networks to embed best practice, implement national frameworks, and advocate for families moving closer to home so their neonatal journey can continue safely. Julia is passionate about removing barriers and ensuring support extends beyond the neonatal unit, helping each family achieve the strongest and most fulfilling dynamic possible.

Rebecca Drescher has been an advanced neonatal nurse practitioner for 7 years. She obtained her bachelor's degree in paediatric nursing and went on to pursue her master of science. She is a dedicated healthcare professional specialising in the care of premature and critically ill newborns. She provides compassionate, evidence-based care while supporting families through every stage of their neonatal journey.

Elen Elias has been qualified as a physiotherapist since 1992, working mostly in paediatrics and specialising in neonates from 2017. She completed her advanced clinical practice master's degree at Bangor University in 2021. Elen works on the neonatal unit at Ysbyty Glan Clwyd in North Wales, demonstrating a strong passion for neonatal physiotherapy and a commitment to delivering the highest quality care for babies and their families. She is a member of the national Association of Paediatric Physiotherapy neonatal committee.

Dr Ramon Fernandez is an associate professor and honorary consultant in neonatology based at the Trevor Mann Baby Unit, University Hospitals Sussex NHS Foundation Trust, Brighton. The Neonatal Department includes the region's tertiary surgical Neonatal Intensive Care Unit, serving the Kent, Surrey, and Sussex network. He has been a consultant neonatologist since 2006 and has held the role of lead for clinical governance for much of his consultant career. Since 2017, he has also worked as a clinical academic at Brighton and Sussex Medical School.

Sarah Fitchett is a neonatal lecturer at the University of Salford. She is the module lead for the QIS (Emergency and Intensive Care of the Newborn Module) and leads on post-registration neonatal education and the development of neonatal education components for the pre-registration midwifery programmes. Her clinical career in neonates commenced in 1999.

Lynette Forsythe leads the dietetic service for newborn care across Manchester University NHS Foundation Trust, overseeing one Level 3 unit and two Level 2 units. She has worked clinically for over 10 years at St Mary's Hospital, the Level 3 surgical NICU. Lynette is also the lead dietitian for the North-West Neonatal ODN. She is passionate about improving the nutritional outcomes for babies in the neonatal unit and longer-term post discharge.

Dr Deanna Gibbs is an occupational therapist and clinical academic for nursing and allied health professional (AHP) research for neonates and children at Barts Health NHS Trust. She is an honorary reader at Queen Mary University London. Her research focuses on the influence of parent psychological wellbeing on engagement in caregiving and parent self-efficacy in the NICU. Deanna is certified as a neonatal therapist and specialises in neonatal touch and massage. She is a senior trainer for the Brazelton Centre of Great Britain and a mentor for the FINE UK programme.

Radica Hardyal is a programme leader and associate subject lead at the University of Hertfordshire. A nurse, midwife, and educator with over 30 years of experience, she has held several clinical and leadership roles across healthcare and higher education. Her research interests focus on maternal critical illness. Alongside her educational leadership, she has led the development and implementation of strategies to advance equality, diversity, and inclusion within higher education. Her professional aims are to ensure that all women, regardless of risk status, have a positive and empowering birth experience, and to reduce and ultimately eliminate awarding gaps in higher education.

Phillip Harniess is a post-doctoral clinical academic physiotherapist with expertise in early identification and early intervention in childhood-onset disability. Apart from his PhD, he holds a BSc in physiotherapy and MSc in neurorehabilitation and is an associate fellow of the Higher Education Academy. Phill's research interests broadly include child neurodisability, family-centred care, and parent carer wellbeing – explored using participatory qualitative methods through an applied health sociological lens. He is currently undertaking a process evaluation study within the CHildren's Early Self-care Support (CHESS) study for children with neurodisability.

Jenni Jones is an advanced neonatal nurse practitioner currently working at Glan Clwyd Hospital in North Wales. She completed her MSc in advanced clinical practice in 2023, during which she developed a particular interest in neonatal pain assessment and management. She divides her clinical time between the neonatal unit and the North Wales neonatal transport service. As part of her work with the Welsh Risk Pool, Jenni has been involved in establishing the Multiprofessional Neonatal Emergency Training course in North Wales.

Tracey Jones has been a qualified nurse since 1996, having roles in education and senior clinical management. She is an independent prescriber educated to master's level and is a senior fellow for the higher education academy. Tracey has worked as a senior lecturer in nursing at the University of Manchester for over 20 years, leading the neonatal intensive care course, the enhancing neonatal nursing course, and the NIPE course. Her publications include *The Student Guide for Newborn Infant Physical Examination*. Tracey is a board member of the Council of International Neonatal Nurses and chair of the education committee.

Lesley Kilby qualified as an advanced neonatal nurse practitioner at Southampton University in 2004 and is currently working at Milton Keynes University Hospital. Prior to this she worked in Level 2 and Level 3 Units in London, East of England, and Thames Valley and Wessex Networks. Lesley also works with the University of Bedfordshire to continue to develop and deliver the QIS course. Lesley has contributed to midwifery textbooks relating to home births. She is a recognised STABLE and newborn life support (NLS) instructor and fellow of the Institute of Higher Education.

Alex Mancini is the National Lead Nurse for Neonatal Palliative Care, leading the UK's National Neonatal Palliative Care Programme. She has played a key role in developing national and international guidelines, including palliative care pathways, and is Co-Chair of the BAPM Framework Recognising Uncertainty. Alex is widely published and lead editor of the *Nurses Textbook in Neonatal Palliative Care*. She is joint chair of an NHSE/BAPM national scoping project on neonatal palliative care in England, Alex provides senior peer support, reflective practice, and wellbeing training, chairs several national networks and collaborates closely with hospice, palliative care and bereavement groups to strengthen shared learning and peer support nationally.

Nicky McCarthy is a senior advanced neonatal nurse practitioner at University Hospitals Sussex NHS Trust with over 20 years' experience in neonatal clinical practice, education and research. She is clinically recognised as an expert in neonatal intensive care and neonatal transport. Her published research explores neonatal life support outcomes, team dynamics, and professional influences on performance, with particular expertise in human factors, debriefing, and civility. An RCUK course director and ERC faculty member, she presents nationally and internationally and is committed to advancing nursing leadership, education, and multidisciplinary collaboration in neonatal care.

Linda McDonald is a senior ANNP who began her nursing career as a critical care children's nurse in Sydney, Australia. After relocating to London, she worked in PICU and CICU at Guy's Hospital before moving into neonatal nursing at St Thomas'. With over 25 years' experience in neonatal care – including 14 years in tertiary centres in London and Cambridge – Linda has held roles such as senior sister, clinical educator, neonatal transport nurse, and lecturer practitioner. She is now based in Worcester, practising as a senior ANNP within the tier 2 medical rota.

Marina Loarce Montero qualified as a nurse in 2013 from the Universidad Autónoma de Madrid. She subsequently completed her training as an advanced neonatal nurse practitioner at the University of Southampton in 2024 and is also a qualified non-medical prescriber. Marina currently holds the role of ANNP lead for the North Wales Neonatal Transport Service, where she contributes to the leadership, coordination, and delivery of specialist neonatal transport care. In addition to her clinical and leadership responsibilities, Marina organises and delivers medical and neonatal transport education, supporting the ongoing development of the regional workforce.

Rebecca Murphy is Clinical Lead Neonatal Speech and Language Therapist specialising in neonatal feeding and early communication development. She is currently completing a PhD investigating feeding decision-making in infants receiving nasal high flow, with the aim of improving outcomes for medically vulnerable neonatal populations. Her work brings together clinical expertise and research to advance evidence-based practice and drive improvements in neonatal care.

Debra Nicholson is an advanced neonatal nurse practitioner at Lancashire Teaching Hospitals NHS Foundation Trust with 24 years of experience in neonatal care. She has worked as a clinical facilitator within her trust and the North West Neonatal Operational Delivery Network supporting education development within neonatal services. Her professional interests include neonatal pain management, optimisation, and point of care ultrasound. She has recently become a peer reviewer for the *Journal of Neonatal Nursing*.

Katherine Noble has been a qualified nurse since 2002 with roles in neonatal clinical nursing, then education and senior clinical management. She is educated to master's level and is a course director for NLS, instructing on both NLS and GIC courses. Katherine has worked in multiple level 3 NICUs within the North West and has previously been a long-standing chair of the managers' and educators' group in Lancashire and South Cumbria, having an active part within the North West Neonatal Operational Delivery Network. Katherine has worked at matron level in a NICU but is currently one of the neonatal nurse education and governance leads.

Jonathan O'Keeffe holds a BSc in adult nursing, a higher diploma in children's nursing, specialist neonatal qualifications, and a MSc in advanced clinical practice (neonatal). With 16 years of neonatal experience, including 10 years as an ANNP, Jonathan has developed extensive expertise in advanced neonatal care. His career has been shaped by a longstanding passion for cardiology, reflected in roles at University Hospitals Sussex NHS Foundation Trust and the Evelina Children's Hospital, where he pursued this specialty interest. Education and knowledge sharing are central to his advanced practice, underpinning his commitment to developing the profession and supporting future clinicians.

Kelly Phizacklea is a previous neonatal parent herself who now works at a local and regional level as the East of England ODN Family Engagement Lead. She also works at a national level as a neonatal service user voice representative within the NHS England Maternity and Neonatal Programme and Specialised Commissioning team. Within her roles, she aims to support the embedding of the neonatal service user voice. She is passionate about supporting staff and services to consider the whole perinatal journey for neonatal families.

Katy Powis is the Lead Neonatal Educator at Northampton General Hospital with 25 years of neonatal nursing experience. She has worked as course lead for the Qualified in Specialty neonatal course at University of Bedfordshire, where she completed a master's degree in medical education. Katy has a deep passion for providing the best possible care to babies but also to develop staff to do the same.

Dr Sabin Roy began his paediatric medical training in 2006 in India, where he completed his master's in paediatrics and fellowship in neonatology. He subsequently undertook further paediatric and neonatal training in the United Kingdom and achieved fellowship of the Royal College of Paediatrics and Child Health. He has been working as a consultant neonatologist in the UK since 2024, with a special clinical interest in neonatal respiratory diseases. His professional focus includes advancing evidence-based respiratory care, optimising ventilation strategies, and improving outcomes in bronchopulmonary dysplasia.

Rhian Smith studied for her bachelor of nursing at the University of Wales College of Medicine in Cardiff and then worked in a variety of paediatric clinical areas before returning to North Wales in 2001 when her neonatal career began. She undertook QIS and enhanced nursing practice courses before her ANNP training at the University of Southampton, subsequently establishing the ANNP service in North Wales in 2011. Her areas of interest are transitional care, MatNeo quality improvement, and teaching on a variety of Resuscitation Council (UK) courses. She was the national lead nurse for the PERIPrem Cymru programme and has contributed to Wales-wide and UK-wide working groups.

Cassie Swire is a neonatal nurse with over 17 years of experience in neonatal care across level 2 and level 3 neonatal intensive care settings. Cassie's clinical background includes neonatal intensive care, neonatal surgery, clinical education, and clinical governance, providing a broad perspective on the delivery and development of high-quality neonatal services. Cassie is currently a children's and young people's lecturer at the University of Manchester, where she leads postgraduate teaching in neonatal care as unit lead for the Intensive Care of the Neonate module. She holds a degree in children's and young people's nursing, a postgraduate certificate in professional education (PGCE), and a master of science in advanced leadership for professional practice (nursing).

Patrick Turton is currently the Lead Nurse for the South West Neonatal Advice and Retrieval (SoNAR) service. Patrick has experience of working in both neonatal and paediatric intensive care, as well as for neonatal and paediatric critical care transport teams.

Peter Venables is a clinical pharmacist based in Wrexham Maelor Hospital. Having qualified from Cardiff University in 2011, he has spent his career to date based in Betsi Cadwaladr University Health Board. For the past decade, amongst other specialties, he has worked in paediatric and neonatal medicine.

He is currently working towards his Advanced Practice accreditation with the Royal Pharmaceutical Society. His particular interests are in nephrology and critical care.

Lynne Wainwright trained as an adult and children's nurse at Great Ormond Street and Hammersmith Hospitals and undertook her neonatal QIS education at King's College London. She worked clinically in NICU and then as a neonatal practice development nurse prior to her current role as a senior lecturer in children's and neonatal nursing and faculty senior tutor at King's College London.

ACKNOWLEDGEMENTS

The rewriting and updating of this book have been a team effort. All the contributors are thanked and commended for their involvement while engaging in work responsibilities and busy personal lives and commitments. We would also like to acknowledge, where applicable, all previous contributors from previous editions of the book, as follows:

1st and 2nd editions: Glenys Boxwell, the previous editor and originator of this book, Fiona Hutchinson; Tilly Reid, Yvonne Freer; Sue Turrill, Pauline Fellows, Simone Jollye; David Summers; Rosarie Lombard; Anja Hale; Jackie Dent; Katie McKenna, Dee Beresford, Elizabeth Harding; Beverley Guard, Rachel Homer; Stevie Boyd, Anne Aspin; Anne Mitchell; Catherine Hall; Peter Mullholland, Joan Cameron, Helen Frizell.

Previous contributors from the 3rd edition: Breidge Boyle, Liam Brennan, Yvonne Cousins, Liz Crathern, Erica Everett, Karen Hoover, Emma Kyte, Marie Lindsay-Sutherland, Alison Mitchell, Heather Maxwell, Sharon Nurse, Katie O'Connell-Binns, Alison O'Doherty, Louise Oduro-Dominah, Ella Porter, Annette Rathwell, Kaye Spence, and Debbie Webster.

Their contributions have formed a vital and valuable basis for subsequent updates.

ABBREVIATIONS

ACP	advance care planning
ACTH	adrenocorticotrophic hormone
ADH	antidiuretic hormone
aEEG	amplitude-integrated electroencephalography
AHP	allied health professional (used interchangeably with HCP)
AKI	acute kidney injury
ANNP	Advanced Neonatal Nurse Practitioner
ANTT	aseptic non-touch technique
AOP	anaemia of prematurity
AP	anterior-posterior
APH	antepartum hemorrhage
APTT	activated partial thromboplastin time
ARM	anorectal malformation
ART	antiretroviral treatment
ASD	atrial septal defect
ATP	adenosine triphosphate
AV(SD)	atrioventricular (septal defect)
BAT	brown adipose tissue
BBB	blood-brain-barrier
BCPAP	bubble continuous positive airway pressure
BiPAP	bi-level positive airway pressure
BP	blood pressure
BPD	bronchopulmonary dysplasia
BGL	blood glucose level
BVM	bag-valve-mask
cAMP	cyclic adenosine monophosphate
C & S	culture & sensitivity
CBF	cerebral blood flow
CCAM	congenital cystic adenomatoid malformation
CCHD	critical congenital heart disease
CDH	congenital diaphragmatic hernia
CFM	cerebral function monitoring
CHD	congenital heart defect

CHF	congestive heart failure
CLD	chronic lung disease
CMV	cytomegalovirus
CMV	continuous mandatory ventilation
CNS	central nervous system
CO	cardiac output
CO	carbon monoxide
CoA	coarctation of the aorta
CoNS	coagulase-negative staphylococcus
CP	cerebral palsy
CPAM	congenital pulmonary airway malformation
CPAP	continuous positive airway pressure
CRP	C-reactive protein
CRT	capillary refill time
CSF	cerebrospinal fluid
CT	computed tomography
CUSS	cranial ultrasound scan
CVL	central venous line
CVP	central venous pressure
CVS	chorionic villi sampling
CVS	cardiovascular system
CXR	chest x-ray
DA	domestic abuse
DAT	direct antibody test
DCC	delayed/deferred cord clamping
DCT	direct Coomb's test
DDH	developmental dysplasia of the hip
DEBM	donor expressed breastmilk
DIC	disseminated intravascular coagulation
DJF	duodeno-jejunal flexure
DM	diabetes mellitus
EBF	erythroblastosis fetalis
EBM	expressed breastmilk
EBP	evidence-based practice
ECG	electrocardiogram
ECHO	echocardiography
ECMO	extracorporeal membrane oxygenation
EDTA	ethylenediaminetetraacetic acid
EEG	electroencephalogram
ELBW	extremely low birthweight
EOI	early-onset infection
ESA	erythropoiesis-stimulating agent

ETT	endotracheal tube
FASP	fetal anomaly screening programme
FBC	full blood count
FCC	family-centred care
FETO	fetal endoscopic tracheal occlusion
FFP	fresh frozen plasma
FGR	fetal growth restriction (see also IUGR)
FiCare	family integrated care
FiO_2	fractional inspired oxygen
FRC	functional residual capacity
FTT	failure to thrive
GA	gestational age
GBS	group B beta-haemolytic streptococcus
GDM	gestational diabetes mellitus
GFR	glomerular filtration rate
GI	gastrointestinal
GMH	germinal matrix haemorrhage
FeNa	fractional excretion of sodium
GOR(D)	gastro-oesophageal reflux (disease)
G6PD	glucose-6-phosphate dehydrogenase
GRV	gastric residual volume
Hb	haemoglobin
HCO3-	bicarbonate
HCP	healthcare professional (used interchangeably with AHP)
HDN	haemorrhagic disease of the newborn; also haemolytic disease of the newborn
HD	Hirschsprung's disease
HDP	hypertensive disorders of pregnancy
HD(U)	high dependency (unit)
NEPDF	nutrient enriched post discharge formula
HFOV	high frequency oscillation ventilation
HFNC	high flow nasal cannula
HI	hypoxic ischaemic
HIC	high-income country
HIE	hypoxic-ischaemic encephalopathy
HIV	human immunodeficiency virus
HLHS	hypoplastic left heart syndrome
HM	human milk
HMF	human milk fortification
HR	heart rate
HRV	heart rate variability
HSV	herpes simplex virus

HUSS	head ultrasound scan
IAA	interrupted aortic arch
IADH	inappropriate (secretion) of antidiuretic hormone
IFCDC	infant family-centred developmental care
Ig	immunoglobulin
ILGF	interleukin growth factor
IM	intramuscular
IMV	intermittent mandatory ventilation
iNO	inhaled nitric oxide
IPPV	intermittent positive pressure ventilation
IO	intraosseous
IUGR	intrauterine growth restriction (see also FGR)
IV	intravenous
IVC	inferior vena cava
IVH	intraventricular haemorrhage
IVIG	intravenous immunoglobulin
IWL	insensible water loss
LBW	low birthweight
LED	light-emitting diode
LFTs	liver function tests; includes alanine aminotransferase (ALT), aspartate aminotransferase (AST), and alkaline phosphatase (ALP)
LGBTQ+	lesbian, gay, bisexual, trans, queer +
LISA	less invasive surfactant administration
LLC	life-limiting condition
LMA	laryngeal mask airway
LMIC	lower and middle income countries
LNU	local neonatal unit
LOI	late-onset infection
LP	lumbar puncture
MAP	mean airway pressure
MAP	mean arterial pressure
MAS	meconium aspiration syndrome
MDT	multidisciplinary team
MEF	minimal enteral feeds
MetHb	methaemoglobin
MgSO4	magnesium sulphate
MIST	minimally invasive surfactant treatment
MOM	mother's own milk
MRI	magnetic resonance imaging
MSAF	meconium-stained amniotic fluid
MV	minute volume
NAS	neonatal abstinence syndrome

NAVA	neurally adjusted ventilatory assist
NE	neonatal encephalopathy
NEC	necrotising enterocolitis
NGT	nasogastric tube
NICU	neonatal intensive care unit
NIDCAP	neonatal individualised developmental care and assessment programme
NIP	nurse independent prescriber
NIPE	newborn infant physical examination
NIPPV	nasal intermittent positive pressure ventilation
NIRS	near-infrared spectroscopy
NIV	non-invasive
NJ	nasojejunal
NLS	newborn life support
NMP	non-medical prescriber
NND	neonatal death
NNS	non-nutritive sucking
NNU	neonatal unit
NO	nitric oxide
NTE	neutral thermal environment
OA	oesophageal atresia
OCM	optimal cord management
ODN	operational delivery network
OGT	orogastric tube
OI	oxygen index
$PaCO_2$	partial pressure of carbon dioxide
PAG	parent advisory group
PaO_2	partial pressure of oxygen
PCR	polymerase chain reaction
PCV	packed cell volume
PD	peritoneal dialysis
PDA	patent ductus arteriosus
PFO	patent foramen ovale
PEEP	positive end-expiratory pressure
PGE1	prostaglandin
PH	pulmonary haemorrhage
PHVD	post-haemorrhagic ventricular dilatation
PICC	peripherally inserted central catheter
PICU	paediatric intensive care unit
PIE	pulmonary interstitial emphysema
PIP	peak inflation pressure
PlGF	placental growth factor

PK	pharmacokinetics
PN	parenteral nutrition
PNA	postnatal age
POCUS	point of care ultrasound
POS	pulse oximetry screening
PPE	personal protective equipment
PPHN	persistent pulmonary hypertension of the newborn
PPV	positive pressure ventilation
PROM	preterm rupture of membranes
PSV	pressure support ventilation
PT	prothrombin
PTV	patient-triggered ventilation
PVH	periventricular haemorrhage
PVHI	periventricular haemorrhage infarction
PVL	periventricular leukomalacia
PVR	pulmonary vascular resistance
RBC	red blood cell
RCT	randomised controlled trial
RDS	respiratory distress syndrome
Rh	rhesus
ROP	retinopathy of prematurity
ROSC	return of spontaneous circulation
RSV	respiratory syncytial virus
$Sa0_2$	saturation of haemoglobin (oxygen)
SBR	serum bilirubin
SC(U)	special care (unit)
SG	specific gravity
SGA	small for gestational age
SIDS	sudden infant death syndrome
SIMV	synchronised intermittent mandatory ventilation
SIP	spontaneous intestinal perforation
S(N)IPPV	synchronised (nasal) intermittent positive pressure ventilation
SOP	standard operating procedure
Sp02	saturation of oxygen
SSC	skin-to-skin
SST	serum separating tube
SUV	service user voice
SV	stroke volume
SVC	superior vena cava
SVT	supraventricular tachycardia
SSB	suck-swallow-breathe
$t_{1/2}$	half-life

TAPS	twin anaemia polycythaemia sequence
TAPVR	total anomalous pulmonary venous return
TAT	transanastomotic tube
TC	transitional care
TB	transcutaneous bilirubinometer
TDM	therapeutic drug monitoring
TEWL	transepidermal water loss
TGA	transposition of the great arteries
TH	therapeutic hypothermia
Ti	inspiratory time
TIC	trauma-informed care
TIS	transport incubator system
TOF	tracheo-oesophageal fistula
ToF	Tetralogy of Fallot
TORCH	Toxoplasmosis, (other), rubella, cytomegalovirus, and herpes
TPN	total parenteral nutrition
TSH	thyroid-stimulating hormone
TTN	transient tachypnoea of the newborn
TTTS	twin-to-twin transfusion syndrome
Us & Es	urea and electrolytes
USS	ultrasound scan
UAC	umbilical arterial catheter
UVC	umbilical venous catheter
UTI	urinary tract infection
VC	volume control
VCSE	voluntary, community and social enterprise
VD	ventricular dilatation
V_D	volume of distribution
VEGF	vascular endothelial growth factor
VILI	ventilator induced lung injury
VKDB	vitamin K deficient bleeding
VLBW	very low birthweight
V/Q	ventilation perfusion
VSD	ventricular septal defect
VT	ventricular tachycardia
VTe	expiratory tidal volume
VTi	inspiratory tidal volume
VTV	volume targeted ventilation
VZV	varicella zoster virus
WCC	white cell count
WMI	white matter injury

GLOSSARY

Selected terms are highlighted in **bold** type in the text on their first occurrence in the book or in key contexts.

abduction	to move (a limb or other body part) away from the midline of the body
acidosis	excessive buildup of acid in body fluids (pH < 7.35)
acquired immunity	defence system developed after exposure to pathogens or vaccines where white blood cells (B and T lymphocytes) form antibodies and build immune memory, allowing for a fast, effective response upon re-exposure to a disease
adduction	to draw (a limb or other body part) into the mid-line of the body
adenosine triphosphate (ATP)	organic molecule in body cells responsible for storage and release of energy
adverse childhood experience	potentially traumatic events occurring before age 18 (e.g. abuse, neglect, parental separation, painful events) that trigger toxic stress
aerobic	processes that require free oxygen to function or produce energy
aganglionic	without ganglia (innervation)
agonist	a substance that binds to a cell receptor and activates it, triggering a biological response
alkalosis	where body fluids have excess base (alkali) or too little acid, causing blood pH to rise above 7.45
amniocentesis	removal of amniotic fluid via the maternal abdominal wall for fetal diagnostic purposes

amnionicity	the number of amniotic sacs (membranes) surrounding fetuses in a multiple pregnancy
amplitude-integrated electroencephalography	a continuous brain monitoring technique used primarily in neonatal intensive care to assess cerebral function over hours or days
anabolic	building phase of metabolism
anaemia of prematurity	physiologic condition in preterm infants, characterised by a rapid decline in haemoglobin (Hb) levels within the few weeks of life
anaerobic	living, acting, or occurring in the absence of oxygen
anastomosis	a union between two structures
aneuploidy	an abnormal number of chromosomes (missing or extra) in cells
anencephaly	neural tube defect occurring when the upper neural tube fails to close, causing the brain and skull to not develop properly in utero
anion	ion carrying one or more negative charges
antagonist	a substance that opposes, inhibits, or blocks the actions of an agonist or physiological process
anterior-posterior	anterior is the front (or ventral) side of the body, while posterior is the back (or dorsal) side
antibody	protein released by plasma cells in response to an antigen
anti-diuretic hormone (ADH)	a hormone produced in the hypothalamus and released by the pituitary gland to regulate water balance and blood pressure
antigen	substance recognised as foreign by the immune system
antepartum haemorrhage	genital tract bleeding from 24+0 weeks gestation to birth; also sometimes termed intrapartum haemorrhage
apnoea	temporary cessation of breathing, either voluntarily or involuntarily, where airflow to the lungs stops
Apnoea of prematurity	A pause in breathing due to immaturity of the brain's control centre, managed with ventilatory support and caffeine to stimulate respiratory drive.

apoptosis	programmed cell death
asphyxia	severe oxygen deprivation (leading to hypoxia)
aspiration	fluid entering the lungs
asymmetrical fetal growth restriction	occurs when a fetus's body grows slower than its head, typically in the third trimester, often caused by placental insufficiency
atelectasis	alveolar collapse
atresia	a blind-ended tube
auscultation	the process of listening with a stethoscope
autonomy	the capacity, right, or state of being self-governing, independent, and free to make one's own decisions without external control
autoregulation	the automatic adjustment of blood flow to a particular body area in response to current need
bag-valve-mask	self-inflating device to provide positive pressure ventilation to neonates who are not breathing or not breathing adequately, covering the nose and mouth to deliver manual breaths
Ballard's (score)	a standardised, validated assessment tool used to estimate a newborn's gestational age (from 20 to 44 weeks) based on their neuromuscular and physical maturity
barotrauma	physical damage to body tissues caused by a difference in pressure
baroreceptors	receptors stimulated by pressure change
beneficence	the ethical principle of acting to benefit others
bilirubinometer	used to estimate bilirubin levels in newborns
bioavailability	the proportion of a nutrient or drug that enters the bloodstream and becomes available for the body to use
bradycardia	slow heart rate, less than 80bpm (term) and 100bpm (preterm)
bronchopulmonary dysplasia	a chronic lung disease primarily affecting premature infants, caused by inflammation, damage, and altered development of the lungs, often following prolonged ventilation

brown adipose tissue (BAT)	specialised, strategically placed tissue (fat) which is capable of generating heat
buccal	the cheek or the area inside the mouth between the teeth and gums
calcaneal	relating to the heel, where the calcaneal nerve is
cardiac output	amount of blood pumped from ventricles in one minute
carina	The bifurcation (division) at the base of the trachea that separates the openings of the right and left main bronchi
catecholamines	compounds that have the effect of sympathetic nerve stimulation
cation	a positively charged ion
caudal	relating to the tail end of the body
cerebral function monitoring	a bedside, amplitude-integrated EEG (aEEG) technique, commonly used in neonatal units to continuously assess brain function in infants
cervical insufficiency	a condition where the cervix weakens, usually during the second trimester, risking miscarriage or preterm birth
chemoreceptors	receptors sensitive to chemical change
chorioamnionitis	an infection of the amniotic fluid, membranes, and placenta, commonly caused by bacteria ascending from the vagina
chorionic villi sampling	a prenatal test performed between 10 and 13 weeks of pregnancy to detect chromosomal or genetic conditions by sampling placenta tissue
chorionicity	the number of chorions (outer membrane/placenta) surrounding fetuses in a multiple pregnancy
choroid plexus	CSF producing a capillary 'knot' within a brain ventricle
chronic lung disease	a respiratory condition primarily affecting premature infants who require prolonged breathing support, such as oxygen therapy
cold stress	skin and internal body temperatures drop significantly, preventing the body from warming itself. Also called thermal stress

colostrum	highly concentrated breast milk produced in the first few days after birth
co-morbidities	two or more chronic diseases or conditions existing simultaneously in one person
conduction	the transfer of heat or electricity through a material via direct physical contact
congenital	develops before birth
congenital diaphragmatic hernia	the diaphragm fails to form fully in utero allowing abdominal organs (stomach, intestines, liver) to move into the chest cavity and restrict lung development
conotruncal	a group of congenital heart defects affecting the heart's outflow tracts and great vessels
continuing care	ongoing care of the neonate after discharge from the neonatal unit
convection	the transfer of heat through the physical movement of circulating air currents
coproduction	a collaborative approach, often used in public services and healthcare, where service users, carers, and communities work in equal partnership with professionals to design, develop, and evaluate services
cord prolapse	the umbilical cord drops through the cervix into the vagina ahead of the baby after membranes rupture during labour, causing compression and restricted oxygen flow
corticosteroids	anti-inflammatory medicines used to treat conditions such as inflammatory lung disease
couplet care	a care model where the mother, parent, or caregiver and their baby are kept together
cryptorchidism	a congenital condition where one or both testes fail to descend into the scrotum
cue-based feeding	a responsive approach where caregivers feed neonates based on behavioural and readiness cues rather than a strict schedule
cyanosis	a bluish or purplish discoloration of the skin, nail beds, or mucous membranes (lips, tongue, mouth) caused by an increase in deoxygenated haemoglobin in the blood

cytochrome	iron containing proteins found on the inner mitochondrial layer of cells which function as electron carriers during oxidative phosphorylation
cytokine	signalling proteins secreted by immune and non-immune cells that act as chemical messengers to regulate immunity and inflammation
debrief	a structured review process used for teams to discuss and reflect on an incident in practice. May be a 'hot' debrief straight after the event or a 'cold' debrief at a later date
decompression	used to relieve elevated pressure within the stomach or intestines by removing accumulated gas and fluids
developmental dysplasia of the hip	a condition where a neonate's hip socket is too shallow to properly cover and hold the top of the thigh bone, causing instability or dislocation
diaphoresis	sweating
diastole	relaxation phase of the cardiac cycle
di-chorionic	twin pregnancy where each fetus has its own placenta and amniotic sac
disseminated intravascular coagulation	an acquired syndrome characterised by widespread, abnormal blood clotting within blood vessels, followed by severe bleeding as clotting factors are depleted
distal	further from the attached limb or the origin of a structure
diuretic	medications that act on the kidneys to remove water from the body through urine
doppler	a non-invasive, painless imaging test that uses sound waves to measure the speed and direction of blood flow through vessels
Dubowitz (score)	a comprehensive clinical assessment used to estimate a newborn's gestational age (between 26 and 44 weeks) based on 21 criteria
duct-dependent	neonatal heart defects that rely on a patent ductus arteriosus (PDA) for survival to maintain pulmonary or systemic blood flow

dysmorphic	an abnormal shape or structure of a body part
dysrhythmia	an abnormality in the heart rhythm
early-onset infection	infection occurring within the first 72 hours of life
embolus	(plural **emboli**) obstruction of a blood vessel by particulate matter, e.g. blood clot or air
encephalitis	inflammation of the brain
endotracheal tube	a flexible, hollow tube inserted through the mouth or nose into the trachea to maintain an open airway for mechanical ventilation
energy triangle	a conceptual framework representing the critical interlinked relationship between body temperature, oxygen, and energy at birth
epiglottis	leaf-shaped cartilage at back of throat that covers the larynx during swallowing
equitable	treating everyone fairly, justly and impartially, according to individual disparities and making individual adjustments where needed, to ensure accessibility for everyone
erythematous	abnormal skin or mucous membrane redness caused by increased blood flow in dilated capillaries, often signalling inflammation, infection, or injury
erythroblastosis fetalis	a severe condition where antibodies in pregnancy cross the placenta and destroy fetal red blood cells, caused by Rhesus (Rh) or ABO blood incompatibility
erythropoietin	hormone released predominantly by the kidney which stimulates red blood cell production (erythropoiesis)
evaporation	the physical process where a liquid, such as water, turns into a gas (water vapour)
evidence-based (care)	the integration of best available clinical evidence with an individual's expertise
extracorporeal membrane oxygenation	a specialised, temporary life-support system for patients with severe, reversible heart or lung failure
extrauterine	anything situated or occurring outside the uterus. Also known as ex utero
extravasation	leakage of fluid from a vessel into the surrounding tissue

extremely low birthweight (ELBW)	infant of less than or equal to 999g
ex utero	see extrauterine
facilitated tucking	supported positioning of a baby to contain the limbs
family integrated care	a neonatal care model partnering parents with staff as primary caregivers, transforming neonatal unit culture from passive observation to active participation
fetal growth restriction	occurs when a fetus fails to reach its genetic growth potential. May be 'symmetrical' or 'asymmetrical'. Also known as intrauterine growth restriction (IUGR)
fistula	unnatural connection between two structures or body cavities
flexed	to curl inwards, as opposite to extended (for example, limbs)
free radicals	highly reactive, unstable atoms or molecules with unpaired electrons, generated naturally by metabolism or external factors like pollution
functional residual capacity	the volume of air remaining in the lungs at the end of a normal, passive exhalation
gastric-residual volume	the amount of fluid aspirated from the stomach through a feeding tube
gastro-oesophageal reflux (disease)	a condition where stomach acid frequently flows back up into the oesophagus, irritating its lining
gestational age	period of time from the first date of last normal menstrual period to the date of birth. Expressed in number of completed weeks or days
glomerular filtration rate	rate of filtrate formation by the kidneys
gluconeogenesis	formation of glucose from a non-carbohydrate source; for example, muscle
glycogen	stored carbohydrate predominantly in muscle
glycogenolysis	breakdown of glycogen to glucose (opposite of **glycogenesis**, which is the formation of glycogen from glucose)
glycolysis	breakdown of glucose to pyruvate

glycosuria	presence of glucose in the urine
golden hour	the critical first hour after birth
governance	a framework of rules, relationships, systems, and processes by which an organisation or society is directed, controlled, and held accountable
ground glass	fine, diffuse, bilateral granular opacities ('white-out' effect) representing widespread alveolar collapse (atelectasis)
haematocrit	the percentage of total blood volume composed of red blood cells (RBCs) also known as packed-cell volume (PCV)
haematuria	presence of blood in the urine
haemolysis	rupture of red blood cells
haemolytic disease of the newborn (HDN)	maternal antibodies cross the placenta and destroy fetal red blood cells, often caused by Rh or ABO incompatibility
half-life	the time required for the concentration of a substance in the blood plasma to decrease by 50% from its maximum initial concentration
hepatomegaly	liver enlargement
heterotaxy	chest and abdominal organs are abnormally arranged or mirrored, often including severe heart defects
holistic	encompassing all aspects of care
homeostasis	a state of equilibrium within the body
hydrocele	a fluid-filled sac in the scrotum causing swelling
hydrocephalus	an abnormal increase in the amount of cerebral spinal fluid within the ventricles of the brain
hyperbilirubinaemia	high levels of bilirubin (either conjugated or unconjugated) in the blood. Also known as jaundice
hypercapnia	high carbon dioxide in the blood
hyperchlorinaemia	high chlorine levels in the blood
hyperglycaemia	high glucose levels in the blood
hyperkalaemia	high potassium levels in the blood
hypernatraemia	high sodium levels in the blood
hyperoxia	high tissue and/or blood oxygenation

hyperthermia high central body temperature

hypocapnia low carbon dioxide in the blood

hypocalcaemia low calcium levels in the blood

hypochlorinaemia low chlorine levels in the blood

hypoglycaemia low glucose levels in the blood

hypokalaemia low potassium levels in the blood

hyponatraemia low sodium levels in the blood

hypospadias congenital condition in biological males where the urethral opening forms on the underside of the penis rather than the tip

hypothermia low central body temperature

hypoxaemic describes low blood oxygenation or **hypoxaemia**

hypoxia low tissue and/or blood oxygenation

hypoxic-ischaemic encephalopathy an umbrella term for a brain injury that happens before, during, or shortly after birth when there is reduced oxygen or blood flow

i-gel a single-use, non-inflatable supraglottic airway device designed to create an anatomical, low-trauma seal for airway management in resuscitation

immunoglobulins antibodies that bind to specific antigens

inferior a directional term meaning below, lower, or away from the head (caudal) in relation to another body part

inflammatory signalling coordinated molecular communication network within tissues that detects pathogens, tissue damage and orchestrates a defensive inflammatory response

innate immunity the body's first, non-specific line of defence present from birth, acting immediately to prevent infection or destroy pathogens

inotrope a drug that changes the force of cardiac contractions

insensible water loss the unmeasured, daily loss of solute-free water from the body

intersectionality a framework for understanding how various identities, such as race, gender, class, and sexuality, overlap and intersect to create unique experiences of discrimination or privilege

intrauterine	anything situated or occurring inside the uterus. Also known as in utero
intrauterine growth restriction	see fetal growth restriction
intraventricular haemorrhage	bleeding into the brain's ventricles
in utero	see intrauterine
ischaemia	a restriction in blood supply to tissues or organs, causing a shortage of oxygen needed for cellular metabolism
jaundice	see hyperbilirubinaemia
justice	treating individuals according to their needs and rights, preventing discrimination, and ensuring equitable access to resources and healthcare
kangaroo care	a method of holding a baby skin-to-skin against a parent's bare chest. Also known as skin-to-skin contact
keratin	a structural protein forming the protective, fibrous layer of hair, skin, and nails, providing strength and reducing damage
kernicterus	yellow staining of the brain stem, cerebellum, and hypocanthus with toxic degeneration of nerve cells due to hyperbilirubinaemia
ketone bodies	water-soluble molecules produced by the liver from fatty acids during periods of low glucose availability, acting as a vital energy source for the brain and muscles
kinaesthetic	learning or experiencing through physical activity, movement, and touch
lactate	an organic compound, produced by body tissues during anaerobic metabolism (low oxygen)
lanugo	a soft, fine, and unpigmented hair that covers a fetus in the womb between 16 and 20 weeks of pregnancy
late-onset infection	infection occurring after the first 72 hours of life
lateral	away from the mid-line of the body
lateral decubitus	lying on one side
linea alba	a fibrous, tendon-like structure running vertically down the midline of the abdomen from the xiphoid process to the pubic bone, separating the left and right rectus abdominis muscles

lipophilic	substance attracted to fatty tissues
loading dose	an initial, high-dose medication administered to rapidly achieve a target therapeutic concentration in the body
low birthweight (LBW)	infant of less than or equal to 2499g
macrophages	principal phagocytes found at specific sites or within bloodstream
macrosomia	a newborn significantly larger than average regardless of gestational age
magnesium sulphate	a chemical compound used medically in premature labour for fetal neuroprotection, to reduce the risk and severity of cerebral palsy in infants
magnetic resonance imaging	a non-invasive medical imaging technique that uses a powerful magnetic field and radio waves to produce detailed images of soft tissues, organs, and bone
malrotation	anomaly of fetal intestinal rotation and fixation resulting in intestinal obstruction
meconium aspiration syndrome	a neonatal condition occurring when a newborn breathes a mixture of meconium and amniotic fluid into their lungs, usually due to stress during labour
medial	towards the mid-line of the body
meningitis	an infection of the membranes that surround the brain and spinal cord (meninges)
mesenteries	extensions of the peritoneum that support abdominal organs
metabolites	small molecules, intermediate, or end products, produced during metabolism
microbiome	microorganisms living on and in the body, particularly in the gut, skin, and oral cavities
micrognathia	lower jaw is underdeveloped or significantly smaller than normal, causing a recessed chin
minimal enteral feeds	or trophic feeds; small volumes of milk, given to preterm or high-risk neonates to stimulate gastrointestinal development rather than provide nutrition
mitochondria	organelles found in all cells responsible for production of adenosine triphosphate (ATP)
mono-chorionic	identical twins that share a single placenta, developing from one zygote

murmur	a whooshing or swishing sound caused by turbulent, rapid blood flow within or near the heart, heard via a stethoscope
myelination	the formation of a fatty insulating sheath surrounding most nerve fibres. See also oligodendrocyte
necrotising enterocolitis	a serious, often fatal gastrointestinal emergency primarily affecting premature infants, where intestinal tissue becomes inflamed
neonatal abstinence syndrome	a condition caused by fetal exposure to addictive substances (prescribed or recreational) antenatally, resulting in withdrawal symptoms in the early postnatal period
nephrotoxic	damaging to nephrons/kidneys
neurodiversity	the concept that neurological differences, such as autism and other conditions are natural variations in human cognition, not deficits to be cured
neuroprotection	proactive strategies to prevent or minimise brain injury in high-risk and/or preterm infants and those with hypoxic-ischemic encephalopathy (HIE)
neutral thermal environment	See thermoneutral zone
nociception	the perception by the nerve centres of painful stimulation. The term used in relation to pain perception in neonates
non-maleficence	a fundamental ethical principle, often summarised as 'do no harm'
non-nutritive sucking	sucking on a pacifier, finger or empty breast for comfort, self-regulation, or pain relief rather than for nutrition
non-shivering thermogenesis	ability to produce heat by activation of BAT
normostasis	the maintenance of normal, healthy physiological states, also known as homeostasis
normothermia	the physiological state where the human body maintains a normal core temperature
nosocomial	an infection that develops within the hospital environment
oedema	excess extracellular (outside cells) fluid in the body, showing as skin puffiness/swelling

oligodendrocyte	specialised glial cells in the central nervous system (CNS) that produce myelin, a fatty substance insulating axons to enable rapid electrical signal transmission
oliguria	diminished urine output, e.g. < 1 ml/kg/hr
Ommaya reservoir	device for cerebrospinal fluid aspiration placed under the scalp
omphalitis	infection of the umbilical stump and surrounding tissues in newborns
opsonisation	process whereby antigens are made more 'attractive' to phagocytes
osmolarity	the measurement of the total concentration of solute particles (ions, molecules) dissolved in a solution, expressed in osmoles per litre
osmotic diuresis	increased urination caused by high concentrations of non-reabsorbed solutes (for example, glucose) in the kidney tubules, which draw water into the lumen inhibiting reabsorption
ototoxic	inner ear or auditory nerve damage caused by specific medications
outreach	community-based nursing care to high-risk neonates transitioning from hospital to home
oxygenation index	a metric measuring the severity of hypoxic respiratory failure by comparing mean airway pressure (MAP) and oxygen concentration to arterial oxygen levels
packed-cell volume	see haematocrit
palliative care	an active and total approach to care from the point of diagnosis or recognition, throughout a neonate's life, death, and beyond. Used synonymously with end-of-life care, supportive care, comfort care
parenteral	administration of medication, fluids, or nutrition through routes other than the mouth and gastrointestinal tract
patent ductus arteriosus	a temporary fetal blood vessel (the ductus arteriosus) fails to close after birth, connecting the aorta and pulmonary artery
percutaneous	accessing an internal body structure or organ through the skin

perinatal	the period surrounding birth and up to the first week of life
peristalsis	involuntary contraction and relaxation of muscles in the digestive tract that moves food, liquids, and waste through the body
periventricular leucomalacia	a brain injury, primarily affecting premature infants, where white matter around the brain ventricles is compromised due to oxygen or blood flow deprivation
petechiae	small haemorrhages in the skin
phagocytes	white blood cells (leucocytes) that destroy pathogens by engulfment
pharmacodynamics	how drugs affect the body
pharmacokinetics	absorption, distribution, metabolism, excretion, or what the body does to a drug
physiological anaemia	a normal, temporary drop in haemoglobin levels occurring from birth
plantar (nerve)	referring to the sole of the foot; the plantar nerve runs across the sole
plasticity	the brain's ability to reorganise its structure, functions, and neural connections in response to experience, learning, or injury
plagiocephaly	a flat spot on one side or the back of the head due to external pressure
pleural effusion	the presence of fluid in the pleural space
plus disease	a severe form of retinopathy of prematurity (ROP) in infants, characterised by significant tortuosity (twisting) and dilation (widening) of retinal blood vessels
pneumonia	an infection that inflames the air sacs (alveoli) in one or both lungs
pneumocyte	epithelial cells lining the alveoli of the lungs
pneumoperitoneum	free air in the peritoneal space
pneumothorax	free air in the pleural cavity
polycythaemia	an abnormal increase in red blood cells, causing thickened blood, poor circulation, and high risks of clots
polyhydramnios	an excess of amniotic fluid. Opposite of oligohydramnios, which is a reduction in amniotic fluid
posterior	towards the back of the body

pre-ductal	blood oxygen saturation measured before it passes through the ductus arteriosus (typically right hand), reflecting oxygen levels leaving the heart/lungs
pre-eclampsia	a serious blood pressure disorder occurring after 20 weeks of pregnancy or postpartum, characterised by high blood pressure protein in the urine
preterm	less than 37 completed weeks of gestation (259 days). Accounts for 8 per cent of births. Also known as premature
primary apnoea	a temporary cessation of breathing in a newborn, often caused by acute hypoxia, where the respiratory centre fails, but they typically respond to stimulation and resuscitation
primigravida	pregnant for the first time or has been pregnant once
probiotics	live, beneficial bacteria that provides health benefits when consumed in adequate amounts
processus vaginalis	a tubular protrusion of the peritoneum that precedes testicular descent into the scrotum during fetal development
prokinetic	agent that increases gastric motility
prone	laying on the front
proprioceptive	a sense providing body awareness in terms of space and position
proteinuria	presence of protein in the urine
proximal	closer to the body or origin of a structure, e.g. the knee is proximal to the ankle
pulmonary interstitial emphysema	air leaks from damaged air sacs (alveoli) and becomes trapped in the connective tissue of the lungs
pulmonary vascular resistance	the resistance the right ventricle must overcome to pump blood through the pulmonary circulation, representing the afterload of the right heart
pulse oximetry	a noninvasive method to measure blood oxygen saturation
radiation	heat loss resulting from a temperature gradient

recession	inward movement of the chest, often seen between in the sternum, between or below the ribs when a neonate uses extra effort to breathe
red reflex	or fundal reflex, is a reddish-orange reflection of light from the retina observed through the pupil during an eye exam
renal agenesis	rare congenital disorder where one (unilateral) or both (bilateral) kidneys fail to develop in a fetus
repatriation	the process of returning a neonate back to their home unit
Replogle tube	a double-lumen suction catheter used in neonates with oesophageal atresia to drain saliva from the blind-ending upper pouch, preventing aspiration pneumonia
respiratory distress syndrome	surfactant deficiency in premature babies, leading to lung collapse (atelectasis) and low oxygen levels
retinopathy of prematurity	abnormal blood vessels grow in the retina
retropleural	a surgical approach or anatomic space located behind (retro-) the pleura
safeguarding	the proactive process of protecting an individual's health, wellbeing, and human rights, enabling them to live free from abuse, harm, and neglect
seizure	over-excitation of the brain neurons. Also termed convulsion or fit. May be subtle, generalised tonic, multifocal clonic, focal clonic, or myoclonic
sepsis	a life-threatening medical emergency caused by the body's extreme, dysfunctional response to an infection, leading to tissue damage, organ failure, and potential death
shoulder dystocia	a rare but critical obstetric emergency where a baby's shoulder becomes trapped behind the pubic bone after the head is delivered
situs inversus	major organs (e.g. heart and stomach) are reversed from their normal positions (as seen on X-ray)

situs solitus	normal position of major organs (as seen on X-ray)
skeletal dysplasia	genetic condition causing abnormal cartilage and bone growth, resulting in restricted growth, short stature (dwarfism), and orthopaedic issues
skin-to-skin contact	placing a neonate directly onto their parent's chest. See also kangaroo care
small for gestational age (SGA)	infant with a birthweight less than the 10th percentile
solute	substance dissolved in solution
specific gravity	a measure of urine concentration, comparing the density of urine to water
steady-state	the rate of drug administration equals the rate of elimination, resulting in stable, therapeutic plasma concentrations
stenosis	an abnormal narrowing
stoma	a surgically created opening in the abdominal wall that connects the bowel or urinary tract to the outside of the body
stratum corneum	the outermost layer of the skin epidermis
stricture	an abnormal narrowing of a bodily passage, usually caused by scar tissue
stridor	a harsh, high-pitched breathing sound indicating a partial airway obstruction
stroke volume	amount of blood pumped from the ventricles with each contraction
superior	towards the head or upper part of the body or a structure
supine	lying on back, face upwards
suprapubic	above the symphysis pubis
surfactant	a vital lipoprotein complex produced by pneumocytes in the lungs which reduces surface tension at the air-liquid interface of the alveoli, preventing lung collapse (atelectasis) during expiration
symmetrical fetal growth restriction	where all fetal biometric parameters (head circumference, abdominal circumference, femur length) are proportionately small
systole	contraction phase of the cardiac cycle
tachycardia	heart rate greater than 160bpm (term) and 180bpm (preterm) at rest

tachypnoea	a high respiratory rate
tension pneumothorax	free air (under pressure) in the chest resulting in a shift in the mediastinum potentially reducing cardiac output
term	from 37 to 42 completed weeks of gestation (259–293 days); see also **preterm**
terminal apnoea	a critical state of breathing cessation following a period of gasping due to severe hypoxia, typically in newborns failing to breathe at birth
therapeutic hypothermia	lowering the body temperature to protect the brain and organs in newborns with brain injury
thermogenic	production of heat
thermoneutral zone	the ambient temperature range where a neonate will maintain a stable core body temperature. Also termed neutral thermal environment (NTE)
thrombocytopaenia	a condition characterised by abnormally low levels of platelets
thrombus	a clot that develops and persists within a blood vessel
tocolytic	drugs used to temporarily suppress premature labour by inhibiting uterine contractions
torsion	twisting, e.g. of gut
torticollis	a painful condition causing the neck to twist and tilt at an odd angle, often due to muscle spasms or tightness, particularly of the sternocleidomastoid muscle
t-piece	a 3-way, T-shaped connector used to divert flow in tubing systems at a 90-degree angle
tracheomalacia	'floppy' trachea
transcutaneous	passing, entering, or acting through the skin
transient tachypnoea of the newborn	a temporary, self-limiting breathing disorder in newborns due to delayed absorption of fetal lung fluid
transillumination	a diagnostic technique involving passing a high-intensity light through body tissues or structures to identify abnormalities
transition	the process of changing from one dependency level or condition to another
transitional care	support allowing parents and neonates to stay together while they receive extra monitoring and care prior to discharge home

trauma-informed care	a universal approach acknowledging the intense stress of the neonatal unit, aiming to prevent re-traumatisation for infants and families
tri-chorionic	triplet pregnancy
trisomy	a genetic disorder characterised by having 47 chromosomes instead of 46, with an extra copy of a specific chromosome
trophic	the processes of nutrition, growth, and nourishment
ultrasound scan	a safe, painless diagnostic test using high-frequency sound waves to create real-time images of the body
urinalysis	a common diagnostic test that analyses a urine sample
vasa praevia	a rare, serious pregnancy complication where fetal blood vessels cross or run near the internal cervical os
vascularisation	forming new blood vessels
ventilation/perfusion mismatch	imbalance between the air reaching the alveoli (ventilation, V) and the blood flowing to them (perfusion, Q)
ventilator-induced lung injury	damage to the lung caused by positive pressure ventilation; may include barotrauma or volutrauma
very low birthweight (VLBW)	infant of less than or equal to 1499g; see also small for gestational age
veteran parent	a parent with previous neonatal care experience
viability	the gestational age at which a fetus has a reasonable chance of surviving outside the uterus
wheeze	a high-pitched sound produced by narrowed or obstructed airways, usually heard on expiration
xiphisternum	the lower part of the breastbone

INTRODUCTION
Neonatal Intensive Care Nursing: 4th edition

Dr Julia Petty and Lisa Kaiser (eds)

DOI: 10.4324/9781003591405-1

This is the 4th edition of *Neonatal Intensive Care Nursing*, first published in 2000 by Glenys Boxwell, with two previous updates since then. During this time, many areas of practice have developed and changed due to the impact of research on healthcare practices in the care of neonates and families. Examples include family integrated care (FiCare), optimal cord management, high flow nasal cannula support, less invasive ventilation and surfactant administration strategies, and the first hour of care, to name but a few. Therefore, it is imperative that a reputable book such as this, which is widely referenced and used by those both learning and working within the clinical area nationally and globally, be fully updated. The update aims to ensure that readers have the most up-to-date information to apply to their practice, in line with the most recent research-based evidence and current practices. The editors were mindful of this in the planning of the new edition to ensure that the fundamental principle of evidence-based practice remains steadfast and of vital importance.

In this 4th edition, the majority of previous chapters have remained with their original titles and are presented in updated forms. Other chapters are new and have been added in response to the robust peer review of the 3rd edition. Details of this current edition are as follows:

- The book is divided into four sections:
    - **Section 1:** An overview of neonatal care, which sets out the broad context of care, how it is organised, and where it sits in the wider arena of the family's future.
    - **Section 2**: The physical and emotional wellbeing of the neonate and family, which places importance on psycho-emotional care as well as the more physical, clinically based care.
    - **Section 3:** Clinical aspects of neonatal care, which includes the majority of the previous chapter topics in the context of a systems approach.
    - **Section 4**: Practices in neonatal care, which focuses on some of the more procedural-based content relevant to practice.
- **New chapters and content:** While the title of the book is *Neonatal Intensive Care Nursing*, we felt that any discussion of neonatal practice must include what went both *before* and *after* the intensive care period, in the context of the whole neonatal care trajectory. Therefore, new chapters are included on antenatal and perinatal aspects of care and continuing care beyond the neonatal unit. In addition, it was felt that some aspects formerly not covered in detail warranted inclusion, so there is now a new chapter on specific diagnostic neonatal practice and more content integrated within the family chapter on psychologically informed care of parents. Greater inclusion of the multidisciplinary team is reflected in the range of allied health

professionals who have authored the chapter updates and/or written new content for the current book. So, while recognising the vital role of neonatal nurses (Neonatal Nurses Association, 2026) represented by a number of key contributors, we now have inclusion of midwifery, psychologist, parent, physiotherapy, occupational therapy, researcher, speech and language therapy, pharmacy, dietician, and medical perspectives, all giving valuable input.

- **Reflective practice and additional 'Think points,' Practice points,' and 'Activities' boxes:** Reading through the chapters, you are encouraged to reflect on the key points and content relating to your practice and engage with this and the relevant literature in an enquiring way. Specific pointers to consider, and questions to reflect on, are therefore posed at the start of each chapter, as well as throughout the text.
- **Case studies:** these are at the end of each chapter, and as before, there will be the opportunity to view suggested answer guides by referring to the relevant webpage on the companion website for each chapter.
- **Web-based companion:** See www.routledge.com/cw/petty This includes the following:
  - **Case study answer guides** (with signposting to additional information and resources as applicable)
  - **Supplementary information** – any extra information relevant to the chapter that is not included in the actual book.
  - **'Test your knowledge'**- multiple choice quizzes and a combination of other self-testing formats for learning reinforcement (such as crosswords, word searches, short answer quizzes) related to each chapter.
  - **Web-based resources** – a selection of open-access articles and web resources will be provided for each chapter.

Importantly, we feel it is vital to emphasise some key underpinning principles that are relevant to each and every chapter, and which will be threaded through the whole book. First, the importance of the family; while certain practices may have changed over time, what has *not* changed is the recognition and value placed on the family, regarding them as essential partners in the care of their baby. We believe that it is paramount to keep the neonate and family together and to treat parents as key members of the multidisciplinary team.

Second, we must never lose sight of the need for inclusive clinical practice and education in neonatal care (NHS Race and Health Observatory, 2024). Ensuring inclusive and equitable care, particularly for marginalised or under-represented populations, is not just important; it is essential. As editors, we strongly advocate diverse and inclusive practices that uphold the principles of non-discrimination and fairness. Culturally sensitive care must acknowledge and respect differences in ethnic background, religious beliefs, gender identity, disability, and sexual orientation, ensuring that neonates and their families receive equitable support. Equity, diversity, and inclusion are fundamental values that must be embraced, celebrated, and integrated into all aspects of care, in alignment with the protected characteristics of the Equality Act 2010. These characteristics include age, disability, gender reassignment, marital or civil partnership status, pregnancy and maternity, race, nationality, ethnic or national origin, religion, sex, and sexual orientation. Additionally, we recognise that some parents may have physical or cognitive disabilities or be neurodiverse, requiring tailored and sensitive communication and care. Furthermore, families come from diverse socio-economic and educational backgrounds, and many belong to under-represented communities. This reality reinforces the necessity of equitable and adaptable care that meets the unique needs of every individual and fosters an environment of true inclusivity.

Third, allied health professionals play a vital role in ensuring comprehensive, multidisciplinary care for neonates and their families (Robertshaw & Dobbin, 2025), contributing expertise across fields such as midwifery, community professionals, physiotherapy, dietetics/nutrition, speech and language therapy, occupational therapy, pharmacy, and psychological support, including parental input. Their collaboration enhances patient outcomes, fosters holistic wellbeing, and underpins the principles of equitable and inclusive care explored throughout the chapters of this book.

Fourth, there is a need to consider the care principles that apply globally. While this book is written within the UK context, we must not forget the necessity to mutually learn from our global partners (Kenner & Boykova, 2019; Petty et al., 2022). We recognise that there are individual differences in practice across countries, regions, and specific units even within the UK itself. The book aims to be universally applicable to anyone caring for neonates and/or infants in the clinical and/or home setting, and the reader should keep this in mind in their own unit or workplace.

Finally, this book uses specific terminology to define stages of early life. The term *neonate* refers to the first 28 days post-term, while *infant* applies to children up to one year old. That said, these terms will be used interchangeably throughout the text. Additionally, the term *baby* specifically refers to the newborn period at birth. We also recognise the importance of inclusive language when referring to our patients (Lennon, 2021; Harvey Bluemel, 2023) and parents. The term 'parent' is used broadly to encompass mothers, fathers, partners, caregivers, and anyone with parental responsibility. While mother and father are included in the text, the terms 'parent' and 'partner' are used alongside to avoid making assumptions about gender. This approach ensures inclusivity for all parents, including cisgender individuals, non-binary people, and transgender men and women, whose gender identity may differ from the sex they were assigned at birth. The term partner is also used to recognise same-sex parents.

Finally, it is essential to recognise the unique contributions of the whole neonatal healthcare team with whom neonatal nurses work. Throughout this book, the terms allied health professional (AHP), healthcare professional (HCP), clinician, and practitioner are used interchangeably to refer to members of the neonatal multidisciplinary team (MDT). It has been a real privilege to edit this valuable textbook that plays an important role in joint learning about the vital elements of current, high-quality neonatal care and support of neonates and families.

References

Harvey Bluemel, A. (2023). The importance of using inclusive language in medical practice. *BMJ*. https://blogs.bmj.com/bmjsrh/2023/03/31/the-importance-of-using-inclusive-language-in-medical-practice/

Kenner, C., & Boykova, M. (2019). Neonatal care from a global perspective. In *Comprehensive neonatal nursing care* (6th ed., Chap. 43). Springer Publishing.

Lennon, E. (2021). *Inclusive language in health and care: Why the words we use matter*. Kings Fund. https://www.kingsfund.org.uk/insight-and-analysis/blogs/inclusive-language-health-care

Neonatal Nurses Association. (2026). *Be a neonatal nurse*. https://nna.org.uk/becoming-a-neonatal-nurse/

NHS Race and Health Observatory. (2024). *The Observatory's mission to ensure equity in neonatal assessments: Latest guidelines*. https://nhsrho.org/blogs/the-observatorys-mission-to-ensure-equity-in-neonatal-assessments-latest-bapm-and-nhse-guidelines/

Petty, J., Jones, T., van den Hoogen, A., Walker, K., & Kenner, C. (Eds.). (2022). *Neonatal nursing: A global perspective*. Springer Publishing.

Robertshaw, L., & Dobbin, S. (2025). The role of occupational therapy and physiotherapy in the neonatal unit. *Paediatrics and Child Health*, *35*(1), 16–22. https://doi.org/10.1016/j.paed.2024.10.003

PART 1

AN OVERVIEW OF NEONATAL CARE

DOI: 10.4324/9781003591405-2

1 THE CONTEXT AND ORGANISATION OF NEONATAL CARE

Julia Petty

CONTENTS

DOI: 10.4324/9781003591405-3

GUIDANCE ON HOW TO ENHANCE PERSONAL LEARNING FROM THIS CHAPTER

Key points covered in this chapter

- The context of neonatal care from both a UK and global perspective relating to organisation and care delivery at different dependency levels.
- An insight into the types of admissions to neonatal care for both term and premature neonates.
- Various roles of the multidisciplinary team and their contribution to an infant's journey through neonatal care.

Reflection

Reading through the chapter, you are encouraged to engage with the key points and related literature in an enquiring way. Ask these questions:

- Why are categories of care important and how do they impact the planning and delivery of neonatal care?
- What are the advantages of extended and enhanced nursing roles? Do they form part of your unit's structure?
- Which specialities of the multidisciplinary team are available for your unit, and how can they benefit your patients?

Implications for nursing care

- Finally: this chapter should facilitate your understanding of how neonatal care is organised. Consider how you can contribute towards the effectiveness of your own neonatal unit in your own country, and what this means for the individual neonates you look after on a day-to-day basis.

INTRODUCTION AND BACKGROUND

Approximately 1 in 7 babies born in England, Scotland, and Wales, or around 105,000 out of 750,000, require specialist neonatal care in a hospital. This includes babies born prematurely or those who are full-term but sick (Office for National Statistics (ONS), 2025). One in twelve babies are born preterm in the United Kingdom (UK; UK Government, 2025), while in Northern Ireland over 1,900 babies are born prematurely or sick, requiring care in a neonatal unit (NNU; TinyLife, 2022). Globally, this rate is higher at one in ten (World Health Organization (WHO), 2023), but rates may be as high as 15% in low to middle-income countries (Imperial College, 2025).

Neonatology is a relatively small speciality, but, owing to continual medical advancements, the survival rates of small, sick, and extremely premature babies have improved. Numerous stakeholders from national organisations and government bodies, such as the National Institute for Health and Care Excellence (NICE), NHS England (NHSE), Neonatal National Audit Programme (NNAP), Neonatal Nurses Association (NNA), British Association of Perinatal Medicine (BAPM), Royal College of Paediatrics and Child Health (RCPCH), Royal College of Nursing (RCN), Scottish Neonatal Nurses Group (SNNG), Bliss, and TinyLife, among others, help shape neonatal care and provide guidance and support for staff and families.

This chapter will explore how neonatal services are structured and coordinated, describing the function of operational delivery networks (ODNs). It examines the role of the neonatal nurse and the multidisciplinary team relating to the care of pregnant and post-partum women, trans, and non-binary people, and their babies. The UK context will be drawn upon but acknowledging the differences that need consideration in relation to premature birth rates, delivery of, and resources, for neonatal care and outcomes worldwide. A discussion of the global neonatal context will therefore also be presented.

CATEGORIES OF NEONATAL CARE

Newborn infants are admitted to the NNU for a variety of clinical conditions, including having been born too early, having a low birthweight, or having a medical or surgical condition that needs specialist treatment. These will determine the levels of care different infants require, and thus the staff who may safely look after them. BAPM (2022a) defines criteria for four categories of care for neonatal patients to ensure every baby is assigned appropriate care levels. These are **transitional care**, **special care**, **high dependency care**, and **intensive care**. Throughout an infant's stay within neonatal services, the category of care may vary due to changes in their condition, e.g. clinical improvement or deterioration (NHSE, 2024a).

Transitional care

The concept of transitional care (TC) has proven its value by preventing unnecessary separation of parent(s) and baby (RCPCH, 2023). It serves infants who require support but do not require NNU admission, until they may be discharged home. This model confers benefits such as reduced length of stay on the NNU, allowing for optimised use of neonatal cots, improved parental confidence, bonding, establishment of breastfeeding with higher success rates, and an overall improvement of the family experience including promotion of sibling bonds (BAPM, 2017). Admissions of term infants in particular were the focus of NHS England (2017) who identified avoidable admissions to neonatal care. These include the number of full-term babies who did not have serious birth defects or disorders, thus leading to stress and trauma for the families and additional financial pressures on neonatal services with finite resources.

The Avoiding Term Admissions into Neonatal Units (ATAIN) project aimed to reduce the number of full-term babies admitted to neonatal units unnecessarily. The focus is on preventing avoidable harm, ensuring that babies born at 37 weeks or later remain with their parents whenever possible (NHSE, 2025a, 2025b). The initiative works to keep admission rates below 5% of births per month (NHSE, 2017). Key strategies include preventing separation between mother/parent and baby to support bonding and breastfeeding; improving fetal monitoring to reduce admissions due to complications; providing transitional care for babies who need extra support but do not require full NNU admission; and addressing common causes of admission, such as hypoglycaemia, jaundice, and respiratory symptoms (Battersby et al., 2017). Therefore, appropriate expertise and early planning are essential if such infants are managed away from specialised neonatal settings.

TC can be delivered by two service models: on a dedicated TC ward or within a postnatal ward, and is facilitated via close cooperation between neonatal and midwifery staff. This may include maternity care assistants, nursery nurses, and other nursing support roles. In either case, the mother or parent must be resident and caring for their baby as the primary caregiver, supported with care activities above those required normally (BAPM, 2017).

Criteria for TC could include:

- Prematurity (≥34 weeks or ≥33 weeks if discharged from the NNU)
- Low birthweight (but >1600 grams)
- Nasogastric tube feeding (≥3 hourly)
- Babies on intravenous (IV) antibiotics, if otherwise stable
- Hypothermia (<36°C) requiring intervention
- Haemolytic jaundice requiring phototherapy
- Maternal substance misuse with the need for oral medication and/or feeding support
- Palliative care following multidisciplinary team discussion with parental agreement

- Congenital malformations resulting in feeding problems, e.g. cleft lip/palate
- Newborn babies readmitted from home with excessive weight loss and requiring nasogastric tube feeding
- Babies transferred from the NNU for further support/observation prior to discharge home.

Other areas of care provision, above routine postnatal care, may be observation of infants at risk of deteriorating health, blood glucose monitoring for those at risk of hypoglycaemia, feeding support, monitoring jaundice, and meeting care needs arising from a baby's social background. These are classed as 'normal care' and should ideally be provided by midwifery staff on the postnatal ward (BAPM, 2017).

Despite the need for TC, there is variation in the provision of facilities nationally alongside care delivery, classification, and commissioning (RCPCH, 2025). While many maternity and neonatal services provide elements of TC, these may not always be formally recognised (BAPM, 2017). McKeon-Carter (2018) reports that many hospitals provide some elements of TC, although provision varies and there is a need for strengthening the effectiveness and equitable delivery of TC services. The importance of investing in appropriately staffed TC facilities is now a priority by commissioners and NHS Trusts, as otherwise, the number of admissions to NNUs resulting in separation of mothers, parents, and babies will continue to rise. The neonatal critical care specification (NHS England, 2024a) sets out expected standards for optimum neonatal care.

ACTIVITIES

Take a look at some of the resources in the reference list for this chapter; for example:

- The BAPM (2022a) document on nurse staffing to see if your NNU is consistent with the guidance.
- In addition, consider the NNA Interactive Careers framework (NNA, 2025) to view the range of options for professional development in neonatal care.
- Finally, register on and access the e-learning for health platform (eLH) (NHS England, 2025a) and search for/plan some e-learning on neonatal modules to support your development.

The following three levels of care require admission to the NNU and therefore result in separation of mother or parent and baby until the infant is fit for discharge home, to the postnatal ward, or to a TC ward.

Special care

Special care (SC) is defined as any care in which a baby does not fulfil the criteria for intensive or high dependency care. Criteria for special care include:

- Oxygen by nasal cannula
- Feeding by nasogastric/nasojejunal tube or gastrostomy
- Continuous physiological monitoring (excluding apnoea monitors only)
- Care of a stoma
- Presence of IV cannula
- Baby receiving phototherapy
- Special observation of physiological variables at least four-hourly.

High dependency care

Infants under the high dependency (HD) care category should be looked after by highly skilled practitioners, but they have lower demands than those under intensive care, from a perspective of nurse-to-patient ratios. Any day where a baby does not fulfil the criteria for intensive care is classed as a high dependency day and may include the following:

- Any form of non-invasive respiratory support (e.g. nasal continuous positive airway pressure (nasal CPAP), biphasic positive airway pressure (BiPAP), humidified high flow nasal cannula (HHFNC))
- Any day receiving any of the following:
  - **Parenteral** nutrition (PN)
  - Continuous infusion of drugs (except prostaglandin and/or insulin)
  - Presence of a (**percutaneous**) central venous catheter
  - Presence of a tracheostomy
  - Presence of a urethral or **suprapubic** catheter
  - Presence of a transanastomotic tube following oesophageal **atresia** repair
  - Presence of nasopharyngeal airway/nasal stent
  - Observation of seizures/cerebral function monitoring
  - Barrier nursing
  - Need for ventricular taps.

Intensive care

This is provided for the most unwell or unstable infants with the greatest needs in relation to staff skills and staff-to-patient ratios. An intensive care day is defined as:

- Any day where a baby receives any form of mechanical respiratory support via a tracheal tube
- *Both* non-invasive ventilation (e.g. nasal CPAP, BiPAP, HHFNC) and PN
- Day of surgery (including laser therapy for retinopathy of prematurity)
- Day of death
- Any day where any of the following applies:
  - Presence of an umbilical arterial line
  - Presence of an umbilical venous line
  - Presence of a peripheral arterial line
  - Insulin infusion
  - Presence of a chest drain
  - Exchange transfusion
  - Therapeutic hypothermia
  - Prostaglandin infusion
  - Presence of a Replogle tube
  - Presence of an epidural catheter
  - Presence of a silo for gastroschisis
  - Presence of an external ventricular drain
  - Dialysis (any type).

THINK POINTS

Can you think of examples of neonates that you have cared for that fit each of the criteria for transitional care, special care, high dependency care, and intensive care? What were the key differences between them? Are there any variations globally between categories of care that you are aware of? You could look up the WHO's 2020 document on quality of care for small and sick newborns at facility levels as well as the Neopedia webpage: https://www.neopedia.org/pregnancy-birth/nicu-preparation/clinic-levels.

LEVELS OF SERVICE PROVISION

Factors such as gestation, weight, clinical condition, and co-morbidities determine the category of care each individual infant requires (BAPM, 2022a). Due to numerous potential clinical conditions discussed throughout this book, levels of care may mean an infant cannot be safely nursed in the NNU at the hospital in which the mother has booked to deliver, or clinical deterioration may result in a need for transfer to another specialist NNU. According to NHSE (2024a) and BAPM (2022a), neonatal care provision can be categorised as outlined in Table 1.1.

TABLE 1.1 CATEGORIES OF NEONATAL CARE IN THE UK

Level 1 **Special Care Unit (SCU)**	Units provide special care (SC) but do not aim to provide any continuing high dependency (HD) or intensive care (IC).
Level 2 **Local Neonatal Unit (LNU)**	Units provide HD care and some short-term IC (as agreed locally), but infants who require complex or longer-term IC would be transferred to a neonatal intensive care unit.
Level 3 **Neonatal Intensive Care Unit (NICU)**	Units provide the entire range of medical neonatal care, including IC. In some units, specialist services such as neonatal surgery are available. These units also provide additional care for babies and their families referred from the neonatal network in which they are based, and from other networks when necessary to deal with peaks of demand or requests for specialist care not available elsewhere.

(adapted from BAPM, 2022a)

Pillay et al. (2025) report that birth and early care for neonates born at 28 weeks and older are safe in both neonatal intensive care units (NICUs) and local neonatal units (LNUs). For anticipated births at extreme prematurity, antenatal transfer to NICU-equipped centres is recommended. If birth occurs in a LNU, clinicians should assess risks for postnatal transfer, considering patient needs, staff expertise, and available resources, while informing parents about the heightened risk of brain injury linked to transfer. Some hospitals may also have a neonatal surgical intensive care unit that, in addition to services provided by NICUs, will provide surgical care as part of an approved ODN pathway. Units providing neonatal surgical care must have staff with appropriate skills and knowledge to deliver care at a high standard (NHSE, 2024a).

Thus, an infant born at 33 weeks' gestation who needs no respiratory support but is clinically well, requiring solely nasogastric feeds while progressing to oral feeding, would be placed under the SC category and could be nursed at a level 1, 2, or 3 NNU. However, if there is a need for respiratory support such as CPAP, this infant would fall under the HD category of care and would thus not be eligible to be nursed on a level 1 special care unit (SCU), requiring transfer to either a level 2 LNU or a level 3 NICU. In another instance, if an infant was born at 24 weeks' gestation with an anticipated ongoing need for mechanical ventilation (i.e. not short-term IC), this infant should be delivered and cared for at a level 3 NICU. However, not all mothers or pregnant people whose babies require level 3 NICU admission book to deliver at such hospitals; therefore, transfer to a suitable hospital is required, ideally antenatally (Watson et al., 2020). Once the infant's progress and clinical condition allow, transfer back to the home unit may be appropriate.

NEONATAL TRANSPORT

Neonatal services depend on the availability of reliable transport facilities to bring babies and their parents to the most appropriate care setting to meet their needs. Prior to birth, if admission to neonatal services is deemed necessary, ideally the level of care required can be anticipated and transport can be ***in utero***. This is safer than ***ex utero*** transfer after a baby is born and is seen as a necessary component of contemporary obstetrics to ensure better health outcomes for the mother and fetus (Watson et al., 2020; Pillay et al., 2025). However, many problems only become apparent at birth or later, and this may necessitate stabilisation and transport to a higher-level NNU from the place of delivery or thereafter, hence the need for an *ex utero* transfer. Unlike some nations where neonatal transport is hospital-based, the UK has dedicated transport teams operating twenty-four hours a day.

Wherever in the world, however, neonatal transport services are highly specialised, with dedicated teams ensuring safe and efficient transfers for critically ill newborns. The UK has standardised national datasets to track transport activity and improve care (Leslie et al., 2024) along with national benchmarks for tracking transport quality, while Europe focuses on regional guidelines, ensuring NICU-level care during transfers (European Standards of Care for Newborn Health, 2025). The UK also tracks ventilation benchmarks and hypothermia treatment availability, ensuring consistent care standards. Chapter 24 will explore this subject in more depth, in line with the current perspective.

THE ROLE OF OPERATIONAL DELIVERY NETWORKS

All NNUs are within geographically determined groups known as a neonatal network or operational delivery network (ODN). As a result, every NNU in the UK is part of an ODN, and each network oversees multiple NNUs within their allocated region, with a responsibility for estimating their population's neonatal care needs. There are allocated numbers of SC, HD, and IC beds in each ODN, which are coordinated with the aim of ensuring that babies receive their required care as close to home as possible where this can be anticipated. Cot capacity issues within an ODN may sometimes result in a baby and family being transferred to the nearest available cot outside their geographical network, to be cared for there until a cot within the network is available and the infant is stable enough for the journey.

ODNs have a duty to benchmark and audit their practice, as well as monitor their workforce with regard to sustainability of neonatal services (Getting It Right First Time [GIRFT], 2022). The continuous drive towards improving care standards and efficiency is facilitated by projects such as the Commissioning for Quality and Innovation (CQUIN) framework and the NNAP delivered by the RCPCH. By evaluating data obtained through the BadgerNet

UK system, the aim of the NNAP is to establish whether there is consistency with regard to the standards of care received by infants admitted to UK NNUs (RCPCH, 2025). The web-based companion contains a number of relevant links for additional information.

STAFFING OF NEONATAL UNITS

Appropriate nurse, medical, and allied health professional staffing on all NNUs is essential to meet the needs of babies at various care levels. It is, however, well documented that there are issues both in recruiting and retaining neonatal nurses (Chant et al., 2024). Based on professional consensus, recommendations for minimum nurse staffing levels are as follows (NHSE, 2024a):

Intensive care: Due to the complex needs of both the baby and their family, the ratio of neonatal nurses who are qualified in specialty (QIS) to baby should be one nurse:one baby. This nurse should have no other (including managerial) responsibilities during the time of clinical care but may be involved in the support of a less experienced nurse working alongside them in caring for the same baby, e.g. a nurse undertaking the QIS course.

High dependency care: The ratio of QIS neonatal nurses responsible for the care of babies requiring HD care is recommended as one nurse:two babies. The more stable and less dependent babies may be cared for by registered nurses who are not QIS but who are under the direct supervision and responsibility of a neonatal nurse who is QIS.

Special care: At a minimum, a ratio of one nurse:four babies is required for infants categorised as SC. It is essential that staffing in SC is sufficient to ensure all discharges are carefully planned and organised, including rigorous parental support. Registered nurses and non-registered clinical staff may care for these babies under the direct supervision and responsibility of a QIS neonatal nurse.

Transitional care: The ratio of neonatal nurses caring for TC babies should be at least one nurse:four babies, while midwifery support must also be available for the mother. There must be joint working between midwifery and neonatal nursing to determine appropriate staffing for the transitional care service (BAPM, 2017).

PRACTICE POINT

Consider how staffing levels, skill mix, and training influence practice in relation to the care given to sick and/or premature neonates and their families. Also consider any variations globally and what influences neonatal care across different world regions.

THE NEONATAL NURSE

In 2018, NHS Improvement on behalf of the National Quality Board summarised the neonatal nursing function in their statement:

> *Neonatal nurses play a key role in the planning and delivery of care to babies and their families. They require a wide skill base as their work ranges from providing care for the sick or premature neonate to teaching parents how to care for their baby, gradually handing over responsibility for this in the lead up to discharge. They also provide care across a whole spectrum of care needs, from intensive care, high dependency care, special care and eventually to care in the home environment.*
>
> (NHS Improvement, 2018, p. 22)

This wide skill base comes from a combination of undergraduate study and ever-growing experience as well as personal characteristics and postgraduate education.

Education and continuing professional development

Neonatal nursing offers the opportunity for a nurse to undertake postgraduate study and become a neonatal nurse who is QIS. Undertaking postgraduate study towards QIS neonatal nursing involves combining theory, which is delivered and fully assessed at a higher educational institute (HEI), and acquiring competency within clinical practice. Standardising neonatal nurse QIS education is important given the variations that have been reported nationally in competency and training (Health Education England, 2021). In England as an example, NHSE (2024b) has established standards to improve neonatal QIS education, ensuring consistency and quality. Developed in collaboration with the NNA, BAPM, and RCN, these standards replace previous guidelines. They define minimum requirements for QIS programmes, promoting uniform knowledge, skills, and behaviours in neonatal care. HEIs, education providers, and neonatal ODNs must align their courses accordingly. While focusing primarily on nurses, the framework also applies to other healthcare professionals delivering cot-side neonatal care.

Furthermore, all neonatal nurses with acquired QIS status must demonstrate competency in a core skill set, to include, for example:

- Respiratory and cardiovascular management
- Fluid, electrolyte, nutrition, and elimination management
- Neurological and pain management
- Skin and hygiene and infection prevention management

- Management of health, safety, and security for neonates and their families
- Complex medicine management
- Investigations and procedures
- Temperature management
- Breastfeeding support
- Supporting the family.

(NHSE, 2024b)

All infants have individual needs, which can often be complex. In addition to core competencies, neonatal nurses who are QIS must undertake assessment in clinical practice and acquire clinical skills to provide high-quality care for sick and/or preterm infants. Irrespective of the level at which a neonatal nurse functions, they are obliged to have evidence of continuous professional development and conform to Nursing and Midwifery Council (NMC) revalidation requirements.

CAREER PROGRESSION

Following completion of postgraduate neonatal nursing QIS study, there will be the opportunity for career progression and the potential to develop skills beyond QIS level, as well as to undertake additional study to work within further neonatal roles. The NNA (2026) outlines a variety of established nursing roles and a full, career pathway; these are not all utilised in every NNU but integrated to match an individual units' requirements.

Extended nursing roles

Senior QIS nurses may have the opportunity to undertake and lead additional non-clinical activities, such as:

- Breastfeeding support
- Family support
- Infant development
- Discharge planning
- Safeguarding children
- Bereavement support and palliative care
- Health, safety, and risk management
- Education and practice development.

Some examples of specific roles include outreach and advanced practice.

NEONATAL OUTREACH NURSE

Following discharge from the neonatal unit, some infants have ongoing care needs (Petty et al., 2018), e.g. due to requiring nasogastric tube feeding or oxygen therapy at home. The role involves providing nursing care, practical and emotional support, parental education, and growth monitoring in the home environment (BAPM, 2017). Chapter 3 has further information on community based neonatal nursing roles and responsibilities.

ADVANCED NEONATAL NURSE PRACTITIONER

The role of the advanced neonatal nurse practitioner (ANNP) was introduced in the UK approximately 33 years ago. Advanced nursing practice is based on the four pillars of advanced practice (see Figure 1.1).

From a clinical perspective, following education at master's level, ANNPs may autonomously and independently manage their own caseload through assessment, diagnosis, and instigation of treatment within the neonatal population. This includes activities such as the attendance of high-risk deliveries and delivery room resuscitation, stabilisation, independent prescribing, ordering and evaluation of investigations and complex procedures, among other aspects of care. With regard to education, ANNPs are frequently involved in teaching resident doctors as well as members of the neonatal nursing team and often participate in quality improvement activities such as audit, research, and the implementation of **evidence-based care** as part of their role.

ENHANCED NEONATAL NURSE PRACTITIONER

The enhanced neonatal nurse practitioner (ENNP) role in the UK offers an alternative career pathway for experienced neonatal nurses and helps address staffing pressures in neonatal intensive care. With a clearly defined scope of practice and alignment to the ANNP MSc pathway, the role supports professional progression

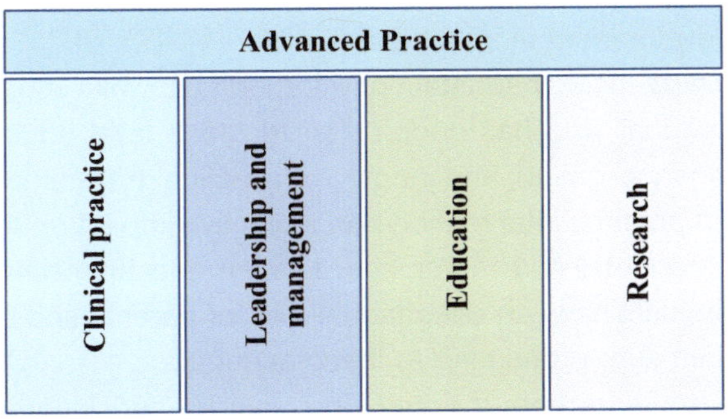

Figure 1.1 Four pillars of advanced practice

while strengthening recruitment and retention. ENNPs enhance service resilience by providing advanced clinical skills that support both medical and nursing teams (Talbert & Keeling, 2019).

THE MULTIDISCIPLINARY TEAM

Neonatology involves working within a multidisciplinary team (MDT) to achieve the best neonatal outcomes. Both medical and nursing teams have various roles and responsibilities, each designed to work in collaboration with the extended multidisciplinary team.

Pharmacy Pharmacists play a vital role in the monitoring and optimisation of neonatal drug therapy and have an important advisory function with regard to safe delivery of complex and often unlicensed medications. Issues unique to the neonatal population such as patient size, limited intravenous access, and uncertain pharmacodynamics and pharmacokinetics mean that specialist training is required before the role of neonatal pharmacist can be safely assumed. Medication practice in the NNU is further discussed in Chapter 21.

Dietetics Neonatal dietitians play an integral role for assessing and improving the nutrition of premature infants and work in collaboration with medical and nursing teams as well as families. There is a requirement for all NNUs to have access to a dietitian who has undergone specialist education in neonatal nutrition (Marlow, 2022). Please refer to Chapter 19 for nutritional management in the NNU for more information.

Diagnostic imaging NHS Improvement (2018) highlights the need for all NNUs to be able to access timely diagnostic imaging and draw on the expertise of professionals with the ability to interpret neonatal imaging.

Occupational therapy The role of the neonatal occupational therapist involves neurobehavioural assessment, advice on sensory issues, and parental education relating to infant behavioural cues. The occupational therapist often works very closely with the physiotherapist, both being vitally important for the wellbeing and development of infant and family.

Physiotherapy The neonatal physiotherapist will usually be a very experienced individual who has undertaken master's level education to enable autonomous, evidence-based, and innovative practice. Physiotherapy in the form of movement and postural intervention has a positive impact on the development of infant musculoskeletal and motor coordination and thus outcomes. Furthermore, physiotherapists have an educational role for parents and staff with regard to optimising infant support relating to these aspects.

Speech and language therapy The speech and language therapist is responsible for the assessment of infant feeding readiness, swallowing ability and formulation of individualised management plans. This is vital to promote successful oral feeding and reduce aversion to feeding. Additionally, the role involves providing education for all professionals on feeding and swallowing problems, as well as supporting parents relating to interventions to promote language development. The feeding MDT is covered in Chapter 19 as well as the web-based companion.

Psychological support It is recognised that emotional outcomes are improved by providing appropriate support for parents and families. Furthermore, parents whose infants are admitted to the NNU may experience significant post-traumatic stress symptoms (Alsallum et al., 2025). Therefore, access to a psychologist through the ODN and/or Trust is essential, alongside a dedicated care coordinator who acts as a vital link between families and healthcare professionals. This role enables parents to become active partners in their baby's care and supports the delivery of Family Integrated Care (FiCare) principles. Parent involvement and engagement representatives also play an important role in providing family support and contributing to the development and implementation of related initiatives. Unfortunately, not all NNUs have around-the-clock access to psychological support for parents. Neonatal charities such as Bliss may assist parents throughout their neonatal journey, and ensuring access to psychological support for families is a criterion for achieving accreditation to the Bliss Baby Charter (Bliss, 2025). Emotional support will be covered in more detail in Chapter 6, relating to families in the NNU.

Social workers in the NNU setting provide social support services to families, providing practical and social-emotional support in particular situations when families may face challenges or when safeguarding issues arise.

SAFEGUARDING IN THE NEONATAL UNIT

A key example of multidisciplinary working is safeguarding, which is a fundamental responsibility for the whole neonatal team, requiring vigilance and sensitivity when working with families (Rogers & Nurse, 2019). Staff should remain alert to signs of postnatal mental health difficulties, including postpartum depression or situations that may potentially delay early bonding, such as the barriers presented by a neonatal admission. If any concerns are raised, observing parent-infant interactions and ensuring sensitive, non-judgemental communication along with facilitation of **family integrated care** (see Chapter 6) is essential. Awareness of potential domestic abuse (DA) is also needed if any relevant concerns are raised, including controlling or erratic behaviours by parents and/or partners or unexplained injuries. A thorough understanding of family history, including substance misuse or complex social circumstances, is vital. Where concerns arise, timely referral to safeguarding teams or social workers is necessary, particularly if antenatal referrals have not occurred or risks have escalated.

> **THINK POINT**
>
> Consider a family with an infant diagnosed with **neonatal abstinence syndrome (NAS),** following maternal alcohol and substance misuse before and during pregnancy, leading to antenatal referral to social services. Reflect on how you would support parents experiencing guilt, anxiety, or stigma. Identify strategies to provide non-judgemental care, promote bonding, and encourage parental involvement in comfort measures. Consider when to involve multidisciplinary teams, including social services, and how to communicate concerns while maintaining trust and prioritising the infant's safety and wellbeing.

NEONATAL OUTCOMES

Over recent decades, the survival rate of preterm infants has rapidly increased with advances in healthcare and medical technology. The UK EPICure study highlighted the rise in survival rates of the extremely premature infant and still continues to inform our knowledge in this area (EGA Institute for Women's Health, 2025). Reports indicate that neonatal mortality rates in the UK have fluctuated, with disparities persisting across ethnic and socio-economic groups (Bliss, 2023; National Maternal and Perinatal Audit (NMPA), 2024; MBRRACE-UK, 2025). Advances in neonatal respiratory care, improved infection control, and neurodevelopmental care have contributed to improved outcomes for preterm infants (BAPM, 2022b). Additionally, national initiatives continue to focus on reducing brain injury and long-term complications through enhanced perinatal care strategies that focus on making maternity and neonatal care safer, more personalised, and more equitable (NHSE, 2023; RCPCH, 2024).

THE GLOBAL PERSPECTIVE

Neonatal healthcare varies significantly worldwide, with disparities in outcomes, service organisation, standards of care, and education. Higher-income countries have well-structured neonatal networks, ensuring specialist transport teams, regional NICUs, and standardised national guidelines. In contrast, many low-income countries struggle with limited NICU access, leading to higher neonatal mortality rates. Globally, neonatal mortality remains a challenge, with sub-Saharan

Africa experiencing the highest rates; 27 deaths per 1,000 live births (World Health Organization, 2024).

Neonatal nursing workforce also varies significantly across the globe, influenced by economic resources, healthcare policies, and workforce availability. The WHO (2025) reports that nursing shortages remain a critical issue, with global disparities in neonatal nurse-to-patient ratios. Efforts to address these disparities include international collaborations, standardised neonatal education programmes, and policy-driven workforce investments. WHO's Global Strategic Directions for Nursing and Midwifery and the Council of International Neonatal Nurses (COINN, 2025) aim to strengthen education, leadership, and service delivery to improve neonatal care worldwide.

Neonatal education also differs worldwide. Some countries such as the UK, United States of America and Australia follow standardised training programmes for neonatal nurses and doctors, ensuring consistent competency levels (Petty et al., 2022; COINN, 2021). In contrast, many countries lack formalised neonatal education, leading to variability in care quality. International efforts, such as WHO guidelines, aim to bridge these gaps, promoting nursing and/or midwife-led continuity of care, which has been shown to reduce neonatal mortality (Fernandez Turienzo et al., 2021). Global disparities highlight the need for continued investment in neonatal health, ensuring equitable access to life-saving interventions worldwide.

Chapter takeaways

- The organisation of neonatal care in the UK is guided by nationally universal standards, with the aim to ensure every neonate is looked after as close to home as possible in the clinical environment their level of care requirement necessitates, by appropriately skilled and educated staff.
- Across the world, neonatal healthcare practice and delivery is organised into 'levels' or 'categories' of care relating to the dependency level required by those neonates born sick and/or small.
- Globally, neonatal care varies with disparities present in the necessary resources, provision of services, education, and training which impact the outcomes of neonates born preterm, sick, or vulnerable.
- The neonatal nurse alongside a range of allied healthcare professionals plays a pivotal role in a neonate's progress, not only through the clinical aspects of their responsibilities, but also by identifying potentially changing care needs, communicating these where necessary to appropriate hospitals and services, enhancing care by timely collaboration, and supporting families on their journey.

CASE STUDY

CASE STUDIES

Case study 1: The 27-week infant in a LNU

You have just commenced your shift at your unit, which is a level 2 LNU. Dylan, the baby you have been allocated today, was born only 2 hours before at 27 weeks' gestation, weighing 1085 grams. He was delivered via emergency C-section due to concerns about fetal wellbeing.

Having received surfactant in the delivery room, he is now stable on CPAP with acceptable blood gases. His other parameters are satisfactory. Dylan is receiving PN via an umbilical venous catheter.

Q.1. Which care category does Dylan fall under in accordance with BAPM guidelines? Is it suitable for him to be cared for on your unit in the longer term – what is the rationale behind your answer?

Q.2. What does the shift leader have to consider with regard to distribution of the workload among staff and whom she allocates to look after Dylan?

The decision is made for Dylan to be transferred to a level 3 NICU for his ongoing care.

Q.3. How would you prepare for Dylan's transfer? Who needs to be contacted to facilitate this happening?

Case study 2: The journey of an extremely preterm infant transferred ex utero

Pavneet was born unexpectedly at 23+2 weeks' gestation without having received antenatal corticosteroids. The SCU at her mother Rashmi's booking hospital stabilised Pavneet and had her transferred to the regional NICU.

Q.1. Could anything have been done to prevent Pavneet's being delivered in an inappropriate setting for her care requirements?

Pavneet is now nine weeks old and has multiple problems: she is still requiring oxygen, has suffered significant intraventricular haemorrhages likely to affect her long-term neurodevelopment, and is failing to thrive, with her current weight on the 0.4th percentile. However, as Pavneet is now stable, there is a

CASE STUDY

plan to transfer her back to the SCU at her booking hospital. Rashmi and her husband Manjunath are feeling extremely anxious about this and express a wish for Pavneet to remain on the NICU instead.

Q.2. In your opinion, is it appropriate for Pavneet to be repatriated to her local SCU, considering the level of care she is now receiving?
Q.3. How would you approach a conversation with Rashmi and Manjunath?
Q.4. What are your considerations for Pavneet's ongoing care and which members of the multidisciplinary team will most likely need to be involved?

Case study 3: Safeguarding in the neonatal unit

Jayden is admitted to the neonatal unit (NNU) at 36 weeks' gestation, born to Leah. This is Leah's fourth child; her previous children are currently in foster care. A referral to social services was made during pregnancy due to longstanding safeguarding concerns, including a history of substance misuse and previous involvement with child protection services.

Leah arrives on the unit alone. She appears withdrawn and anxious, frequently checking her phone. During initial conversations, she discloses that her partner has been 'staying nearby' and becomes visibly unsettled when discussing him. Staff are aware from handover that there are concerns regarding ongoing domestic abuse.

The allocated nurse, Sarah, introduces herself and spends time building rapport with Leah, using a calm and non-judgemental approach. She explains Jayden's care and gently encourages Leah's involvement, including nappy changing and skin-to-skin contact. Leah is hesitant but agrees with reassurance. Sarah is mindful of Leah's emotional state and avoids overwhelming her with information.

During the shift, Sarah observes fluctuating engagement and low mood. She documents her observations and shares relevant information during handover, ensuring continuity of care. She also liaises with the safeguarding team and neonatal social worker to confirm that appropriate support and risk assessments are in place.

Q1. How can staff balance a non-judgemental, supportive approach with the need to prioritise safety and wellbeing?
Q2. What safeguarding concerns are present, and how should staff respond?

CASE STUDY

Q3. How can Sarah support Leah to engage in her baby's care while being mindful of her emotional wellbeing and past experiences?

Q4. What multidisciplinary input is required in this case, and how can effective communication between services be maintained?

Case study 4: The 26-week unstable infant requiring trauma-informed care

You have just started your shift on your Level 3 NICU. Aisha, a baby you have been allocated today, was born 3 hours ago at 26 weeks' gestation, weighing 820 grams. She is a small, extremely preterm infant born to parents from a Black African ethnic background, via emergency caesarean section due to severe placental insufficiency and maternal pre-eclampsia. At birth, Aisha required intubation, surfactant administration, and ongoing ventilatory support. She is currently ventilated with high oxygen requirements and has labile blood gases. She has hypotension requiring inotropic support and is receiving parenteral nutrition via an umbilical venous catheter.

Her parents arrived on the unit shortly after delivery. Both appear distressed and overwhelmed. Her mother is recovering from surgery and has expressed fear about touching Aisha due to all the equipment. Her father is asking frequent questions but appears anxious and uncertain. There are cultural considerations the family wishes to be respected, including involvement of extended family and spiritual practices.

Q1. Which care category does Aisha fall under according to BAPM guidelines? What specific clinical factors contribute to her categorisation?

Q2. Considering Aisha's instability and her parents' emotional state, what factors should the nurse in charge consider when allocating staff to care for Aisha?

Q3. Using principles of trauma-informed care, how would you support Aisha's parents during this early stage of admission while ensuring safe and effective clinical care for Aisha?

For suggested answer guides to the questions posed in these case studies, please refer to the web-based companion site specific to this chapter. See www.routledge.com/cw/petty

References

Alsallum, F. S., Boyle, B., McLaughlin, D., & McGowan, I. (2025). The risk factors of post-traumatic stress disorder among parents of neonatal intensive care unit infants: A systematic review. *Journal of Neonatal Nursing*, *31*(2), 101620. https://doi.org/10.1016/j.jnn.2025.101620

Battersby, C., Michaelides, S., Upton, M., & Rennie, J. M., Jaundice Working Group of the ATAIN (Avoiding Term Admissions Into Neonatal units) programme, led by the Patient Safety team in NHS Improvement. (2017). Term admissions to neonatal units in England: A role for transitional care? A retrospective cohort study. *BMJ Open*, 7(5), e016050. https://doi.org/10.1136/bmjopen-2017-016050

Bliss. (2023). *New reports show poorer neonatal outcomes for babies already facing inequalities, highlighting urgent need for action*. https://www.bliss.org.uk/news/2024/two-new-reports-show-poorer-outcomes-for-babies-already-facing-inequalities

Bliss. (2025). *Bliss baby charter*. https://www.bliss.org.uk/health-professionals/bliss-baby-charter/what-is-the-baby-charter

British Association of Perinatal Medicine. (2017). *Neonatal transitional care – A framework for practice*. www.bapm.org/resources/framework-neonatal-transitional-care

British Association of Perinatal Medicine. (2022a). *Service standards for hospitals providing neonatal care* (4th ed.). BAPM. https://www.bapm.org/resources/service-and-quality-standards-for-provision-of-neonatal-care-in-the-uk

British Association of Perinatal Medicine. (2022b). *New GIRFT national report outlines measures to improve neonatal care*. https://www.bapm.org/articles/new-girft-national-report-for-neonatology

Chant, K., Latour, J. M., Booth, N., Viola, L., Crofts, K., Nishimura, Y., & Gallagher, K. (2024). Job satisfaction and intent to stay in neonatal nursing in England and Wales: A study protocol. *BMC Health Services Research*, *24*(1), 913. https://doi.org/10.1186/s12913-024-11379-0

Council of International Neonatal Nurses (COINN). (2021). *COINN core competencies*. https://www.coinnurses.org/competencies

Council of International Neonatal Nurses (COINN). (2025). *Unifying neonatal nurses globally*. https://www.coinnurses.org/about-us

EGA Institute for Women's Health. (2025). *EPIcure study publications*. https://www.ucl.ac.uk/womens-health/research/neonatology/epicure/publications

European Standards of Care for Newborn Health. (2025). *Newborn transport*. https://newborn-health-standards.org/standards/standards-english/birth-transfer/neonatal-transport/

Fernandez Turienzo, C., Rayment-Jones, H., Roe, Y., Silverio, S. A., Coxon, K., Shennan, A. H., & Sandall, J. (2021). A realist review to explore how midwifery continuity of care may influence preterm birth in pregnant women. *Birth*, *48*(3), 375–388.

Getting It Right First Time. (2022). *Neonatology – workforce*. GIRFT Programme National Specialty Report. https://gettingitrightfirsttime.co.uk/wp-content/uploads/2025/01/Neonatology-workforce-report-09-12f-FINAL.pdf

Health Education England. (2021). *Neonatal qualified in specialty (QIS) education and training review*. https://www.hee.nhs.uk/sites/default/files/documents/RSM%20Neonatal%20QIS%20Review.pdf

Imperial College. (2025). *Preterm birth, labour and delivery*. https://www.imperial.ac.uk/metabolism-digestion-reproduction/research/reproductive-developmental-biology/clinical-themes/preterm-birth

Leslie, A., Harrison, C., Jackson, A., Broster, S., Clarke, E., Davidson, S. L., Devon, C., Forshaw, B., Philpott, A., Tinnion, R., Whiston, J., Fenton, A. C., & Sharkey, D. (2024). Tracking national neonatal transport activity and metrics using the UK Neonatal Transport Group dataset 2012–2021: A narrative review. *Archives of Disease in Childhood – Fetal and Neonatal Edition*, *109*, 460–466.

Marlow, N. (2022). *Dietitian staffing on neonatal units: Neonatal sub-group recommendations for commissioning.* https://www.bda.uk.com/static/ab614d3e-e095-4e4f-96ae1458204e8810/391a27be-69a0-4b43-a52d54a731da7f01/BDA-Formatted-Staffing-Recc.pdf

MBRRACE-UK. (2025). *MBRRACE-UK perinatal mortality surveillance-UK perinatal deaths of babies born in 2023.* https://timms.le.ac.uk/mbrrace-uk-perinatal-mortality/surveillance/

McKeon-Carter, R. (2018). Neonatal transitional care – a concept not a place. *Infant, 14*(3), 98–102.

National Maternal and Perinatal Audit. (2024). *Evaluating hospital and crisis care for perinatal mental health.* https://maternityaudit.org.uk/FilesUploaded/REF%20480%20Perinatal%20Mental%20Health%20Report_Final.pdf

Neonatal Nurses Association UK. (2026). *Interactive careers framework.* https://nna.org.uk/neonatal-nurse-career-framework/

NHS England. (2017). *Reducing harm leading to avoidable admission of full-term babies into neonatal units.* https://www.england.nhs.uk/wp-content/uploads/2021/03/reducing-harm-leading-to-avoidable-admission-of-full-term-babies-into-neonatal-units.pdf

NHS England. (2023). *Update from the maternity and neonatal programme.* https://www.england.nhs.uk/long-read/update-from-the-maternity-and-neonatal-programme/

NHS England. (2024a). *Service specification: neonatal critical care.* https://www.england.nhs.uk/publication/service-specification-neonatal-critical-care/

NHS England. (2024b). *National standards for neonatal qualified in specialty (QIS) education.* https://www.england.nhs.uk/long-read/national-standards-for-neonatal-qualified-in-specialty-qis-education/

NHS England. (2025a). *E-learning for health portal.* https://portal.e-lfh.org.uk/

NHS England. (2025b). *Reducing admission of full-term babies to neonatal units.* https://www.england.nhs.uk/mat-transformation/reducing-admission-of-full-term-babies-to-neonatal-units/

NHS Improvement. (2018). *An improvement resource for neonatal care.* https://www.england.nhs.uk/wp-content/uploads/2021/04/safe-staffing-neonatal.pdf

Office for National Statistics. (2025). *Births in England and Wales: 2023.* https://www.ons.gov.uk/peoplepopulationandcommunity/birthsdeathsandmarriages/livebirths/bulletins/birthsummarytablesenglandandwales/2023

Petty, J., Jones, T., van den Hoogen, A., Walker, K., & Kenner, C. (Eds.). (2022). *Neonatal nursing: A global perspective*. Springer Publishing.

Petty, J., Whiting, L., Green, J., Fowler, C., Rossiter, C., & Elliott, D. (2018). Parents' views on preparation to care for extremely premature infants at home. *Nursing Children and Young People, 30*(4), 22–27.

Pillay, T., Rivero-Arias, O., Armstrong, N., Seaton, S. E., Yang, M., Banda, V. L., Dawson, K., Ismail, A. Q., Bountziouka, V., Cupit, C., Paton, A., Manktelow, B. N., Draper, E. S., Modi, N., Campbell, H. E., & Boyle, E. M. (2025). Optimising neonatal services for very preterm births between 27+0- and 31+6-weeks' gestation in England: The OPTI-PREM mixed-methods study. *Health and Social Care Delivery Research, 13*(12), 1–126. https://doi.org/10.3310/JYWC6538.

Rogers, A., & Nurse, S. (2019). Child protection in the neonatal unit. *Journal of Neonatal Nursing, 25*(2), 99–101.

Royal College of Paediatrics and Child Health. (2024). *National neonatal audit programme (NNAP) summary report on 2023 data.* https://www.rcpch.ac.uk/sites/default/files/2024-10/nnap_summary_report_on_2023_data_0.pdf

Royal College of Paediatrics and Child Health. (2025). *About the National Neonatal Audit Programme (NNAP).* https://woww.rcpch.ac.uk/work-we-do/clinical-audits/nnap/about

Royal College of Paediatrics and Child Health – Neonatal Partnership Board. (2023). *Report from the UK Neonatal Partnership Board national reviews of maternity and neonatal care: Supporting the perinatal team to implement recommendations related to neonatal care.* https://www.rcpch.ac.uk/sites/default/files/2023-08/Report-UK-Neonatal-Partnership-Board-2023.pdf

Talbert, J., & Keeling, D. (2019). The development and impact of the ENNP role in the NICU. *Infant*, *15*(6), 234–236.

TinyLife. (2022). *Tiny Life cares: Strategic plan 2022–2025.* https://www.tinylife.org.uk/app/uploads/2022/08/stat-plan-WEB.pdf

UK Government. (2025). *Preterm birth.* https://view-health-screening-recommendations.service.gov.uk/preterm-birth/

Watson, H., McLaren, J., Carlisle, N., Ratnavel, N., Watts, T., Zaima, A., Tribe, R. M., & Shennan, A. H. (2020). All the right moves: Why in utero transfer is both important for the baby and difficult to achieve and new strategies for change. *F1000Research*, *9*, F1000 Faculty Rev-979. https://doi.org/10.12688/f1000research.25923.1

World Health Organization. (2023). *Preterm birth.* https://www.who.int/news-room/fact-sheets/detail/preterm-birth

World Health Organization. (2024). *Newborn mortality.* https://www.who.int/news-room/fact-sheets/detail/newborn-mortality

World Health Organization. (2025). *Nursing workforce grows, but inequities threaten global health goals.* https://www.who.int/news/item/12-05-2025-nursing-workforce-grows--but-inequities-threaten-global-health-goals

2 ANTENATAL AND PERINATAL ASPECTS OF CARE

Radica Hardyal, Julia Petty, Sarah Fitchett, and Rhian Smith

CONTENTS

DOI: 10.4324/9781003591405-4

GUIDANCE ON HOW TO ENHANCE PERSONAL LEARNING FROM THIS CHAPTER

Key points covered in this chapter

Antenatal aspects of care

- The impact of maternal health and illness on the fetus and neonate.
- Fetal and antenatal screening.
- Antenatal and genetic counselling.
- Decision-making during pregnancy.

Perinatal aspects of care

- Perinatal management and optimisation of high-risk conditions in pregnancy, including, for example, antenatal steroids, magnesium sulphate, optimal cord management and birthing room care.
- The importance of interprofessional teamwork.
- Inequalities in maternal and neonatal outcomes.

Reflection

Reading through the chapter, you are encouraged to engage with the key points and related literature in an enquiring way. Ask these questions:

- Why is care of the pregnant woman/person important, and how does this impact the planning and care provision for the neonate?
- What are the antenatal and perinatal aspects of care that impact fetal and neonatal wellbeing?

Implications for nursing care

- Optimum care is essential to ensure positive maternal and neonatal outcomes.
- Inequalities exist in outcomes, so it is vital that antenatal and perinatal care is inclusive, considering diversity across all demographics and protected characteristics.

INTRODUCTION AND BACKGROUND

Stillbirths and neonatal deaths (NNDs) have steadily declined globally over the last decade; however, ethnic and socioeconomic disparities persist (Saberian et al., 2025). The leading causes of **perinatal** mortality have consistently been reported to be placental issues, **congenital** anomalies, umbilical cord complications, and extreme prematurity. These findings emphasise the importance of personalised antenatal care to address risk factors such as preterm birth, socioeconomic deprivation, and congenital anomalies (Gallimore et al., 2025).

Maternity care provision during pregnancy and birth and the early postpartum period plays a vital role in determining neonatal health outcomes, particularly for infants needing neonatal intensive care. In the United Kingdom (UK), early recognition of congenital disorders through genetic screening and counselling, coupled with informed decision-making during pregnancy, encourages healthcare professionals and parents to optimise care pathways before and during birth.

This chapter examines the evolving landscape of antenatal care, with a focus on advancements in fetal and genetic screening, managing maternal health conditions, and exploring the complexities of decision-making during pregnancy. Additionally, it examines the impact of maternal circumstances on neonatal outcomes, such as medical **co-morbidities**, lifestyle, and psychosocial factors, and discusses evidence-based perinatal practices, including optimal cord management. By integrating these aspects, neonatal nurses can enhance their understanding of the transition from fetal to neonatal life and be equipped with the knowledge to support parents and contribute to improved outcomes for at-risk newborns.

The terms *woman, women*, *mother*, and *maternal* are used throughout this chapter alongside the term *pregnant person(s)*. We recognise that pregnancy, birth, and the postnatal period may be experienced by trans men, non-binary people, and others who do not identify as women but who may become pregnant. These terms are therefore intended to be inclusive, referring to all individuals who are pregnant or have the potential to be pregnant, while also reflecting the terminology widely used in clinical guidelines and national datasets.

IMPACT OF MATERNAL HEALTH ON THE FETUS AND NEONATE

Several maternal risk factors influence perinatal morbidity and mortality in the antenatal period, including medical, lifestyle, psychosocial factors, and demographic variables. Therefore, optimising maternal wellbeing and provision of quality care in the antenatal period can influence fetal and neonatal wellbeing. Maternal health directly influences fetal growth, placental function, and neonatal transition. The National Institute for Health and Care Excellence (NICE, 2021) antenatal care guideline emphasises early access to antenatal care, systematic risk assessment, and provision of information on modifiable factors (smoking cessation, alcohol avoidance, and supplements such as folic acid and vitamin D) to reduce poor neonatal outcomes.

Hypertensive disorders of pregnancy

Hypertensive disorders of pregnancy (HDP), including chronic hypertension, gestational hypertension, and **pre-eclampsia**, are a leading cause of maternal and perinatal morbidity and mortality in the UK. These conditions are associated with increased risks of fetal growth restriction (FGR), placental abruption, preterm birth, stillbirth, neonatal morbidity, and neonatal unit (NNU) admission (Conti-Ramsden et al., 2025). Hypertensive disorders of pregnancy, including pre-eclampsia, increase risks of fetal growth restriction, preterm birth, and neonatal morbidity. NICE (2023) provides recommendations on diagnosis and management, including placental growth factor (PlGF)-based testing to identify pre-eclampsia prediction and pathways, aiming to decrease severe disease and adverse neonatal outcomes. The Royal College of Obstetricians and Gynaecologists (RCOG) guidance reinforces the burden and potential neonatal impact of pre-eclampsia (e.g. growth restriction), and the need for timely birth when maternal and/or fetal indications arise. When a fetus does not achieve its growth potential or is compromised in some way, this is associated with stillbirth, preterm birth, and increased risk of neonatal morbidity and mortality. Although several factors can cause FGR, it is predominantly related to poor placental function. Maternal hypertensive disorders, either pre-existing or developed during pregnancy, often co-exist with FGR, and pregnancies affected by both usually have poorer outcomes (Chmielewska et al., 2025).

Diabetes

Diabetes in pregnancy affects neonatal outcomes through risks associated with elevated maternal blood glucose, including hypoglycaemia, respiratory distress, and cardiomyopathy. NICE (2020) covers preconception optimisation, diagnosis and management of gestational diabetes, intrapartum and neonatal care pathways to mitigate risks. Recent evidence from a large UK single-centre cohort study (Karkia et al., 2023) highlights the significant impact of diabetes mellitus (DM) on pregnancy outcomes. The study found that the severity of perinatal complications is closely linked to the severity of maternal hyperglycaemia. Pregnancies complicated by pre-existing DM, whether type 1 or type 2, are associated with increased risks of adverse outcomes across the antenatal, intrapartum, and neonatal periods. These include congenital anomalies, stillbirth, preterm birth, hypertensive disorders, and neonatal complications such as hypoglycaemia, jaundice, and increased neonatal unit admission.

Gestational DM (GDM) is primarily associated with third-trimester complications. These include preterm birth, pre-eclampsia, increased rates of caesarean births, and neonatal morbidity. While GDM does not appear to increase the risk of stillbirth or NND to the same extent as pre-existing DM, it nonetheless contributes to a higher burden of neonatal care needs, particularly in terms of respiratory support and metabolic monitoring (Fotă & Petca, 2025). These findings highlight the importance of early screening, multidisciplinary antenatal management, and close glycaemic control to mitigate risks. Multidisciplinary teams must understand the neonatal complications associated with different types of maternal diabetes to anticipate care needs and improve outcomes.

Cardiac conditions

Maternal cardiac conditions during pregnancy increase the risk of adverse outcomes for both the fetus and newborn. These outcomes include higher rates of preterm birth, small-for-gestational-age (SGA) infants, and low birthweight. A cohort study from specialised pregnancy heart clinics in the UK found that pregnancies in women with pre-existing structural heart disease frequently lead to adverse outcomes, including a high prevalence of medically indicated preterm deliveries (Huang et al., 2025). Neonatal complications associated with these conditions include respiratory distress, feeding difficulties, and a higher likelihood of neonatal intensive care admissions (Eggleton et al., 2023). Although the national surveillance programme MBRRACE-UK does not currently track specific adverse perinatal outcomes attributed to maternal cardiac disease, the 2025 maternal report indicates that cardiovascular conditions remain a major contributor to maternal mortality. This highlights the importance of multidisciplinary antenatal care and careful perinatal planning to optimise outcomes for both mother and baby (Knight et al., 2025).

Maternal infections

Adverse fetal and neonatal outcomes associated with maternal infection vary according to the gestational timing of exposure, ranging from miscarriage (infections in early pregnancy) to congenital malformations (infection during fetal development), and fetal or neonatal morbidity (infection later in pregnancy or during labour). Viral infections such as cytomegalovirus, rubella, varicella, and parvovirus B19 may cross the placenta and lead to congenital infection, structural abnormalities, fetal growth restriction, or long-term neurodevelopmental impairment (see also Chapter 20) (Al Beloushi et al., 2024).

Bacterial infections in pregnancy, such as group B streptococcus (GBS), are associated with miscarriage, stillbirth, preterm birth, and early-onset neonatal sepsis (Manuel et al., 2025). Pregnant women should receive intrapartum antibiotics if they have GBS colonisation or bacteriuria, a previous baby with GBS disease, intrapartum fever or suspected infection, preterm labour, or prolonged rupture of membranes, as these factors increase the risk of early-onset neonatal infection (NICE, 2024a).

Parasitic infections, including *Toxoplasma gondii*, can cause congenital disease affecting the brain and eyes (Auriti et al., 2022). Studies have also found that maternal covid infection is associated with increased risk of preterm births, low birthweight, and neonatal respiratory complications, as well as an increased rate of admission to NNU and SGA (Ali et al., 2023; Sturrock et al., 2023).

Effective interventions to reduce the impact of maternal infections on fetal and neonatal outcomes focus on prevention, early detection, and timely management. Strategies include antenatal screening, targeted vaccination where available, and the appropriate use of antimicrobial or antiparasitic therapy during pregnancy. Combined with enhanced maternal and fetal surveillance, these measures can significantly reduce the risk of miscarriage, congenital disease, preterm birth, and neonatal morbidity, supporting safer pregnancy and optimum neonatal outcomes (Baguiya et al., 2021).

Maternal obesity

Maternal obesity is associated with GDM, hypertensive disorders, thromboembolism, operative birth, and increased risks for the baby such as macrosomia, preterm birth, and stillbirth. RCOG (2018) outlines risk stratification and interventions before and during pregnancy. Moreover, patient information materials provide practical counselling points. A recent longitudinal cohort study investigated the relationship between maternal body mass index (BMI) and hospital admission for infections in the neonate. They found that maternal obesity (BMI over 35) was positively associated with rates of hospital admissions for infections (Coathup et al., 2025).

PRACTICE POINT

Early, inclusive booking, targeted screening (PlGF test for pre-eclampsia risk; oral glucose tolerance test for GDM), weight and thromboembolism risk management, and continuity of carer reduce preventable neonatal compromise (NICE, 2021).

Maternal smoking

Smoking during pregnancy remains a significant public health concern and is associated with a wide range of adverse maternal, fetal, and neonatal outcomes. Tobacco smoke contains numerous harmful substances, including nicotine and carbon monoxide, which cross the placenta and impair oxygen delivery to the fetus. This can disrupt placental function and fetal development, increasing the risk of miscarriage, placental complications, preterm birth, fetal growth restriction, and stillbirth. Smoking during pregnancy is also associated with low birthweight and increased infant mortality, highlighting the importance of early identification and intervention within antenatal care (NICE, 2021).

In the UK, national guidance emphasises the role of routine antenatal screening and targeted interventions to reduce smoking during pregnancy. According to current recommendations, maternity services should assess smoking status at the booking appointment and offer routine carbon monoxide (CO) monitoring to identify exposure to tobacco smoke. CO testing should be performed at the first antenatal appointment and again at around 36 weeks' gestation, with additional testing offered during pregnancy when indicated (NICE, 2021).

Reducing smoking in pregnancy is also a key component of national maternity safety initiatives. The NHS England Saving Babies' Lives Care Bundle (2025) highlights smoking cessation as an important strategy for reducing stillbirth, fetal growth restriction, and neonatal morbidity. Interventions include advice from healthcare professionals, behavioural support, and consideration of nicotine replacement therapy when appropriate. Midwives and other maternity professionals play a central role in delivering these interventions through routine antenatal contacts, using a supportive, non-judgemental approach to encourage engagement with cessation services and improve maternal and neonatal outcomes.

Maternal mental health disorders

Mental health disorders in pregnancy and the perinatal period can range from mild anxiety and depression to severe conditions such as bipolar disorder, schizophrenia, or postpartum psychosis. Maternal mental health disorders during pregnancy have been associated with increased risks of adverse maternal and neonatal outcomes, including hypertensive disorders of pregnancy, preterm birth and low birthweight infants, highlighting the importance of early identification and integrated perinatal mental health support within antenatal care (Runkle et al., 2023).

NICE (2021) recommends routine assessment of mental health at the antenatal booking appointment and throughout pregnancy to identify anyone who may require additional support. Early screening allows timely referral to specialist services and facilitates the development of personalised care plans. Those with moderate to severe mental health conditions benefit from coordinated multidisciplinary care involving midwives, obstetricians, general practitioners, and specialist perinatal mental health teams. Such collaborative approaches aim to ensure that both psychological and physical health needs are addressed during pregnancy.

Maternal medication and recreational substance use

Maternal use of prescribed or illicit substances during pregnancy is increasingly common and poses significant risks to fetal and neonatal health. Prolonged *in utero* exposure to opioids and other substances can result in **neonatal abstinence syndrome** (NAS), a complex neurobehavioural condition characterised by disturbances in autonomic regulation, feeding, sleep-wake control, and motor tone. The severity of NAS varies widely and is influenced by the type and timing of maternal substance use, polysubstance exposure, prematurity, and genetic factors. Diagnosis can be challenging due to under-reporting of maternal drug use and limitations of biological testing; therefore, structured clinical observation remains central. Historically, tools such as the Finnegan score have guided treatment, though lack of consistency in scoring contributes to variation in practice. Non-pharmacological care including rooming-in, breastfeeding, low-stimulus environments, and parental involvement is now recognised as first-line management and reduces the need for medication. When required, morphine or methadone are commonly used, though evidence for optimal pharmacotherapy remains limited. Effective antenatal support, transitional care, and coordinated community follow-up are essential to minimise maternal–infant separation and improve outcomes for families affected by NAS (Kumar & Garg, 2019).

ACTIVITIES

Consider how maternal health conditions can impact the growing fetus and neonate

- Diabetes
- Hypertension
- Cardiac conditions

You may wish to access the various National Institute for Care Excellence (NICE) and Royal College of Obstetricians and Gynaecologists (RCOG) guidelines to add to your knowledge on these areas (see reference list).

MULTIPLE GESTATION

Multiple pregnancy is associated with significantly increased neonatal morbidity and mortality compared with singleton pregnancy, with the associated risk increasing proportionally as fetal number rises (Bell et al., 2024; NICE, 2024b). Preterm birth, fetal growth restriction/low birthweight, and complications specific to **monochorionic** placentation (e.g. **twin-to-twin transfusion syndrome (TTTS)**) are identified as the key factors underlying increased perinatal morbidity and mortality in multiple pregnancy.

According to national guidance from NICE (2024) and RCOG (2026), those with multiple pregnancies should be cared for within a specialist multidisciplinary team and offered a first-trimester ultrasound to estimate **gestational age** and determine **chorionicity** and **amnionicity**. These individuals should also be offered information on screening for Down's, Edwards', and Patau's syndromes as outlined in the fetal anomaly screening programme (FASP) handbook (Gov.uk, 2024). Screening for structural abnormalities and advice on diet, lifestyle, and nutritional supplements should be offered as routine. Information to women should be communicated sensitively.

Diagnostic monitoring for fetal growth restriction in **dichorionic** twin and **trichorionic** triplet pregnancies should occur after 24 weeks of gestation in an interval of 28 days for a dichorionic twin pregnancy and 14 days for those with a trichorionic triplet pregnancy. Monochorionic pregnancies should be monitored for TTTS, FGR, and advanced-stage twin anaemia-polycythaemia sequence (TAPS; see Box 2.1) at every ultrasound assessment, every 14 days from 16 weeks until birth.

BOX 2.1 TAPS (TWIN ANAEMIA-POLYCYTHAEMIA SEQUENCE)

This condition involves a slow, uneven blood transfer through very small placental vessels, whereas twin-to-twin transfusion syndrome is caused by larger vascular connections that create rapid, unbalanced blood flow and clear amniotic fluid differences.

To prevent preterm birth, a single cervical length scan is recommended between 16 and 20 weeks and progesterone 200 mg capsules until 34 weeks of gestation if the woman has a short cervix (25mm or less; NICE, 2024b). The team may seek advice from a tertiary-level fetal medicine centre if complications are confirmed. Timing, planning, mode, and place of birth should also be discussed with the expectant parent(s) and their family.

ANTENATAL CARE AND SCREENING

Antenatal care provides an important opportunity to identify and manage risks that may affect maternal and fetal outcomes. Any woman or pregnant person with complex medical and mental health needs require enhanced assessment, monitoring, and coordinated multidisciplinary support throughout pregnancy. Antenatal screening programmes are designed to detect maternal conditions, fetal anomalies, and genetic disorders at an early stage, enabling timely intervention, informed decision-making, and appropriate care planning. For those with pre-existing physical illness, severe mental health conditions, or social vulnerability, screening and surveillance pathways may need to be adapted to ensure that care is personalised, equitable, and responsive to individual needs. Effective antenatal screening, integrated within comprehensive maternity care, is therefore essential to optimise outcomes for both mother and baby (NICE, 2021).

NICE (2021) guidelines provide an evidence-based framework for antenatal care, ensuring the early identification of maternal and fetal conditions and the delivery of personalised care pathways. These guidelines emphasise the importance of routine screening, risk assessment, and timely interventions to support maternal and fetal wellbeing throughout pregnancy.

Routine screening offered at the booking appointment includes blood tests for infectious diseases such as HIV, hepatitis B, and syphilis, screening for haemoglobinopathies such as sickle cell disease and thalassaemia. The NHS FASP offers combined first-trimester screening and a 20-week ultrasound screening scan for 11 structural conditions, with national standards and quality assurance pathways to ensure equity and timeliness. This programme is embedded within routine antenatal care and is continuously updated.

Key conditions screened at 18+0–20+6 weeks include **anencephaly**, neural tube defects, major cardiac anomalies, **diaphragmatic hernia**, abdominal wall defects, severe **skeletal dysplasia**, and bilateral **renal agenesis**, each with established care pathways aiming to optimise perinatal planning and neonatal outcomes. For anyone pregnant and who has complex medical, psychological, or social needs, these screening pathways are often supplemented with enhanced surveillance and multidisciplinary care to support optimal maternal and neonatal outcomes (NICE, 2021).

Antenatal counselling and decision-making

Open and honest communication between families and healthcare professionals constitutes a foundational element of ethical decision-making and the delivery of family integrated care (FiCare). Antenatal counselling is essential, ensuring that parents are fully included in informed decision-making and the planning of a high-risk birth through honest, compassionate, and realistic discussions about perinatal care and their hopes and expectations. The NICE (2021) antenatal care guideline emphasises that pregnant women should be supported to make informed decisions about their care through clear, evidence-based information and shared decision-making in line with professional standards. Involved in these discussions should be senior practitioners from obstetric, midwifery, and neonatal teams who will be caring for the birthing parent and their baby before, during, and after the birth (Mactier et al., 2020). Input should also be sought from the referral centre if a transfer is being considered.

Individualised discussion and decision-making with parents should be factual, based upon the best evidence for prognosis and being mindful of the baby's best interests, avoiding generalisations and assumptions. Statistics and information given should be in a format that can be understood by parents, personalised, and address prognosis based on all available data, not gestational age alone, including the impact on later life (Thivierge et al., 2025). Discussions must be documented but may remain open, and wishes can be further discussed and renegotiated when needed, including decisions based upon clinical condition before, at, or after birth, or subsequently on the NNU.

If possible, when active care is planned, an opportunity for parents to visit the NNU should be facilitated to meet staff and receive both verbal and written information and support regarding expressing breastmilk (British Association of Perinatal Medicine (BAPM), 2019b, 2026). Where possible, all this information should be supported in a written format to allow parents to revisit it whenever required.

Where appropriate, discussions with parents should include the practical considerations surrounding the initiation, withholding, or withdrawal of intensive care, as well as the beneficial role of palliative care strategies. Such communication is essential in preparing parents for potential postnatal outcomes. During this period, many parents may gain significant support from family members, friends, spiritual advisors, and relevant local or national support organisations, to whom they should be appropriately referred (BAPM, 2019b).

Shared decision-making and FiCare should underpin antenatal counselling, fostering a sense of partnership from the outset and preparing parents for the potential need for neonatal care in line with FiCare principles (BAPM, 2021). Parents report that effective antenatal counselling when undertaken before a preterm delivery was important. This has demonstrated many benefits for parents, such as reducing parental anxiety, increased trust and knowledge, facilitation of informed decision-making, and establishing a rapport with the neonatal team prior to birth (Fish et al., 2021).

An understanding of how information may affect parents should guide the approach to communication, with the aim of minimising distress wherever possible. It is important to recognise that some parents may respond with anger or aggression, which often reflects a physiological reaction to fear and the emotional impact of receiving difficult news. Such situations require sensitive management, maintaining a calm demeanour, and non-threatening body language, while also remaining alert to any need to withdraw to ensure personal safety.

Genetic counselling

Prenatal diagnosis by **chorionic villus sampling** (CVS) or **amniocentesis** and post-screen counselling must be timely, accurate, and non-directive to support informed parental choices. RCOG guidance on amniocentesis and CVS provides procedural standards, while the FASP handbook outlines diagnostic pathways and standards, including **aneuploidy** testing. Genetic counselling is integral to discussing residual risk, test limitations, and implications for pregnancy management or neonatal care (e.g. readiness for cardiac surgery for certain anomalies), emphasising equitable access and respect for parental autonomy.

PERINATAL CARE

Perinatal management of high-risk conditions in pregnancy

The maternal factors discussed above can potentially affect neonatal outcomes at birth, so it is essential to manage these situations in a timely and evidence-based manner in line with current recommendations.

- *Obesity*: As there is an increased risk of **macrosomia** and **shoulder dystocia**, operative birth, and difficulties with fetal monitoring, RCOG (2018) advocates preconception weight optimisation, thrombosis prophylaxis as indicated, and tailored intrapartum care (equipment/positioning), each influencing neonatal safety at birth.
- *Hypertensive disorders*: Targeted maternal monitoring, antihypertensive therapy, seizure prophylaxis should be considered when indicated, and timing of birth based on maternal and fetal indications. These measures reduce stillbirth, growth restriction, and severe neonatal morbidity by preventing maternal deterioration and by planning delivery in appropriately resourced settings (NICE, 2023).
- *Diabetes in pregnancy*: NICE (2020) provides intrapartum glycaemic targets to minimise neonatal hypoglycaemia and guides neonatal surveillance post-birth (e.g. early feeding, glucose monitoring). Implementation decreases NNU admissions for hypoglycaemia and respiratory issues.

- *Antenatal corticosteroids*: A course of steroids for imminent preterm birth (24^{+0}–34^{+6} weeks; targeted use for multiples), reduces NND and respiratory distress. Timing within 48 hours of birth is notably beneficial (RCOG, 2025a).
- *Infections*: RCOG guidance on identification and management of maternal sepsis stresses early recognition and treatment to mitigate fetal compromise and neonatal sepsis. GBS prevention standards further reduce early-onset disease.

Perinatal optimisation for premature birth

There are a number of evidence-based interventions available to reduce neonatal mortality and short and long-term morbidities associated with preterm birth, when it cannot be prevented. Perinatal optimisation (PO) refers to the process of reliably delivering these interventions in the antenatal, intrapartum, and neonatal period to improve preterm outcomes (BAPM, 2026). BAPM and the National Neonatal Audit Programme (NNAP) are working collaboratively on a PO quality improvement initiative that aligns with national workstreams, including NHS England's Maternity and Neonatal Safety Improvement Programme (NHS England, 2026) and the Saving Babies' Lives Care Bundle (SBLCB, 2025). The PO pathway (see Figure 2.1) includes seven key elements that are divided into antenatal optimisation: (1) optimising place of birth, (2) optimal antenatal steroids, (3) magnesium sulphate, and (4) intrapartum antibiotics, and peripartum optimisation: (5) optimal cord management (OCM), (6) normothermia, and (7) early maternal breastmilk. Other areas of focus include volume-targeted ventilation and caffeine administration. Collectively, these aim to provide preterm babies with the best possible start in life (BAPM, 2019a, 2026).

BAPM (2019a, 2019b) recommends that education about preterm birth begins early in pregnancy and is revisited at every antenatal appointment. This should include: (1) the importance of preventing or identifying preterm labour

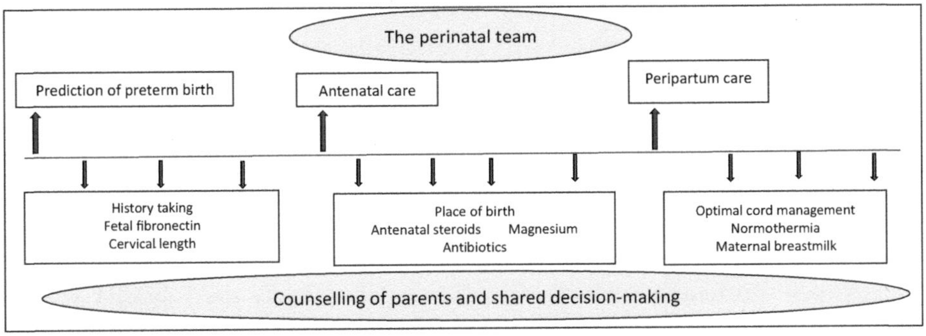

Figure 2.1 The BAPM framework for perinatal optimisation

early to enable timely and beneficial interventions, (2) risk factors for preterm birth and how these can be modified or monitored, and (3) the possibility of NNU admission following preterm birth. Individuals at high risk of preterm labour should be identified promptly and considered for timely *in utero* transfer to a maternity service co-located with a neonatal intensive care unit (NICU), as outcomes are significantly better for babies transferred before birth than for those transferred postnatally, and antenatal transfer also reduces parental-infant separation (Watson et al., 2020). Although birth during transport is rare, decisions about the appropriateness of transfer must be made by the responsible consultant obstetrician, based on an assessment of risks, benefits, travel distance, and the likelihood of imminent birth. All discussions with parents should be clearly documented and communicated with the multidisciplinary teams at both the referring and receiving centres, and management plans should be reviewed regularly with parents (BAPM, 2019a). Providing written information from charities such as BLISS can support families during this time, and information sharing between units can be further enhanced through the use of a parent-held passport detailing interventions undertaken.

TOCOLYTICS

Tocolytics are medications to halt uterine contractions aiming to prolong the pregnancy for up to 48 hours, to allow for the administration of antenatal corticosteroids and transfer to a tertiary centre for ongoing care, thus improving neonatal outcomes. Nifedipine is a calcium channel blocker, and one of the main tocolytics used. The inhibition of the return of calcium ions across cell membranes decreases smooth muscle tone. It is given orally, and doses are adjusted in line with the observed response of uterine activity. If nifedipine is contraindicated, oxytocin receptor antagonists are offered for tocolysis (RCOG, 2026).

ANTIBIOTICS

Preterm birth has been associated with infection; commonly, transvaginal ascending infection. The most common cause of severe early-onset infection in the newborn is GBS. As intrapartum antibiotics reduce the risk of neonatal GBS sepsis in colonised individuals by 86% (Panneflek et al., 2024; Health Innovation West of England, 2026), it is recommended that anyone in preterm labour at less than 37 weeks' gestation should receive intravenous intrapartum antibiotic prophylaxis at least 4 hours prior to birth, as there is no universal screening in the UK, compared to some other countries globally. This excludes planned caesarean births without labour (NICE, 2022). For further information on GBS and its treatment, see Chapter 20.

ANTENATAL CORTICOSTEROIDS

Corticosteroid administration in threatening preterm birth is well established and among the most important interventions to improve neonatal outcomes (Stock et al., 2022; RCOG, 2025a). Documented benefits include improved survival by up to 40%, decreased risk of severe **intraventricular haemorrhage** (IVH) by 45% and **necrotising enterocolitis** (NEC) by 50% (BAPM, 2019a), decreased risk of a **patent ductus arteriosus (PDA)**, reduced need for respiratory support, and reduced systemic infections in the first 48 hours of life. Corticosteroids enhance fetal surfactant production by maturing type II pneumocytes and accelerating fetal lung maturity, increasing the volume of terminal air sacs, allowing closer alignment to the blood vessels for gaseous exchange. In addition, corticosteroids activate epithelial sodium channels and commence the process of lung fluid resorption.

A complete course of antenatal corticosteroids should be administered to all pregnant women between 24+0 and 33+6 weeks who are in suspected, diagnosed, or established preterm labour, accompanied by clear discussion of the benefits. For pregnancies between 22+0 and 23+6 weeks, corticosteroids should also be offered when preterm labour is suspected or established, when a planned preterm birth is anticipated, or in the presence of preterm rupture of membranes (PROM), with counselling tailored to the individual clinical circumstances. Timing is critical: the greatest benefit occurs when birth takes place 24 hours to 7 days after administration. Birth should not be delayed solely for corticosteroid completion if delivery is required for maternal or fetal wellbeing. A repeat course may be considered if delivery is likely within 48 hours and a significant interval has passed since the first course, but no more than two courses should be given (NICE, 2022). In pregnancies under 33+0 weeks, or when FGR is suspected, corticosteroids should still be administered, although clinicians should be aware that they may slightly reduce fetal growth and subsequent birthweight. Betamethasone or dexamethasone remain the recommended corticosteroid preparations.

The rates of administration of corticosteroids have been negatively affected by recent RCOG advice regarding adverse neurodevelopmental outcomes for babies born at term who have been exposed to antenatal corticosteroids between 22–37 weeks, although this is not fully proven, and there are still many positive effects for babies whose mothers have had antenatal corticosteroids, especially where birth takes place prior to 34 weeks (Liauw et al., 2025). However, the administration of antenatal corticosteroids prior to planned caesarean section at greater than 37 weeks is generally no longer recommended.

MAGNESIUM SULPHATE

Preterm birth is the leading cause of cerebral palsy (CP), with lifelong consequences for children and their families. Magnesium sulphate ($MgSO_4$) has been shown to offer significant **neuroprotection** for infants born prematurely, reducing both mortality and the incidence of CP (Crowther et al., 2017). The PReCePT perinatal quality improvement (QI) programme (Burhouse et al., 2017) has enhanced adherence to NICE recommendations by increasing awareness of $MgSO_4$ as a neuroprotective intervention, standardising clinical pathways, and providing structured QI support and training. Evidence demonstrates that magnesium sulphate is a low-cost yet highly effective intervention, reducing the risk of CP in infants born before 30 weeks' gestation by approximately 50% while also lowering mortality rates. Its widespread global implementation before imminent preterm birth therefore has the potential to deliver a substantial public-health benefit (Health Innovation West of England, 2026).

ACTIVITIES

Take a look at the following resources and note key learning points:

- The PReCePt Programme (Health Innovation West of England, 2022) – https://www.healthinnowest.net/our-work/transforming-services-and-systems/precept/ and https://www.healthinnowest.net/our-work/case-study/precept-preventing-cerebral-palsy-in-preterm-babies/
- BAPM (2019a) Perinatal Management of Extreme Preterm Birth Before 27 weeks of Gestation: A BAPM Framework for Practice – https://www.bapm.org/resources/80-perinatal-management-of-extreme-preterm-birth-before-27-weeks-of-gestation-2019
- BAPM (2026) Perinatal Optimisation Pathway. https://www.bapm.org/pages/perinatal-optimisation-pathway and PeriPrem (2026) https://www.healthinnowest.net/our-work/transforming-services-and-systems/periprem/

OPTIMAL CORD MANAGEMENT

Optimal cord management (OCM) is one of the key evidence-based peripartum interventions of the perinatal optimisation care pathway (BAPM, 2026). See also Chapter 13 for further information. Effective cord management relies on proactive planning and clear communication between the attending clinical teams and the parents. It is essential to confirm the plan to perform OCM with the obstetric team in the delivery room. Deferring (or delayed) cord clamping (DCC) by at least one minute (BAPM, 2020; World Health Organization, 2023) allows for continued blood flow from the placenta to the newborn and is more representative of a physiological process. This is the preferred method unless undertaking this would prevent immediately necessary resuscitation measures. Documented benefits of OCM in the preterm population include: improved survival; improved cardiovascular stability in the first 24 hours of life with reduced requirement for inotropic support and higher mean blood pressure (BP) measurements; reduced need for blood transfusions due to better red cell volume (Seidler et al., 2023); and lower incidence of IVH and NEC. There appears to be no increased risk in adverse maternal complications such as postpartum haemorrhage (Arora et al., 2025).

However, BAPM (2020) recognises that immediate cord clamping may occasionally be required in rare circumstances, such as when the mother requires urgent resuscitation due to massive acute haemorrhage, in the presence of ruptured **vasa praevia**, if the cord has torn, or sustained vascular trauma leading to significant fetal bleeding. In these situations, early clamping is justified to preserve maternal or neonatal safety. Cord milking should solely be considered for babies born above 28 weeks' gestation and only when it is not feasible to provide at least 60 seconds of OCM (BAPM, 2020; Hogeveen et al., 2025). Crucially, the rationale for deviating from optimal cord management must be clearly documented.

PRACTICE POINT

Given the strong evidence supporting the benefits of optimal cord management, neonatal teams need to ensure that systems, equipment, and workflows are designed to enable cord-intact resuscitation wherever possible. This necessitates appropriate setup, for example, mobile resuscitation platforms, suitably positioned surfaces, and longer T-piece resuscitator tubing to allow stabilisation with the cord left unclamped.

FURTHER EARLY CARE INTERVENTIONS FOR THE PRETERM NEONATE

There are a range of other interventions in the early care of the neonate who is admitted to the NNU. These are also covered in Chapter 12 and summarised in Box 2.2.

BOX 2.2 EARLY INTERVENTIONS IN THE IMMEDIATE POSTNATAL PERIOD

- *Birthing room care*: NICE antenatal and intrapartum guidance emphasises preparedness (equipment, staffing, clear escalation/transfer protocols) and person-centred birth planning. Birthing-room priorities include ensuring **normothermia** and optimum thermoregulation, airway support, skin-to-skin (when feasible), timely identification of infants needing NNU care, and coordination with fetal medicine/surgical teams for prenatally diagnosed anomalies.
- *Delivery room cuddles*: Although not strictly a part of perinatal optimisation bundles, the facilitation of delivery room cuddles for babies who are to be admitted to neonatal care is gaining in popularity (Bates et al., 2019) linking with the philosophy of FiCare. Benefits include improved cardiovascular stability, long-term cognitive benefits for the neonate, improved breastmilk supply, and parental psychosocial wellbeing. This requires planning by the multidisciplinary team around how thermoregulation and respiratory needs can be supported.
- *Maternal early breastmilk*: Supporting early expression and delivery of colostrum/breastmilk is vital, to reduce NEC and sepsis and improve neurodevelopment.
- *Caffeine*: A loading dose caffeine given within 6 hours of birth for babies who are born at less than 30 weeks gestation has positive effects such as reduced bronchopulmonary dysplasia (BDP) and extubation failure, reduced number of days of ventilation, lower incidence of CP, and improved white matter development, which helps to reduce neurodevelopmental impairment at 18–21 months (NICE, 2019; Marques et al., 2023; Sweet et al., 2023).
- *Continuous positive airway pressure*: Support of the preterm infant using continuous positive airway pressure (CPAP) from the time of delivery during OCM can be considered. Implementation of this as an intervention will depend on local resources. The continuation of CPAP via mask or prongs for transfer to the NNU is associated with a reduction in respiratory distress syndrome and lung injury leading to BPD (NICE, 2019; Sweet et al., 2023).
- *Probiotics*: The use of a multiple-strain probiotics is associated with the reduction of mortality through a decrease in NEC and the

sequalae associated with it. This intervention forms a part of some perinatal optimisation bundles with the cohort of babies where it is indicated is less than 32 weeks and/or less than 1500 grams (Wang et al., 2023).

- *Hydrocortisone*: Some perinatal optimisation bundles include administration of prophylactic low-dose hydrocortisone to babies who are born at extremely low gestations (24–25 weeks) and who are thought to have adrenal insufficiency due to their gestational age. The intention of this is to prevent death and BPD. Some areas have reported an increase in spontaneous intestinal perforation in cohorts of babies who have been treated with low-dose hydrocortisone (Baud et al., 2025).

THE IMPORTANCE OF INTERPROFESSIONAL TEAMWORK

High-reliability maternity and neonatal systems depend on coordinated, multidisciplinary teamwork that is visible and embedded in governance. National oversight continues to highlight the same pillars of safe, equitable care, for examples, the need for clear escalation policies, compassionate practice, and data-driven quality improvement (NHS England, 2023).

The key areas to address are as follows:

- Team structure, roles, and shared situational awareness: Effective teamwork hinges on explicit role definition across obstetrics, midwifery, anaesthesia, neonatal care, fetal medicine, theatres, and transport with clear communication between all areas. National reviews and inspection findings have found failures in listening, escalation and teamworking link to avoidable harm particularly prominent in specific ethnic groups (Care Quality Commission (CQC), 2024). Consistent, compassionate communication is a vital safety intervention.
- Interprofessional teamwork should join up antenatal screening and counselling with intrapartum readiness and neonatal transition. NHS England's maternity and neonatal programme emphasises *safer, more personalised and more equitable care* through: (1) listening to parents and families, (2) workforce growth and support, (3) cultures of learning, and (4) standards/structures that underpin safety.
- Using national datasets to drive improvement. NNAP reports optimal perinatal care such as ideal birthplace for preterm neonates, antenatal steroids

and magnesium sulphate, OCM, normothermia on admission, and early maternal breastmilk (RCPCH, 2026). Teams should ensure optimisation elements are consistently recorded.

- All stillbirths and NNDs should have a standardised, multidisciplinary review, with feedback shared compassionately with parents (National Perinatal and Epidemiology Unit (NPEU), 2026).
- Perinatal optimisation as a team: The BAPM perinatal optimisation pathway specifies the aforementioned evidence-based elements. Reliable delivery depends on cross-disciplinary planning. National QI programmes (e.g. PReCePT) show what good teamwork can achieve; for example, $MgSO_4$ administration to eligible mothers in England rose from 66% in 2017 to 86% in 2022 with structured, multi-professional implementation (Edwards et al., 2025).
- Networked care, levels, and transport readiness: Maternity and neonatal teams must collaborate with neonatal transport services from antenatal *in utero* transfer planning through to time-critical *ex utero* transfers.
- Culture, kindness, and equity as team competencies: CQC's national maternity reviews emphasise that compassion, listening and inclusion are not soft skills but core competencies which reduce harm and inequity. Multi-professional teams should embed co-produced information, professional interpreting, and objective newborn assessment tools (e.g. **bilirubinometers** and **pulse oximetry** to avoid bias in visual assessments, particularly important for babies with darker skin tones). Leaders must monitor equity metrics (ethnicity, deprivation) and make them part of routine team reviews (CQC, 2024; RCOG, 2025b).

INEQUALITIES IN MATERNAL AND NEONATAL OUTCOMES

Overall, interprofessional teamwork is essential for translating national standards into safer clinical practice, helping to reduce mortality, brain injury, infection, NEC, and BPD while also strengthening family trust in the care provided. However, marked and persistent inequalities in maternity and neonatal outcomes remain a central concern in the UK as well as globally (Peng et al., 2023; Roberts et al., 2024). In the UK, the national maternity and neonatal investigation (NMNI), led by Baroness Amos, has interim findings of systemic failures, ranging from racism and discrimination to staff shortages, weak accountability, and a 'postcode lottery' of care, while it continues evidence-gathering ahead of final national recommendations set in 2026. These national themes echo high-profile inquiries: the Ockenden exposed two decades of failures in leadership, learning, and listening to families, with clear system-wide immediate and essential actions; Kirkup's *Reading the Signals* identified avoidable harms and called for better identification of poorly performing units, compassionate care, teamworking, and honest responses to challenge (NMNI, 2025).

Surveillance data continue to show inequity. MBRRACE-UK reports (NPEU, 2026) persistent gaps in perinatal mortality by ethnicity and deprivation. Black and Asian babies face significantly higher stillbirth and NND rates and families in the most deprived areas experience worse outcomes than the least deprived. CQC's national review similarly highlights higher risks for Black and South Asian women (including maternal mortality, preterm birth, SGA, and severe morbidity) and inconsistent local action to address inequality. The NHS Race and Health Observatory (2024) has shown that standard neonatal assessments (Apgar, jaundice, cyanosis) relying on skin-colour cues are not fit for purpose for infants of ethnic minority backgrounds, recommending device-based assessment and curriculum change to mitigate diagnostic delay.

Policy responses emphasise prioritising and reducing inequalities alongside safety and compassion, using a family focused methodology and local investigations to inform a national plan. The NHS England's three-year maternity and neonatal delivery plan and Core20PLUS5 framework aim to embed equity through personalised care, workforce growth, safer cultures, better data, and targeted action in deprived and ethnic minority populations. For clinical teams, this means operationalising equity by robust listening and escalation; culturally safe, co-produced care; routine use of objective monitoring for jaundice/cyanosis; complete and timely ethnicity/deprivation data; and relentless learning from incidents. Sustained national leadership and local accountability are essential to close the gap and prevent further avoidable harm to women/pregnant persons, babies, and families.

THINK POINTS

- Think about the inequalities that exist in outcomes . . .
- Think of key interventions that are recommended from national guidance, to optimise care and outcomes for pregnant women/ pregnant persons and neonates.
- Consider early and inclusive booking, risk assessment, accessible entry points to care, provision of tailored information on modifiable risks, screening, and diagnostic pathways, maternal condition management, antenatal corticosteroids, care of imminent preterm birth, optimal cord management, and team-based perinatal readiness.

Chapter takeaways

- Maternal health (for example, hypertension disorders in pregnancy, diabetes, cardiac disease), lifestyle, and psychosocial factors directly affect fetal growth, prematurity risk, and neonatal morbidity.
- Early, inclusive booking; systematic risk assessment; and personalised, shared decision-making underpin safer antenatal pathways and screening/counselling choices.
- Perinatal optimisation (appropriate place of birth, antenatal steroids, magnesium sulphate, intrapartum antibiotics, optimal cord management, normothermia, early breastmilk) reduces mortality and severe morbidity in preterm infants.
- Multiple pregnancy requires specialist surveillance (chorionicity-led), preterm birth prevention strategies, and planned intrapartum care to mitigate risks.
- Birthing-room preparedness, clear escalation, and coordinated multidisciplinary teamwork are essential for safe transition and timely neonatal interventions.
- Addressing inequalities in maternal and neonatal outcomes through culturally safe care, objective assessment tools, complete equity data, and co-produced services is critical to closing outcome gaps.

CASE STUDY

CASE STUDIES

Case study 1: Late booking, multiple risks, and equity focused antenatal planning

Fatima, 29, attends her first antenatal appointment at 24+2 weeks. She recently moved area and has not previously engaged with maternity services. Her BMI is 36, she smokes 5–7 cigarettes/day, reports intermittent headaches, and has a family history of pre-eclampsia (her sister). She lives in temporary accommodation with limited access to cooking facilities. Fundal height is small for dates; BP is 148/96; urinalysis shows 1+ protein. English is her second language; a family member acts as an *ad hoc* interpreter. Fatima is anxious about scans.

Q1. What risk assessment steps and screening are priorities at this visit, and how will you organise inclusive communication to support informed decision-making?

CASE STUDY

Q2. Which modifiable factors should be addressed now, and how will you follow up?
Q3. Outline a plan for Fatima for the rest of the pregnancy.
Q4. How will you identify and mitigate inequalities and how will you document and share the plan with the multidisciplinary team?

Case study 2: Imminent extreme preterm birth

Aisha, 26+4 weeks with threatened preterm labour, arrives contracting every 4 minutes. Cervix is 3cm dilated; membranes intact. Fetal heart rate is reassuring. She has received one dose of steroids at a local hospital; magnesium sulphate is not yet commenced. GBS status is unknown. The tertiary NNU has a cot; *in utero* transfer is being considered. Theatre, obstetric anaesthetics, and neonatal teams are on standby. The delivery room has an intact cord resuscitation trolley, polyethylene wrap, temperature probes, and breast pump kit available.

Q1. Map the perinatal optimisation bundle you aim to deliver before, during, and immediately after birth.
Q2. What factors determine *in utero* transfer versus on site birth, and how will the MDT reach and document a time critical decision?
Q3. Detail your delivery room setup.
Q4. Which data must be recorded to evidence care against the NNAP and perinatal optimisation measures to support continuous quality improvement?

Case study 3: Suspected fetal cardiac anomaly

At the 20-week scan, a male fetus (planned name Noah) is suspected to have a significant congenital cardiac anomaly. The finding is confirmed by fetal cardiology. Parents, Sam and Lee, are shocked and request clear, balanced information. They ask about prognosis, place and mode of birth, immediate neonatal care, and the possibility of surgery. English is their first language, but they prefer written material to take home. The local unit is a LNU; the regional NICU has on-site paediatric cardiac services and neonatal transport support. Parents also ask about the option of not pursuing surgery if Noah's condition is more complex than expected at birth.

CASE STUDY

Q1. Outline an evidence-based counselling approach.

Q2. What is the interprofessional care necessary for timing/place of birth, stabilisation, and transfer?

Q3. How will you support the family before birth and how will you document preferences?

Q4. Identify key elements for safe birthing room readiness.

For suggested answer guides to the questions posed in these case studies, please refer to the web-based companion site specific to this chapter. See www.routledge.com/cw/petty

References

Al Beloushi, M., Saleh, H., Ahmed, B., & Konje, J. C. (2024). Congenital and perinatal viral infections: Consequences for the mother and fetus. *Viruses*, *16*(11), 1698. https://doi.org/10.3390/v16111698

Ali, S., Mactier, H., Morelli, A., Hurd, M., Placzek, A., Knight, M., Ladhani, S. N., Draper, E. S., Sharkey, D., Doherty, C., Kurinczuk, J. J., Quigley, M. A., & Gale, C. (2023). Neonatal outcomes of maternal SARS-CoV-2 infection in the UK: A prospective cohort study using active surveillance. *Pediatric Research*, *94*(3), 1203–1208.

Arora, A., Pollack, B., Babajanian, M., Friedman-Ciment, R., Glass, M., Kasoff, M., Bibi, M., Magovern, M., Soto, R., Hirani, R., Nussbaum, O., Steinhart, A., Drugge, E. D., Silber, A., & Grimes, C. L. (2025). Maternal and neonatal outcomes after delayed vs early cord clamping at cesarean delivery: A systematic review and meta-analysis. *American Journal of Obstetrics & Gynecology MFM*, 7(6), 101680.

Auriti, C., Bucci, S., De Rose, D. U., Coltella, L., Santisi, A., Martini, L., Maddaloni, C., Bersani, I., Lozzi, S., Campi, F., Pacifico, C., Balestri, M., Longo, D., & Grimaldi, T. (2022). Maternal–fetal infections (cytomegalovirus, toxoplasma, syphilis): Short-term and long-term neurodevelopmental outcomes in children infected and uninfected at birth. *Pathogens*, *11*(11), 1278.

Baguiya, A., Bonet, M., Cecatti, J. G., Brizuela, V., Curteanu, A., Minkauskiene, M., Jayaratne, K., Ribeiro-do-Valle, C. C., Budianu, M.-A., Souza, J. P., & Kouanda, S. (2021). Perinatal outcomes among births to women with infection during pregnancy. *Archives of Disease in Childhood*, *106*(10), 946–953.

Bates, S., Edwards, L., Peters, C., Morrish, P., Ashton, K., Nicholas, H., & Sullivan, C. (2019). Delivery room cuddles for preterm babies: Should we be doing more? *Infant*, *15*(2), 52–56.

Baud, O., Torchin, H., Butin, M., Flamant, C., & Nuytten, A. (2025). Prophylactic low-dose hydrocortisone in neonates born extremely preterm: Current knowledge and future challenges. *Pediatric Research*, *98*(1), 65–71. https://doi.org/10.1038/s41390-024-03756-6.

Bell, A., Carter, B., Davies, C., Evans, D., Foster, E., Green, F., Harris, G., Irving, H., Jones, J., Knight, M., Lewis, L., Morgan, N., Patel, P., Quinn, R., Smith, S., Turner, T., & Williams, W. (Eds.). (2024). *Saving lives, improving mothers' care: Lessons learned to inform maternity care from the UK and Ireland confidential enquiries into maternal deaths and morbidity 2022–24* [Online]. National Perinatal Epidemiology Unit. https://www.npeu.ox.ac.uk/mbrrace-uk-reports

British Association of Perinatal Medicine. (2019a). *Perinatal management of extreme preterm birth before 27 weeks of gestation: A framework for practice.* https://www.bapm.org/resources/80-perinatal-management-of-extreme-preterm-birth-before-27-weeks-of-gestation-2019

British Association of Perinatal Medicine. (2019b). *Enhancing shared decision making in neonatal care. A BAPM framework for practice.* https://www.bapm.org/resources/158-enhancing-shared-decision-making-in-neonatal-care

British Association of Perinatal Medicine. (2020). *Optimal cord management in preterm babies. A quality improvement toolkit.* https://www.bapm.org/pages/197-optimal-cord-management-toolkit

British Association of Perinatal Medicine. (2021). *Family integrated care; A BAPM framework for practice.* https://www.bapm.org/resources/ficare-framework-for-practice

British Association of Perinatal Medicine. (2026). *Perinatal optimisation pathway; resources to help improve preterm outcomes.* https://www.bapm.org/pages/perinatal-optimisation-pathway

Burhouse, A., Lea, C., Ray, S., Bailey, H., Davies, R., Harding, H., Howard, R., Jordan, S., Menzies, N., White, S., Phillips, K., & Luyt, K. (2017). Preventing cerebral palsy in preterm labour: A multiorganisational quality improvement approach to the adoption and spread of magnesium sulphate for neuroprotection. *BMJ Open Quality*, *6*(2), e000189. https://doi.org/10.1136/bmjoq-2017-000189

Care Quality Commission. (2024). *State of care 2023/24.* https://www.cqc.org.uk/publications/major-report/state-care/2023-2024

Chmielewska, B., Pegorie, C., Jie, M., Mehta, N., McStay, D., Bhide, A., & Thilaganathan, B. (2025). Impact of hypertensive disorders on disease progression in pregnancies affected by early-onset fetal growth restriction. *Acta Obstetricia et Gynecologica Scandinavica*, *104*(11), 2122–2128. https://doi.org/10.1111/aogs.70049

Coathup, V., Carson, C., Ashdown, H. F., Santorelli, G., & Quigley, M. A. (2025). Association between maternal body mass index and hospital admissions for infection in offspring: Longitudinal cohort study. *BMJ Medicine*, *4*(1), e001050. https://doi.org/10.1136/bmjmed-2024-001050

Conti-Ramsden, F., Fleminger, J., Lanoue, J., Chappell, L. C., Battersby, C., & UK Neonatal Collaborative. (2025). The contribution of hypertensive disorders of pregnancy to neonatal unit admissions and iatrogenic preterm delivery at< 34+ 0 weeks' gestation in the UK: A population-based study using the National Neonatal Research Database. *BJOG: An International Journal of Obstetrics & Gynaecology*, *132*(3), 306–317.

Crowther, C. A., Middleton, P. F., Voysey, M., Askie, L., Duley, L., Pryde, P. G., Marret, S., Doyle, L. W., & AMICABLE Group. (2017). Assessing the neuroprotective benefits for babies of antenatal magnesium sulphate: An individual participant data meta-analysis. *PLoS Medicine*, *14*(10), e1002398. https://doi.org/10.1371/journal.pmed.1002398

Edwards, H. B., Sillero-Rejon, C., McLeod, H., Hill, E. M., Opmeer, B. C., Peters, C., Odd, D., De Vocht, F., & Luyt, K. (2025). Implementation of national guidelines on antenatal magnesium sulphate for neonatal neuroprotection: Extended evaluation of the effectiveness and cost-effectiveness of the National PReCePT Programme in England. *BMJ Quality & Safety*, *35*, 95–105.

Eggleton, E. J., Bhagra, C. J., Patient, C. J., Belham, M., Pickett, J., & Aiken, C. E. (2023). Maternal left ventricular function and adverse neonatal outcomes in women with cardiac disease. *Archives of Gynecology and Obstetrics*, *307*(5), 1431–1439. https://link.springer.com/article/10.1007/s00404-022-06635-9

Fish, R., Weber, A., Crowley, M., March, M., Thompson, C., & Voos, K. (2021). Early antenatal counseling in the outpatient setting for high-risk pregnancies: A randomized control trial. *Journal of Perinatology*, *41*(7), 1595–1604. https://doi.org/10.1038/s41372-021-00933-x.

Fotă, A., & Petca, A. (2025). Gestational diabetes mellitus: The dual risk of small and large for gestational age: A narrative review. *Medical Sciences*, *13*(3), 144. https://doi.org/10.3390/medsci13030144.

Gallimore, I. D., Matthews, R. J., Page, G. L., Smith, L. K., Fenton, A. C., Knight, M., Smith, P. W., Redpath, S., & Manktelow, B. N., on behalf of the MBRRACE-UK Collaboration. (2025). *MBRRACE-UK perinatal mortality surveillance: UK perinatal deaths of babies born in 2023 – State of the nation report*. TIMMS, Department of Population Health Sciences, University of Leicester.

Gov.uk. (2024). *NHS fetal anomaly screening programme (FASP): Programme overview*. https://www.gov.uk/guidance/fetal-anomaly-screening-programme-overview

Health Innovation West of England. (2026). *PeriPrem*. https://www.healthinnowest.net/our-work/transforming-services-and-systems/periprem/

Hogeveen, M., Monnelly, V., Binkhorst, M., Cusack, J., Fawke, J., Kardum, D., Roehr, C. C., Rüdiger, M., Schwindt, E., Solevåg, A. L., Szczapa, T., Te Pas, A., Trevisanuto, D., Wagner, M., Wilkinson, D., & Madar, J. (2025). European resuscitation council guidelines 2025 newborn resuscitation and support of transition of infants at birth. *Resuscitation*, *215*, 110766.

Huang, Q., Franklin, R. C. G., Seale, A. N., Jowett, V., Pagel, C., Crowe, S., & Brown, K. L. (2025). Congenital heart disease in England: A national cohort study from fetal diagnosis to end of infancy. *Heart*, *112*(9), 495–503. https://doi.org/10.1136/heartjnl-2025-326369

Karkia, R., Giacchino, T., Shah, S., Gough, A., Ramadan, G., & Akolekar, R. (2023). Gestational diabetes mellitus: Association with maternal and neonatal complications. *Medicina*, *59*(12), 2096. https://doi.org/10.3390/medicina59122096

Knight, M., Bunch, K., Felker, A., Patel, R., Kotnis, R., Kenyon, S., & Kurinczuk, J. J. (Eds.). (2025). *Saving lives, improving mothers' care: Lessons learned to inform maternity care from the UK and Ireland confidential enquiries into maternal deaths and morbidity 2021–23*. National Perinatal Epidemiology Unit, University of Oxford. https://www.npeu.ox.ac.uk/assets/downloads/mbrrace-uk/reports/maternal-report-2025/MBRRACE-UK%20Maternal%20Report%202025%20-%20Main%20ONLINE%20v1.0.pdf

Kumar, R., & Garg, S. (2019). Neonatal abstinence syndrome: A current update. *Infant*, *15*(4), 132–136.

Liauw, J., Campbell, K. S. J., Foggin, H., Grunau, R. E., Petrie, J., Qasim, A., Brignardello-Petersen, R., Mishaal, R. A., & Hutcheon, J. A. (2025). Antenatal corticosteroids and child neurodevelopment: A systematic review and meta-analysis. *Obstetrics & Gynecology*, *146*(3), 360–376. https://doi.org/10.1097/AOG.0000000000005950.

Mactier, H., Bates, S. E., Johnston, T., Lee-Davey, C., Marlow, N., Mulley, K., Smith, L. K., To, M., Wilkinson, D., & BAPM Working Group. (2020). Perinatal management of extreme preterm birth before 27 weeks of gestation: A framework for practice. *Archives of Disease in Childhood: Fetal and Neonatal Edition*, *105*(3), 232–239. https://doi.org/10.1136/archdischild-2019-318402.

Manuel, G., Twentyman, J., Noble, K., Eastman, A. J., Aronoff, D. M., Seepersaud, R., Rajagopal, L., & Adams Waldorf, K. M. (2025). Group B streptococcal infections in pregnancy and early life. *Clinical Microbiology Reviews*, *38*(1), e0015422. https://doi.org/10.1128/cmr.00154-22.

Marques, K. A., Bruschettini, M., Roehr, C. C., Davis, P. G., Fiander, M., & Soll, R. F. (2023). Methylxanthine for the prevention and treatment of apnea in preterm infants.

Cochrane Database of Systematic Reviews, *2025*(5). https://doi.org/10.1002/14651858.CD013830.pub2

National Institute for Health and Care Excellence. (2019). *Specialist neonatal respiratory care for babies born preterm*. https://www.nice.org.uk/guidance/ng124/chapter/Recommendations

National Institute for Health and Care Excellence. (2020). *Diabetes in pregnancy: management from preconception to the postnatal period*. https://www.nice.org.uk/guidance/ng3

National Institute for Health and Care Excellence. (2021). *Antenatal care*. https://www.nice.org.uk/guidance/ng201

National Institute for Health and Care Excellence. (2022). *Preterm labour and birth*. https://www.nice.org.uk/guidance/ng25

National Institute for Health and Care Excellence. (2023). *Hypertension in pregnancy: Diagnosis and management*. https://www.nice.org.uk/guidance/NG133

National Institute for Health and Care Excellence. (2024a). *Neonatal infection QS75*. Quality statement 1: Intrapartum antibiotics | Neonatal infection | Quality standards | NICE.

National Institute for Health and Care Excellence. (2024b). *Twin and triplet pregnancy*. NICE.

National Maternity and Neonatal Investigation. (2025). https://www.matneoinv.org.uk/

National Perinatal and Epidemiology Unit/EMBRRACE-UK. (2026). *Perinatal mortality surveillance reports*. National Perinatal Epidemiology Unit. https://www.npeu.ox.ac.uk/mbrrace-uk/reports/perinatal-mortality-surveillance

NHS England. (2023). *Three year delivery plan for maternity and neonatal services*. https://www.england.nhs.uk/publication/three-year-delivery-plan-for-maternity-and-neonatal-services/

NHS England. (2025). *Saving babies lives care bundle (SBLCB)*. https://www.england.nhs.uk/long-read/saving-babies-lives-version-3-2/

NHS England. (2026). *Maternity and neonatal safety improvement programme*. https://www.england.nhs.uk/mat-transformation/maternal-and-neonatal-safety-collaborative/

NHS Race and Health Observatory. (2024). *Review of neonatal assessment and practice in Black, Asian and minority ethnic newborns: Exploring the Apgar score, the detection of cyanosis, and jaundice*. https://nhsrho.org/research/review-of-neonatal-assessment-and-practice-in-black-asian-and-minority-ethnic-newborns-exploring-the-apgar-score-the-detection-of-cyanosis-and-jaundice/

Panneflek, T. J. R., Hasperhoven, G. F., Chimwaza, Y., Allen, C., Lavin, T., Te Pas, A. B., Bekker, V., & van den Akker, T. (2024). Intrapartum antibiotic prophylaxis to prevent Group B streptococcal infections in newborn infants: A systematic review and meta-analysis comparing various strategies. *EClinicalMedicine*, *74*, 102748. https://doi.org/10.1016/j.eclinm.2024.102748

Peng, R., Tong, Y., Yang, M., Wang, J., Yang, L., Zhu, J., Liu, Y., Wang, H., Shi, Z., & Liu, Y. (2023). Global burden and inequality of maternal and neonatal disorders: Based on data from the 2019 Global Burden of Disease study. *QJM*, *117*(1), 24–37. https://doi.org/10.1093/qjmed/hcad220

Roberts, J. M., Abimbola, S., Bale, T. L., Barros, A., Bhutta, Z. A., Browne, J. L., Celi, A. C., Dube, P., Graves, C. R., Hollestelle, M. J., Hopkins, S., Khashan, A., Koi-Larbi, K., Lackritz, E., Myatt, L., Redman, C. W. G., Tunçalp, Ö., Vermund, S. H., & Gravett, M. G. (2024). Global inequities in adverse pregnancy outcomes: What can we do? *AJOG Global Reports*, *4*(3), 100385. https://doi.org/10.1016/j.xagr.2024.100385

Royal College of Obstetricians and Gynaecologists. (2018). *Care of women with obesity in pregnancy (Green-top Guideline No. 72)*. https://www.rcog.org.uk/guidance/browse-all-guidance/green-top-guidelines/care-of-women-with-obesity-in-pregnancy-green-top-guideline-no-72/

Royal College of Obstetricians and Gynaecologists. (2025a). *Antenatal corticosteroids to reduce neonatal morbidity and mortality*. https://www.rcog.org.uk/guidance/browse-all-guidance/green-top-guidelines/antenatal-corticosteroids-to-reduce-neonatal-morbidity-and-mortality-green-top-guideline-no-74/

Royal College of Obstetricians and Gynaecologists. (2025b). *Standards for maternity care.* RCOG. https://www.rcog.org.uk/guidance/browse-all-guidance/other-guidelines-and-reports/standards-for-maternity-care/

Royal College of Obstetricians and Gynaecologists. (2026). *Green-top guidelines.* https://www.rcog.org.uk/guidance/browse-all-guidance/green-top-guidelines/

Royal College of Paediatrics and Child Health. (2026). https://www.rcpch.ac.uk/work-we-do/clinical-audits/nnap

Runkle, J. D., Risley, K., Roy, M., & Sugg, M. M. (2023). Association between perinatal mental health and pregnancy and neonatal complications: A retrospective birth cohort study. *Women's Health Issues*, *33*(3), 289–299. https://doi.org/10.1016/j.whi.2022.12.001

Saberian, S., Gale, C., Subhedar, N., Gallagher, N., Esan, O. B., Sinha, I., Harvey, K., Schlüter, D. K., & Taylor-Robinson, D. (2025). Inequalities in neonatal unit mortality in England and Wales between 2012 and 2022: A retrospective cohort study. *The Lancet Child & Adolescent Health*, *9*(12), 857–867.

Seidler, A. L., Libesman, S., Hunter, K. E., Barba, A., Aberoumand, M., Williams, J. G., Shrestha, N., Aagerup, J., Sotiropoulos, J. X., Montgomery, A. A., Gyte, G. M. L., Duley, L., Askie, L. M., Seidler, A. L., Libesman, S., Hunter, K. E., Barba, A., Aberoumand, M., Williams, J. G., . . . & Askie, L. M. (2023). Short, medium, and long deferral of umbilical cord clamping compared with umbilical cord milking and immediate clamping at preterm birth: A systematic review and network meta-analysis with individual participant data. *The Lancet*, *402*(10418), 2223–2234.

Stock, S. J., Thomson, A. J., & Papworth, S. (2022). Antenatal corticosteroids to reduce neonatal morbidity and mortality: Green-top guideline no. 74. *BJOG: An International Journal of Obstetrics & Gynaecology*, *129*(8).

Sturrock, S., Ali, S., Gale, C., Battersby, C., & Le Doare, K. (2023). Neonatal outcomes and indirect consequences following maternal SARS-CoV-2 infection in pregnancy: A systematic review. *BMJ Open*, *13*(3). https://pubmed.ncbi.nlm.nih.gov/36921946/

Sweet, D. G., Carnielli, V. P., Greisen, G., Hallman, M., Klebermass-Schrehof, K., Ozek, E., & Halliday, H. L. (2023). European consensus guidelines on the management of respiratory distress syndrome: 2022 update. *Neonatology*, *120*(1), 3–23. https://doi.org/10.1159/000528914

Thivierge, E., Luu, T. M., Bourque, C. J., Pearce, R., Jaworski, M., Barrington, K. J., Duquette, L. A., & Janvier, A. (2025). Function over diagnoses: Parents of extremely preterm infants give recommendations to clinicians about their information needs. *Archives of Disease in Childhood – Fetal and Neonatal Edition*, *111*(1), F67–F73. https://doi.org/10.1136/archdischild-2024-328249

Wang, Y., Florez, I. D., Morgan, R. L., Foroutan, F., Chang, Y., Crandon, H. N., Zeraatkar, D., Bala, M. M., Mao, R. Q., Tao, B., Shahid, S., Wang, X., Beyene, J., Offringa, M., Sherman, P. M., El Gouhary, E., Guyatt, G. H., & Sadeghirad, B. (2023). Probiotics, prebiotics, lactoferrin, and combination products for prevention of mortality and morbidity in preterm infants: A systematic review and network meta-analysis. *JAMA Pediatrics*, *177*(11), 1158–1167. https://doi.org/10.1001/jamapediatrics

Watson, H., McLaren, J., Carlisle, N., Ratnavel, N., Watts, T., Zaima, A., Tribe, R. M., & Shennan, A. H. (2020). All the right moves: Why in utero transfer is both important for the baby and difficult to achieve and new strategies for change. *F1000Research*, *13*(9), F1000 Faculty Rev-979. https://doi.org/10.12688/f1000research.25923.1

World Health Organization. (2023). *Optimal timing of cord clamping for the prevention of iron deficiency anaemia in infants.* https://www.who.int/tools/elena/interventions/cord-clamping

3 CONTINUING CARE BEYOND THE NEONATAL UNIT

Jo Bennett, Deanna Gibbs, Elen Elias, and Phillip Harniess

CONTENTS

DOI: 10.4324/9781003591405-5

GUIDANCE ON HOW TO ENHANCE PERSONAL LEARNING FROM THIS CHAPTER

Key points covered in this chapter

- The principles and strategies of continuing care following discharge and transition from neonatal unit and/or transitional care.
- The importance of neurodevelopmental follow up.
- The consideration of the family unit as a whole in continuing care.

Reflection

Reading this chapter, you are encouraged to engage with the key points and related literature in an enquiring way. Ask these questions:

- What aspects of continuing care do you need to consider when a baby is ready to transition from neonatal inpatient services, and are you aware of the teams delivering these areas of care in your locality?
- How does communication support continuing care for the family and neonate?
- What guidance is available to support this area of practice?

Implications for nursing care

- Finally: how will this chapter enable you to consider and implement supporting parents in preparing for transition from neonatal inpatient services and continuing care at home or paediatric inpatient services?

INTRODUCTION AND BACKGROUND

For most families, continuing care after a neonatal service admission will be at home with, where available, specialist support from a neonatal **outreach** service or when required, a children's community nursing team alongside universal services such as the health visitor. For a few infants, however, care will need to continue as an inpatient on a paediatric intensive care unit (PICU) or a children's ward and for some, their discharge from neonatal care may be to a children's hospice. Throughout, there needs to be consideration not just for the infant's ongoing care needs but also the psychological impact of the **transition** on the parents and helping them to be practically and emotionally ready for it. Effective communication and consistency in information sharing between clinical staff and parents will support this (Aydon et al., 2018).

This chapter will explore these different areas of **continuing care** on transition from neonatal unit and/or neonatal **transitional care** (TC) services, the importance of comprehensive discharge planning to facilitate a smooth transition for the family and how greater equity of services is required to ensure all families can access the same level of support in the community. Follow up assessments and preparation for potential readmission to paediatric services will also be discussed.

Discharge from the neonatal unit (NNU) should be considered as a transition in care for the baby and family rather than a final point. However, for the purposes of this chapter we will use the term discharge planning to describe the process used to support the transition from the NNU to home or ongoing care with inpatient paediatric services or, when required, children's hospice services (refer to Chapter 9).

DISCHARGE PLANNING

Discharge planning should be facilitated and coordinated from admission to discharge date, to ensure the appropriate support and resources are in place for the baby and family on leaving the neonatal unit (NHS England, 2024). A number of key areas should be discussed (see Table 3.1). This can be facilitated by a dedicated discharge coordinator, the neonatal outreach service or other allocated personnel. On admission to the NNU, the named health visitor should be informed, as well as social care when required. This will enable the health visitor to contact the family as part of the first steps in discharge preparation.

Effective discharge planning requires constant and consistent communication with parents throughout. Parents or other named carers need to have time to prepare for this transition, which includes the sharing of information, time to ask questions and learn the necessary skills to care for their baby at home. The National Institute for Health and Care Excellence (NICE, 2017) recommends that all parents of preterm babies have an agreed discharge plan. This could be further extended to include all parents of infants admitted to a NNU or neonatal TC facility. For those whose admission was shorter and who have no ongoing nursing care needs, the plan may be agreed on a ward round discussion with parents and written information in the discharge letter. For others who have had a longer NNU stay and may also have ongoing nursing care needs, a more formal discharge planning meeting may be required. This planning and preparation enable parents the chance for anticipatory guidance as to what to expect when they are at home, based on their baby, his/her ongoing healthcare needs, and the family situation (Smith, 2020).

The following people might be required at a discharge planning meeting:

- Parents or other named carers
- Neonatal consultant

- Neonatal nurse representative
- Neonatal outreach nurse and/or children's community nurse
- Health visitor
- General practitioner (GP)
- Allied health professionals (AHPs) as required
- Social care when required
- Interpreter
- Learning disability advocate or other advocate/family member if needed

THINK POINTS

What is your role in a discharge planning meeting as a healthcare professional? How does your role support parents/carers in ensuring their voice is heard, their questions answered, and understanding gained throughout the meeting?

TABLE 3.1 DISCHARGE PLANNING MEETING

Nutrition	Method of feeding, any dietitian involvement, feeding plan if required, any supplements or formulas prescribed as required. If on formula feeds, do parents know how to prepare these?
Medication	Review what is required on discharge and ensure all ordered in time, parents are taught and practising how to administer medications.
Oxygen	If oxygen is required, is the infant on a prescribed set amount following a pulse oximetry study? Has a home assessment been completed and oxygen ordered?
Other specific needs	For example, if a baby has a **stoma**, management and supplies for this will need consideration; or if a baby requires treatment for **neonatal abstinence syndrome**, then a treatment plan will need to be agreed upon.
Screening	Discharge cranial ultrasound scan, screening for **retinopathy of prematurity** (ROP), hearing screening.
Immunisations	Where is the baby in the schedule, ensure parents know when and where any pending immunisations will be given.

TABLE 3.1 (Cont.)

Infant basic life support training	All parents should be offered the chance to have this training prior to discharge.
Follow-up appointments	Are these required, when and where?
Open access to children's assessment unit or other suitable escalation pathway	Ensure open access arranged if required, e.g. if an infant is on oxygen, and parents know when and who to call and have been to see the ward.
Rooming in	Offer parents the chance to room in with their baby prior to discharge home, either on the NNU or TC.
Community support	Discuss who will be supporting them at home, when first home visit will be, and how to contact community teams.

A planning meeting will also be required for those infants transitioning to PICU or to a children's hospice, although these may be slightly different. For those transitioning to PICU, all the above ongoing care needs will be discussed, alongside respiratory support, any surgical care needs, or other specific treatment requirements. Some of the other points such as infant basic life support training may not be appropriate at this time, however. For those transitioning to a children's hospice or home with children's community palliative care nursing team support, discussion of an advance care plan along with a symptom management plan should be considered at this point.

All families transitioning to home with their baby will require assessment of readiness (Box 3.1) and will need:

- The offer of infant basic life support training.
- Safe sleep guidance.
- Information for minimising the risk of traumatic head injury to babies through advising parents on infant crying and how to cope.
- Information on signs of infection and what to do if they are concerned that their baby is unwell. This may include discussion on hospital paediatric services and the possibility of admission after discharge. Data identified an admission rate to PICU for infants born <32 weeks gestation after discharge home from neonatal care, before 2 years of age as 5.7% (van Hasselt et al., 2023).
- Preparation with practical skills, such as how to administer medication, bathing and milk storage guidance.

For those families taking their baby home on oxygen, phototherapy, or with a nasogastric tube still in-situ, parents/carers will also complete the relevant skills acquisition for these.

BOX 3.1 READINESS FOR DISCHARGE HOME

This is indicated when:

- Infant is physiologically stable and able to maintain body temperature in an open cot; has a stable and positive growth trajectory; and shows no significant infection markers, apnoeas, bradycardias, or desaturations for 48 hours.
- Infant is breathing in air or in a prescribed rate of low flow oxygen.
- Infant is feeding effectively by preferred method for 48–72 hours, which may include top ups by nasogastric tube.
- Parents are integrated in care and have completed appropriate skills frameworks, e.g. giving medicines or tube feeding.
- Ensuring families feel psychologically supported during the transition period.

(Adapted from the British Association of Perinatal Medicine (BAPM) Neonatal Outreach Framework (2025a))

SUPPORTING PARENT WELLBEING IN THE TRANSITION TO HOME

Bringing a preterm or high-risk infant home from the NNU is an activity that is longed for and anticipated by parents throughout the hospital admission. The transition from NNU to home can be momentous. Depending on the design and facilities of a NNU, parents may only have had the opportunity to be with their baby for a continuous period immediately preceding discharge, and this is only the case if hospital accommodation supports parents rooming-in. Therefore, despite considerable hours spent at their infant's bedside, parents may still feel ill equipped to care for their infant in the days following discharge (Gibbs et al., 2015). Ensuring that families feel psychologically supported during the transition period is a key factor in planning continuing care (BAPM, 2025a). A stressful perinatal experience for parents and infants may begin during pregnancy and can persist for months to years after NNU discharge (Griffith et al., 2022). Following discharge, approximately 1 in 3 parents report high levels of anxiety, depression, and post-traumatic stress syndrome, often with symptoms from two or more conditions (Pace et al., 2016; van Wassenaer-Leemhuis et al., 2016; Axelin et al., 2022; Haeusslein et al., 2021).

Such an overwhelming and prolonged stressful experience may potentially have a negative impact on the developing parent-infant relationship (Purdy et al., 2015; Axelin et al., 2022; Griffith et al., 2022). These early days, weeks, and months post-discharge may be further complicated as the behavioural cues of the infants are often more difficult to read, and there may be ongoing medical and neurodevelopmental concerns that require ongoing input and monitoring (van Wassenaer-Leemhuis et al., 2016), which will also cause potential challenges to the parents striving to develop a sensitive and nurturing relationship with their baby.

One of the most prominent concerns for parents as they prepare to take their baby home is a concern that they will not be able to provide the appropriate care for their baby without the help of professional caregivers (Jiménez-Palomares et al., 2021). As a result, a range of potential interventions aimed at supporting parental wellbeing during this period of transition to home have been evaluated. These include in-person home visits, follow-up phone/video calls or text messages, and telehealth apps (Griffith et al., 2022). These interventions have been demonstrated to be beneficial for families during the transition from the NNU to home, serving to decrease parental stress and anxiety, as well as supporting parental competency, self-efficacy, and a sense of security in caring for their infants (Griffith et al., 2022).

THINK POINTS

Consider the experiences of parents caring for their babies while they are admitted to the NNU. How is family integrated care delivered to enable parent engagement in caregiving for their baby to support the developing parent-infant relationship? What approaches might we use which recognise the stress and anxiety that parents experience and build their confidence as they prepare for transition to home? How do we ensure that our approach is individualised to specific family situations and cultural beliefs and values?

SAFE SLEEP ADVICE FOR PARENTS

Preparing families for discharge from a NNU should provide clear, evidence-based safe sleep education aligned with UK guidance to reduce the risk of sudden infant death syndrome (SIDS). Current recommendations from the National Health

Service (NHS) and The Lullaby Trust (2025) emphasise **supine** positioning and parents should be advised that **prone** or side sleeping, often used in neonatal care, must be discontinued at home. Therefore, once infants are medically stable, neonatal nurses should support parents with establishing a safe sleep environment compliant with infant safe sleep guidance (Hickling et al., 2025).

Education should reinforce the importance of a firm, flat mattress in a clear cot, free from loose bedding or soft objects. While room-sharing remains encouraged, advice around bed-sharing should acknowledge that it can be a preferred option for some families; however, it is not recommended for babies born <2.5 kg or <37 weeks and therefore is generally unsuitable for the NNU population (Lullaby Trust, 2025). Thermal regulation advice is essential, including avoiding overheating and promoting appropriate clothing. Nurses and healthcare professionals should also address modifiable risk factors such as smoking and promote breastfeeding where possible, ensuring consistent, comprehensible messaging prior to discharge with signposting to advice and resources.

NEONATAL OUTREACH

Whether the NNU is the best environment for a baby once they no longer require intensive care and are at the stage of 'feeding and growing' is an important question (see Chapter 7). Apart from this, a NNU stay can add significant financial and practical pressures on a family, along with the psychological burden. A Bliss (2022) parent survey found the average additional cost that parents faced whilst their baby was in hospital was £405 per week. There has been much research which highlights the negative psychological impact that a NNU stay can have on the family, affecting bonding and an increased incidence of anxiety and post-traumatic stress in parents when compared with the general perinatal population (Malouf et al., 2021). Taking all these factors into consideration, as well as the need to improve patient flow and facilitate cot capacity, consideration of early discharge home with neonatal outreach support has benefits for the baby, family and NNU capacity.

Earlier discharge home may be facilitated by offering hospital at home services with neonatal outreach support. These may include:

- part nasogastric tube feeding
- neonatal abstinence syndrome treatment
- home iv antibiotics
- home phototherapy.

To support with this, some neonatal outreach services are now introducing a virtual ward system. This means that infants discharged from the NNU or TC ward under the care of the outreach team are admitted to a virtual ward. This system enables a combined approach of home visits by the outreach nurse and remote monitoring by the outreach and wider multidisciplinary team (MDT). AHPs are able to meet with families and the outreach nurse virtually to support those infants discharged home with outreach support who would otherwise have remained in hospital. Virtual wards should be seen as a method of building system resilience to safely support care and not as a way of reducing bed numbers (Royal College of Paediatrics and Child Health (RCPCH), 2023).

However, neonatal outreach service provision is not solely for the purpose of facilitating earlier discharge home but is to support the transition from hospital to home. One of the key recommendations of the BAPM Neonatal Outreach Framework is that 'All babies and families who have experienced specialist neonatal care should have equitable access to a multidisciplinary, robust 7-day a week neonatal outreach service to support their transition from hospital to home' (BAPM, 2025a).

In supporting the transition to home, neonatal outreach teams offer:

- Support with the discharge process
- Growth monitoring and feeding support
- Wellbeing checks on baby and where required observations, e.g. temperature, oxygen saturation
- Liaising with the neonatal consultant, allied health professionals, health visitor, and GP
- Medicine management
- Checking on how parents are and where necessary signposting to mental health support services
- **Safeguarding** support and liaison with social care
- When there are continuing nursing needs, the team will affect a smooth handover to the children's community nursing service.

Where required they will also offer:

- Blood sampling in the home, e.g. for newborn screening, bilirubin levels, or medication monitoring and titration
- Support for transitioning from tube to full oral feeds
- Pulse oximetry studies
- Other monitoring as requested and agreed with the neonatologist; e.g. regular head circumference measurements when infant has an **Ommaya reservoir** in-situ and ventricular taps may be required
- Palliative care at home in collaboration with other community services
- Bereavement support (if appropriately trained).

Unfortunately, at the time of writing this, there is disparity in provision of neonatal outreach services. A recent survey found that 72% of neonatal units in England, Wales, and Scotland offer dedicated neonatal outreach services. This ranged from 95% of neonatal intensive care units to just 56% of special care units (Lee et al., 2025) However, where there is provision, this too ranges from 2–7 days/week and the services offered vary, with not all currently supporting home tube feeding and just a small proportion offering home phototherapy. This picture is reflected globally with varying levels of neonatal outreach provision.

A neonatal outreach team consists of nurses and non-registered staff, all of whom will be experienced in NNU and/or TC nursing. The team liaise closely with the neonatal consultant and AHPs, as recommended in the Getting It Right First Time (GIRFT, 2022) Neonatology report, ensuring that all aspects of the baby's care and development are supported. It is essential that neonatal outreach do not replace health visitor input, which is a universal service, but instead the two services work in coordination with each other. Health visitors provide a minimum of five home visits up to a developmental assessment at 2 years. The first of these visits is in late pregnancy, which means that when a baby is born preterm, the parents might not have met a health visitor yet. The health visitor is a registered nurse or midwife who has undergone further training in public health. Their expertise can provide early help and support to babies and their families (Appleton, 2021). However, unless they also have neonatal nursing experience, some health visitors may not be equipped with the specialist clinical expertise to appropriately support families on discharge from neonatal care. A recent survey of parents conducted by the Neonatal Networks Outreach Group (NNOG) found from 396 responses of the 57% who received outreach support on discharge, 81% felt adequately supported compared to the 43% who received no outreach support, with only 44% of these feeling adequately supported.

As well as working closely with health visitors, the outreach team will liaise with social care as the need arises. Safeguarding children is everyone's responsibility, and as such there needs to be an awareness of this with all families. Where there are safeguarding concerns, then interagency communication and collaboration is essential to identify and respond to the needs of the neonate and their family (HM Government, 2023). To support with this, neonatal outreach nurses will liaise with social care prior to and after discharge home, where there are child protection concerns.

The safety of the outreach nurse as a lone worker in the community also needs to be considered and it is therefore important that the service has a lone worker policy to support with this. Staff should have access to a lone worker safety device for use on each community visit, which can be activated if they have any concerns for their safety. They should also have access to a work mobile phone and ensure that someone at their base knows where they are going to be for the duration of their time out of the hospital. Planned joint visits with another healthcare or social care professional can be helpful when there is a known risk.

In areas where there is no neonatal outreach provision, length of stay on the NNU may be longer as there is little or no provision for early discharge support in the community. Infants will be supported on discharge by health visiting teams, and where the infant has an ongoing nursing need such as low flow oxygen, they will have children's community nursing input too.

A neonatal outreach service may support families with phone contact, clinic attendance and home visits. During any face-to-face contact either in clinic or in the family home, the outreach nurse will take time for in-depth discussions with parents/carers. The psychological impact of a NNU admission on parents/carers can continue after discharge, as demonstrated by the recent NNOG parent survey which found the number one area that parents would like additional information provision on discharge was further mental health support.

At each contact, the nurse will talk with parents to find out how they feel their baby is, how they have been feeding and sleeping, for example. On a home visit or clinic attendance they will also assess the baby, which may include weight, head circumference, skin integrity and colour, temperature, respiratory effort, and response to handling. If the infant is still at the age where they may become jaundiced the nurse will also assess for this. The NHS Race and Health Observatory has issued guidance on assessing for jaundice in infants with darker skin tones (see Chapters 4 and 17) and the use of transcutaneous bilirubinometer alongside visual assessment.

Depending on the specific needs of the infant, further assessments or interventions may be required. If on low flow oxygen, oxygen saturation monitoring should be recorded on each contact. Overnight pulse oximetry studies will be undertaken and oxygen reduced as per local oxygen weaning guidance. It is recommended that all infants are transitioned to children's community nursing services where there is a continuing nursing need such as low flow oxygen, within 6 months of discharge home (BAPM, 2025a). Infants with chronic lung disease and home oxygen should have open access to the children's assessment unit or other suitable escalation pathway, so that they can be seen by a paediatrician promptly without the need for going through the GP or emergency department.

When a baby has been discharged early while having short-term tube feeding, they will be usually be taking approximately 50% of their feeds orally, with the remainder being administered via a nasogastric tube. The parents will have been completing tube feeds in hospital and taught tube feed administration safety checks. The outreach nurse will liaise with the parents as to how the baby is feeding and alongside their weight gain and general wellbeing and will guide as to when to remove the tube to enable full oral feeding. Research has shown that this can save about 8 inpatient cot days and no readmissions related to home tube feeding (Schuler et al., 2020).

Retinopathy of prematurity (ROP) screening may still be required on discharge. This will be discussed at the discharge planning meeting and follow up screening appointments made. On occasion the infant may require treatment if the degree of ROP dictates this. In this case, they may be readmitted as an in-patient and referred to an ophthalmologist to support any necessary treatment.

Those infants who required gastrointestinal surgery during their neonatal admission may require further specialist support when transitioning to home. This may be through a neonatal surgical specialist nurse, the local outreach team (in liaison with the tertiary surgical unit), dietitian, speech and language therapist, and neonatologist. The neonatal surgical unit team will ensure the parents have the necessary information and training prior to discharge to meet any additional needs their baby's condition requires and surgical follow-up has been arranged. The National Neonatal Surgical Interest Group recommend in their Framework for Best Practice (2024), that each family has a dedicated single point of contact from the specialist centre in case of any problems. At home, the family and outreach nurses will closely monitor weight gain, feeding and observe for any signs of feed intolerance, potential problems such as strictures, adhesions causing bowel obstruction, diarrhoea, and constipation (see Chapter 22).

DEVELOPMENTAL FOLLOW-UP

Child development is a complex orchestration between experience within environments and genetics. Preterm birth is considered a neurological life course event. The disruption caused by the mismatch of the NNU environment to the requirements of the developing brain impacts emergent neurological connectivity. Aberrant connectivity can have a profound long-term functional impact across different domains of a child's development. For example, preterm infants often present with early reduced movement variability and gross motor delay (e.g. in early postural control and reaching), which is associated with later cognitive delays (Hadders-Algra, 2018).

Co-morbidities of prematurity place infants at higher risk of developing childhood-onset disabilities and other presentations of **neurodiversity**, with potentially multiple developmental areas affected to varying levels (Moore et al., 2012) including:

- Cognitive (e.g. learning disability, poor working memory, or dyscalculia)
- Motor (e.g. cerebral palsy (CP), developmental coordination disorder)
- Sensory (e.g. visual and hearing impairments)
- Behavioural and psychological (e.g. autism, attention deficit hyperactivity disorder, emotional disorders, and other mental health problems)
- Communication and feeding delays

The most relevant predictor of CP in preterm infants born before 30^{+0} weeks' gestation are cerebral lesions, such as focal **periventricular leukomalacia** and severe intraventricular haemorrhage (Beaino et al., 2010). In addition, infants who experience **hypoxic ischaemic encephalopathy** (HIE) are at risk of adverse developmental outcomes (Jacobs et al., 2013).

Early presentation of difficulties may be clear in some cases, but frequently subtleties and the transient or emergent nature of neurodevelopmental concerns causes complexity in prediction, diagnosis, and prognosis (Hadders-Algra, 2018). Often preterm infants may experience delay in development trajectories as more complex socio-environmental challenges are presented, for example, when children encounter new environments such as nursery or school settings. Therefore, good developmental care for the infant is essential beyond discharge from the NNU. The British Association for Neonatal Neurodevelopmental Follow up (BANNFU, 2021) recommends that every baby discharged from a NNU in the UK has the right to a purposeful comprehensive medical and developmental service that addresses their needs, from discharge for as long as they need. Developmental follow-up programmes play a critical role in screening and triaging infants who would benefit from more targeted early intervention with AHPs. In addition, tracking longitudinal cohorts of infant developmental outcomes provides an important audit and quality improvement tool for neonatal networks.

Post-discharge follow-up needs to be systematic and coordinated in the long-term with the MDT, in partnership with families (National Neonatal Discharge Planning and Follow-up Framework, 2019). NICE guidelines recommend a minimum standard for the 'Developmental follow-up of children and young people born preterm' (NICE, 2017). These include criteria for enhanced developmental support and surveillance up to 2 years (corrected age), for infants:

- born before 30^{+0} weeks' gestation or
- born between 30^{+0} and 36^{+6} weeks' gestation and has or had one or more of the following risk factors:
  - a brain lesion on neuroimaging likely to be associated with developmental problems or disorders (for example, grade 3 or 4 intraventricular haemorrhage or cystic periventricular leukomalacia)
  - grade 2 or 3 HIE in the neonatal period
  - neonatal bacterial **meningitis**
  - herpes simplex **encephalitis** in the neonatal period.

Further consideration is needed for children born preterm who do not meet these criteria but are suspected of being at increased risk of developmental problems or disorders, taking into account the presence and severity of risk factors. For all children born before 28^{+0} weeks' gestation, a face-to-face developmental assessment at 4 years (uncorrected age) is recommended. Nevertheless, it has been highlighted that there is a lack of standardisation and so service delivery models may vary locally (Merchant et al., 2022). Specific Operational Delivery Networks, and equivalent networks within the devolved nations and individual NNUs, have accessible published developmental follow-up guidelines specifying the structure and content of their follow-up service provision. Many units provide an information leaflet for parents describing the support framework available following discharge, an opt-in service requiring proactive consent from the family. It is considered essential that parents are aware of what developmental follow-up and their ongoing access to professional support entails, as an additional means of mitigating the stressful experiences of parenting a preterm or sick baby within a NNU setting (Hutchon et al., 2019; Merchant et al., 2022).

Different members of the MDT may be involved within development follow-up, and require extensive knowledge of infant development, an enhanced skill set to provide specialised assessments and sensitivity to detect subtle early indicators of delay (Elliot-Smith et al., 2024). Along with nursing roles, clinicians may include neonatologists, hospital or community paediatricians, paediatric neurologists together with AHPs, such as physiotherapists, occupational therapists, speech and language therapists, and dieticians. The follow-up setting may be in a hospital outpatient or within children's community settings (e.g. child development centres). A combination of more specialist assessments is advised for early and accurate prediction, diagnosis and prognosis of CP (Novak et al., 2017). In addition to cranial ultrasound, **magnetic resonance imaging** (MRI) has a strong predictive value. Assessing an infant's early movement repertoire can be a strong predictor of developmental outcome. The General Movements Assessment is a reliable predictive clinical assessment, which often involves the physiotherapist, occupational therapist, paediatricians, and in some cases parents videoing the infant's movements at key developmental windows at corrected term age and 11–16 weeks. The Hammersmith Infant Neurological Examination is used to identify infants between 3 and 24 months of age with high probability of CP. It assesses cranial nerves, posture, movements, tone and reflexes, and includes assessment of motor asymmetry score. At 12- and 24-months corrected age, further comprehensive multi-developmental domain assessments can be used to evaluate an infant's cognition, socioemotional, sensory and motor development (NICE, 2017).

It should also be highlighted that while late preterm infants are often not included in developmental follow-up programmes because of a lower risk, their risk of long-term developmental sequelae is still higher relative to term born peers (Woythaler, 2019). Hence, awareness is needed amongst universal services such as health visitors and GPs to ensure proper attention is given to arising developmental concerns.

ACTIVITY

List the possible follow-up appointments/additional services that an infant who has spent time in neonatal care may require. Consider too, support groups – can you list support groups and charities available in your area which you may be able to signpost families to on transitioning from neonatal care?

COMPLEX NEURODEVELOPMENTAL DISABILITY

Some preterm infants can present early on with a clear, complex neurodevelopmental disability. These infants and their parents are likely to experience profound interconnected developmental challenges including postural control, oral feeding, socialisation, and emotional regulation. These families benefit from targeted early intervention provided by AHPs to offer treatment strategies to improve function and manage challenging activities, such as feeding in a developmentally appropriate and graded manner. Relational approaches have been shown to be crucial within this early therapeutic support for building sensitivity within the parent and infant dyad, as well as with the therapists with whom long-term continuity is advocated for as they also navigate a disrupted transition to parenthood (Harniess et al., 2022; 2023).

TRANSITIONING TO PAEDIATRICS OR THE PAEDIATRIC INTENSIVE CARE UNIT

Whilst most babies are discharged home from the NNU, a small but growing number have complex healthcare needs that require ongoing medical care and are transitioned directly to a paediatric intensive care unit (PICU). The majority are aged 36 weeks corrected gestational age and above, with the most frequent medical diagnosis being respiratory disease such as severe bronchopulmonary dysplasia, with many presenting with multimorbidity. There is a high rate of mortality and morbidity in this population, all of which require significant PICU resources (van Hasselt et al., 2023). Nearly half of the admissions of children aged under 2 years to a PICU had previously been cared for in a NNU, with a third admitted on more than one occasion (Seaton et al., 2025).

Historically, there has been a lack of data identifying the number of babies who transition directly to PICU, together with a paucity of research exploring the needs of this cohort of babies and their families, as they negotiate a new environment, medical team, and delivery of care (van Hasselt et al., 2023). Challenges reported by parents in a PICU included the heterogeneity of patients in comparison to the neonatal cohort. Others experienced less participation in the care of their baby due to a less prominent family integrated care-based partnership between families and staff (Crossley et al., 2022; family integrated care is covered in more depth in Chapters 6 and 7). Some parents describe more positive accounts, such as gaining better access to PICU hospital-based accommodation enabling greater cot side presence, and better shared care of their baby by both parents with the mother physically recovered from her post-partum period (Seaton et al., 2025). An anticipated addition to facilitate a well-planned and coordinated transition with multidisciplinary and parental collaboration is the practice guidelines entitled the BAPM Framework for 'Transition from neonatal to paediatric care for babies with long term or complex healthcare needs,' which is still in draft at the time of writing this chapter (BAPM, 2025b).

PRACTICE POINT

The parents of neonates born prematurely or who require additional care after the NNU may have specific support needs from primary care professionals, for example, relating to advice on expected developmental milestones, growth, feeding, oxygen therapy, and emotional support (Lopez et al., 2012; Smith et al., 2022; BAPM, 2025a). Consider these needs of families at home. In addition, what tailored advice and resources are available to them? Identify examples of good practice that have supported families in your area.

Chapter takeaways

- Continuing care for the baby and family post hospital discharge from the neonatal unit/neonatal transitional care service is multifaceted, requires multidisciplinary support from community and hospital professionals, and should be individualised to meet the needs of the baby and their family.
- Consideration is required for the ongoing healthcare needs and developmental needs for the baby, the wellbeing for the parents/carers, and appropriate training and skills of the health and social care professionals meeting these needs.
- Communication is crucial between services to ensure the smooth transition of continuing care either in the community or in hospital for those infants who require ongoing hospital care with paediatric services.

CASE STUDY

CASE STUDIES

Case study 1: A 20-week-old baby born extremely preterm with complex needs on discharge home

Male infant Jordan is born at 24 weeks gestational age and is the first child for Kate and Derek. During his neonatal course, he is intubated and ventilated for a prolonged period. He has different episodes of sepsis and concerns of necrotising enterocolitis managed with cessation of feeds and parenteral nutrition, though he did not require surgery. He has difficulty weaning from ventilation until eventually he can cope with high flow oxygen at approximately 30 weeks post-menstrual age. A few weeks later he is able to be weaned onto low flow oxygen.

Establishing oral feeds is a significant challenge for him and his parents, which slows his progression on the special care unit in preparation for discharge. His parents are keen to establish breastfeeding – however, during feeding opportunities at the breast, he has difficulty establishing a latch. When he is able to establish a latch and begins feeding, his oxygen levels quickly drop and his respiratory rate increases significantly.

During this period, cranial ultrasounds indicate that he has evidence of post-haemorrhagic ventricular dilatation (PHVD) and emerging brain parenchymal lesions (grade 4 intraventricular haemorrhage). He requires surgery for the placement of a subgaleal shunt for ongoing hydrocephalus which is subsequently converted into a ventriculo-peritoneal shunt around term. On assessment his trunk and neck tone appear lower than his peers' and there are subtle indications of increased tone in all four limbs, with persistent hand fisting which is worse on his right side.

When he can be discharged at 4 weeks corrected age, he goes home with long term oxygen therapy and a nasogastric tube as he has not yet established full oral feeding.

Jordan's parents do not have family locally for support and are particularly anxious regarding managing his feeding to ensure his growth is on track, as there have been a lot of concerns articulated by the neonatal team before discharge.

Q1. How would you go about preparing this family for discharge?

Q2. What would you consider in relation to follow-up, specifically?

- What areas of need would you expect require follow up for Jordan post-discharge?

CASE STUDY

- Which members of the MDT might continue to be involved for this child and family from the neonatal services and/or be referred to within the community setting?

Q3. Are there any neurodevelopmental risks that he faces and what domains of development might be affected and how?

Q4. Beyond addressing the medical concerns, what else would you think about for this family?

Case study 2: A term baby requiring therapeutic cooling

Santiago was born at 39+6 weeks' gestation in poor condition, with the onset of seizure activity from 4 hours of life. He required mechanical ventilation and underwent therapeutic hypothermia for 72 hours. His magnetic resonance imaging revealed subdural haematomas, and he was subsequently diagnosed with hypoxic-ischaemic encephalopathy, grade 2. He was discharged home at 44+1 weeks.

His mother Camila had difficulty being present with Santiago on the NNU due to being a single mother and needing to care for Santiago's 3-year-old brother. Camila also experienced an ongoing anxiety disorder. Before Santiago's discharge, she expressed her fears to the care team about his ongoing development.

Q1. According to the NICE guidelines regarding 'Developmental follow-up of children and young people born preterm' (2017) why would Santiago be entitled to neurodevelopmental follow up?

Q2. How can the care team staff support and prepare Santiago's mother for his discharge home?

Q3. Which members of the MDT should provide developmental follow-up for Santiago and his family, and why?

Q4. Name the three gold standard assessments for early and accurate diagnosis of cerebral palsy.

Case study 3: Six-week-old premature twins discharged home short-term tube feeding

Twins Adeola and Obi were born at 29+6 weeks gestation. They both received high flow respiratory support for under 1 week each before weaning off and spent the remainder of their time in the NNU breathing in air, establishing

CASE STUDY

feeds, and developing. They moved to transitional care at 34+5 and were discharged home 10 days later, both part breast and part tube feeding. These are the first babies for their parents, who have recently moved to the area, with the closest relatives living an hour away. The neonatal outreach team visit regularly monitoring feeding, weight gain, the babies' general physical health, and family wellbeing.

Q1. What information and physical indicators would you be looking for to indicate when to remove the nasogastric tube for each twin?
Q2. What other community practitioners will it be important to ensure the family are engaged with to support them, particularly as they are new to the area with little support nearby?

After 2 weeks at home, parents call you as they are concerned that Obi has not been feeding so well for the last 24 hours and is becoming quite sleepy. A home visit is promptly conducted. On examination, Obi appears fractious and pale and has marked respiratory effort.

Q3. What would be your immediate actions and what observations would you carry out?
Q4. Who would you escalate your concerns too?
Q5. What would you say to parents about your concerns and escalation?

For suggested answer guides to the questions posed in these case studies, please refer to the web-based companion site specific to this chapter. See www.routledge.com/cw/petty

References

Appleton, J. V. (2021). Vulnerable children and early intervention – what about health visiting? *Child Abuse Review*, *30*, 89–97.

Axelin, A., Feeley, N., Campbell-Yeo, M., Silnes Tandberg, B., Szczapa, T., Wielenga, J., Weis, J., Pavicic Bosnjak, A., Jonsdottir, R. B., George, K., Blomqvist, Y. T., Bohlin, K., & Lehtonen, L., Separation, Closeness Experiences in Neonatal Environment (SCENE) Research Group. (2022). Symptoms of depression in parents after discharge from NICU associated with family-centred care. *Journal of Advanced Nursing*, *78*(6), 1676–1687. https://doi.org/10.1111/jan.15128

Aydon, L., Hauck, Y., Murdoch, J., Siu, D., & Sharp, M. (2018). Transition from hospital to home: Parents' perception of their preparation and readiness for discharge with their preterm infant. *Journal of Clinical Nursing*, *27*, 269–277

Beaino, G., Khoshnood, B., Kaminski, M., Pierrat, V., Marret, S., Matis, J., Ledésert, B., Thiriez, G., Fresson, J., Rozé, J.-C., Zupan-Simunek, V., Arnaud, C., Burguet, A., Larroque, B., Bréart, G., Ancel, P.-Y., & EPIPAGE Study Group. (2010). Predictors of cerebral palsy in very preterm infants: The EPIPAGE prospective population-based cohort study. *Developmental Medicine & Child Neurology*, *52*(6), e119–e125. https://doi.org/10.1111/j.1469-8749.2010.03612.x

Bliss. (2022). *Bliss briefing: Impact of cost-of living crisis in neonatal care*. Bliss.

British Association for Neonatal Neurodevelopmental Follow-Up (BANNFU). (2021). *Terms of reference*. Retrieved March 12, 2025, from https://hubble-live-assets.s3.amazonaws.com/bapm/redactor2_assets/files/975/BANNFU_TOR_16.06.2021.pdf

British Association of Perinatal Medicine. (2025a). *Neonatal outreach service: A framework for practice*. British Association of Perinatal Medicine.

British Association of Perinatal Medicine. (2025b). *Transition from neonatal to paediatric services framework*. https://www.bapm.org/articles/help-shape-bapm-s-transition-from-neonatal-to-paediatric-services-framework

Crossley, N., Leake, N., & Deierl, A. (2022). Family integrated care – what, why and how? *Infant*. https://www.infantjournal.co.uk/pdf/inf_103_7266.pdf

Elliot-Smith, A., Sammut, A., Hutchon, B., Merchant, N., O'Brien, F., & Huertas-Ceballos, A. (2024). Early intervention to improve neurodevelopmental outcomes for high-risk infants. *Paediatrics and Child Health*. https://doi.org/10.1016/j.paed.2023.12.003

Getting It Right First Time. (2022). *Neonatology: Getting It Right First Time (GIRFT)*.

Gibbs, D., Boshoff, K., & Stanley, M. (2015). Becoming the parent of a preterm infant: A meta-ethnographic synthesis. *British Journal of Occupational Therapy*, *78*(8), 475–487. https://doi.org/10.1177/0308022615586799

Griffith, T., Singh, A., Naber, M., Hummel, P., Bartholomew, C., Amin, S., White-Traut, R. & Garfield, L. (2022). Scoping review of interventions to support families with preterm infants post-NICU discharge. *Journal of Pediatric Nursing*, *67*, e135–e149. https://doi.org/10.1016/j.pedn.2022.08.014

Hadders-Algra, M. (2018). Early human motor development: From variation to the ability to vary and adapt. *Neurosci Biobehav Rev*, *90*, 411–427. https://doi.org/10.1016/j.neubiorev.2018.05.009

Haeusslein, L., Gano, D., Gay, C. L., Kriz, R. M., Bisgaard, R., Vega, M., Cormier, D. M., Joe, P., Walker, V., Kim, J. H., Lin, C., Sun, Y., & Franck, L. S. (2023). Relationship between social support and post-discharge mental health symptoms in mothers of preterm infants. *Journal of Reproductive and Infant Psychology*, *41*(3), 260–274. https://doi.org/10.1080/02646838.2021.1984404

Harniess, P. A., Basu, A. P., Bezemer, J., & Gibbs, D. (2023). How do parents frame their engagement experience in early intervention? A grounded theory study. *Disability and Rehabilitation*, *46*(14), 3067–3076. https://doi.org/10.1080/09638288.2023.2242788

Harniess, P. A., Gibbs, D., Bezemer, J., & Basu, A. (2022). Parental engagement in early intervention for infants with cerebral palsy – A realist synthesis. *Child: Care, Health and Development*, *48*(3), 359–377. https://doi.org/10.1111/cch.12916

Hickling, A., Mason, L., Chapman, V., & Barnes, D. (2025). Differences in infant safe sleep practice between the neonatal unit and the home environment: A systematised review. *Journal of Neonatal Nursing*, *31*(2), 101622.

HM Government. (2023). *Working together to safeguard children 2023: A guide to multi-agency working to help, protect and promote the welfare of children*. Crown Copyright.

Hutchon, B., Gibbs, D., Harniess, P., Jary, S., Crossley, S., Moffat, J. V., Basu, N., & Basu, A. P. (2019). Early intervention programmes for infants at high risk of atypical neurodevelopmental outcome. *Developmental Medicine & Child Neurology*, *61*(12), 1362–1367. https://doi.org/10.1111/dmcn.14187

Jacobs, S. E., Berg, M., Hunt, R., Tarnow-Mordi, W. O., Inder, T. E., & Davis, P. G. (2013). Cooling for newborns with hypoxic ischaemic encephalopathy. *Cochrane Database of Systematic Reviews*, *1*, Article CD003311. Retrieved June 13, 2025, from https://doi.org/10.1002/14651858.CD003311.pub3

Jiménez-Palomares, M., Fernández-Rejano, M., Garrido-Ardila, E. M., Montanero-Fernández, J., Oliva-Ruiz, P., & Rodríguez-Mansilla, J. (2021). The impact of a preterm baby arrival in a family: A descriptive cross-sectional pilot study. *Journal of Clinical Medicine*, *10*(19), 4494. https://doi.org/10.3390/jcm10194494

Lee, C. W., Snook, J., & Salgin, B. (2025). Current practice of neonatal community outreach teams in England, Wales and Scotland. *Archives of Disease in Childhood-fetal and Neonatal Edition*. https://doi.org/10.1136/archdischild-2024-327865

Lopez, G. L., Anderson, K. H., & Feutchinger, J. (2012). Transition of premature infants from hospital to home life. *Neonatal Network: NN*, *31*(4), 207–214.

Lullaby Trust. (2025). *Safer sleep advice for babies*. https://www.lullabytrust.org.uk/baby-safety/safer-sleep-information/safer-sleep-overview/

Malouf, R., Harrison, S., Burton, H., Gale, C., Stein, A., Franck, L., & Alderdice, F. (2021). prevalence of anxiety and post-traumatic stress among the parents of babies admitted to neonatal units: A systematic review and meta-analysis. *EClinicalMedicine*. https://doi.org/10.1016/j.eclinm.2021.101233

Merchant, N., Shekhar, L., Huertas-Ceballos, A., Johnson, S., & Arasu, A. (2022). Neurodevelopmental care following neonatal discharge. *Paediatrics and Child Health*, *32*(9), 324–331. https://doi.org/10.1016/j.paed.2022.07.002

Moore, T., Hennessy, E. M., Myles, J., Johnson, S. J., Draper, E. S., Costeloe, K. L., & Marlow, N. (2012). Neurological and developmental outcome in extremely preterm children born in England in 1995 and 2006: The EPICURE studies. *BMJ*, *345*, 1–13. https://doi.org/10.1136/bmj.e7961

National Institute for Health and Care Excellence. (2017). *Developmental follow-up of children and young people born preterm*. https://www.nice.org.uk/guidance/qs169/resources/developmental-followup-of-children-and-young-people-born-preterm-pdf-75545608839109

National Neonatal Discharge Planning and Follow-up Framework. (2019). https://perinatalnetwork.scot/wp-content/uploads/2020/01/2019-11-Nat-Neo-Disch-Plan-FU-Framework-v1.0-for-printing.pdf

National Neonatal Surgical Interest Group. (2024). *Holistic feeding and nutritional management for the near term/term neonate following bowel surgery*. Framework for Practice Endorsed by BAPM.

Neonatal Networks Outreach Group. *Parent survey Supporting families at home*, cited in British Association of Perinatal Medicine. (2025). *Neonatal outreach service: A framework for practice*. British Association of Perinatal Medicine.

NHS England. (2024). *Neonatal critical care service specification*. https://www.england.nhs.uk/wp-content/uploads/2015/01/Neonatal-critical-care-service-specification-March-2024.pdf

NICE. (2017). *Developmental follow-up of children and young people born preterm*. NICE. https://www.nice.org.uk/guidance/indevelopment/gid-cgwave0752

Novak, I., Morgan, C., Adde, L., Blackman, J., Boyd, R. N., Brunstrom-Hernandez, J., Cioni, G., Damiano, D., Darrah, J., Eliasson, A.-C., De Vries, L. S., Einspieler, C., Fahey, M., Fehlings, D., Ferriero, D. M., Fetters, L., Fiori, S., Forssberg, H., Gordon, A. M., . . . Badawi, N. (2017). Early, accurate diagnosis and early intervention in cerebral palsy: Advances in diagnosis and treatment. *JAMA Pediatrics*, *171*(9), 897–907. https://doi.org/10.1001/jamapediatrics.2017.1689

Pace, C. C., Spittle, A. J., Molesworth, C. M., Lee, K. J., Northam, E. A., Cheong, J. L., Davis, P. G., Doyle, L. W., Treyvaud, K., & Anderson, P. J. (2016). Evolution of depression and anxiety symptoms in parents of very preterm infants during the newborn period. *JAMA Pediatrics*, *170*(9), 863–870. https://doi.org/10.1001/jamapediatrics.2016.0810

Purdy, I. B., Craig, J. W., & Zeanah, P. (2015). NICU discharge planning and beyond: Recommendations for parent psychosocial support. *Journal of Perinatology*, *35*(Suppl 1), S24–S28. https://doi.org/10.1038/jp.2015.146

Royal College of Paediatrics and Child Health. (2023). *Paediatric virtual wards – position statement.* https://www.rcpch.ac.uk/resources/paediatric-virtual-wards-position-statement

Schuler, R., Ehrhardt, H., & Mihatsch, W. (2020). Safety and parental satisfaction with early discharge of preterm infants on nasogastric tube feeding and outpatients clinic follow-up. *Frontiers in Pediatrics*, *8*, 505.

Seaton, S. E., Manning, J. C., Colville, G., & Mackintosh, N. (2025). Creating a home with a critically ill child: A qualitative study exploring the experiences of parents of children admitted to paediatric critical care following treatment in neonatal care. *Australian Critical Care.* https://doi.org/10.1016/j.aucc.2024.07.082

Smith, V. (2020). Discharge planning considerations for the neonatal intensive care unit. *Archives of Diseases in Childhood Fetal Neonatal Edition*, *106*(4), 442–445.

Smith, V. C., Love, K., & Goyer, E. (2022). NICU discharge preparation and transition planning: Guidelines and recommendations. *Journal of Perinatology*, *42*(S1), 7–21. https://doi.org/10.1038/s41372-022-01313-9

van Hasselt, T. J., Gale, C., Battersby, C., Davis, P., Draper, E., & Seaton, S. (2023). Paediatric intensive care admissions of preterm children born <32 weeks gestation: A national retrospective cohort study using data linkage. *Archives of Diseases in Childhood Fetal Neonatal Edition*, *109*(3), 265–271.

van Wassenaer-Leemhuis, A. G., Jeukens-Visser, M., van Hus, J. W., Meijssen, D., Wolf, M. J., Kok, J. H., Nollet, F., & Koldewijn, K. (2016). Rethinking preventive post-discharge intervention programmes for very preterm infants and their parents. *Developmental Medicine & Child Neurology*, *58*(Suppl 4), 67–73. https://doi.org/10.1111/dmcn.13049

Woythaler, M. (2019). Neurodevelopmental outcomes of the late preterm infant. *Seminars in Fetal and Neonatal Medicine*, *24*(1), 54–59. https://doi.org/10.1016/j.siny.2018.10.002

4 ASSESSMENT OF THE NEONATE

Linda McDonald

CONTENTS

DOI: 10.4324/9781003591405-6

GUIDANCE ON HOW TO ENHANCE PERSONAL LEARNING FROM THIS CHAPTER

Key points covered in this chapter

- How history taking, including a background of maternal health problems in pregnancy, can improve the quality of an assessment.
- A systematic approach to assessment of the neonate.
- Practical considerations for neonatal assessment.

Reflection

Reading through the chapter, you are encouraged to engage with the key points and related literature in an enquiring way. Ask these questions:

- How do you incorporate assessment into your daily nursing care and the planning of this?
- Do you understand the potential implications maternal and family health problems including psychosocial needs may have for the neonate?
- Following a systems approach, which aspects do you need to incorporate into the assessment of a neonate to ensure this is thorough and complete?
- How can do you involve parents and primary care givers in all elements of the assessment process?

Implications for nursing care

- Finally: how will this chapter enable you to plan your approach to assessment of the neonate? Will what you learn affect your current practice?

INTRODUCTION AND BACKGROUND

Assessment of the neonate is a fundamental aspect of nursing in the neonatal unit (NNU). Familiarisation with the clinical status of a neonate at the beginning of a shift, and constant re-evaluation throughout, is essential and frequently occurs unconsciously. This continuous assessment facilitates the detection of often subtle changes and thus makes the neonatal nurse's role crucial in the timely recognition, escalation and management of the deteriorating infant. This chapter aims to provide a theoretical background as well as a practical approach to the comprehensive assessment of the neonate. As individual pathologies commonly seen in the neonatal population are explored in other chapters within the book, it should be considered how the principles of assessment discussed over the next few pages can be applied in the context of various conditions. The psychosocial needs of the parents and family should also be considered as an intrinsic part of assessment. These considerations should include but are not limited to financial, spiritual, cultural, mental health and safeguarding status. Historical issues should be known, and current needs should be frequently assessed by the neonatal team including associated health care professionals to provide **holistic** care planning for the baby and their family.

HISTORY TAKING

The foremost aim of history taking is to identify neonates who may be at risk of difficulties following birth and potential health issues extending into childhood, which require ongoing monitoring and management. Good-quality history taking is a fundamental element in assessing possible short and long-term outcomes including potential mortality. Whether history taking and assessment take place in chronological sequence will depend on the immediate needs of the baby. For example, providing time critical interventions for a hypoxic neonate requiring resuscitation at delivery will take precedence over acquiring an in-depth family history. The nature and depth of details explored will also depend on the situation. While clinicians caring for a term neonate born in poor condition just admitted from the labour ward need to establish the significant elements of maternal, familial, antenatal, and perinatal history, such details should be known and updated regularly for the 6-week-old preterm neonate in the NNU at the point in time when he/she is deteriorating (see Table 4.1 for the necessary components of a comprehensive history).

Thus, history taking may occur at various points in a neonate's care episode:

- At delivery by midwives and obstetricians.
- On admission to the NNU (whether from labour ward or the postnatal ward).
- Following a referral from the community or another NNU.
- During antenatal screening for probable neonatal admission post birth.
- Specialist consultation referral to a tertiary centre.
- During daily ward rounds.
- During allied health professionals review e.g. physiotherapy, dieticians.
- At any time, a change in the neonate's condition requires reassessment.
- At any time, a parent or carer expresses a concern requiring reassessment.

See Table 4.1 for history-taking components

TABLE 4.1 HISTORY-TAKING COMPONENTS

Identification	Name, sex, date of birth, gestational age, corrected gestational age
Presenting problem(s)	What are the primary concerns with the infant at this time?
History of current illness or presenting problem(s)	When did current problem(s) commence?
Current treatment	Current diagnoses/treatments?
Previous medical history	Using a systems approach (see below), inquire about the baby's journey so far; any previous diagnoses/treatments?
Medications	Relevant medications the infant has received in the past? What medication is the baby currently receiving and why? Any known drug allergies/reactions?
Maternal history	Long-term conditions or medications? (Maternal problems are further discussed in Chapter 2.)
Antenatal history	Maternal health during pregnancy? Results of investigations – blood group, serology, ultrasound scans? Problems in pregnancy/hospital admissions?
Perinatal history: labour	Onset of labour – spontaneous/induced/none? Signs of infection? Antenatal corticosteroids/magnesium sulphate received?
Perinatal history: birth	Presentation? Mode of delivery (vaginal/instrumentally assisted/caesarean section)? Condition at birth? Resuscitation required?
Family medical history	Is there a family history of note, particularly of first-degree relatives during infancy or early childhood? Any known genetic abnormalities in the family?
Family psychosocial history	What are the individual elements that make up this family and may influence care decisions? Consider ethnicity, culture, religion, economic factors, primary caregivers and family dynamics (see Chapter 6).
Safeguarding concerns	Are there any social concerns, including maternal substance misuse, other children in care, parental disability?
Parents	Ask parents and primary care givers to share their baby's history as this can provide vital information.

PARENTAL INVOLVEMENT WITH THE ASSESSMENT PROCESS

The process of history taking should seek to establish an open discussion between parents and practitioner. Parents are crucial to the assessment process as they can provide unique insight of any familial history of note and any observed changes in their baby's behaviour. While the order of history taking may differ, each element outlined above should be established to form a comprehensive understanding of the neonate's background, working with parents and care givers to form an appropriate care plan for their baby. Parents should be encouraged to be present during any assessment and any findings should be openly discussed and questions answered.

MATERNAL CONDITIONS AND THEIR POTENTIAL IMPACT

There are numerous maternal medical conditions which commonly precipitate the need for planned or unplanned neonatal care (Baston & Durward, 2025). Antenatal maternal conditions which may affect the neonate include maternal substance misuse, pre-eclampsia, preterm rupture of membranes (PROM) and diabetes mellitus including gestational and type one or type two. Maternal conditions which may impact the neonate at delivery may include antepartum haemorrhage (APH) and malpresentation. Having a basic understanding of these is essential to contextualise assessment findings. Please review Chapter 2 to increase your understanding of antenatal and perinatal issues which may require NNU admission.

ASSESSMENT AT BIRTH

Virginia Apgar was an anaesthesiologist who developed the Apgar tool to assess well infants' recovery from anaesthesia (Apgar et al., 1958). Despite it being designed for term babies, Apgar scoring remains the most universally used tool in the assessment of all newborn babies regardless of gestation. Scored at 1 minute, 5 minutes, and 10 minutes of age, 10 is the highest score, whereas a score of 0 would indicate a baby requiring emergency assistance (see Table 4.2). The system has been recognised to have major limitations; usually scores are recorded retrospectively and are very subjective (Fawke et al., 2025). Various research studies have identified poor correlation between low Apgar scores and cord gases reflecting perinatal compromise or adverse neurodevelopmental outcome (Olofsson, 2023). Furthermore, Apgar scoring does not aid assessing appearance for neonates from ethnic minority backgrounds with darker skin pigmentation (National Health Service Race and Health Observatory (NHS RHO), 2023). It is generally now accepted that the Apgar score should be used in conjunction with other assessment criteria. When using this scoring system, it is important to recognise that adaptation of the evaluation criteria may be necessary. For example, when assessing colour in babies of ethnic minority background, colour should be assessed around the lips, mouth, and tongue with

TABLE 4.2 APGAR SCORING

Score	*0*	*1*	*2*
Colour	Pale/blue	Pink centrally (lips, tongue)*, blue extremities	Pink centrally (lips, tongue)*
Heart rate	Absent	Below 100bpm	Above 100bpm
Response to stimulation	None	Some movement	Cry
Muscle tone	Floppy	Some flexion of extremities	Well flexed
Respiratory effort	Absent	Slow and irregular	Vigorous cry/ regular respiratory effort

**Note: Skin colour is no longer a reliable indicator of adequate central oxygenation due to the difficulties of identifying hypoxia and cyanosis in babies with dark skin tones. Therefore, it is essential to assess lips, gums, and tongue (National Health Service Race and Health Observatory (NHS RHO), 2023).*

increased reliance on preductal pulse oximetry to ascertain sufficient oxygenation or cyanosis (NHS RHO, 2023). Furthermore, the tone of a preterm neonate is less **flexed** than that of a term neonate. Therefore, in an extremely preterm infant, flexed arms and legs would be abnormal.

PHYSICAL ASSESSMENT AFTER BIRTH – A SYSTEMS APPROACH

There are many approaches to physical assessment, and these may vary dependent on the situation. For example, an airway, breathing, circulation, disability, exposure approach and neonatal life support (NLS) algorithm would be appropriate during an emergency situation (Fawke et al., 2025) A knowledge of neonatal-specific anatomy and physiology combined with a systems approach will help guide a holistic and comprehensive assessment. As discussed in the history taking section, it also provides a systematic method for collecting and communicating information between staff members and family members.

Table 4.3 suggests a practical approach to assessment of the neonate.

Respiratory system

Respiratory problems soon after birth may be due to delayed adaptation to extrauterine life, congenital pneumonia, congenital (surgical) conditions, meconium aspiration, but also non-respiratory causes such as cardiac conditions. Normal

TABLE 4.3 THE LOOK-LISTEN-FEEL APPROACH TO PHYSICAL ASSESSMENT OF THE NEONATE

Look

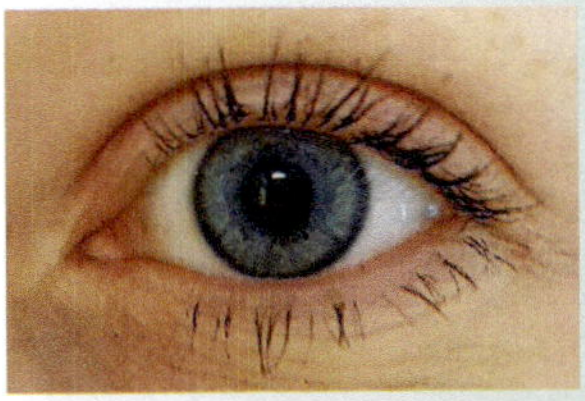

LOOK: Looking first without disturbing the neonate can provide a valuable starting point for assessing at rest. Examples: Is the neonate's posture appropriate for gestation? Are there visual signs of increased work of breathing? Is the colour pale, plethoric, or jaundiced? Does the abdomen appear distended, loopy, or discoloured? Is there evidence of distress or pain?

Listen

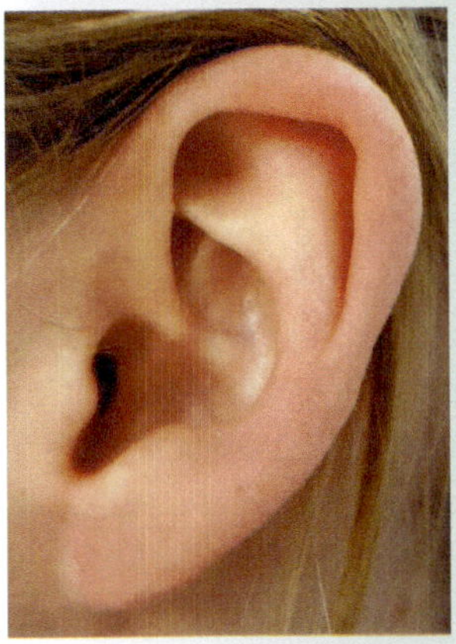

LISTEN: Complete an auditory assessment without and then with a stethoscope. Examples: Are there audible noises such as grunting or stridor that you can hear without a stethoscope? A stethoscope should be used to listen to the baby's breath sounds, heart sounds, and abdomen for active or absent bowel sounds.

Feel

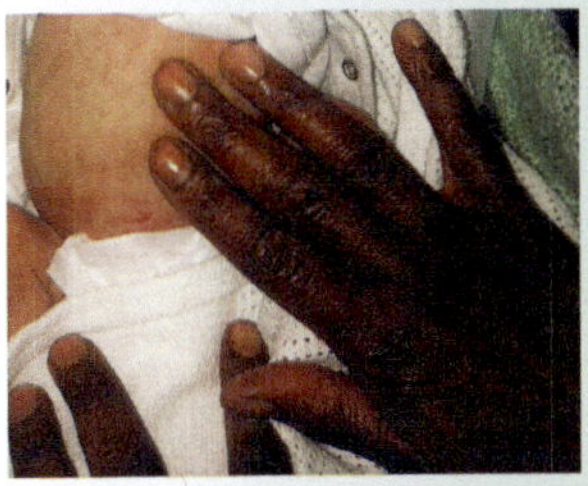

FEEL: Finally, assess by gentle purposeful touch. Examples: Does the neonate feel warm, hot, or cold to touch? Is the anterior fontanelle tense/normotensive/sunken? Does the abdomen feel soft or firm? Is there hepatomegaly or a palpable spleen?

neonatal breathing may be periodic with bilateral chest movement and clear chest sounds. No extra oxygen should be required, and saturations should be within the normal range (Table 4.4). Signs of respiratory distress may include **tachypnoea** (with a breathing rate above 60 breaths per minute), nasal flaring, chest **recession**, **apnoea**, oxygen requirement, **cyanosis**, abnormal chest sounds including **stridor** or **wheezing** (Hogden et al., 2021) and grunting, a noise occurring during exhalation resulting from the baby's breathing against a partially closed glottis. It warrants reiterating that assessment of cyanosis for neonates from ethnic minority backgrounds should include the mucous membranes including the lips, mouth, gums and tongue. Pink mucous membranes would signify adequate perfusion and oxygenation, whereas a pale appearance suggests cyanosis and poor perfusion. Increased reliance on pulse oximetry to ascertain adequate oxygenation is needed with this neonatal group (NHS RHO, 2023) and should be used with any neonate with cyanotic concerns. Abnormal respiratory effort is a key symptom of neonatal disease and requires urgent review. An in-depth respiratory assessment should include oxygen saturations, a blood gas, chest X-ray with consideration for infection screening such as a nasopharyngeal viral panel, and blood cultures. If ventilation is required, bilateral chest movement should be visible, and clear breath sounds with no audible secretions should be heard. Increased oxygen requirement with poor oxygen saturation must be observed for and escalated. Absent breath sounds on one or both sides may be indicative of a **pneumothorax** or other conditions such as diaphragmatic hernia (Walsh, 2023).

Cardiovascular system

It is not just **auscultation** of the heart and determination of the heart rate which give information about the neonate's cardiovascular system status. A full assessment, as is carried out, for example, during the Newborn Infant Physical Examination (NIPE), takes into account several other aspects. Easily and quickly appreciated is the neonate's colour. Facial congestion and peripheral cyanosis of the hands and feet are common in the early postnatal period, but must be differentiated from central cyanosis, which is evident as blue discolouration of the mucous membranes and indicates the presence of blood insufficiently saturated with oxygen. As this can be a sign not only of congenital heart defects but respiratory problems, the immediate management of checking saturation levels (ideally pre- and post-ductal) and oxygen supplementation as indicated is the same for both cases (Walsh, 2023). Pulse oximetry is a safe, non-invasive, inexpensive, and reasonably sensitive test that will detect many cases of critical congenital heart disease (Menahem et al., 2021).

Abnormal work of breathing may not only reflect respiratory problems, but underlying cardiac pathology, so this should form part of the cardiovascular assessment and must be borne in mind as a potential cause (Walsh, 2023). On auscultation, the neonates heart rate, heart rhythm and heart sounds can be appreciated. This may reveal murmurs, additional noises caused by the blood flowing through the heart. **Murmurs** warrant further investigation as they may be indicative of congenital heart defects. The heart rhythm should be regular, although **dysrhythmias** are not uncommon in the neonatal period and are often benign.

Multiple reasons may be causative of a heart rate outside normal limits (Menahem et al., 2021); **tachycardia** can be secondary to stress, pain, hyperthermia, congestive heart failure, but is also a common side effect of inotrope infusions. **Bradycardia** can be a sign of hypothermia, significant acidosis, or problems in the cardiac conduction pathways. When the neonate's pulses are palpated, they should be easy to feel, and equal in upper and lower limbs on both sides. Weak, 'thready' pulses are indicative of shock, while a 'bounding' quality can be noted in the presence of a ductus arteriosus.

Blood pressure (BP) evaluation is very liable to measurement errors, so that it is important to ensure that the infant is settled, and the correct cuff size is selected; the BP will appear high if the cuff is too small, while inappropriately large cuffs will give falsely low readings (Dionne et al., 2020). Normal limits for the BP vary depending on the current gestational age. The efficacy of using current gestational age for ideal neonatal mean BP to ensure adequate organ and tissue perfusion has been previously questioned; however, it is still widely used in neonatal care (van Zadelhoff et al., 2023).

Finally, abdominal palpation also forms part of the cardiovascular assessment: **hepatomegaly**, a liver edge palpable more than 1 cm below the costal margin, may be a sign of cardiac failure (Menahem et al., 2021). More details about management of cardiovascular disorders, including hypotension, can be found in Chapter 15.

Hepatic system

Assessment of **jaundice** is a core nursing role in neonatal care and early recognition of jaundice is vital for treatment of any underlying condition. Bilirubin is a product of red blood cell decay and is conjugated in the liver prior to excretion. An increased turnover of fetal erythrocytes compared to adult red blood cells, combined with hepatic immaturity at birth, makes jaundice, the deposition of yellow pigment in the neonate's sclera and skin, a common occurrence. This should usually become apparent from 48 hours of age and resolve by the end of 2 weeks. Neonates who are preterm or bruised following delivery, for example, breech presentation, are more likely to develop jaundice. An assessment of the gums and sclerae should be undertaken in babies of ethnic minorities, as visual examination of the skin may be inaccurate or misleading (NHS RHO, 2023). Any indication of jaundice from physical examination should be followed up with serum and/or transcutaneous bilirubin levels to identify neonates who require treatment with phototherapy. For example, many breastfed neonates appear jaundiced in the first few weeks of life. Physiological jaundice is a normal occurrence and usually does not require intervention. Routine observations for any jaundiced neonate should include adequate feeding, urine output and passage of meconium. Conversely, pathological jaundice is defined as jaundice occurring during the first 24 hours of life. Maternal history should be explored as risk factors for early jaundice may be identified antenatally with maternal blood group screening, diabetes, and congenital infection. Pathological jaundice should trigger neonatal investigations for haemolytic causes of jaundice, congenital infections, hereditary enzyme deficiency (glucose-6-phosphate dehydrogenase (G6PD) deficiency), and neonatal sepsis. Beyond the first 24 hours of life, any neonate with prolonged unconjugated or conjugated hyperbilirubinaemia may require regular monitoring and investigations. For example, biliary atresia is a rare condition that is associated with dark urine and pale stools. Conjugated **hyperbilirubinaemia** is commonly seen in preterm neonates who have received parenteral nutrition, but other causes should be investigated in any neonate presenting with jaundice which has not resolved after 2 weeks.

Gastrointestinal system

The neonate's abdomen should be pink, soft, not distended, and non-tender with active bowel sounds present. Dusky or **erythematous** discolouration, or periumbilical redness extending beyond the cord stump, are abnormal and may indicate necrotic/inflamed bowel or **omphalitis**. On palpation, no enlargement of the abdominal organs should be noted (Baston & Durward, 2025). The majority of term infants will pass meconium within 24 hours of birth. If a gastric tube is in situ, stomach aspirates should be clear or milky and minimal in volume. In all gestational ages, symptoms of feed tolerance including abnormal gastric aspirates or vomiting, as well as an abnormal abdominal examination may be indicative of infection or surgical problems, further discussed in Chapter 22. Dependent on the degree of prematurity, preterm neonates' first passage of meconium can be delayed to more than 48 hours, and the transition to changed/normal stools also occurs later. Assessment of nutritional status is also important in relation to inclusion of weight and other growth parameters, which will be covered in Chapter 19.

External genitalia

A newborn assessment should include the examination of neonatal genitalia. Preterm infants' genitalia will be underdeveloped at birth and differences in physical appearance depend on current gestational age. The clitoris in preterm female infants may appear more prominent as the labia majora have not fully developed to enclose the clitoris, labia minora, vaginal opening, and urethra. In extremely preterm male infants, the scrotum may be smooth, and the testes will not yet be palpable. In preterm male infants, the testes may not have descended into the scrotum; however, they may be palpable in the inguinal canals. Parents should be counselled that their baby's genitalia will continue to develop outside the womb and will be assessed as part of the NIPE from 34 weeks corrected gestational age (Baston & Durward, 2025). Undescended or absent testes will be assessed during the first NIPE and should be referred.

There are several abnormalities of both female and male genitalia that may be ascertained during physical examination. Vaginal skin tags may be found in 10% of female infants. The presence of maternal oestrogen in the newborn infant causes swelling of the hymen, resulting in the presence of vaginal skin tags.

These self-resolve in the first few weeks of life without treatment. Assessment of swelling in the groin area requires further investigation (Basta et al., 2015). Inguinal hernias are usually unilateral and occur predominantly in male infants, with a higher risk associated with preterm birth. The hernia swelling may become more prominent when the infant is crying or straining and should be reducible when gentle pressure is applied. A non-reducible hernia that is discoloured requires urgent medical review. A unilateral or bilateral swelling of the scrotum may indicate the presence of a hydrocele (Baston & Durward, 2025). This is caused by fluid moving into the scrotum during birth. Positive **transillumination** of the scrotum using a non-heated light source can confirm the presence of a **hydrocele**. Hydroceles self-resolve within the first year of life without treatment and do not affect testicular function. Torsion of the testes is caused by perinatal twisting of the spermatic cord. The affected testicle may appear darkened due to lack of blood supply, feel firm on palpation, and will not transilluminate. This rare condition requires urgent surgical review to preserve testicular function. If physical examination is inconclusive for any of these conditions, additional imaging, such as ultrasound scanning, should be undertaken to aid diagnosis.

The urethra should be visualised at the tip of the penis in male genitalia and between the clitoris and vaginal opening in female genitalia. **Hypospadias** is a relatively common malformation found during postnatal assessment of male genitalia where the urethral opening (meatus) is incorrectly positioned down the ventral shaft. Hypospadias can be classed as mild to severe dependent on the meatus position. In mild presentations, the meatus can be seen just under the glans with an incomplete or hooded foreskin. In the most severe cases, the meatus may be positioned at the base of the scrotum or perineum. If hypospadias is present, the presence of testes must also be assessed, as the absence may be indicative of disorders of sex development. Hypospadias is sometimes associated with chordee, which is curvature of the penile shaft in normally erect states including urination. Both hypospadias and chordee require referral to paediatric surgery (Mole et al., 2020). In all hypospadias, a visual assessment of the neonate passing a good urine stream is essential. An urgent referral is required if urine cannot be passed. Parents should be counselled not to circumcise their baby prior to surgical review, as the foreskin is utilised for the repair. Early circumcision is a common practice within many cultures, and therefore the importance of delaying this should be explained promptly and with sensitivity. Please see the web companion for diagrams and further information on hypospadias presentation and assessment.

Renal system

Most healthy newborns pass some urine in the first 24 hours of life, and failure to do so requires holistic assessment including feeding, general wellbeing, and physical examination (Abitbol et al., 2016). It is important to consider that urination may be difficult to assess if passed with meconium. The renal tract is not functioning fully at birth, meaning that neonates have poor urine concentration ability in the early postnatal period (Doherty et al., 2023). In preterm neonates particularly, this can result in dehydration necessitating careful fluid balance assessment and individualised fluid management plans based on clinical hydration status as well as biochemical indicators such as serum sodium. Evaluation of renal health on the NNU may include dipstick **urinalysis** to monitor **glycosuria, haematuria**, and **proteinuria** and determination of specific gravity. This substitutes measurements of urine osmolality, which indicates whether fluid intake is adequate by reflecting hydration status and urine concentration. Normal specific gravity in the neonate is 1020–1030. Colour should also be documented; dark appearance of urine may be due to conjugated hyperbilirubinemia or haematuria. If urine output falls below 1mL/kg/hour in the newborn or 2mL/kg/hour from 48hours, known as **oliguria**, this could be indicative of acute renal failure, which can result from sepsis, respiratory disease, or necrotising enterocolitis or following a perinatal hypoxic-ischaemic event (Goldstein, 2020). This requires further investigation and careful management. Fluid management will be covered in Chapter 18.

Neurological system

Inspection alone of the neonate's posture, tone, and movements can be very helpful in the evaluation of the neurological status. The mainstay of neurological assessment remains the **Dubowitz** Neurological Examination (Dubowitz et al., 2005) or, alternatively, **Ballard's** score. Differentiating premature infants from those born small for gestational age is an essential aspect to anticipate different clinical scenarios and intervene accordingly. A normal response to external stimuli should be gestational age appropriate and includes alertness such as waking for feeds and/or crying when in pain. Neonates should be observed for excessive wakefulness and irritability as well as excessive quiet, as both can be indicative of neurological problems. Unresponsiveness or subdued response to stimuli may indicate neurological dysfunction or injury as does hypotonia. Depending on the neonate's gestational age at time of assessment, reflexes such as suck, gag, and Moro reflex may be evaluated as part of a neurological examination (Baston & Durward, 2025). This would, however, not be appropriate for very preterm neonates. In any gestation, there should be no signs of pain or stress, and the infant should appear comfortable and be settled between feeding and cares. The presence of pain or stress will be exhibited by tense continual movements, facial expressions, excessive crying, grimacing, changes to vital signs, colour change, apnoea, and desaturations. Maternal medications and psychosocial issues including substance misuse should be considered for potential neonatal abstinence syndrome (Jansson & Patrick, 2019). The web-based companion has various links to resources on neurological assessment tools.

THINK POINT

Can you think of an example of a neonate that you have cared for that appeared behaviourally or physically younger or older than their documented birth gestation? What were the key differences you noted? What was the antenatal history? Were there any psychosocial issues that may have contributed? Were there any underlying neonatal pathologies? Use the web-based companion to review the Dubowitz or Ballard Score to add to your reflections.

Skin and general appearance

The maturity of the skin should match the neonate's gestational age. For example, an extremely preterm infant's skin evolves in the first few weeks of life from red, shiny, and translucent to a thicker appearance as the **stratum corneum** of the epidermis develops in response to the extrauterine environment (Marissen et al., 2023). It is important to explain to parents of ethnic minority backgrounds that all preterm neonates' skin will initially have a reddened appearance regardless of ethnicity, and true skin pigmentation will begin to develop over the first few months of life (NHS RHO, 2023).

There are several normal skin variations and rashes which occur particularly in the term population and must be differentiated from abnormal skin lesions (see activity below). Symptoms of inflammation should always be investigated for cause and potential treatment options (Marissen et al., 2023). Regardless of gestational age, breakdown of skin is always abnormal. In neonates with indwelling cannulas, venous catheters, and chest drains, the insertion sites must be regularly observed for swelling, erythema, and evidence of **extravasation**. Given the fragility of preterm skin, regular skin assessments should be completed with a specific focus on pressure areas such as the nasal septum in a neonate requiring continuous positive airway pressure (Pascual & Wielenga, 2023). Early identification of pressure areas should be escalated for review and assessment by tissue viability health care professionals may be warranted.

ACTIVITY

Take a look at this webpage to identify common skin variations and rashes in the term neonatal population.

- https://www.nhs.uk/symptoms/rashes-babies-and-children/.

Thermoregulation

Assessment of thermal stability and temperature is a fundamental area of assessment, as it is an essential part of transition and adaptation to extrauterine life at birth and thereafter. Mild temperature fluctuations are difficult to interpret in the first few hours after birth, as they can be subject to changing environmental conditions. Persistently abnormal or unstable temperature measurements, however, warrant further investigation as they may be indicative of other issues such as infection (see Table 4.4). Furthermore, hypothermia has been identified as causative factor for intracranial haemorrhage, hypotension, and hypoglycaemia. Neonatal thermoregulation, including the importance of maintaining normothermia, will be covered in greater depth in Chapter 13.

TABLE 4.4 VITAL SIGNS ASSESSMENT

Measurement: Respiratory	Method: Visual, ECG, stethoscope	Preterm Values: 40–60 resp. rate/min	Term Values: 30–60 resp. rate/min
Respiratory assessment: Observe the movement of the chest for symmetry and bilateral air entry via stethoscope. Work of breathing should also be assessed, making note of the rate per minute and any substernal or intercostal recession.			
Measurement: Heart rate	Method: ECG, pulse oximetry, auscultation	Preterm values: 120–180bpm	Term values: 90–160bpm
Cardiac assessment: Place bell of the stethoscope to the immediate left of sternum between the originating from the sinoatrial node located in the right atrium of the heart, this electrical impulse travels throughout the heart causing the heart to contract, thus creating each heartbeat.			
Measurement: Blood pressure	Method: cuff or invasive via arterial access. The transducer should be zeroed to the right atrium of the heart before measurement.	Preterm values: Mean: current gestational age Systolic: 50–62mmHg Diastolic: 25–47mmHg	Term values: Mean: current gestational age Systolic: 46–94mmHg Diastolic: 31–63mmHg
Blood pressure assessment: Recorded measurements are systole, mean and diastole. The systolic pressure reflects the arterial pressure resulting from the ejection of blood during ventricular contraction. The diastolic pressure represents the arterial pressure of blood during ventricular relaxation. Mean blood pressure is of particular significance within the neonatal period as desirable blood pressure should be gestational age or greater.			
Measurement: capillary refill time (CRT)	Method: apply gentle pressure by the pad of a finger to sternum	Term values: <3seconds indicates adequate perfusion	Preterm values: <3seconds indicates adequate perfusion
Perfusion assessment: Apply gentle pressure by the pad of the finger onto the middle chest and hold for 5 seconds. Release and count seconds the area takes to return to normal colour. This will be the capillary refill time. It is important to remember that many factors can influence perfusion particularly in the newborn period, including immature or changing pulmonary, cardiac, and renal function.			

TABLE 4.4 (Cont.)

Measurement: Oxygen saturation	Method: pulse oximetry probe on foot, hand or wrist	Preterm values: 89%–100% Titrate supplemental O_2 as indicated	Term values: 95%–100% Titrate supplemental O_2 as indicated
Oxygen saturation assessment: Analysis of how much the haemoglobin is saturated with oxygen. Measurement is taken from capillary blood, which provides a close representation of arterial blood oxygen saturation.			
Measurement: Carbon dioxide and oxygen	Method: transcutaneous probe, end-tidal CO_2, blood gas	Preterm values: pO_2 7.5–10kPa pCO_2 4.5–6.5kPa	Term values: pO_2 8–12kPa pCO_2 4.5–6kPa
Both oxygenation and carbon dioxide can be assessed by application of a calibrated heated skin probe applied to skin preferably the abdomen. Another alternative to blood gases is the use of end-tidal CO_2 monitoring attached to endotracheal tubes. If neither of these equipment options is available, blood gases continue to provide the most common form of pCO_2 and pO_2 measurement.			
Measurement: Temperature	Method: intermittent axilla, continuous abdominal and rectal probe	Preterm values: 36.5–37.5°C (97.7–99.5°F)	Term values: 36.5–37.5°C (97.7–99.5°F)
Assessment of temperature: While axilla thermometers may be appropriate for stable babies, continuous monitoring may be useful for babies that are unwell or for servo-control modes. Toe-core gap monitoring provides a useful indicator for perfusion. While hyperthermia indicates a higher than normal body temperature, hypothermia forms part of the three H triangle for metabolic adaption (hypoxia, hypothermia, hypoglycaemia).			
Measurement: Blood sugar	Method: Glucometer, blood gas or laboratory	Preterm values: 2.6–6mmol/L (46.8–108.0mg/dL)	Term values: 2.0–6mmol/L (36.0–108.0mg/dL)
Assessment of blood sugar: Ensure a neonatal lancet is used choosing the appropriate puncture depth for a preterm or term neonate. Frequency of blood sugar assessment may differ between units and on individual needs, therefore, check local guidelines for instruction.			
Measurement: Urine output	Method: calculate all fluid intake and output, including insensible water losses	Preterm values for urine output: Newborn:>1ml/kg/hr >24hours: >2ml/kg/hr	Term values for urine output: Newborn: >1ml/kg/hr >24hours: >2ml/kg/hr
Assessment of fluid status: Expected urine output is dependent on time since birth, gestational age and underlying condition. For example, perinatal hypoxia can reduce renal function, as can prematurity.			

Metabolism

Following birth, the neonatal metabolism must adapt to intermittent nutritional delivery having been accustomed to a constant placental supply of glucose and other nutrients. In well term neonates, the utilisation of fatty fuels and ketones compensates for interruptions in glucose availability (Baston & Durward, 2025). However, in preterm and low birthweight neonates, the immaturity of such metabolic processes results in a propensity for **hypoglycaemia**. Similarly, unwell term neonates may not be able to meet their heightened metabolic demands with such alternative fuels. Maternal conditions including diabetes mellitus and medications such as beta blockers may result in initial hypoglycaemia. As a result, glucose levels need to be carefully monitored in neonatal patients and treated with early feeding and glucose solutions or infusions as needed (Harding et al., 2024).

Hyperglycaemia is commonly transient, and an issue more commonly observed in the extremely preterm and low birthweight population. This may be due to immaturity-related insulin resistance or the inability to down-regulate gluconeogenesis in the presence of the infusion of glucose solutions such as parenteral nutrition. While the abovementioned postnatal changes affect the neonatal metabolic system and must contend with the necessity for close observation of glucose levels early on, it is also important to recognise changes in glucose homeostasis, as they can indicate problems such as sepsis (Beardsall, 2021).

ASSESSMENT OF THE DETERIORATING NEONATE

Whilst preterm birth and congenital anomalies may account for neonatal deterioration in the early hours and days of life, the most common causes of deterioration are respiratory conditions and infection. Signs of infection may be non-specific and difficult to distinguish from other issues; for example, changes to vital signs such as increased respiratory rate and heart rate may be indicative of infection but may also be signs of environmental hyperthermia, pain or progressing lung disease requiring increased respiratory support. Neonatal infection should, however, always be considered as part of holistic assessment of the neonate due to the potential impact both short and long term. Assessment for infection is discussed in detail in Chapter 20. Where clinical concerns arise, a systematic approach to assessment is required including vital signs (Table 4.4) and physical examination. It is essential to place the time of systems observations in the context of events preceding assessment. Ideally, the assessment should take place when the infant has not been disturbed recently, as this will provide a baseline of observations when the baby is at rest. Wherever possible throughout the assessment process, parents' views must be included as they can provide valuable information about their baby's normal status quo and any changes that may have occurred.

> **PRACTICE POINT**
>
> Assessment is the beginning point of recognising a neonate's potential issue or condition and is understandably anxiety provoking for parents. Discussions with parents should be conducted as soon as feasible in a professional and empathetic manner. The information discussed with parents should be transparent and as accurate as possible, providing information about the assessment findings, planned investigations with their consent, and timely updates as available. Parents should be involved in planning care for their baby.

NEWBORN INFANT PHYSICAL EXAMINATION

The NIPE programme is endorsed by the UK Screening Committee (Public Health England, 2025) and aims to reduce mortality and morbidity through the identification of neonates with congenital abnormalities of four key areas (see below). It differs from systematic assessment in that it is a physical screening tool for all babies. All eligible neonates greater than 34 weeks corrected gestational age should be examined within the first 72 hours of life, unless they are too unwell. The NIPE is repeated at 6–8 weeks of age in the community, at which point previously undetected issues may have emerged (Public Health England, 2025). The examination can be carried out by a doctor, nurse, or midwife who has undertaken a university-accredited NIPE module.

The minimum NIPE examination components are these four key areas:

- *Eyes* These are primarily assessed for congenital cataracts, but conditions such as aniridia, coloboma, or retinoblastoma are also excluded. With the aid of an ophthalmoscope, the fundus reflex is assessed by observing light reflecting off the back the of the eye (the fundus). The fundus reflex has been historically referred to as the **'red' reflex**; however, this can be misleading as the Caucasian orange/red colour may appear significantly paler in minority ethnicities (Kelly et al., 2025). This may lead to the incorrect diagnosis of congenital cataracts which presents as a clouding of the eye. For accuracy, the clarity and symmetry of both corneas should be assessed in all neonates and ethnicity should be considered when assessing the fundal colour. If uncertainty exists, a biological parent's fundal reflex can be completed for comparison, with their permission (Public Health England, 2025).
- *Heart* Examination of the cardiovascular system aims to identify critical or major serious heart defects which require timely (surgical) intervention. While not currently an essential component of the UK NIPE standards, consideration of pulse oximetry (pre- and post ductal saturations) can be

beneficial in identifying previously undiagnosed duct dependent lesions. All neonates should undergo cardiovascular assessment of inspection, palpation, and auscultation as described above. Any abnormalities should be escalated for senior medical review.

- *Hips* **Developmental dysplasia of the hips** (DDH) is a congenital problem associated with serious long-term morbidity. Dislocatable hips found on examination need to be referred for ongoing management to allow for normal mobility later in life. The condition is identified by performing the Galeazzi, Barlow and Ortolani manoeuvres (see companion website for a video demonstration). If the screen is positive, an urgent hip ultrasound and orthopaedic review is arranged. Neonates with a normal examination but with first degree relative history of DDH or other risk factors such as breech presentation will automatically be referred for a non-urgent ultrasound of the hips.
- *Testes* Both testes are assessed to determine whether they have descended into the scrotum at birth. The testes of neonates who are still preterm at time of examination may not have descended into the scrotum but should palpable just above the scrotum in the inguinal canals. Bilaterally undescended testes (**cryptorchidism**) must raise the possibility of ambiguous genitalia and trigger relevant investigations. As cryptorchidism has been associated with reduced fertility and the potential for malignancies, even unilaterally undescended testes must be referred for ongoing monitoring and intervention.

ACTIVITIES

- Take a look at this webpage for further guidance and videos on how to complete a comprehensive physical examination of the healthy newborn: https://geekymedics.com/newborn-baby-assessment/.
- Take a look at this webpage for an approach to assessment for dysmorphism. This includes the steps recommended in this chapter starting with gaining maternal and familial history, systematic physical assessment, investigations, and discussion with parents: https://www.safercare.vic.gov.au/best-practice-improvement/clinical-guidance/neonatal/dysmorphology-assessment-in-neonates.

Chapter takeaways

- The neonatal nurse plays a crucial role in promoting neonatal wellbeing and improving outcomes. Assessment of the neonate, a continuous and sometimes unconscious process, forms the basis of neonatal nursing care and contributes to the timely identification of potentially serious problems.

- Taking a thorough history can identify valuable information about risk factors, hereditary problems, and the baby's wider psychosocial context.
- A comprehensive understanding of the theoretical and practical principles behind the assessment process allows for a systematic approach (Look – Listen – Feel, applied to each body system).
- Parent involvement is crucial throughout the assessment and care planning process.

CASE STUDY

CASE STUDIES

Case study 1: Assessing a neonate who is not feeding well

Priya was born at 37 weeks at 3.21kg and is now 3 days old. She has been admitted from the postnatal ward for further investigation. Her parents originate from India and report that her frequency and length of feeding have decreased over the past 24 hours. She has had one wet nappy in the past 12 hours and appears very sleepy. You are asked to undertake an initial assessment.

Q.1. What information would you like to know from Priya's history?
Q.2. What information would you like to know about maternal and family history?
Q.3. Using the vital signs parameters and the systematic approach, how would you undertake a physical assessment of Priya?
Q.4. Which investigations would you like to do?
Q.5. Reviewing the information you have collected, list possible causes (differential diagnoses) for Priya's lethargy, reduced breastfeeding, and urine output.
Q.6. How would you communicate your assessment process and findings with the parents?

Case study 2: Assessing a neonate with low oxygen saturations

Leo was born at 39 weeks at 3.78kg and is now 12 hours old. He has been admitted from delivery suite for suboptimal pulse oximetry which was obtained as a routine part of the newborn examination. The midwife handover is that the rest of the examination was normal. His parents are of black African ethnicity and are understandably concerned.

CASE STUDY

Q.1. What are your immediate steps, and which investigations would you like to do?
Q.2. What information would you like to know from Leo's history?
Q.3. What information would you like to know about maternal and family history?
Q.4. Using the vital signs parameters and the systematic approach, how would you undertake a physical examination of Leo?
Q.5. Reviewing the information you have collected, list possible causes (differential diagnoses) for Leo's low oxygen saturations.
Q.6. How would you communicate your assessment process and findings with parents?

Case study 3: Assessing a neonate with neonatal abstinence syndrome

Nathan is admitted to the neonatal unit at 8 hours of age following birth at 36 weeks' gestation, weighing 2.8 kg. He was transferred from the delivery suite for observation due to signs consistent with neonatal abstinence syndrome. On admission, Nathan is noted to be jittery, irritable, and difficult to settle. Nathan's mother, Fran, is 19 years old and remains on the postnatal ward. She appears anxious and tearful, expressing guilt about Nathan's condition.

Q1. What key components should be included in the physical assessment of a baby with NAS?
Q2. Why is the use of a structured NAS scoring tool important in guiding care and management, and what does this include?
Q3. What pharmacological and non-pharmacological strategies can be used to support Nathan's symptoms, and why are they effective?
Q4. How can staff support Fran in a non-judgemental way while promoting her confidence and involvement in Nathan's care?
Q5. What additional assessment, support services or multidisciplinary input may be beneficial for Fran and Nathan?

For suggested answer guides to the questions posed in these case studies, please refer to the web-based companion site specific to this chapter. See www.routledge.com/cw/petty

References

Abitbol, C. L., DeFreitas, M. J., & Strauss, J. (2016). Assessment of kidney function in preterm infants: Lifelong implications. *Pediatric Nephrology*, *31*(12), 2213–2222.

Apgar, V., Holaday, D. A., James, L. S., Weisbrot, I. M., & Berrien, C. (1958). Evaluation of the newborn infant-second report. *Journal of the American Medical Association*, *168*(15), 1985–1988.

Basta, A. M., Courtier, J., Phelps, A., Copp, H. L., & MacKenzie, J. D. (2015). Scrotal swelling in the neonate. *Journal of Ultrasound in Medicine*, *34*(3), 495–505.

Baston, H., & Durward, H. (2025). *Examination of the newborn: A practical guide* (4th ed.). Routledge.

Beardsall, K. (2021). Hyperglycaemia in the newborn infant. Physiology verses pathology. *Frontiers in Pediatrics*, *9*, 1–9.

Dionne, J. M., Bremner, S. A., Baygani, S. K., Batton, B., Ergenekon, E., Bhatt-Mehta, V., Dempsey, E., Kluckow, M., Koplowitz, L. P., Apele-Freimane, D., & Iwami, H. (2020). Method of blood pressure measurement in neonates and infants: A systematic review and analysis. *The Journal of Pediatrics*, *221*, 23–31.

Doherty, T. M., Hu, A., & Salik, I. (2023). *Physiology, neonatal*. StatPearls Publishing.

Dubowitz, L., Ricciw, D., & Mercuri, E. (2005). The Dubowitz neurological examination of the full-term newborn. *Mental Retardation and Developmental Disabilities Research Reviews*, *11*(1), 52–60.

Fawke, J., Alexander-Elborough, E., Benson Clarke, A., Bradfield, M., Cusack, J., Hamilton-Bower, I., Madar, J., Monnelly, V., Reeves, N., Tinnion, R., Wood, T., & Wyllie, J. (2025). *Newborn life support* (6th ed.). Resuscitation Council (UK).

Goldstein, S. L. (2020). Urine output assessment in acute kidney injury: The cheapest and most impactful biomarker. *Frontiers in Pediatrics*, *7*, 565.

Harding, J. E., Alsweiler, J. M., Edwards, T. E., & McKinlay, C. J. (2024). Neonatal hypoglycaemia. *BMJ Medicine*, *3*(1), e000544.

Hogden, L., Munger, K., & Duffek, S. (2021). Neonatal respiratory distress. *South Dakota Medicine*, *74*(1).

Jansson, L. M., & Patrick, S. W. (2019). Neonatal abstinence syndrome. *Pediatric Clinics of North America*, *66*(2), 353.

Kelly, C., Anderson, M., & Smith, H. (2025). Decolonising the "red" reflex test: Transitioning from terminology based on colour to anatomy. *Eye*, *39*, 379–381.

Marissen, J., Gomez de Agüero, M., Chandorkar, P., Reichert, L., Glaser, K., Speer, C. P., & Härtel, C. (2023). The delicate skin of preterm infants: Barrier function, immune-microbiome interaction, and clinical implications. *Neonatology*, *120*(3), 295–307.

Menahem, S., Sehgal, A., & Meagher, S. (2021). Early detection of significant congenital heart disease: The contribution of fetal cardiac ultrasound and newborn pulse oximetry screening. *Journal of Paediatrics and Child Health*, *57*(3), 323–327.

Mole, R. J., Nash, S., & MacKenzie, D. N. (2020). Hypospadias. *British Medical Journal*, *369*.

NHS Health and Race Observatory. (2023). *Review of neonatal assessment and practice in Black, Asian and minority ethnic newborns: Exploring the Apgar score, the detection of cyanosis, and jaundice*. National Health Service.

Olofsson, P. (2023). Umbilical cord pH, blood gases, and lactate at birth: Normal values, interpretation, and clinical utility. *American Journal of Obstetrics & Gynecology*, *228*(5), S1222–S1240.

Pascual, A., & Wielenga, J. M. (2023). Nasal pressure injuries among newborns caused by nasal CPAP: An incidence study. *Journal of Neonatal Nursing*, *29*(3), 477–481.

Public Health England. (2025). *Newborn and infant physical examination screening programme handbook*. Public Health England.

van Zadelhoff, A., Poppe, J., Willemsen, S., Mauff, K., van Weteringen, W., Goos, T., Reiss, I., Vermeulen, M., & de Graaff, J. (2023). Age-dependent changes in arterial blood pressure in neonates during the first week of life: Reference values and development of a model. *British Journal of Anaesthesia*, *130*(5), 585–594.

Walsh, B. (2023). Assessment and monitoring of the neonatal and paediatric patient. In *Neonatal and paediatric respiratory care* (6th ed.). Eselvier.

5 THE PREMATURE AND LOW BIRTHWEIGHT INFANT

Lesley Kilby and Katy Powis

CONTENTS

DOI: 10.4324/9781003591405-7

GUIDANCE ON HOW TO ENHANCE PERSONAL LEARNING FROM THIS CHAPTER

Key points covered in this chapter

- An overview of prematurity and low birthweight.
- Common conditions affecting premature and/or low birthweight infants, their underlying pathophysiology and clinical management.
- Aspects to be considered antenatally, on the neonatal unit and in preparation for discharge when caring for infants born prematurely and/or low birthweight.

Reflection

- What are your considerations when caring for an extremely/very preterm infant? How do these differ from when you are planning your care of a late preterm infant?
- Are you confident in recognising presenting signs of most of the issues preterm and/or low birthweight infants can encounter during their journey through the neonatal unit?
- How do you need to focus your support to the parents depending on the gestation/weight their baby was born at?

Implications for nursing care

- Finally: this chapter should facilitate your understanding of your approach to the assessment and management of neonates born prematurely or at a low birthweight. Consider how you incorporate your understanding of the care of the preterm and/or low birthweight infant within your provision of family integrated care.

INTRODUCTION AND BACKGROUND

The World Health Organization (WHO, 2023) define prematurity as birth before 37 weeks completed gestation. This, however, is a broad definition, as outcomes and management can vary significantly across this spectrum. There are sub-categories of preterm birth based on gestational age (GA):

- Moderate to late preterm (32–37 weeks)
- Very preterm ($28–31^{+6}$ weeks)
- Extremely preterm (<28 weeks)

Infants who are small for their gestation may experience issues not unlike those faced by preterm infants, so that there are similarities in the approach to their care. This chapter will identify contributing factors, care in the delivery setting, common associated conditions, and key physiological aspects of prematurity and low birthweight. It will also explore the impact this may have on the baby and their family and form a basis for topics discussed in other chapters.

ASSESSMENT OF GESTATIONAL AGE

GA refers to the time elapsed since the beginning of the last menstrual period and is counted in weeks and days. Antenatally, GA is most accurately determined by menstrual history or ultrasound scanning in the first trimester. The earlier the dating ultrasound is performed, the more accurate the predicted GA (Morgan & Cooper, 2022). However, not all mothers have a regular cycle, and some may not receive antenatal care, so exact information regarding GA may not be available at the time of birth.

Infants who are small for GA (SGA) may initially appear to be more premature, and conversely infants who are large for GA may appear more mature, therefore estimation of gestation based on weight can be inaccurate (Petty, 2024). Preterm

TABLE 5.1 DIFFERENCES BETWEEN PRETERM INFANTS AND SGA INFANTS

	Preterm Infant	*SGA infant*
Characteristics	**Physical** Small in size Thin, shiny, and sometimes red or transparent skin **Lanugo** often present Very little body fat Soft, underdeveloped ear cartilage Genitals may appear small and underdeveloped; in boys, the testes might be undescended and the scrotum has few folds, while in girls, the labia minora may not be covered by the labia major **Behavioural and functional** Poor muscle tone and posture Weak sucking and swallowing reflexes Poor temperature regulation Immature breathing reflex pathways	**Physical** Low birthweight for GA Little subcutaneous fat and muscle resulting in loose skin Skin development appropriate for GA Umbilical cord often thin and dull In many cases, the head may be relatively large compared to the rest of the body, or the anterior fontanelle can be larger than normal **Behavioural and functional** May not achieve adequate catch-up growth Despite their size, developmentally, their behaviour and function should meet expectations for their GA Sometimes associated with other congenital/chromosomal presentations
Primary problems	Immature organs leading to poor adaptation High risk for infection Jaundice Neurological sequelae Respiratory distress syndrome Disrupted retinal vascularisation Nutritional/feeding immaturity and intolerance	Risk for hypoglycaemia Poor temperature control **Polycythaemia** and jaundice Breathing difficulties, including **Meconium aspiration** Increased risk for infection Slow adaptation to feeding

infants and those who are SGA differ in their characteristics and primary problems in the neonatal period (see Table 5.1).

Tools to determine GA accurately in the immediate postnatal period are useful in situations where there is uncertainty. The New Ballard Score has widely replaced the Dubowitz Assessment of Gestational Age and the original Ballard Score to encompass preterm infants born before 28 weeks GA and remains in common use. It enables the practitioner to estimate GA through the assessment of neuromuscular control as well as physical characteristics (Lee et al., 2017).

LONG-TERM OUTCOMES OF PREMATURITY

The outcome for infants delivered prematurely has been investigated widely. Previous robust studies about long-term outcomes and survival rates include EPICure and EPICure 2; however, a more recent retrospective analysis collected information on survival rates at 28 days preterm infants born in the United Kingdom (UK) and British Crown Dependencies between 22 and 31^{+6} weeks' gestation. It was concluded that all infants with a birthweight over 1000g, survival was 90% or higher (Seaton et al., 2023)

Disability and survival statistics are seen to improve with greater GA.

The main categories of disability identified are:

- Severe cognitive impairment
- Cerebral palsy
- Blindness or profound hearing impairment

Internationally, various tools have been developed to assist in predicting outcomes, including the Extremely Preterm Birth Outcomes Tool. Users of such tools should be aware that every infant is an individual and that factors beyond those described within the tool can influence survival and neurodevelopmental outcomes.

There is a continuing global drive to enhance antenatal care, monitor the incidence of preterm deliveries, investigate their causes, and implement evidence-based strategies to avoid premature births and improve the outcomes of infants born too early (WHO, 2023).

ACTIVITY: PREDICT AND COMPARE

Instructions:

Below are three children, each born at a different gestational age. Based on what you've learned about outcomes of prematurity, write down what short-term and long-term outcomes you might expect for each child.

Profiles:

1. Baby A: Born at 24 weeks gestation, weighing 600 grams.
2. Baby B: Born at 30 weeks gestation, weighing 1.2kg.
3. Baby C: Born at 36 weeks gestation, weighing 2.4kg.

Questions:

What neurodevelopmental or physical challenges might each baby face?
What factors could improve or worsen their outcomes?
How might early intervention strategies differ between these babies?

THE LOW BIRTHWEIGHT INFANT

With regard to birthweight, the WHO (2022) differentiate **extremely low birth weight** (ELBW) <1000g, **very low birthweight** (VLBW) 1000g–1500g, and **low birthweight** (LBW) <2500g.

It is important to recognise that these weight categories can relate to any gestation. LBW can be the result of premature birth, genetic abnormalities, or **fetal growth restriction** (FGR), sometimes also called intra-uterine growth restriction (IUGR). SGA refers to infants with a birthweight <10th percentile and includes infants who are constitutionally small. There are multifactorial causes contributing to SGA. FGR is defined as a fetal size or abdominal circumference <3rd centile or <10th centile with **Doppler** abnormalities identified. The term SGA also includes those with FGR, which means that for a number of possible reasons, a baby may not achieve their growth potential *in utero*. While the terms SGA and FGR are often used synonymously, they are in fact not interchangeable but refer to different conditions (Morris et al., 2024).

Factors contributing to fetal growth restriction

FGR infants (see Figure 5.1) have historically been subcategorised into symmetrical and asymmetrical FGR. Asymmetrical FGR was considered the most common form of growth restriction with disruption to fetal growth occurring mainly in the third trimester. Symmetrical FGR has been characterised by a global growth restriction throughout pregnancy. Asymmetrical FGR was defined as weight below the 10th percentile, but head circumference preserved within the normal range, whereby symmetrical FGR was defined as both weight and head circumference <10th percentile (Morris et al., 2024). FGR occurs when demands for oxygen and nutrition outstrip placental supply. The main causes are congenital infections, maternal hypertension, suboptimal maternal health and weight gain, drug misuse/smoking, chromosomal and genetic factors, and multiple pregnancy. Monitoring the quality of placental blood flow has been beneficial in identifying fetal wellbeing and early detection of FGR. A Cochrane meta-analysis showed that the monitoring of umbilical artery blood flow reduces the risk of perinatal deaths as it detected those at risk of developing reduced fetal growth and compromise (Alfirevic et al., 2017).

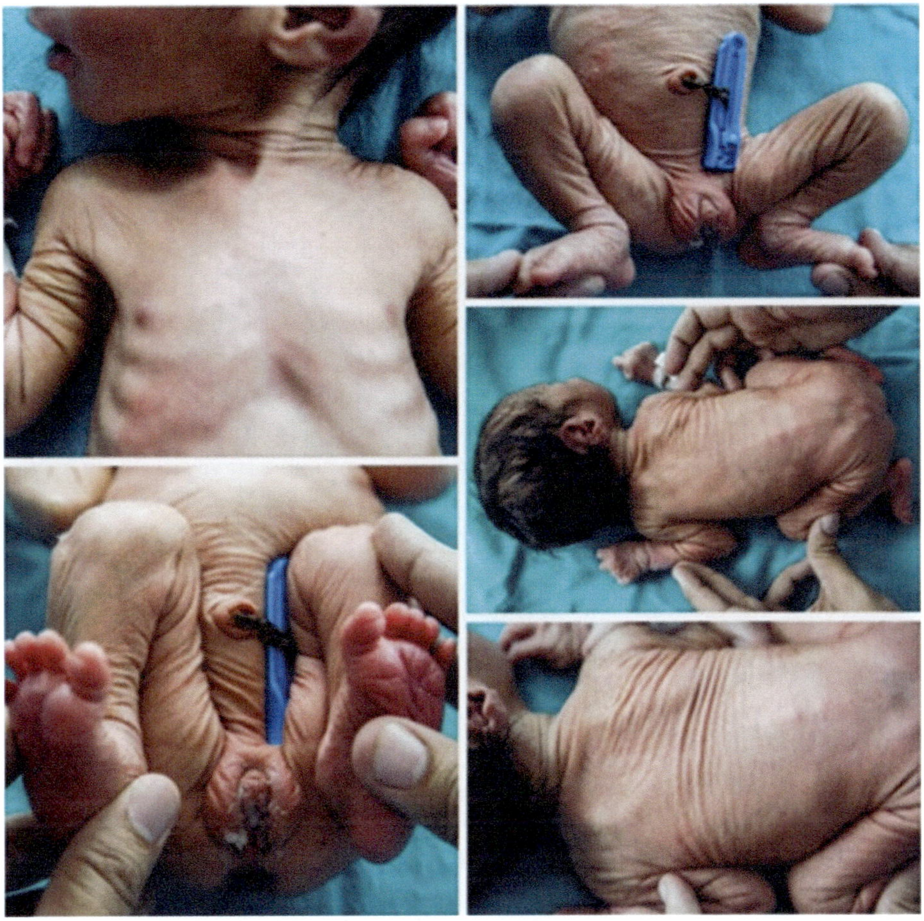

Figure 5.1 The typical appearance of a growth-restricted neonate. This was a 36-week female infant born to a mother with severe pre-eclampsia with a birthweight of 1600 grams. This baby was asymmetrically growth restricted. Note loss of fat all over the body, visible rib cage, excessive skin folds especially over inter-scapular and gluteal areas, and relatively large head compared with the rest of the body.

CARE IN THE DELIVERY SETTING

Common causes of prematurity include pregnancy-induced hypertension, multiple pregnancy, maternal health (including weight, drug misuse, smoking, and stress), infection/**chorioamnionitis**, uterine/placental conditions, and **cervical insufficiency**, among others. There are many circumstances whereby the underlying cause is unknown; however, genetic causes have been suggested (Dauengauer-Kirlienė et al., 2023).

Pre-delivery considerations

Attempts to optimise maternal and fetal health should start before conception and continue throughout a woman's pregnancy. Adequate antenatal management is of crucial importance, particularly for the preterm population, and has a direct impact on long-term outcomes (BAPM, 2019a).

BAPM has guidance for perinatal management at less than 27 weeks' gestation in light of increasing evidence around improving outcomes, and the evolving national and international approaches to care and management strategies. It is acknowledged that care should be individualised and led by senior, experienced neonatal, midwifery and obstetric staff. Decision-making for babies born at extremely low GA should not be based on this alone, but on assessment of the baby's prognosis, taking into account multiple factors which are associated with increased or decreased risk of absolute survival and survival without severe impairment. These factors include:

- *Fetal factors* which may increase risk include male sex, multiple pregnancy, congenital anomaly, and poor fetal growth.
- *Clinical conditions* which pose additional risk and have been associated with increased mortality and morbidity are prolonged pre-labour rupture of membranes before 24 weeks' gestation and clinical evidence of chorioamnionitis.
- *Therapeutic strategies* such as the administration of antenatal **corticosteroids** and **magnesium sulphate** are associated with improved survival, neonatal outcomes, and reduced risk of childhood impairment, even before 24 weeks gestation.
- *Clinical setting* should be considered so that infants at lower gestations are admitted to centres equipped for higher dependency care with experienced staff. Antenatal transfer before 27 weeks' gestation is recommended to ensure delivery occurs in a maternity unit with a co-located neonatal intensive care unit (NICU).

Following full history taking and assessment of both fetal and maternal health, the chances of an unacceptably poor outcome will generally fall into one of the following categories: extremely high risk, high risk, or moderate risk. Discussion with the family should be led by a senior neonatologist where possible and decisions for active management or palliative care based on prognosis should be agreed and documented fully prior to the birth.

Where delivery at borderline viability is likely, the role of the joint neonatal and obstetric team under the guidance of the most senior clinician is to discuss the likely outcome with the family, and to provide support in their informed decision-making (see Box 5.1).

1. Assess gestational age – estimate risk of poor outcome

Gestational age	Outcome
22/23	Extremely high risk
24	High risk
25	Moderate risk
26	Less risk

2. Assess non-modifiable factors – adjust risk of poor outcome

	Increased risk	Decreased risk
Gestational week	Start of week	End of week
Fetal growth	Growth restriction	Normal estimated weight
Fetal sex	Male	Female
Plurality	Multiple	Singleton

3. Modifiable risk factors – adjust risk of poor outcome

	Increased risk		Decreased risk
Antenatal steroids	None	Incomplete course	Complete course
Setting for birth	Local hospital		Hospital with NICU

Figure 5.2 Visual tool for refinement of risk (adapted from BAPM, 2019a)

BOX 5.1 A SUGGESTED APPROACH TO SHARED DECISION-MAKING

- Focus on building a partnership and including parents in the process
- Determine parents' desired role in decision-making
- Define the required decision
- Avoid over-simplistic presentation of options such as 'do everything' vs 'do nothing' (include benefits and risks of potential actions)
- Provide balanced and individualised information
- Support parents' decision-making with enough time to carefully reflect and ask questions
- Ensure consent is valid, informed, and voluntary

(BAPM, 2019b; Krick et al., 2022)

Long-term developmental outcomes of babies born at the borderline of viability remains useful evidence for counselling parents on their individualised prognosis alongside BAPM's infographic 'Outcomes for babies born alive between 22–26 weeks' gestation' (BAPM, 2019a).

> **THINK POINT**
>
> - In the UK, national guidelines recommend transferring women at risk of extremely preterm birth (before 27 weeks) to a hospital with a Level 3 NICU.
> - Consider this:
>   What challenges – both logistical and emotional – might families and healthcare teams face when trying to arrange such a transfer quickly? How could these challenges affect the outcome for the baby and the experience of the parents?

Corticosteroid and magnesium sulphate administration

Please refer to Chapter 2 for details about the benefits, evidence, and practice considerations of antenatal corticosteroid and magnesium sulphate administration.

Delivery room management

PREPARATION

Delivery room preparation for a preterm baby includes gathering clear and relevant history, conversations with parents regarding management and expectations of the care of their baby, adjusting equipment for the appropriate gestation, and ensuring the necessary personnel are present.

When evaluating maternal notes and discussing the history with maternity professionals, it is essential to have a clear understanding of any risk factors, relevant medical history, and indications for delivery to effectively plan for the birth. A conversation with the parents can assist with this information gathering whilst also providing information and support for them. In providing clear explanations, the aim is to minimise adverse psychological effects associated with preterm birth (Carr et al., 2023).

Ensuring a warm environment is critical, with preheated resuscitation areas, and plastic wrapping for very preterm infants (Fawke et al., 2025). Essential equipment, such as a **T-piece** resuscitator, an appropriately sized **endotracheal tubes (ETT)**, and **surfactant** for early administration, should be readily available

(BAPM, 2019a). Adjustment for premature births will need to be made to the airway pressures and oxygen to avoid **barotrauma** and **hyperoxia**.

A multidisciplinary team, including neonatal and obstetric practitioners, should be present. The Neonatal Life Support (NLS) algorithm as recommended by the Resuscitation Council UK should be followed. Early communication with the neonatal team ensures a well-coordinated approach to ongoing care. A more detailed breakdown of delivery room preparation can be found in Chapter 12.

OPTIMAL CORD MANAGEMENT

Delaying clamping of the umbilical cord by 1–3 minutes has been recommended in the term population (with the initial heart rate >60bpm and not requiring positive pressure ventilation), and is known to increase neonatal blood volume and iron stores, whilst preventing a sudden drop in the baby's blood pressure by allowing the extra blood to replace the blood that flows into the baby's lungs when they take their first breaths (Fawke et al., 2025). In preterm infants, deferring clamping of the cord for a minimum 60 seconds has been shown to reduce the risk of IVH, late onset sepsis, and death (Rabe et al., 2019) and is now common practice. Contraindications to deferred clamping include maternal resuscitation or ruptured vasa previa, snapped cord, or other trauma to the cord vessels (BAPM, 2020). During stabilisation, a flat, stable surface may be needed where the head position and mask fit can be controlled. In most delivery units in the UK currently, this will be the traditional Resuscitaire® which should be positioned close to the mother's bed, if additional respiratory support is to be provided. Although not a physiological process, milking the umbilical cord 2–4 times toward the baby has been investigated as an alternative to waiting at least 60 seconds before clamping. Meta-analyses of studies on cord milking suggest comparable benefits. However, there are very few circumstances where waiting for a full minute is not possible and should only be used when delayed clamping is not feasible, in neonates born at 28 weeks gestation or more. (BAPM, 2020).

THINK POINT

- Optimal cord management is recommended in the UK for most preterm and low birthweight babies, unless immediate resuscitation is needed.
- Consider this:
  How do clinicians balance the potential benefits of delayed cord clamping such as improved circulatory stability and reduced risk of IVH, with the need for urgent neonatal care in very preterm or compromised infants? What practical factors might influence this decision in the delivery room?

ASSESSMENT

Initial assessment includes evaluating colour, tone, breathing, and heart rate, following the NLS algorithm (Fawke et al., 2025. This is discussed in detail in Chapter 12). Preterm infants are at high risk of RDS, so assessment of breathing effort and the need for respiratory support, such as high flow nasal cannula (HFNC), continuous positive airway pressure (CPAP), or intubation, is crucial (BAPM, 2019a; Sweet et al., 2023).

Pre-ductal oxygen saturations should be obtained by placing the saturation probe on the right hand or wrist. Hyperoxia is particularly damaging to the preterm infant, therefore a low concentration of oxygen (21–30%, depending on GA) should be used in the first instance and until oxygen saturation levels can be assessed (see Table 5.2; Fawke et al., 2025).

THERMAL MANAGEMENT

There is a strong association between hypothermia on admission and increased mortality in preterm infants. It may furthermore have a significant impact on long-term outcomes, as hypothermia is known to increase the risk of morbidities such as RDS, IVH, sepsis, and disturbances of haemostasis, among others. Heat loss can be rapid without intervention due to a large surface area to weight ratio, reduced brown fat stores and thin, un**keratin**ised skin, leading to increased **transepidermal** water loss (TEWL) and other evaporative losses.

Thermoregulation is an area where the experienced neonatal nurse can proactively contribute to the optimisation of the baby's start to life and their individual risk of mortality and morbidity. At delivery, neonatal nurses are often well placed to support temperature control whilst other practitioners focus on the management of airway and cardiovascular systems.

Thermal delivery room management is discussed in further detail in Chapter 13.

AIRWAY MANAGEMENT

In spontaneously breathing preterm infants, non-invasive respiratory support rather than tracheal intubation should be offered. The use of these have been

TABLE 5.2 TARGET OXYGEN SATURATIONS AFTER BIRTH

Time from birth	*Acceptable (25th centile) right arm saturation*
3 minutes	70–75%
5 minutes	80–85%
10 minutes	85–95%

(Fawke et al., 2025)

found to maximise functional residual capacity (FRC) of the lungs, reduce numbers of infants receiving oxygen at 28 days and to reduce the use of surfactant without increasing the incidence of **bronchopulmonary dysplasia** (BPD; Sweet et al., 2023).

HFNC has been reported to be as effective as CPAP as a primary intervention for RDS in infants >28 weeks' gestation and compared to CPAP, reduced abdominal distension and nasal trauma (Wilkinson et al., 2016). If intubation is required for insufficient respiratory effort, surfactant should be administered prophylactically in the delivery room, preferably within 15 minutes of birth. Less invasive methods of administration of surfactant have been found to be effective for those infants with RDS who are spontaneously breathing and requiring surfactant, such as infants with increasing oxygen requirements on HFNC or CPAP (Aldana-Aguirre et al., 2017).

Delivery room management is discussed in further detail in Chapter 12.

PARENTS

Parental involvement and communication in the delivery room following a preterm birth are essential for reducing anxiety and fostering a sense of involvement in their baby's care. BAPM and Bliss, the UK charity for premature babies, emphasise the importance of clear, compassionate, and honest communication with parents from the moment of birth (BAPM, 2021; Bliss, n.d.). Parents should be informed about their baby's condition in simple, understandable language, avoiding unnecessary medical jargon. Where possible, they should be encouraged to see and touch their baby, even if immediate medical interventions are required. Skin-to-skin contact, where clinically appropriate, can provide comfort to both the baby and parents (WHO, 2022). Healthcare professionals should provide regular updates on the baby's progress and explain any interventions, ensuring parents are active participants in decision-making (BAPM, 2021). Psychological support should also be offered, recognising the emotional impact of preterm birth. Establishing trust and a partnership between parents and the neonatal team improves parental confidence and long-term bonding with their baby (see also Chapter 6).

TRANSFER TO THE NEONATAL UNIT

The safe transport of a preterm baby from the delivery suite to the NNU requires planning to minimise stress and physiological instability of the baby (see Chapter 24). Parents should be given time and contact with their baby prior to transport. The use of a chemical mattress should be considered when Resuscitaires® do not have an integral battery, to avoid thermal stress as well as ensuring that gas supplies are adequate before moving. Allocation of roles to the team is important, for example, airway management, steering, equipment management, and monitoring. The same applies for transport incubators. These may be a preferable option as they provide a more stable thermal environment and airway support delivery systems.

COMMON CONDITIONS ASSOCIATED WITH PREMATURITY AND/OR LOW BIRTHWEIGHT

Premature and some LBW infants are at risk of conditions which can affect long-term health or are life-limiting. The more preterm the infant, the more likely there is a lasting impact; each physiological system will be affected by the interruption of normal embryological development. The following is a brief overview of these potential conditions; more detailed information can be found within the relevant chapters.

Surfactant insufficiency

Surfactant insufficiency is one of the major causes of **respiratory distress syndrome** (RDS) associated with prematurity. Surfactant production in the human fetal lung begins around 24 weeks of gestation, with type II pneumocytes initiating secretion at this time. However, the production of adequate amounts to prevent atelectasis is not present until 32 weeks (Rehman & Bacha, 2023). Therefore, the greater the gestation, the better the lung compliance, as larger quantities of surfactant become available.

This process continues to term, with surfactant levels reaching full maturity close to birth.

Other risk factors for surfactant deficiency include maternal diabetes in pregnancy, perinatal hypoxia-ischaemia, and LBW. The lack of surfactant availability results in increased surface tension and alveolar **atelectasis**. Clinical presentation includes worsening signs of respiratory distress and respiratory **acidosis**, which result in **ventilation/perfusion mismatch** that may require management with varying levels of ventilatory support. The advent of exogenous surfactant administration has resulted in a reduction of mortality and morbidity. Refer to Chapter 14 for more detail about RDS and its management.

Chronic lung disease

Chronic lung disease (CLD), or BPD, is commonly seen in preterm infants who have required mechanical ventilation and oxygen therapy for treatment of respiratory distress (NICE, 2020a). BPD is the most common CLD in infants and is associated with increased mortality, respiratory morbidity, neurodevelopmental impairment, and increased healthcare costs (Gilfillan et al., 2021). There have been significant changes in practice with regard to antenatal corticosteroid administration, surfactant administration, early caffeine administration, early extubation, and the use of non-invasive respiratory support over the past few decades. Despite this, however, CLD remains a persistent issue, and National Neonatal Audit programme (NNAP) data from 2021 showed that in the UK 38.8% of infants born at less than 32 weeks' gestation developed BPD or died, with the occurrence of the condition varying from 33.5% to 46% across all neonatal networks (Royal College of Paediatrics and Child Health (RCPCH), 2022). Further information about BPD can be found in Chapter 14.

Apnoea of prematurity

Apnoea of prematurity is a common condition in preterm neonates, characterised by pauses in breathing of more than 15–20 seconds, associated with bradycardia and oxygen desaturation. It occurs because the immature brainstem and respiratory control systems are not fully developed, resulting in unstable breathing patterns with incidence increasing with decreasing gestational age. Treatment includes administering caffeine citrate as the standard pharmacological treatment which stimulates the central nervous system, improves respiratory drive, reduces apnoeic episodes, and can decrease the need for mechanical ventilation.

Retinopathy of prematurity

Retinopathy of prematurity (ROP) is recognised as one of the preventable causes of childhood blindness. The highest risk group constitutes infants born at less than 32 weeks GA or less than 1500g birthweight and preterm babies that receive supplemental oxygen. Further risk factors include, chorioamnionitis, IVH, RDS, sepsis, a white or Asian ethnic background, and multiple births. Most premature infants will develop some degree of ROP, which will resolve spontaneously. Some, however, will develop a more severe form of the disease which requires intervention (Kim et al., 2018; RCPCH et al., 2024).

The retina requires a continuous blood supply to provide oxygen and support function. Retinal blood vessels normally develop between 16 and 36 weeks' gestation, with rapid eye development occurring during the final 12 weeks of pregnancy. **Vascularisation** begins at the optic nerve and extends towards the retinal periphery. In preterm neonates, this process is disrupted because exposure to higher oxygen levels after birth alters the balance of vascular endothelial growth factor (VEGF) and insulin-like growth factor (IGF), both essential for normal vessel growth. Consequently, retinal vascular development is delayed, leaving areas of the growing retina inadequately supplied. This can trigger abnormal vasoproliferation, forming retinal ridges and abnormal vessel growth into the vitreous or retinal surface. Progressive disease may cause scarring, retinal traction, detachment, and blindness (Fevereiro-Martins et al., 2023).

ROP is categorised in stages 1–4 and the presence of **plus disease** (see Figure 5.3 and Table 5.3). Plus disease is recognisable by the tortuosity and dilation of the blood vessels, and, if left untreated, will result in partial or total detachment of the retina.

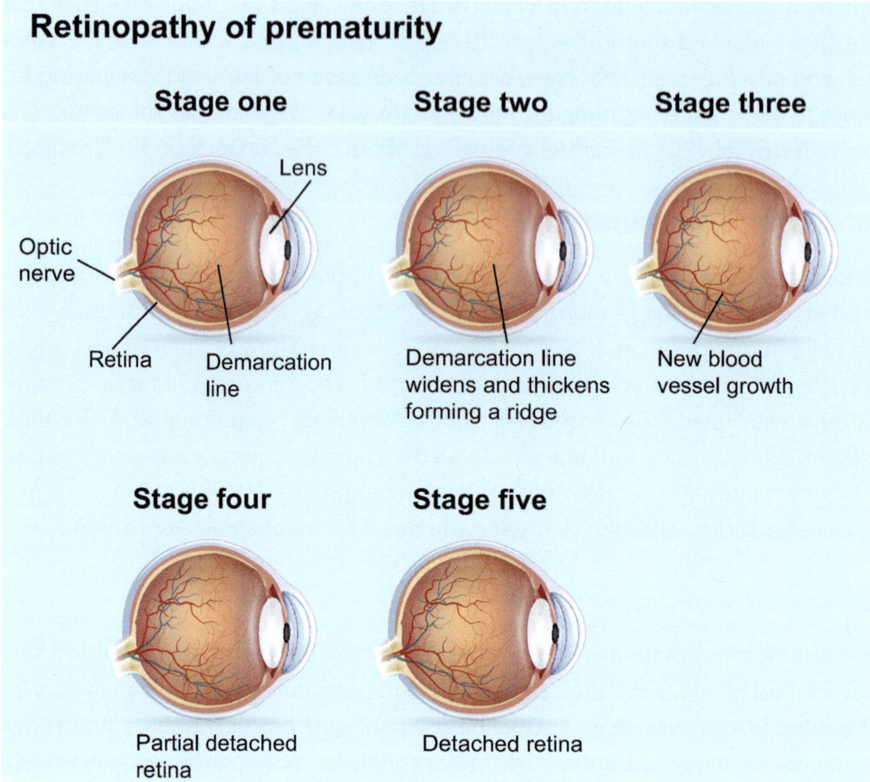

Figure 5.3 Stages of retinopathy of prematurity (adapted from Chiang et al., 2021)

TABLE 5.3 CATEGORIES OF RETINOPATHY OF PREMATURITY

Stage One	A demarcation line within the retina between vascularised and avascularised regions
Stage Two	Ridge or elevation develops at the junction of vascular and avascular regions of the retina
Stage Three	Blood vessels in the ridge which grow, multiply, and are visible within the ridge.
Stage Four	Partial retinal detachment
Stage Five	Total retinal detachment

(adapted from RCPCH et al., 2024)

Treatment of ROP depends on disease progression. It will be required at any stage if plus disease is present, or stage 3 with or without plus disease. The most effective proven treatments for ROP are anti-VEGF injections or laser therapy (Royal College of Ophthalmologists, 2022) which both aim to interrupt the abnormal proliferation of vascular growth. The anti-VEGF injection also promotes less pathological vascularisation beyond treatment.

Outcomes for infants with ROP can be greatly improved locally by the implementation of strict oxygen saturation guidelines. Hyperoxia increases the risk of severe ROP, as the additional oxygen increases vascular endothelial growth factor. A number of research trials have shown that the safest target range for oxygen saturations which affect patient morbidity and mortality, as well as a reduction of ROP, appears to be around 90–95% (Fevereiro-Martins et al., 2023).

Due to the importance of timely diagnosis and treatment, robust pathways to ensure on-time screening and treatment of ROP need to be implemented. The NNAP report for 2023 showed that only 78.4% of babies were screened on time for ROP (RCPCH, 2024), despite target figures of 100%. This is one aspect where the neonatal nurse can contribute towards improving ROP-related morbidity. Perhaps more importantly, it is the nurse's responsibility to continuously ensure that their patients' oxygen saturations are within evidence-based limits, which means close observation, prompt response to monitor alarms, and often frequent adjustments to supplemental oxygen delivery rates for infants on respiratory support. Comfort care needs to be considered throughout the screening process. This includes reduction of light stimuli once drops are instilled and for the duration of their effects, non-pharmacological pain management during and after screening, and supportive positioning or skin to skin to encourage a comfortable return to **normostasis**, all whilst working in partnership with parents.

Anaemia of prematurity

All infants experience a decrease in haemoglobin (Hb) concentration after birth. The physiological transition from a relatively hypoxic state *in utero* to an environment where oxygen is readily available, triggers a suppression in erythropoietin which results in a physiological decrease in red blood cell (RBC) production.

Following delivery, a term infant has a natural drop in Hb levels at a few months of age. This is referred to as **physiological anaemia** and does not require treatment. However, this event occurs earlier and with a more dramatic decline at around 4–6 weeks for the preterm infant, hence the commencement of iron supplementation at 28 days. The process is exacerbated by frequent blood samples, the missed opportunity of transplacental iron transfer which occurs in the third trimester, and the rapid growth requiring good oxygenation undergone by infants born prematurely. Furthermore, the erythropoietin response to reduced

RBC in the plasma is slower than that of the term infant (Cibulskis et al., 2021). Chapter 17 discusses the management of anaemia of prematurity in more detail.

Intraventricular haemorrhage and periventricular leukomalacia

Intraventricular haemorrhage (IVH) is a common neuropathological consequence of preterm birth. Unfortunately, despite significant advances in the management of these babies, which have dramatically reduced mortality for the population, the incidence of IVH has remained static (Rees et al., 2024). There is now, however, increasing evidence that even low-grade IVH results in an increased risk of neurodevelopmental impairment at 2 to 3 years of age, above and beyond the risks posed by prematurity alone (Rees et al., 2022). Periventricular leukomalacia (PVL) is a type of brain injury, most common in premature babies, characterised by the death or softening of the white matter surrounding the brain's ventricles, which can lead to various neurological problems. It is often caused by a lack of oxygen or perfusion to the periventricular area of the brain. Some cases of PVL may occur because the bleeding in IVH can disrupt blood flow and oxygen supply to the surrounding brain tissue, leading to PVL (Starr et al., 2023).

The pathophysiology, grading, management, and prognosis of these significant sequelae of prematurity is described in Chapter 16.

Necrotising enterocolitis

NEC is a severe gastrointestinal condition that primarily affects preterm infants. It is marked by inflammation, ischaemia, and necrosis of the intestinal wall, which can result in perforation, sepsis, and death. Typically emerging within the first few weeks of life, NEC is particularly common in VLBW infants. It initially presents with non-specific symptoms that can quickly escalate, including feeding intolerance, abdominal distension, bilious vomiting, lethargy, and temperature or cardiorespiratory instability. As the disease progresses, additional signs such as bloody stools, apnoea, metabolic acidosis, and sepsis may develop. Abdominal x-rays often reveal pneumatosis intestinalis, the hallmark radiographic indicator of NEC. The condition arises from multiple contributing factors, including prematurity; enteral feeding, especially with formula; intestinal immaturity; dysbiosis (imbalanced gut microbiota); hypoxia-ischaemia; and an exaggerated inflammatory response (Quigley et al., 2024). See Chapter 22 for further details on the condition and its management.

Suboptimal postnatal growth

Suboptimal postnatal growth in preterm or LBW babies can result from multiple factors. Inadequate nutrition is a primary cause, as preterm infants have higher caloric and protein needs but may struggle with feeding due to immature suck-swallow coordination or intestinal immaturity. Some fetal complications may contribute to poor postnatal growth in preterm and low birthweight babies, including FGR, chronic hypoxia, fetal infections, genetic or chromosomal disorders, and fetal malformations (Roggero et al., 2024). Medical complications such as NEC, infections, and chronic lung disease can further hinder growth as well as poor thermoregulation, hypoglycaemia, and other causes of increased energy expenditure.

Many studies have demonstrated that poor nutrition in the early stages of life will impact long-term development and brain growth (Silveira et al., 2023). Therefore, it is vital to ensure the correct amount of protein and energy is delivered, in order to promote growth and good developmental outcome whilst minimising the risk of concerning complications such as NEC. Delayed initiation of enteral feeding and prolonged reliance on parenteral nutrition (PN) may lead to nutrient deficiencies. Early enteral feeding has been associated with improved gut development and metabolic adaptation and optimised postnatal weight gain (Walsh et al., 2020). There have been varying views regarding the speed at which full enteral feeds should be established, with the SIFT (Speed of Increasing Milk Feeds Trial) concluding that no clear advantage was identified for the important outcomes in very preterm or very LBW infants when milk feeds were advanced in daily volume increments of 30 or 18mL/kg/day (Dorling et al., 2020). Freshly expressed breastmilk (EBM) is recommended as first choice for establishing feeds as it contains higher amounts of macronutrients, and immunoactive and trophic factors than pasteurised donor milk. In cases of insufficient EBM availability, fortified donor milk is conditionally recommended over preterm formula milk in preterm infants born <32 weeks' gestation or with a birthweight <1500 g (Embleton et al., 2023).

In circumstances where enteral feeding is not appropriate, PN is a useful adjunct while enteral nutrition is achieved. It is now common practice to commence PN within a few hours of life in both term and preterm infants where enteral feeding is not likely to be achieved within a reasonable timeframe (NICE, 2020b).

Preterm infants in their first weeks of life require a high-protein high-energy diet, starting shortly after birth. Subsequent adjustments in nutritional composition, aimed at achieving optimal body composition and minimising the long-term cardiometabolic risks without jeopardising the brain development and should be guided by the linear growth pattern as opposed to weight only (Ruys et al., 2021). Ongoing monitoring of growth and development in the early stages of life is therefore vital for the preterm and LBW population. For more details on nutrition and feeding in the NNU, see Chapter 19.

Immunological immaturity

Like many body systems, the immune system is not fully functional at birth. It is particularly immature in infants born prematurely or at LBW, predisposing them to a high risk of infection. This risk is related to the immunosuppressive environment of the womb and the lack of immunological memory, which is followed by overwhelming exposure after delivery. The immune system subsequently reduces its response in order to prevent over-activation of the immune response (Machado et al., 2021). Once born, the preterm infant is exposed to a multitude of invasive medical procedures, such as insertion of central lines, cannulas, and intubation, all of which increase the risk of infection. The mechanisms of the immune system and immunity in the neonate are discussed in more detail in Chapter 20.

Skin integrity issues

A preterm baby's skin is thinner, more fragile, and less developed than that of a full-term baby, making it more susceptible to injury, heat loss, and infection. Preterm birth requires an accelerated adaptation of the skin due to the differences between the *in utero* environment and the dry *ex utero* environment.

Preterm skin has an underdeveloped barrier layer, known as the stratum corneum (Figure 5.4), dependent on what gestation the baby is born. The

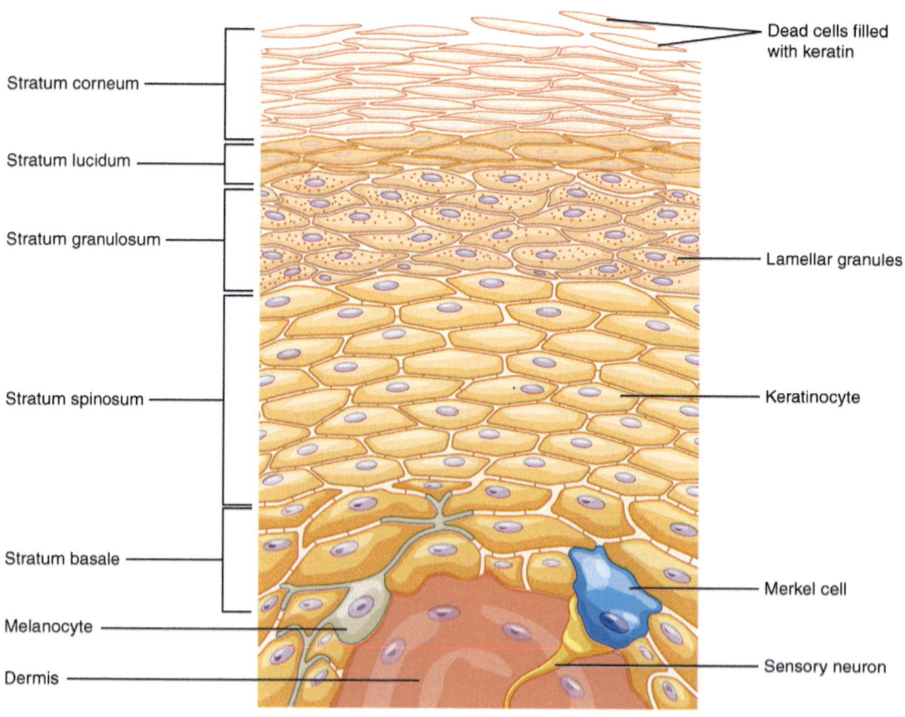

Figure 5.4 The layers of the epidermis at term (Source: Creative Commons)

TABLE 5.4 SUMMARY OF INCUBATOR HUMIDITY PRACTICES WITHIN THE UK

Gestation	*Commence*	*Wean*	*Stop*
<28 weeks GA	80–85% for 7 days	5% per day as long as temperature and electrolyte stability is achieved.	At 40–45% or 21 days or 32 weeks GA, whichever comes first
28–30/32 weeks GA	70–85% for 24–48 hours	5% per day as long as temperature and electrolyte stability is achieved.	At 40–45% or 21 days or 32 weeks GA, whichever comes first

stratum corneum is layered with epithelial cells filled with keratin, which prevents transepidermal water loss (TEWL). Therefore, the more preterm the baby is, the less keratinised the skin, and subsequent high degrees of TEWL will occur if not managed appropriately. Multiple cellular layers with a thin keratin layer on the skin surface can be observed by the 21st week of gestation, and by the 37th week, all layers of the epidermis are visible with a thick keratin layer (Bhat et al., 2025). Optimising humidity within the incubator can reduce TEWL, dehydration and hyponatraemia and aid thermoregulation. Practices slightly vary between units, but recommendations are similar (see Table 5.4 and Chapter 13 for further detail).

In order for skin to function as a protective barrier, there is a need for robust cohesion between the layers of the epidermis and dermis. Not only are these layers thinner in the preterm infant than in the term population, there is also a reduction in the elastin fibres and a lack of cohesion between the layers, which contributes to its fragility and increased permeability. The lower the GA, the more challenging assessment and care of the skin can be. For this reason, specially designed assessment tools are needed for such patients. Skin integrity assessment tools are important in the recognition of potential issues, guiding timely interventions, and ensuring optimal skin health. These issues may include dry, cracked skin, puncture wounds, nappy rash, oedema, pressure injuries, and friction injuries from the use of adhesive dressings and tapes. For further information, see the web companion.

THE MODERATE TO LATE PRETERM INFANT

Babies born between 34^{+0} to 36^{+6} weeks' gestation are referred to as late preterm infants, and those born between 32^{+0} and 33^{+6} weeks' gestation are considered moderate preterm infants. In 2022, this group was noted to constitute 84% of all preterm births in England and Wales (Office for National Statistics, 2024). This large percentage may be due to elective preterm deliveries and advances in obstetric care. Evidence has shown that neonates born before 37 weeks of gestation face increased risks of adverse health outcomes and poorer long-term development compared to those born at or beyond full term. Common neonatal complications in this group include hypothermia, hypoglycaemia, jaundice, feeding difficulties, and a higher incidence of respiratory conditions.

Moderate to late preterm infants are also more vulnerable to infections and are more frequently screened for sepsis. Additionally, they face an elevated risk of adverse neurodevelopmental outcomes. These infants miss critical *in utero* opportunities for brain and body growth, as well as the accumulation of essential nutrient stores needed for perinatal survival. While their precise nutritional needs for optimal growth and development remain uncertain, they are believed to exceed those of term infants (BAPM, 2023). Growth velocity should be evaluated through regular monitoring (head circumference, weight, and possibly length) to ensure adequate nutrition. Additional supplements such as vitamins, iron, folic acid, and breastmilk fortification may be required within this group of infants. Due to immature sleep-wake patterns and coordination of the suck-swallow-breathe reflex, thorough assessment of feeding readiness is required. The establishing of oral feeding may require support from the multidisciplinary team (infant feeding team, dietician, speech and language therapist).

It is now well recognised that the moderate to late preterm infant should not be treated in the same way as a well term infant, as doing so can increase the risk of neonatal morbidity and thus NNU admission. The model for care of moderately preterm infants is reasonably clear, with recognition that the majority of these babies require at least special care because of their immaturity. Late preterm infants, however, may be managed on postnatal wards with specialist input by the multidisciplinary postnatal team, in order to keep mother and baby together. The implementation of transitional care is one such model, which enables the mother to provide normal care to her baby with support from professionals in relation to, for example, nasogastric feeding, establishing breastfeeding, or observation for infection.

THE IMPACT OF PREMATURITY AND/OR LOW BIRTHWEIGHT ON PARENTAL BONDING

The significantly improved survival of premature and LBW infants necessitates an acknowledgement of the impedance of parental bonding with a potential impact on the socio-emotional stress regulation of the infant as a result (Shaw et al., 2023). Developments in neonatal care technologies and strategies in the extreme preterm are related to improved survival rates, without increased proportions of survivors with neurodevelopmental impairment at 1.5 to 2.5 years (Morgan & Cooper, 2022). However, the impact of this intensive approach alongside separation from their baby, and the NNU setting itself, can cause significant distress, negative feelings, and fear for the parents, especially as there is limited ability to predict outcomes. Parents can feel overwhelmed by the physical condition of their baby and the environment that they find themselves in (Shaw et al., 2023).

The set-up and routines of the NNU affect interactions between parent and baby, so it is crucial for the neonatal nurse to promote a family integrated approach to care. This includes facilitation of sharing in what they regard as important events; such as first-time attending to care activities, integrating the baby into the family, and experiencing a feeling of closeness and interaction with their baby (Kutahyalioglu & Scafide, 2022). The bonding process that has begun in pregnancy would ordinarily be cemented in the first hour of life with skin-to-skin contact. However, many preterm and LBW infants require medical stabilisation and intervention that means this critical time is replaced by a traumatic and sometimes life-altering experience. This then leads to a potentially long-term physical separation, which can have a significant negative impact on a parent's mental health and can lead to misunderstandings of behavioural cues, adversely affecting the long-term parent-infant relationship. It has furthermore been suggested that the preterm child is significantly more likely to experience insecure attachment patterns.

When a baby requires medical care that causes separation from the parents, sole responsibility of their child is lost to strangers. Effective and empathetic communication is pivotal in rapidly forming a partnership that enables the parents to maintain a sense of involvement and empowerment. Equally, communication between healthcare professionals should aim to minimise any separation that could disrupt parental bonding during a critical period of brain organisation (Shaw et al., 2023). Individualised parent-professional communication should focus on building and maintaining relationships, exchanging of information, sharing decision-making, and parental empowerment to self-manage whilst adapting to the emerging needs of the baby and their family (Wreesmann et al., 2021).

There are now many video and livestreaming technologies that can support and enhance parental communication and contact and, overall, have demonstrated a positive impact on stress reduction for the parents (Gallagher et al., 2023).

Fundamentally, parents need to be recognised as important collaborative members of the neonatal team and as facilitators of the developmental needs of their babies. This can have long-lasting positive effects on parental bonding and the life-changing experience of having a baby on the NNU. This topic will be covered in more detail in Chapter 6.

DISCHARGE PLANNING

This topic is covered in detail in Chapter 3.

ACTIVITY

Using your local discharge checklist, carefully review each item and then answer the following questions.

- Which items on the checklist do you think are most critical for a safe discharge of a neonate born preterm or small, and why?
- How might a the neonatal care experience of been born early impact the baby's health or development after discharge?
- What additional support could be offered to families of preterm neonates with limited social or emotional resources in your local area?

Chapter takeaways

- Prematurity is defined as birth before 37 weeks. This broad definition encompasses a wide spectrum of developmental maturity and clinical risk, which is why prematurity is further sub-classified based on gestational age: extremely preterm (<28 weeks), very preterm (28–31^{+6} weeks), moderate preterm (32–33^{+6} weeks), and late preterm (34–36^{+6} weeks). Accurate gestational age assessment, especially when antenatal data is limited, is essential for guiding neonatal care and prognosis.
- Delivery room strategies such as thermal regulation, respiratory support, and optimal cord management are critical to reducing morbidity and mortality.
- Preterm and LBW infants are vulnerable to serious conditions including RDS, BPD, ROP, NEC, IVH, PVL, and anaemia of prematurity. Early detection, evidence-based interventions, and multidisciplinary care are essential to improving outcomes.
- Suboptimal growth is linked to inadequate nutrition, medical complications, and increased energy demands. Early enteral feeding with EBM, careful use of PN, and high-protein, high-energy diets support brain development and long-term health.
- Preterm skin is fragile and poorly keratinised, leading to high trans-epidermal water loss. Optimising humidity and using skin integrity assessment tools are essential. Immature immune systems heighten infection risk, requiring vigilant care.

- Infants born between 32+0 and 36^{+6} weeks face increased risks of hypothermia, hypoglycaemia, jaundice, and neurodevelopmental challenges. Transitional care models help maintain parent-baby bonding while addressing feeding and infection risks.
- Prematurity and separation can disrupt bonding and increase parental distress. Family integrated care, empathetic communication, and technologies such as livestreaming help maintain connection and support emotional wellbeing.

CASE STUDIES

CASE STUDY

Case study 1: Impending birth of a preterm infant

Labour ward has contacted your unit to alert them to a new admission. Josheen is a 26-year-old **primigravida** who is 27 weeks pregnant and has attended the assessment unit with ruptured membranes and signs of preterm labour.

Q.1. What else would you like to know at this stage?

Q.2. Josheen is not able to attend the NNU for a look around, so you go and speak to her on the labour ward. What information does she require at this stage? Is there anything in particular you would like to discuss with her?

Josheen's labour is progressing rapidly. She is expected to deliver within the next 30 minutes, but has only received one dose of corticosteroids 2 hours ago. Magnesium sulphate was commenced soon after admission.

Q.3. Consider the prematurity-associated problems Josheen's baby is likely to encounter, both based on gestation and antenatal events. How can you contribute to their early recognition and minimisation of their impact on outcomes in the short term and long term?

Case study 2: Management of an infant with fetal growth restriction (FGR)

Florence is a 34-week gestation infant born via spontaneous vaginal birth weighing 1.1kg. Her mother Kate had been well throughout her pregnancy with the exception of pregnancy-induced hypertension from 26 weeks' gestation, for

CASE STUDY

which she was treated with labetalol. Fetal growth began to slow from 28 weeks' gestation. This was noted to be static in the week prior to birth, with normal diastolic flow noted on ultrasound.

There were no risk factors for sepsis identified. Florence's mother wishes to breastfeed.

Q.1. What could be potential causes for Florence's poor growth?
Q.2. How would Florence's care differ from infants at 34 weeks who are born at an appropriate weight for gestational age?
Q.3. What are your thoughts about Kate's wish to exclusively breastfeed Florence? Will this be feasible?

Case study 3: At the borderline of viability

Alice is a 42-year-old woman who was admitted to the labour ward with abdominal pain at 22^{+5} weeks' gestation. She is a gravida 5, para 2^{+2}, having had two early miscarriages and two extremely preterm babies, both of whom survived less than 24 hours. This pregnancy is the result of *in vitro* fertilisation using a donor egg. On admission Alice is assessed to be in established labour. Alice and her partner Liam agree that they would like the neonatal team to attempt full resuscitation following delivery.

Q.1. What are your thoughts about Alice's and Liam's wishes? Do you think this is in the best interest of their baby?
Q.2. Using one or more available prognostic tools, try and establish their baby's prognosis for survival and long-term outcomes. How would you counsel Alice and Liam?

For suggested answer guides to the questions posed in these case studies, please refer to the web-based companion site specific to this chapter. See www.routledge.com/cw/petty

References

Aldana-Aguirre, J. C., Pinto, M., Featherstone, R. M., & Kumar, M. (2017). Less invasive surfactant administration versus intubation for surfactant delivery in preterm infants with respiratory distress syndrome: A systematic review and meta-analysis. *Archives of Disease in Childhood: Fetal and Neonatal Edition*, *102*(1), F17–F23.

Alfirevic, Z., Stampalija, T., & Dowswell, T. (2017). Fetal and umbilical Doppler ultrasound in high-risk pregnancies. *Cochrane Database of Systematic Reviews*, *6*, Article CD007529. https://doi.org/10.1002/14651858.CD007529.pub4

Bhat, K. M. R., Febina, F. K., & Prasanna, L. C. (2025). Analysis of the skin layers and its appendages of developing human fetuses at different trimesters of pregnancy. *Translational Research in Anatomy*, *38*, 100369. https://doi.org/10.1016/j.tria.2024.100369

Bliss. (n.d.). *Communication*. Retrieved July 11, 2025, from https://www.bliss.org.uk/health-professionals/family-integrated-care/ficare-pilot-updates/communication-updates

British Association of Perinatal Medicine. (2019a). *Perinatal management of extreme preterm birth before 27 weeks of gestation: A framework for practice*. https://www.bapm.org/resources/80-perinatal-management-of-extreme-preterm-birth-before-27-weeks-of-gestation-2019

British Association of Perinatal Medicine. (2019b). *Enhancing shared decision making in neonatal care. A BAPM framework for practice*. https://www.bapm.org/resources/158-enhancing-shared-decision-making-in-neonatal-care

British Association of Perinatal Medicine. (2020). *Optimal cord management in preterm babies. A quality improvement toolkit*. https://www.bapm.org/pages/197-optimal-cord-management-toolkit

British Association of Perinatal Medicine. (2021). *Family integrated care: A BAPM framework for practice*. https://www.bapm.org/resources/ficare-framework-for-practice

British Association of Perinatal Medicine. (2023). *Early postnatal care of the moderate-late preterm infant: A framework for practice*. https://www.bapm.org/resources/framework-early-postnatal-care-of-the-moderate-late-preterm-infant

Carr, J., Bates, S., & Mactier, H. (2023). Perinatal communication in extreme preterm birth: What can we learn from the British Association of Perinatal Medicine framework? *Paediatrics and Child Health*, *33*(3), 73–77.

Chiang, M. F., Quinn, G. E., Fielder, A. R., Ostmo, S. R., Paul Chan, R. V., Berrocal, A., Binenbaum, G., Blair, M., Peter Campbell, J., Capone, A., Jr., Chen, Y., Dai, S., Ells, A., Fleck, B. W., Good, W. V., Elizabeth Hartnett, M., Holmstrom, G., Kusaka, S., Kychenthal, A., . . . Zin, A. (2021). International classification of retinopathy of prematurity, third edition. *Ophthalmology*, *128*(10), e51–e68.

Cibulskis, C. C., Maheshwari, A., Rao, R., & Mathur, A. M. (2021). Anemia of prematurity: How low is too low? *Journal of Perinatology*, *41*, 1244–1257.

Dauengauer-Kirlienė, S., Domarkienė, I., Pilypienė, I., Žukauskaitė, G., Kučinskas, V., & Matulevičienė, A. (2023). Causes of preterm birth: Genetic factors in preterm birth and preterm infant phenotypes. *The Journal of Obstetrics and Gynaecology Research*, *49*(3), 781–793.

Dorling, J., Hewer, O., Hurd, M., Bari, V., Bosiak, B., Bowler, U., King, A., Linsell, L., Murray, D., Omar, O., Partlett, C., Rounding, C., Townend, J., Abbott, J., Berrington, J., Boyle, E., Embleton, N., Johnson, S., Leaf, A., . . . & Juszczak, E. (2020). Two speeds of increasing milk feeds for very preterm or very low-birthweight infants: The SIFT RCT. *Health Technology Assessment*, *24*(18), 1–94.

Embleton, N. D., Jennifer Moltu, S., Lapillonne, A., van den Akker, C. H. P., Carnielli, V., Fusch, C., Gerasimidis, K., van Goudoever, J. B., Haiden, N., Iacobelli, S., Johnson, M. J., Meyer, S., Mihatsch, W., de Pipaon, M. S., Rigo, J., Zachariassen, G., Bronsky, J., Indrio, F., Köglmeier, J., . . . & Domellöf, M. (2023). Enteral nutrition in preterm infants (2022): A position paper from the ESPGHAN Committee on Nutrition and invited experts. *Journal of Pediatric Gastroenterology and Nutrition*, *76*, 248–268.

Fawke, J., Alexander-Elborough, E., Benson Clarke, A., Bradfield, M., Cusack, J., Hamilton-Bower, I., Madar, J., Monnelly, V., Reeves, N., Tinnion, R., Wood, T., & Wyllie, J. (2025). *Newborn life support* (6th ed.). Resuscitation Council (UK).

Fevereiro-Martins, M., Marques-Neves, C., Guimarães, H., & Bicho, M. (2023). Retinopathy of prematurity: A review of pathophysiology and signaling pathways. *Survey of Ophthalmology*, *68*(2), 175–210.

Gallagher, K., Hayns-Worthington, R., Marlow, N., Meek, J., & Chant, K. (2023). Parental experiences of live video streaming technology in neonatal care in England: A qualitative study. *BMC Pediatrics*, *23*, 107. https://doi.org/10.1186/s12887-023-03907-4

Gilfillan, M., Bhandari, A., & Bhandari, V. (2021). Diagnosis and management of bronchopulmonary dysplasia. *British Medical Journal*, *375*. https://doi.org/10.1136/bmj.n1974

Kim, S. J., Port, A. D., Swan, R., Campbell, J. P., Chan, R. V. P., & Chiang, M. F. (2018). Retinopathy of prematurity: A review of risk factors and their clinical significance. *Survey of Ophthalmology*, *63*(5), 618–637.

Krick, J. A., Feltman, D. M., & Arnolds, M. (2022). Decision-making for extremely preterm infants: A qualitative systematic review. *The Journal of Pediatrics*, *251*, 6–16.

Kutahyalioglu, N. S., & Scafide, K. N. (2022). Effects of family-centered care on bonding: A systematic review. *Journal of Child Health Care*, *27*(4), 721–737.

Lee, A. C., Panchal, P., Folger, L., Whelan, H., Whelan, R., Rosner, B., Blencowe, H., & Lawn, J. E. (2017). Diagnostic accuracy of neonatal assessment for gestational age determination: A systematic review. *Pediatrics*, *140*(6), e20171423. https://doi.org/10.1542/peds.2017-1423.

Machado, J. S., Ferreira, T. S., Lima, R. C. G., Vieira, V. C., & Medeiros, D. S. (2021). Premature birth: Topics in physiology and pharmacological characteristics. *Revista Da Associação Médica Brasileira*, *67*(1), 150–155.

Morgan, J. A., & Cooper, D. B. (2022). Pregnancy dating. In *StatPearls*. StatPearls Publishing. Retrieved July 11, 2025, from https://www.ncbi.nlm.nih.gov/books/NBK442018/

Morris, R. K., Johnstone, E., Lees, C., Morton, V., Smith, G., & Royal College of Obstetricians and Gynaecologists. (2024). *Investigation and care of a small-for-gestational-age fetus and a growth restricted fetus (Green-top Guideline No. 31)*. https://www.rcog.org.uk/guidance/browse-all-guidance/green-top-guidelines/small-for-gestational-age-fetus-and-a-growth-restricted-fetus-investigation-and-care-green-top-guideline-no-31/

National Institute for Health and Care Excellence. (2020a). *Specialist neonatal respiratory care for babies born preterm*. Quality Standard QS193. https://www.nice.org.uk/guidance/qs193/chapter/Quality-statement-1-Respiratory-support-soon-after-birth

National Institute for Health and Care Excellence. (2020b). *Neonatal parenteral nutrition*. NG154. https://www.nice.org.uk/guidance/ng154

Office for National Statistics. (2024). *Birth characteristics in England and Wales – data for 2022*. https://www.ons.gov.uk/peoplepopulationandcommunity/birthsdeathsandmarriages/livebirths/bulletins/birthcharacteristicsinenglandandwales/2022

Petty, J. (2024). The preterm baby and the small baby. In S. MacDonald & G. Johnson (Eds.), *Mayes midwifery* (16th ed., pp. 987–1010). Elsevier.

Quigley, M., Embleton, N. D., Meader, N., & McGuire, W. (2024). Donor human milk for preventing necrotising enterocolitis in very preterm or very low-birthweight infants. *The Cochrane Database of Systematic Reviews*, *9*(9), CD002971. https://doi.org/10.1002/14651858.CD002971.pub6

Rabe, H., Gyte, G. M., Diaz-Rossello, J. L., & Duley, L. (2019). Effect of timing of umbilical cord clamping and other strategies to influence placental transfusion at preterm birth on maternal and infant outcomes. *Cochrane Database of Systematic Reviews*, *9*(9). https://doi.org/10.1002/14651858.CD003248.pub4.

Rees, P., Callan, C., Chadda, K. R., Diviney, J., Harnden, F., Gardiner, J., Battersby, C., Gale, C., & Sutcliffe, A. (2024). Childhood outcomes after low-grade intraventricular haemorrhage: A systematic review and meta-analysis. *Developmental Medicine and Child Neurology*, *66*, 282–289.

Rees, P., Callan, C., Chadda, K. R., Vaal, M., Diviney, J., Sabti, S., Harnden, F., Gardiner, J. Battersby, C., Gale, C., & Sutcliffe, A. (2022). Preterm brain injury and neurodevelopmental outcomes: A meta-analysis. *Pediatrics, 150*(6), e2022057442. https://doi.org/10.1542/peds.2022-057442

Rehman, S., & Bacha, D. (2023). Embryology, pulmonary. In *StatPearls*. Retrieved May 30, 2025, from https://www.ncbi.nlm.nih.gov/books/NBK544372/

Roggero, P., Ryumina, I., Gunier, R. B., Winsey, A., Rauch, S. A., Zarco, I. A. C., Ariff, S., Rego, M. A. S., Conti, C. S., Ochieng, R., Tuzun, F., Asibey, J., Giuliani, F., Renau, M. I., Shekharappa, C. B., Lapillonne, A., Tavcioska, G., Ismail, L. C., Menis, C., . . . Villar, J. (2024). Postnatal growth of etiologically characterized preterm newborns according to gestational age at birth. *Pediatric Research*. https://doi.org/10.1038/s41390-024-03735-x

Royal College of Ophthalmologists. (2022). *Treating retinopathy of prematurity in the UK*. https://www.rcophth.ac.uk/wp-content/uploads/2022/03/Treating-Retinopathy-of-Prematurity-in-the-UK-Guideline-Exec-Summary.pdf

Royal College of Paediatrics and Child Health. (2022). *National Neonatal Audit Programme (NNAP) 2021 data results*. https://www.rcpch.ac.uk/sites/default/files/2022-11/appendix_a_nnap_2021_data_results_0.pdf

Royal College of Paediatrics and Child Health. (2024). *National Neonatal Audit Programme – Summary report on 2023 data*. https://www.rcpch.ac.uk/resources/NNAP-summary-report-2023-data#downloadBox

Royal College of Paediatrics and Child Health, Royal College of Ophthalmologists, British Association of Perinatal Medicine. (2024). *UK screening of retinopathy of prematurity guideline*. https://www.rcpch.ac.uk/resources/screening-retinopathy-prematurity-rop-clinical-guideline

Ruys, C. A., van de Lagemaat, M., Rotteveel, J., Finken, M. J. J., & Lafeber, H. N. (2021). Improving long-term health outcomes of preterm infants: How to implement the findings of nutritional intervention studies into daily clinical practice. *European Journal of Pediatrics, 180*, 1665–1673.

Seaton, S. E., Agarwal, R., Draper, E. S., Fenton, A. C., Kurinczuk, J. J., Manktelow, B. N., & Smith, L. K. (2023). Estimated neonatal survival of very preterm births across the care pathway: A UK cohort 2016–2020. *Archives of Diseases in Child Fetal and Neonatal Edition, 108*, F562–F568.

Shaw, R. J., Givrad, S., Poe, C., Loi, E. C., Hoge, M. K., & Scala, M. (2023). Neurodevelopmental, mental health, and parenting issues in preterm infants. *Children, 10*(9), 1565. https://doi.org/10.3390/children10091565

Silveira, R. C., Corso, A. L., & Procianoy, R. S. (2023). The influence of early nutrition on neurodevelopmental outcomes in preterm infants. *Nutrients, 5*(21), 4644. https://doi.org/10.3390/nu15214644

Starr, R., De Jesus, O., Shah, S. D., & Borger, J. (2023). Periventricular and intraventricular hemorrhage. In *StatPearls*. StatPearls Publishing. https://www.ncbi.nlm.nih.gov/books/NBK538310/

Sweet, D. G., Carnielli, V. P., Greisen, G., Hallman, M., Klebermass-Schrehof, K., Ozek, E., Te Pas, A., Plavka, R., Roehr, C. C., Saugstad, O. D., Simeoni, U., Speer, C. P., Vento, M., Visser, G. H. A., & Halliday, H. L. (2023). European consensus guidelines on the management of respiratory distress syndrome: 2022 update. *Neonatology, 120*(1), 3–23.

Walsh, V., Brown, J. V., Copperthwaite, B. R., Oddie, S. J., & McGuire, W. (2020). Early full enteral feeding for preterm or low birth weight infant. *Cochrane Database of Systematic Reviews, 12*, Article CD013542. https://doi.org/10.1002/14651858.CD013542.pub2.

Wilkinson, D., Andersen, C., O'Donnell, C. P. F., De Paoli, A. G., & Manley, B. J. (2016). High flow nasal cannula for respiratory support in preterm infants. *Cochrane Database of Systematic Reviews, 2*, Article CD006405. https://doi.org/10.1002/14651858.CD006405.pub3

World Health Organization. (2022). *WHO recommendations for care of the preterm or low-birth-weight infant.* Retrieved May 30, 2025, from https://www.who.int/publications/i/item/9789240058262

World Health Organization. (2023). *Preterm birth.* Retrieved May 30, 2025, from www.who.int/en/news-room/fact-sheets/detail/preterm-birth

Wreesmann, W. W., Lorié, E. S., van Veenendaal, N. R., van Kempen, A., Ket, J., & Labrie, N. (2021). The functions of adequate communication in the neonatal care unit: A systematic review and meta-synthesis of qualitative research. *Patient Education and Counseling, 104*(7), 1505–1517.

PART 2

THE PHYSICAL AND EMOTIONAL WELLBEING OF NEONATE AND FAMILY

DOI: 10.4324/9781003591405-8

6 NURTURING SUPPORTIVE FAMILY RELATIONSHIPS IN NEONATAL PRACTICE

Rebecca Chilvers, Julia Cooper, and Kelly Phizacklea

CONTENTS

DOI: 10.4324/9781003591405-9

GUIDANCE ON HOW TO ENHANCE PERSONAL LEARNING FROM THIS CHAPTER

Key points covered in this chapter

- The significant psychological impact of a neonatal admission on the baby, parents, and wider family and the importance of mitigating this impact.
- The importance of supporting parents to be equally included in their baby's care team through family integrated care (FiCare; as distinct from family-centred care).
- Strategies to enhance inclusion and the benefits FiCare delivers both short and long term.
- The research, development and background around FiCare, including the use of frameworks used to implement it in the neonatal setting.
- The key role of peer support, working with veteran parents, and coproduction in the design and implementation of FiCare.

Reflection

Reading through the chapter, you are encouraged to engage with the key points and related literature in an enquiring way. Ask these questions:

- How can you facilitate parents to be truly integrated partners in care and reduce separation of babies from their parents as much as possible?
- We look after babies and parents from a range of backgrounds, beliefs, cultures, and circumstances. How can you embed principles of FiCare to be inclusive of all babies and families?
- Which aspects of FiCare do you recognise in your unit, and how can you enhance them in keeping with the philosophy of care?
- Which members of the multidisciplinary team (MDT) are available on your unit, and what is their role in facilitating FiCare?

Implications for nursing care

- Using every opportunity to help parents take the role of primary care giver for their baby infuses routine practice with the principles of FiCare.
- Nurturing relationships are essential; holding parents emotionally and scaffolding their developing connections with their baby lays the foundation for good FiCare and future relationships.

INTRODUCTION AND BACKGROUND

> *A neonatal intensive care unit is akin to a trauma centre for all participants. Fragile babies struggle to survive and grow. Parents and families worry constantly while trying to maintain optimism and hope. Staff attempt to avoid burnout while both encouraging distraught parents and acknowledging the times of poor prognosis. Distress is the companion of everyone.*
>
> (Hynan & Hall, 2015, p. S1)

The admission of a baby to neonatal care is often a traumatic and unexpected event that has significant and long-lasting implications for the baby, parents and wider family. Parents find the neonatal unit (NNU) a daunting and unfamiliar place leading to anxiety, uncertainty, and fear about the future of their baby. This chapter focuses on the impact of neonatal care on babies and parents, with a particular emphasis on **family integrated care** and ensuring care is trauma-informed, along with the role of co-production, peer support and family engagement. The terms 'mother,' 'father,' 'birthing parent,' and/or 'partner' are used throughout this chapter where appropriate; however, these terms are intended to be inclusive of all individuals with a parenting or primary caregiving role, including same-sex parents and those who are transgender or non-binary.

NEONATAL CARE AS AN ADVERSE CHILDHOOD EXPERIENCE AND ITS IMPACT ON PARENTS

Parents have significant emotional needs in relation to assisting them to cope with their neonatal experience (Petty et al., 2019). For the baby, a neonatal admission can be considered an **adverse childhood experience** (ACE) due to the traumatic events a baby experiences including prolonged separation from their parent/caregiver, numerous painful procedures and multiple and inconsistent caregivers. Whilst the intention in providing life sustaining care is admirable, in reality, from the baby's perspective, this does not change the harmful experience or impact. Prolonged separation from a caregiver is a highly significant aversive experience for a baby, removing the opportunity for coregulation and attuned caregiving, which helps the baby to cope with stress. An environment of pervasive 'toxic stress' also has a significant impact. Shonkoff et al. (2012) state "*toxic stress, can result from strong, frequent, or prolonged activation of the body's stress response systems in the absence of the buffering protection of a supportive, adult relationship*" (p. 236). This can disrupt the development of brain structures and other physical systems during sensitive developmental periods which can lead to long-term changes that have a lifelong impact. It also reduces opportunities to lay the foundations for early bonding and attachment (alongside many of the unique features of a neonatal admission which also create barriers for parents and babies). The global 'zero separation' campaign (Global Foundation for the Care of the Newborn Infant (GFCNI), 2026) originated in the COVID-19 pandemic when there was a catastrophic reduction in contact between babies in neonatal care and their parents. The campaign advocates for keeping babies and parents together. Astonishingly, whilst the cultural shift to ensure children being cared for in paediatrics were not separated from their parents began in the 1950s, neonatal care has been *three quarters of a century behind.*

The psychological context and impact for parents must be considered. Parents who have experienced social adversity, domestic violence, mental health problems, chronic stress, and previous ACEs are more at risk of premature birth (Hardcastle et al., 2022). Experiences of pregnancy loss, fertility difficulties, and the multiple life stressors associated with high-risk pregnancies can have a significant impact on parents before they come to hospital to deliver. Each parent also comes with their unique set of life experiences which interact with their pregnancy, birth, and neonatal experiences.

Events that take place during birth such as a traumatic delivery, which can include experiences of helplessness, horror and abandonment, unmet needs for pain relief, and in some cases reactivation of previous traumatic experiences and distressing life events (such as sexual assault) mean that parents often arrive on the NNU already highly distressed and vulnerable. Both birthing and non-birthing parents can have experiences in pregnancy and birth that have a significant psychological impact.

Once parents are on the NNU, they face multiple challenges in an environment that is inherently infused with risk, uncertainty, unpredictability, and distress. The emotional landscape for each parent is unique, but anxiety, sadness, anger, guilt, shame, and fear are common. Parents are also navigating changes in identity and role (e.g. adjusting to becoming a parent or being a parent of a medically unwell baby), stress on their personal relationships, often challenges to their belief systems and sense of control in the world and a myriad of secondary stressors (such as financial and housing worries). At a time of emotional turmoil recovery from birth, managing pain, sleep deprivation, and the requirements of expressing milk for their baby can leave even the most 'robust' and well supported parent feeling overwhelmed.

As a result of the growing evidence and knowledge about these impacts, principles of **trauma-informed care** (TIC) have evolved in an attempt to mitigate them (Groden, 2026). Importantly, family integrated care (FiCare) is a model advocated across all NNUs in the UK (England, Scotland, Wales, and Northern Ireland) as well as some countries globally. Each of the UK devolved governments promote the philosophy through their perinatal health services (NHS England, 2023; Gov.Wales, 2025; Health & Social Care, 2026; Scottish Perinatal Network, 2026). Worldwide an increasing number of countries are working within a FiCare model of practice with some notable leaders and innovators that drive new approaches and methods of implementation.

WHAT IS FAMILY INTEGRATED CARE?

In the NNU, babies are often separated from their parents for prolonged periods, which can have physical, psychological, and emotional health impacts on both parents and baby. FiCare is a philosophy of care where parents are partners in their baby's care in the neonatal intensive care unit. Parents are facilitated to be the primary caregiver participating directly in caregiving. Key aspects of closeness such as **skin-to-skin** contact, sometimes called **'Kangaroo care,'** are integral to this approach due to the substantial benefits for the baby and parents. A collaborative relationship between parents and staff is fostered to help promote parent-infant interactions, sharing of information and reduce feelings of helplessness and lack of control. Parents are involved in all possible aspects of care for example feeding, nappy changing, bathing, providing oral medication, taking and recording observations, and tracking weight and progress.

FiCare also fosters an approach of encouraging, supporting and empowering parents to participate in decision-making from an early onset of their parenting journey when they feel ready to do so. This includes taking part in medical/multidisciplinary rounds, which increases involvement in their baby's care and helps to build relationships with the multidisciplinary team, thus empowering parents to become true partners in care within the neonatal setting. Parents have support and education in the care of their baby to allow them to grow into the role of primary caregiver for their infants within a medical setting, integrated with healthcare professionals. This shift in staff becoming mentors and coaching parents from caregivers requires support from the wider healthcare system to prepare teams for this change in culture. While nursing professionals still provide medical care for the infants, parents are empowered to 'parent' their baby, as they would have done without the need of neonatal care. FiCare is a relational model, and empowering parents to become partners in care and facilitating success is dependent on the relationship of health care professionals and parents establishing a mutual trust. Being facilitated to grow in autonomy and exploration in caring for and building a connection with their baby whilst also being able to return to the neonatal professionals for help, support, and growing a shared understanding when needed enables parents to grow in confidence. This partnership can also extend to **coproduction** of service development, quality improvement, and innovations in care.

THE ORIGINS OF FICARE

The family integrated model of care was first developed as a humanistic approach (Levin, 1994) in the 1970s as a direct result of staff shortages in Estonia where there were generally four nursing staff looking after seventy mothers and neonates. Mothers were encouraged from the earliest stages of interaction to take an active role in caring for their babies and were expected to remain in the hospital with them 24 hours a day until discharge. Importantly, the findings indicated that reduced reliance on medical and nursing interventions, together with less use of technology, was associated with lower infection rates. This was thought to result from decreased exposure to harmful environmental pathogens transmitted by healthcare professionals, alongside increased exposure to the maternal microbiome, which may enhance infant immunity. Levin (1994) also identified maternal care optimised weight gain and saw a positive improvement in social and psychological development. The psychological impact also benefitted the mother as a stronger mother-baby bond was observed building a greater confidence in mothering. The combination of the above actions in turn led to a decreased length of stay. Levin (1994) describes the style of care as designed to 'maintain the psychological and biological umbilicus.'

Many studies since have found the benefits of FiCare (short and long term) extend to all involved in caring for the neonate improving the baby outcomes along with their family, professionals, and the wider society moving forward. The following list is not exhaustive.

The benefits of FiCare to babies

- Reduced mortality.
- Reduced infection rates, which in turn leads to reduced antibiotic usage.
- Increased breastmilk feeding (including at discharge), earlier suck feeding, and greater weight gain.
- Earlier discharge, with parents feeling better prepared, and a reduced rate of readmissions to hospital.
- Sustained effect on the baby's behaviour, with improved self-regulation observed at 18–21 months (corrected age).

The benefits of FiCare to the family

- Facilitation of bonding, which in turn improves parental wellbeing and reduces parental anxiety.
- Increased breastfeeding rates improves maternal health and financial benefits to the family.
- Reduces parental anxiety, stress, and depressive symptoms.
- Enhances parental confidence at discharge and has benefits for the long-term outcomes of babies and their families.

The benefits of FiCare to healthcare professionals

- Empowering them to lead change in their unit, which in turn contributes to team cohesion and satisfaction (Kirolos et al., 2021).
- Greater consistency in care contributes to increased job satisfaction for staff, and greater service user satisfaction, which results in fewer complaints and reduced incident reporting.
- Support for professionals which recognises the distress inherent in a neonatal healthcare professional role.

The benefits of FiCare to neonatal facilities

- Earlier discharge reduces expensive hospital care.
- Reduction in re-admission rates reduces financial burden on hospitals.
- Fewer complaints reduce litigation costs.
- Increased staff satisfaction increases retention and reduces financial implications of recruitment.

The benefits of FiCare to society

- Reduction in financial cost of childhood behavioural challenges with the improvement in self-regulation. This may reduce necessity for additional teaching staff in schools.
- Reduction in medical intervention and management required through the benefits of breast feeding, for example, eczema or asthma.

RECENT DEVELOPMENTS OF THE FICARE MODEL

A subsequent study in 2011 over 1 year and across nineteen sites was conducted by a team of healthcare professionals and parents which previously had babies in neonatal care and developed a model of care in Mount Sinai Hospital, Toronto (O'Brien et al., 2013). Past parents, known as '**veteran parents**,' played a pivotal role in the development of the model and are essential in the implementation of the model's use on NNUs.

The implications of FiCare on the role of a neonatal nurse

The shift for nursing professionals from wholly active caregivers to care facilitators and mentors who care for the more holistic needs of the infant and the whole family poses a potential challenge to the perceptions of the traditional nursing role and may lead to the question 'What is my role?' (Leake et al., 2025). Whilst there are a range of specialist nursing skills and tasks essential for the care of a baby in neonatal care, particularly in the NNU, the role of a neonatal nurse in a FiCare unit also involves mentoring parents in taking on various aspects of their caregiving role, which can include medical care as well as key parenting roles. This has seen challenges for staff in adopting a new role, with some feeling threatened fewer nurses would be required, and a concern that FiCare is a way of saving costs with a reduction in nurses (McKechnie, 2016). However, there is no reported evidence that nursing ratios change when FiCare is in place. Job satisfaction in nurses has been reported to increase in some studies, although the mechanisms and contextual factors have not been rigorously explored, and the focus remains largely on outcomes for babies and families indicating an area for further nuanced research.

Working with other healthcare professionals in the multidisciplinary team

Care of the neonate is often complex, with a multidisciplinary team (MDT) providing expert knowledge to achieve the best outcome for the baby and family. Each of the specialised disciplines is required to be part of the change process to enable successful implementation and to infuse knowledge and approaches from overlapping approaches (such as developmental care, neuroprotective care). Parental teaching from allied health professionals (AHPs) is essential on both a formal and individualised basis. They also oversee universal interventions that benefit all babies and parents as well as provide specialised interventions within a FiCare approach.

THINK POINT

- How does FiCare differ from family-centred care (FCC)?
- Before progressing, think about the subtle differences between FiCare and FCC – what are the main elements that require change?
- How may those changes be facilitated?
- Which elements can you use in practice?

Healthcare professionals are key drivers of cultural change and can model the importance of working relationally and thinking about the broader needs of the baby and family that extend beyond their medical care. It is important to ensure healthcare practitioners have the required skills for additional coaching and support of parents and ensure time and funding is allocated as well as valued as a key skill set. Supportive management will be required to lead the change process for the ethos of the ward to shift to a successful family integrated facility.

HOW FICARE DIFFERS FROM FAMILY-CENTRED CARE

The evolvement of the philosophy of FiCare differs subtly to FCC. In FCC the family are informed of the care path that is directed by the medical and nursing teams, ensuring understanding and the family wishes taken into consideration, but most of the caregiving is completed by the health professionals. Conversely in FiCare, the decisions are jointly made with the family, and the majority of caregiving is completed and at times led by the parents. The FiCare model is an extension of FCC, where parents are provided with support and education to become their baby's care-giver and to become a central part of the neonatal care team, instead of passive observers of their infant's care. A combination of education, physical support, and psychological support are provided to ensure that parents become confident to provide most of their infant's daily care (O'Brien & Franck, 2019). The shift to move from FCC to FiCare requires cultural change within the NNU and specialities that work within it. Support and 'buy in' from staff at every level, from administrative and housekeeping to unit leads and senior management, are essential.

Table 6.1 shows some selected features/foci of care, how this differs between FCC and FiCare, and some areas to consider:

The FiCare model outlines a strategy for changing the culture of a unit to embrace true integration of the family in care, in a workable and meaningful way. The paradigm consists of four pillars which form the foundations of care, staff education & support, parent education, neonatal unit environment and psychosocial support. Threaded throughout each aspect is the engagement of veteran parents (Box 6.1).

Providing the principles outlined above are followed, the model is adaptive to the available resources and population demographic enabling many centres around the word to implement the approach. The study identified similar baby benefits to the Estonia study, faster growth, decreased length of stay (decreased infection rates), longer breastfeeding rates (providing a multitude of benefits), and decreased stress levels (lower cortisol levels, induced by skin-to-skin kangaroo care). The family benefits were identified as improved confidence in parenting skills, leading to a quicker readiness for transition to home, increased bonding, and lower parental anxiety, leading to lower readmission rates (O'Brien et al., 2018).

TABLE 6.1 FAMILY-CENTRED CARE VERSUS FAMILY INTEGRATED CARE

Feature	*Family-centred care (FCC)*	*Family integrated care (FiCare)*	*Consider*
Role of family	Partner in care **Example**: 'What time can you be here for tomorrow?'	Primary caregiver in clinical care **Example:** Family resident (or present on NNU for an extended time) with facilities to enable them to provide care/make decisions in an informed way. Respecting experience through an understanding of the family dynamics. 'Please tell us about yourself/what a day looks like for you to enable us to help remove any barriers to you being able to care for your baby.'	■ The environment/language is accessible for the family, including information and facilities, empowering them to be the best they can be.
Veteran parents	Access to liaise with veteran parents Example: NNU hosts a community peer support group and welcomes veteran parents in addition to recent parents.	Access to peer support is offered on the NNU to all families. Example: Veteran parents visit the unit to offer families the opportunity for peer support, which could be as a group – for example a cake and chat session, or on an individual basis, either at or away from the cot side.	■ How veteran parents could be utilised to provide peer support to current families. This could be via recruiting as hospital volunteers or via a voluntary organisation. · ■ Be mindful of the need to follow the hospital's volunteer process including appropriate training and disclosure and barring service checks, etc. ■ Veteran parents will require access to psychological support.

TABLE 6.1 (Cont.)

Feature	*Family-centred care (FCC)*	*Family integrated care (FiCare)*	*Consider*
Involvement in rounds	Invited to participate **Example**: Medical practitioner: 'It looks as though Jenny isn't coping so well without the oxygen – I think we need to see how today goes. Have you noticed the changes?'	Actively encouraged to participate and supported to do so **Example**: Medical practitioner: 'Hello John, I'm Khalid; please can you tell me about Jenny?' Father 'Since coming off oxygen yesterday, Jenny has been working harder at breathing, with about four heart rate drops an hour. Also, she isn't feeding as well – she is too tired. Maybe she could have a smaller amount of oxygen rather than removing it completely?'	■ Families lead the discussions with the MDT on how their baby has been since last review rather than informed of the decisions the MDT have made in relation to care of their baby. ■ Important discussions are not limited to ward round specific times, but discussion times are facilitated to ensure the family is available to lead them if they wish/feel able.
Education & training	General orientation and information **Example:** 'Welcome to the ward, I'll show you around and here is an information booklet about the ward, routines, with details of what to bring, and how to do cares, shall we go through those together now?'	Formal training and structured education **Example:** 'Hi, congratulations, would you like me to show you where everything is, or would you prefer to explore later? I can show you around if you like – whenever you are ready. If you prefer, I can link you to one of our veteran parents who run care sessions for families. There is a QR code wall with information for you to explore in your own time.' Veteran parent may be a new father or partner who can be advised to explore how he can provide skin to skin and the benefits to himself and baby.	■ Families receive opportunities provided by the ward to learn about caregiving on NNU, leading the pace they feel confident to provide cares. This may be individual or group activities – often run by past parents (veterans) or AHPs. ■ Opportunities to explore how the NNU feels with the support of veteran and peer groups. Families gain hope in hearing other families have been in similar situations and are able to share experience enabling others to recognise where they are on their own journey, rather than being told by professionals as experts (often with no experience of parental care) 'it will get easier.'

TABLE 6.1 (Cont.)

Feature	*Family-centred care (FCC)*	*Family integrated care (FiCare)*	*Consider*
Care delivery, planning and decision-making	Professionals lead, families assist **Example:** Staff 'What time are you able to get here as Alfred is due a feed at 3pm?'	Families lead daily care with professional support **Example:** Mother 'Hi, I've changed and fed Robyn– all the records have been updated, but please can I speak to the physiotherapist about how to support Robyn in their cot.'	■ Where a family is in their journey. Do they need support? ■ Have they previously been delivering care without supervision? ■ How confident do they feel?
Philosophy	Collaboration **Example:** 'Let's change this nappy together'	Integration and empowerment **Example:** 'Here is the information for you to be able to change this nappy for your baby, I am here to answer any questions you may have and support you where you feel you need it.'	■ Ensure information is available and accessible when families are ready to hear and learn. ■ Providing opportunities and becoming an advocate for baby and family as one. ■ Be curious about the individuals, what do they want to know, when do they want to know, how do they want to know. ■ Guide parents in care, transferring care giving and decision-making to them as they indicate through the sharing of knowledge at a pace dictated by them.
Application	Broad (paediatrics, chronic care, etc.)	Often neonatal-specific, but expanding to other settings	■ How will the change occur? ■ Who will lead the change? ■ Who is required for implementation? ■ What skills and training do staff require?

BOX 6.1 THE FOUR PILLARS OF FICARE

Staff education and support

- Providing education and tools for professionals to enable them to educate, mentor, and support parents in caring for their baby in the NNU.
- Allowing professionals to feel comfortable with the model of care and embrace their role as key facilitators of FiCare and feel supported in their work.

Parent education

- Providing parents with the knowledge, skills, and confidence required to care for their infants in the NNU setting.
- Enabling parents to be part of the healthcare team by offering small group education and the opportunity to participate in medical rounds while being supported by individual bedside learning.

NNU environment

- Ensuring that unit policies and procedures are supportive of the model.
- Creating a physical and social environment that is conducive to the implementation of FiCare.

Psychosocial support

- Providing adequate psychosocial support for families to enable their participation in FiCare.
- Creating and supporting opportunities for peer-to-peer support.

Adapted from FamilyIntegratedCare.com (2026)

TOOLS AND AIDES FOR FICARE IMPLEMENTATION

Implementation in the UK has been broken down further to assist teams to operationalise the paradigm of FiCare. The British Association of Perinatal Medicine (BAPM) in 2021, produced a framework for use in NNUs, comparable to the Toronto model. The BAPM framework has five principles (Figure 6.1): empowerment, wellbeing, culture, and environment wrapped around the central concept of partnership with families (BAPM, 2021).

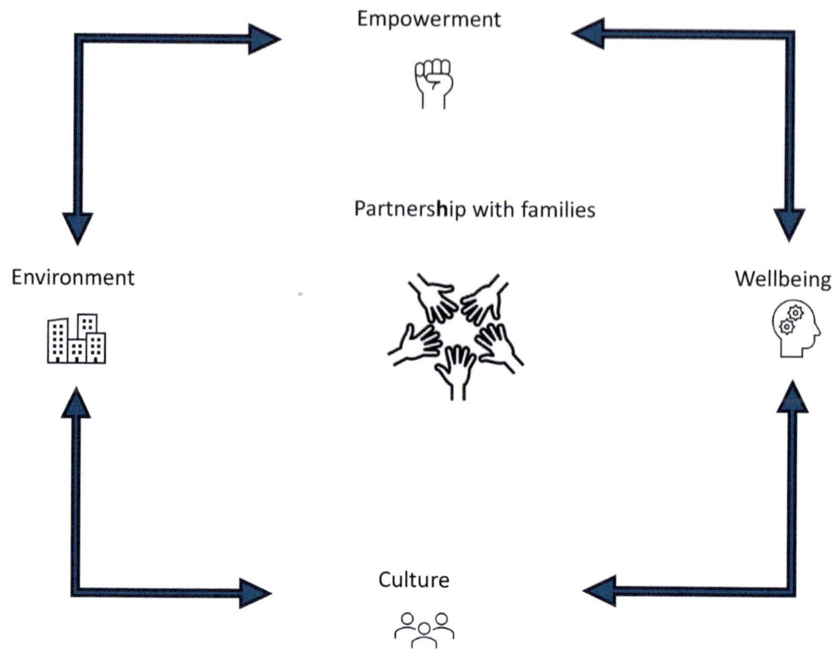

Examples of partnership

1. Parents being actively involved in decisions made at the ward round, working alongside professionals
2. Facilities for siblings
3. Families taught nasogastric feeding
4. Language accessibility including signs in multiple languages and translators

Figure 6.1 Family integrated care: a framework for practice (BAPM, 2021)

Additional recognised tools to aid the cultural change required in implementation of FiCare include a national accreditation process through Bliss – a charity for babies born premature or sick (Bliss, 2026). The Bliss Baby Charter, has an origin in FCC, evolving to reflect the move to FiCare. Bliss is an advocate for families, offering family support, strategic unit support, conducting research, and lobbying in parliament to change/introduce policies improving outcomes and experiences of babies and their families.

PRACTICE POINT

What aspects of each of the principles set out in Figure 6.1 can you implement in your unit?

Look around your unit to identify aspects of care and which principles they fit into; do they merge or interact with each other?

Accreditation is through an audit of seven domains spanning clinical, psychological, developmental, relational, and strategic elements of care provided. The United Nations Children's Fund (UNICEF) also have an international accreditation programme in partnership with The World Health Organization (WHO), Baby Friendly Initiative (BFI). BFI upholds the United Nations Convention on the Rights of the Child (UNCRC), which outlines the right of every child to health. The programme underpins FiCare through assessing units on the care they provide to support families with infant feeding and building close and loving relationships. It is split to focus on specific areas providing standards that are assessed, maternity, neonatal, community, hospital-based children's services, and university standards (UNICEF UK, 2025).

PRACTICE POINT

Which tools/initiatives in relation to FiCare have you encountered in your practice?

Other initiatives have been designed to help units achieve FiCare, some in digital format, reflecting a move to use available technology within health.

BARRIERS AND FACILITATORS OF FICARE

Whilst FiCare has amassed a growing body of evidence to support its use as an overarching model of care, there are many barriers to its implementation. Some of these barriers concern systems (which can also include practical constraints, policies, and procedures as well as cultural attitudes) and others exist at a family and individual level.

Practical, physical, and systems barriers

In each of the studies and frameworks discussed above the element of environment is identified as crucial. Whilst the physical space needs to be inclusive and facilitate ease of access for families to be resident on the NNU, often the physical area is accessible, but the underpinning policies of a unit prevent families from staying for lengths of time required to become partners in care. The physical space, policies, economic support, and culture are all dependent on each other to facilitate success in FiCare. Changing the physical space to look more welcoming is not sufficient; FiCare is not on the walls but in the culture of a unit.

That said, making the environment comfortable and set up for families to stay for long periods of time is important. Facilities for parents to avoid separation can be achieved relatively easily. Comfortable cot-side chairs to promote skin to skin (Figure 6.2) and rest, a kitchen for ease of food and drink preparation, and shower facilities can all encourage parents to stay with their baby for extended times.

ACTIVITY

Case study of interdependence of principles of FiCare

A unit is redecorated to look less clinical, with kitchen, wash, and sleeping facilities all designed to be more homely. Comfortable reclining chairs are placed at the cot-side.

Anna and partner Kai are resident on the unit. They make lunch, provided by the ward, and take their cups of tea into the ward area where baby Ren is in an incubator. They are approached by a nurse who will be supporting them, introducing herself as 'your nurse for the afternoon.' After a conversation about what support Anna and Kai would like her to provide, she leaves them to confidently change and feed Ren independently. During this time the nurse attends another family. A second member of staff enters the nursery and quietly asks Anna and Kai to take their drinks out of the nursery as hot drinks are a danger to the babies.

Questions to consider

How has the ward facilitated FiCare?

The physical space is accessible, welcoming and facilities are good, but is there an outdated policy in place to prevent hot drinks in the nursery?

Have all staff been trained in the philosophy of FiCare?

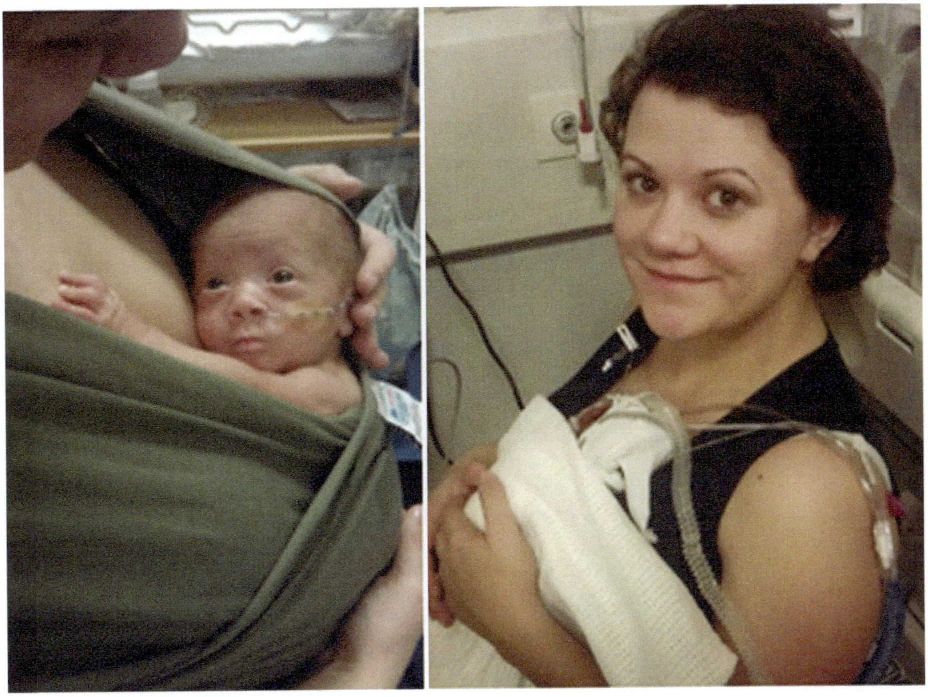

Figure 6.2 Skin-to-skin contact

Policies need to align with FiCare philosophy to remove barriers. The removal of physical barriers of a unit is often achieved first as they are more tangible and visible. Changing policies which may be set in tradition will help to change the culture of a unit but change in belief systems and work routines is more challenging. Listening to parents that have been through the experience (veteran parents) has been shown through the previously discussed studies to be the most effective way of understanding how systems and policies can include parents as partners in care. The parental voice is powerful and has the greatest impact on challenging beliefs.

Education on FiCare for all staff is crucial to maintain a cohesive workforce initially with regular updates of changes. This should be delivered in collaboration with parents to have the greatest effect. However, as FiCare becomes embedded as the philosophy of a unit, it will be threaded through all systems seamlessly with veteran parents included as experts or advisors. Many regions in the UK have access to a parent advisory group who are helping to shape family care within the neonatal service.

Psychological barriers to FiCare: key areas to consider and formulating how to help

Whilst there are many practical barriers to FiCare within units, it is also important to recognise that there are psychological barriers and factors which play a significant role and are often less visible. These may change and play a variably prominent role at different stages in the neonatal journey. Whilst some issues may naturally resolve through changes in exposure, confidence and experience (such as the ability to accurately read baby's cues), others can become more significant over time (for example, avoidance of certain tasks that are essential to master before discharge).

Activity

Consider some of the psychological challenges facing parents in neonatal care based on what you have read so far and on your own clinical experience. Consider how they might impact the different components in the 5 domains of FiCare. Here are some examples:

Domain	Psychological barrier
Empowerment: showing parents how to become confidence with everyday cares such as nappy changing, mouth care	Ruth feels that if she is anxious, she might injure her baby if she touches them despite reassurance. Her anxiety has been misinterpreted as reluctance by the care team, and she is starting to be talked about as 'disengaged.' She feels ashamed to be anxious over 'small tasks' and this makes it harder to discuss, and as time goes on, she begins to feel like she has failed as a neonatal parent on a well-established 'FiCare unit.'
Partnership with families: involving parents in shared decision-making	Darren has gone to great lengths to rearrange his day so he can be present for ward rounds 2–3 times a week. He has been happy to talk with healthcare professionals about the care of his son, but his lack of confidence in reading and writing has made keeping track of details difficult including filling in parent booklets. When he was invited to a meeting about potential surgery, he felt overwhelmed and embarrassed when given written information and felt he was letting his son down when he had a specific responsibility.
My example/s from practice	Take notes on any examples from your own practice, to consider alongside those above.

Asking parents careful questions around FiCare tasks and activities can help develop a shared understanding of these invisible challenges and barriers. This requires sensitive, attuned, and compassionate enquiry, particularly if the reasons may evoke guilt or shame. Of further importance is the use of active listening skills (using open questions, summarising what has been told, taking a non- judgemental and open approach, validation of parents' experiences, responding with empathy and compassion). Maintaining a stance of curiosity for how a parent may be experiencing something which may be very different to ourselves or other parents. We may also be able to contribute our own

TABLE 6.2 A PROCESS TO IDENTIFY AND WORK WITH PSYCHOLOGICAL BARRIERS

Step
1. Identify distress/challenges
2. Ask open questions to identify and characterise challenges
3. Develop a shared understanding (formulation) of what's happening
4. Plan to address challenges and build on strengths and what matters most to the parent/family and what helps
5. Implement the plan with regular review, involving the MDT when and where indicated

observations such as patterns we have noticed and continue to use these skills even when planning or working towards a potential solution, doing this 'with' parents rather than 'to.' Table 6.2 outlines a suggested process to work with psychological barriers.

Examples of questions to understand potential psychological barriers:

- 'What's running through your mind as you x?' (lift her legs to change a nappy, bring her to the breast, read these leaflets)
- Is there anything about this that worries or concerns you?
- What things make this easier/harder that aren't necessarily obvious?
- What makes a good day with your baby? What are the 'key ingredients?'
- What's important for us to know about you to be the most supportive we can be?
- How confident/comfortable/connected do you feel when doing x – what's that about?

Further detailed resources for parents that can also be used with neonatal staff to shape care and help work through the psychological aspects of FiCare are available (Chilvers, 2025) and signposted in the web based companion.

COPRODUCTION WITH PARENTS, PEER SUPPORT, AND THE ROLE OF VETERAN PARENTS

Every neonatal parent will have their personal lived experience of neonatal care, with no two experiences being replicas of one another. However, there are shared characteristics of having a baby in neonatal care, and families often report feeling a connection to those who have also had a baby requiring an admission.

Peer support involves the bringing together of people that have shared similar experiences to offer each other psychosocial support in a non-clinical format. It can help to validate feelings, reduce isolation, and even provide a sense of hope. However, peer supporters must remain mindful that each experience is unique, and variation in outcomes exist; therefore, they must not encourage a false sense of hope that the outcome will definitively be positive.

In the original FICare model, peer support was identified as one of the principles within the psychosocial pillar, highlighting how this type of support is beneficial alongside input from psychological professionals. In 2021, BAPM published a toolkit for FICare (see Figure 6.1), where peer support features in both the empowerment and wellbeing principles. Being embedded within these documents demonstrates the importance of peer support and that it is a recommended element of achieving a true FICare ethos.

PEER SUPPORT

How peer support is provided

The format of peer support can vary and does not always require formal and structured offerings. By offering the opportunity for peer support on the NNU, organic progression of relationship development may occur between families. Peer support may be offered in-house which could be supported, but not led, by the unit's local maternity and neonatal voices partnership (MNVPs) or local third-sector organisations, such as unit-based or local charities, or national schemes, such as champions provided by Bliss.

There are specific requirements that need to be considered whatever route is utilised to provide peer support. Peer supporters need to receive appropriate training to fulfil their role. Ideally the training received should include knowledge and skills in relation to engaging with neonatal families, in addition to the hospital's mandatory training. This may include safeguarding, trauma-informed care, working with vulnerable people, to minimise the risk of causing compounded harm. Protective measures such as a criminal record check, a knowledge of trust policies, and relevant immunisations are essential. Access to psychological support is key, as engaging with vulnerable families can be emotionally challenging to hear and may trigger feelings from their personal lived experience. Psychological support may be provided externally if working in collaboration with a voluntary, community, and social enterprise (VCSE) or offered by an embedded psychology team on the unit.

> **PRACTICE POINT**
>
> Good FiCare means all families are included; consider how your practices help all families feel empowered to be partners in care. Think about how families in your region can be involved in coproduction of their services.

Types of peer support

In-hospital support:

- Informal support offered to parents at cotside (providing a listening ear) usually by parents who have also had a neonatal experience.
- Facilitators/co facilitators of parent unit groups; these can be unstructured such as 'Cake and Chat' or be part of a specific FiCare teaching programme (e.g. sessions on feeding, discharge).

Online support

- Through social media groups that may be linked to a unit, region, or specific medical diagnosis.
- Telephone, texts, and video calls.
- Online forums that are moderated by trained veteran parents and/or members of neonatal staff.

Community-based support

- Follow-up groups in the community (such as 'Stay and Play,' baby massage, or coffee mornings).
- Attendance at unit follow up clinics where parents are invited to stay for groups.
- Ongoing support and signposting post discharge.

Specialist peer support

- Bereavement
- Multiples
- Specific conditions
- Specific groups of parents (e.g. those whose baby is diagnosed with a genetic condition, or are experiencing domestic violence)

Peer support vs service user voice

It is vital to be clear on the distinction between peer support and service user voice (SUV). As described in the previous sections, peer support involves bringing together people that have shared similar experiences to offer psychosocial support. Whereas service user voice focuses on obtaining feedback and involving service users to inform, design, and deliver service improvements. In addition, service user voice should be embedded throughout safety, quality, and assurance processes, with the aim of improving experiences and outcomes for all families. The mechanism for supporting SUV at a local level are MNVPs. They lead on engagement with maternity and neonatal service users, are recognised as a key stakeholder within the MDT and have a strategic role working at trust and integrated care board level. At a regional level, there are regional maternity SUV representatives who are embedded within the regional maternity teams, and parent and family engagement leads, who are an integral part of the neonatal operational delivery networks (ODNs). The parent and family engagement leads work closely with the parent advisory groups (PAGs). PAGs are made up of a group of parents who have lived experience of having a baby who has had a neonatal care stay. Nationally, there are several SUV representatives to ensure service user voice is embedded throughout national policy workstreams.

In relation to FiCare, the BAPM toolkit recognises the requirement of SUV in their partnership with family's principle, by stating the following;

- Families have opportunities to give feedback about their babies' care while on the unit and after discharge
- Families' experiences and feedback are actively sought, to inform and improve the quality of services
- Local FiCare steering groups comprising families, parent advisory groups, and members of the multidisciplinary team are established to drive improvement.

TACKLING HEALTH INEQUALITIES AND MEETING THE NEEDS OF ALL FAMILIES IN NEONATAL CARE

Despite increasing awareness, stark inequalities in outcomes for babies and women in maternity and neonatal care remain. These inequalities are multifaceted and often reflect structural inequalities (such as poverty, racism, and poor housing). Whilst they can manifest in different ways at multiple points in a family's journey, it is important to consider what factors families can be supported with during their baby's admission and discharge. For care to be **equitable**, neonatal systems need to be responsive to each person's unique health and social situation. Individuals hold multiple and overlapping/intersecting identities and factors (**intersectionality**) which means they have a particular profile of discrimination and privilege and the impact of one factor can depend on the presence or absence of another. For example, non-white gay parents may face challenges of both homophobia and racism. Some factors are visible and others invisible, and this is true both for parents and for neonatal professionals. The Social GGRRAAACCEEESSS framework (Figure 6.3) provides a structure to consider areas of social difference and our own ability to reflect on sameness and difference (Burnham, 2012).

ACTIVITY

Consider how each of these domains are relevant to your own experiences of discrimination and privilege. Be mindful that having privilege doesn't mean than you haven't experienced difficulties or earned your success. However, privilege within a certain domain often means you haven't had to consider it a factor in your success, acceptance by others, or experience it as a cause of adversity.

It is important to be aware of the demographics of the population served by the NNU and to develop a shared broad understanding of their needs at a population level, as well as considering the different composition of families you will be working with (e.g. different sexualities, ages) and individual differences (e.g. **neurodiversity**). However, it is also key to understand the individual needs of each family and individuals within a family that may be different to those assumed

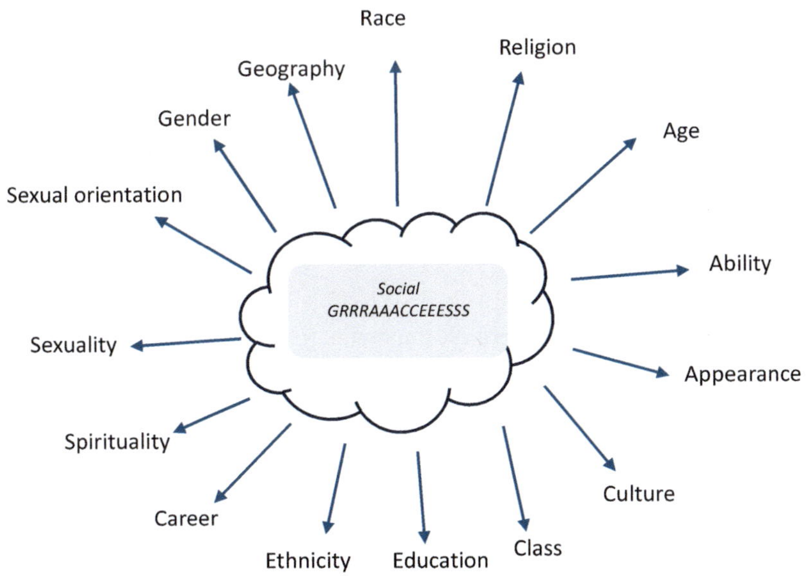

Figure 6.3 The Social GRRRAAACCEEESSS model (adapted from Julia Young, based on Burnham, 2012)

by areas of visible identity, e.g. assumptions about beliefs can be made on the basis of a certain religion; however, religious beliefs vary enormously within even one branch of a religion. Ultimately, good relationships where there are true collaboration, compassion, and care help establish the foundation needed to be curious about parents and understand their context and experience.

PRACTICE POINT

Care is more likely to be culturally and socially relevant, attuned, and sensitive to need if it is coproduced with families who use services. What ways do you coproduce your services with all families, and what steps do you take to ensure all voices are heard?

Are there any groups you feel are underrepresented in your service/practice development?

What domains/differences are more and less visible?

Which religious or community leaders can you build relationships within your community?

How representative is your staff team of the diversity of your neonatal families?

THINK POINT

Consider what you understand by the term 'trauma-informed care' (TIC). It may be helpful to read the paper by Sanders and Hall (2018) to find out more. Reflect on how you implement the principles of TIC in your unit, in line with FiCare.

Chapter takeaways

- Neonatal admission is inherently traumatic; for babies due to separation, pain, and stress and for parents who often arrive already distressed from pregnancy and birth trauma. Trauma-informed care principles should be adhered to and applied to all families as well as to healthcare professionals who are often working under emotional strain.
- FiCare shifts neonatal culture from professionals 'doing to' families toward parents as partners and primary caregivers, promoting closeness, confidence, shared decision-making and improved outcomes for babies, families, staff, and systems.

- Effective FiCare requires cultural, environmental, and systemic change, not just physical improvements; policies, staff training, relational practice, and veteran parent involvement are essential to truly embed the model.
- Psychological barriers are common yet often invisible; anxiety, shame, trauma, literacy challenges, and identity changes, meaning staff must use compassionate enquiry, collaboration, and tailored support to help families participate confidently.
- Equity, inclusion, and coproduction are vital; care must recognise social inequalities, intersecting identities, and diverse needs.
- The service user voice, peer support, and representative staff–family partnership are all key to delivering meaningful, culturally attuned FiCare.

CASE STUDY

CASE STUDIES

Case study 1: Care of the family with same-sex parents

Kaysha and Abbie are the parents of 26-week-old Harry who was transferred from his local neonatal unit to a tertiary centre for surgery. They found the move to a new hospital very stressful and were away from their usual support network. Abbie spent most of the time at the cot side with Harry during the week and didn't feel confident or comfortable in the new unit – everything she thought she knew how to do was different. The staff were friendly but repeatedly asked questions about his 'father' and parental responsibility every time there was a staff change. The unit had developed a pizza night for fathers which was popular and well attended, but Kaysha and the staff were unsure about whether she'd be welcome, and she found herself feeling on edge and anxious every time she came to be with Harry. This wasn't helped by other parents on the unit, who sometimes made them feel uncomfortable when they were affectionate with each other. All the reading materials, education materials and resources available gave a very particular sense of what 'family' in FiCare was considered to be, but they didn't see their family represented.

Q1. What unit culture considerations are important to hold in mind for same-sex parents? (Think about policies and procedures, representation and visibility, staff and family attitudes/approaches, and possible discrimination.)

Q2. How could unit culture influence the ability for same sex couples to participate in FiCare?

CASE STUDY

Q3. How could you work with Abbie and Kaysha to help them develop their roles as parents (both individually and as a couple)?

Q4. What peer support and broader social support might you consider offering/facilitating for them? (Consider who is represented in your peer support programmes, and the set-up of parent groups)

Case study 2: Caring for parents whose first language is not English

Mahi and Advik are brought to the NNU by a midwife for the first time to see their daughter Myra, who was born at 33 weeks whilst visiting family in the UK. The ward has an intercom system that the midwife demonstrates to the couple. Advik speaks some English, but Mahi speaks very little. The word 'Welcome' is translated above the intercom in different languages, along with a staff board with country flags on, representing staff origins. On arrival to reception, they are greeted with a smile and asked what their preferred language is. The video translation system is set to their first language, even though Advik says he understands a little English. The nurse (Jane) allocated to the family sits down with Mahi and Advik next to Myra's cot. Using the translator, Jane asks if Mahi or Advik would like Myra skin to skin. Mahi looks apprehensive and refers to Advik; Jane registers the exchange and asks if Mahi would feel more comfortable with some privacy screens in place. Once Myra is transferred to Mahi, with an explanation through the translator that Jane is on hand should they need her, the family have time privately. After 15 minutes Advik comes out to find Jane and tries to explain Mahi is worried. Jane asks if it is ok to come round the screens and talk to Mahi. Through the video translator Jane asks Mahi what concerns she has and offers reassurance; Mahi asks Advik questions to ask rather than asking directly. Jane shows Mahi and Advik on her phone how to access the ward information through the website in their own language. With mutual agreement Jane helps Mahi to place Myra into her cot and shows Mahi and Advik the layout of the ward, including the facilities available. During the tour, Jane asks the couple about their home life and family and asks what a usual day would look like for them, including noting down what they would like to be called and how Mahi would like to feed Myra. At the end of her shift Jane hands over to the next nurse all the information she has learnt about the family.

CASE STUDY

Q1. What unit culture considerations are important to hold in mind for parents whose first language is not English? (think about systems, routines, policies and procedures, representation and visibility, unit demographic representation, staff and family attitudes/approaches, and possible discrimination)

Q2. How did this ward demonstrate the philosophy of FiCare?

Q3. How could you work with Mahi and Advik to help them develop their roles as parents (both individually and as a couple) in a culturally sensitive way?

Q4. Why did Jane use the question 'What does a usual day look like for you?' How is the information useful?

Q5. What peer support and broader social support might you consider offering/facilitating for them? (Consider who is represented in your peer support programmes, the set-up of parent groups)

For suggested answer guides to the questions posed in these case studies, please refer to the web-based companion site specific to this chapter. See www.routledge.com/cw/petty

References

BLISS. (2026). *What is the BLISS Baby Charter*? https://www.bliss.org.uk/health-professionals/bliss-baby-charter/what-is-the-baby-charter

British Association of Perinatal Medicine (BAPM). (2021). *Family integrated care: A BAPM framework for practice*. BAPM.

Burnham, J. (2012). Developments in social GGRRAAACCEEESSS: Visible–invisible and voiced–unvoiced. In I.-B. Krause (Ed.), *Culture and reflexivity in systemic psychotherapy: Mutual perspectives* (pp. 139–160). Karnac.

Chilvers, R. (2025). *Not alone in NICU: A compassionate companion for parents with a baby in neonatal care*. Jessica Kingsley Press.

Family Integrated Care. (2026). *The FiCare approach: Program development*. Retrieved March 22, 2026, from https://familyintegratedcare.com/the-ficare-approach/program-development/

Global Foundation for the Care of Newborn Infants (GFCNI). (2026). *Zero separation: Together for better care*. https://www.gfcni.org/campaigns/zero-separation

Gov. Wales. (2025). *Quality statement for maternity and neonatal services*. https://www.gov.wales/sites/default/files/pdf-versions/2025/5/3/1747814705/quality-statement-maternity-and-neonatal-services.pdf

Groden, C. M. (2026). Trauma-informed care in the neonatal intensive care unit: Infants, families, and care teams. *NeoReviews*, *27*(2), e62–e72.

Hardcastle, K., Ford, K., & Bellis, M. A. (2022). Maternal adverse childhood experiences and their association with preterm birth: Secondary analysis of data from universal health visiting. *BMC Pregnancy Childbirth*, *22*(1), 129. https://doi.org/10.1186/s12884-022-04454-z

Health and Social Care. (2026). *Neonatal Network Northern Ireland.* https://online.hscni.net/partnerships/neonatalni/#:~:text=The%20Neonatal%20Network%20Northern%20Ireland,and%20the%20Royal%20Maternity%20Hospital

Hynan, M. T., & Hall, S. L. (2015). Psychosocial program standards for NICU parents. *Journal of Perinatology, 35*(Suppl 1), S1–S4. https://doi.org/10.1038/jp.2015.141

Kirolos, S., Sutcliffe, L., Giatsi Clausen, M., Abernethy, C., Shanmugalingam, S., Bauwens, N., Orme, J., Thomson, K., Grattan, R., & Patel, N. (2021). Asynchronous video messaging promotes family involvement and mitigates separation in neonatal care. *Archives of Disease in Childhood – Fetal and Neonatal Edition, 106*, 172–177.

Leake, N., Edney, S., Embleton, N., Berrington, J., & Rankin, J. (2025). Facilitators and barriers to the practice of neonatal family integrated care from the perspectives of healthcare professionals: A systematic review. *Archives of Disease in Childhood – Fetal & Neonatal Edition*, F1–F7.

Levin, A. (1994). The Mother-Infant Unit at Tallin Children's Hospital, Estonia: A truly baby-friendly unit. *Birth, 21*(1), 39–44.

McKechnie, L. (2016). Family-integrated care in the neonatal unit. *Infant, 12*(3), 79–81.

NHS England. (2023). *Three-year delivery plan for maternity and neonatal services.* https://www.england.nhs.uk/long-read/three-year-delivery-plan-for-maternity-and-neonatal-services/

O'Brien, K., Bracht, M., Macdonell, K., McBride, T., Robson, K., O'Leary, L., Christie, K., Galarza, M., Dicky, T., Levin, A., & Lee, S. K. (2013). A pilot cohort analytic study of Family Integrated Care in a Canadian neonatal intensive care unit. *BMC Pregnancy and Childbirth, 13*(Suppl 1), S12.

O'Brien, K., & Franck, L. S (2019). The evolution of family-centred care: From supporting parent-delivered interventions to a model of family integrated care. *Birth Defects Research, 111*(15), 1044–1059.

O'Brien, K., Robson, K., Bracht, M., Cruz, M., Lui, K., Alvaro, R., Da Silva, O., Monterrosa, L., Narvey, M., Ng, E., Soraisham, A., Ye, X. Y., Mirea, L., Tarnow-Mordi, W., Lee, S. K., O'Brien, K., Lee, S., Bracht, M., Caouette, G., . . . Hales, D. (2018). Effectiveness of family integrated care units on infant and parent outcome: A multicentre, multinational, cluster-randomised controlled trial. *The Lancet Child & Adolescent Health, 2*(4), 245–254.

Petty, J., Jarvis, J., & Thomas, R. (2019). Understanding parents' emotional experiences for neonatal education: A narrative, interpretive approach. *Journal of Clinical Nursing, 28*(9–10), 1911–1924.

Sanders, M. R., & Hall, S. L. (2018). Trauma-informed care in the newborn intensive care unit: Promoting safety, security and connectedness. *Journal of Perinatology, 38*(1), 3–10. https://doi.org/10.1038/jp.2017.124

Scottish Perinatal Network. (2026). *Discharge planning.* https://www.perinatalnetwork.nhs.scot/professionals/neonatal-discharge/

Shonkoff, J. P. (2012). The lifelong effects of early childhood adversity and toxic stress. *Pediatrics, 129*(1), e232–e246. https://doi.org/10.1542/peds.2011-2663

UNICEF UK. (2025). *Baby friendly standards.* https://www.unicef.org.uk/babyfriendly/about/standards/

7 DEVELOPMENTALLY FOCUSED NEONATAL CARE

Deanna Gibbs

CONTENTS

DOI: 10.4324/9781003591405-10

GUIDANCE ON HOW TO ENHANCE PERSONAL LEARNING FROM THIS CHAPTER

Key points covered in this chapter

- Underpinning theory of developmentally focused care in the neonatal unit.
- The aims, benefits and outcomes of developmental care.
- The vital link between parent integration and involvement in care with developmentally focused strategies.

Reflection

Reading through the chapter, you are encouraged to engage with the key points and related literature in an enquiring way. Ask these questions:

- Why is developmental care so important in the care of preterm infants and their families?
- What are the key components of developmental care?
- What is the relationship between family integrated care and developmental care?
- Do you want to change how your work environment provides developmental care?

Implications for nursing care

- Finally: how will this chapter enable you to consider and implement supporting parents to interact with their baby to optimise his or her developmental outcomes?

INTRODUCTION AND BACKGROUND

Infant- and family-centred developmental care (IFCDC) is a holistic healthcare model focused on supporting the developmental needs of infants, particularly those born prematurely or with critical health conditions, while ensuring active participation of their families in the care process (Global Foundation for the Care of Newborn Infants (GFCNI), 2025). Implementing the IFCDC approach helps establish a nurturing environment that minimises stress and enhances the infant's growth and development by involving family members in both decision-making and daily caregiving activities (GFCNI, 2025). Integrating IFCDC into neonatal care offers numerous advantages for both infants and their families. These benefits include better neurodevelopmental outcomes in areas such as cognition, motor function, and language; increased family involvement; reduction of stress and pain experiences for infants, contributing to overall wellbeing; and reduced length of hospital stays (Maatman et al., 2020; Nourah Alsadaan et al., 2023).

This chapter covers key issues, theory, and principles in infant care, highlighting practices and interventions for healthcare professionals and parents to enhance infant development. Importantly, the preceding chapter on families and the key messages of family integration and inclusion apply also to this chapter.

THEORETICAL APPROACHES TO DEVELOPMENTAL CARE

Over the last 30 years, advancement in the field of neonatology has improved survival and decreased the incidence of major long-term disabilities among the preterm population. However, the increasing survival of low birthweight infants, particularly those at the limits of viability, has created new challenges and neurodevelopmental outcomes for preterm infants and remains a significant concern for health professionals (Boland et al., 2021). Therefore, there remains a genuine need to explore strategies which support outcomes in the neonatal unit (NNU) so that these are optimised during and after transition to home (Dusing et al., 2018) to ensure the best future for our vulnerable patients.

Premature birth disrupts the process of fetal maturation; preterm infants are developmentally unprepared for the experiences they are exposed to in the NNU. While illness and treatments may have adverse effects on the rapidly developing brain, it is the environment of care which is often intensive, stressful, and sometimes traumatic to both preterm infants and their families (Cheong et al., 2020; see Figure 7.1). From birth, the premature infant is subjected to fluctuations in temperature, touch, sound, light, interrupted sleep, parental separation, and a multitude of painful procedures, along with repetitive, non-nurturing handling. The preterm infant's rapidly developing but immature brain is particularly vulnerable within this stressful environment (Bröring et al., 2017).

Family involvement is a foundational principle of IFCDC, recognising the essential role families play in neonatal care. Over the past ten years there has been increasing recognition of the importance of viewing parents as partners in care and allowing parents to take on roles and responsibilities as primary

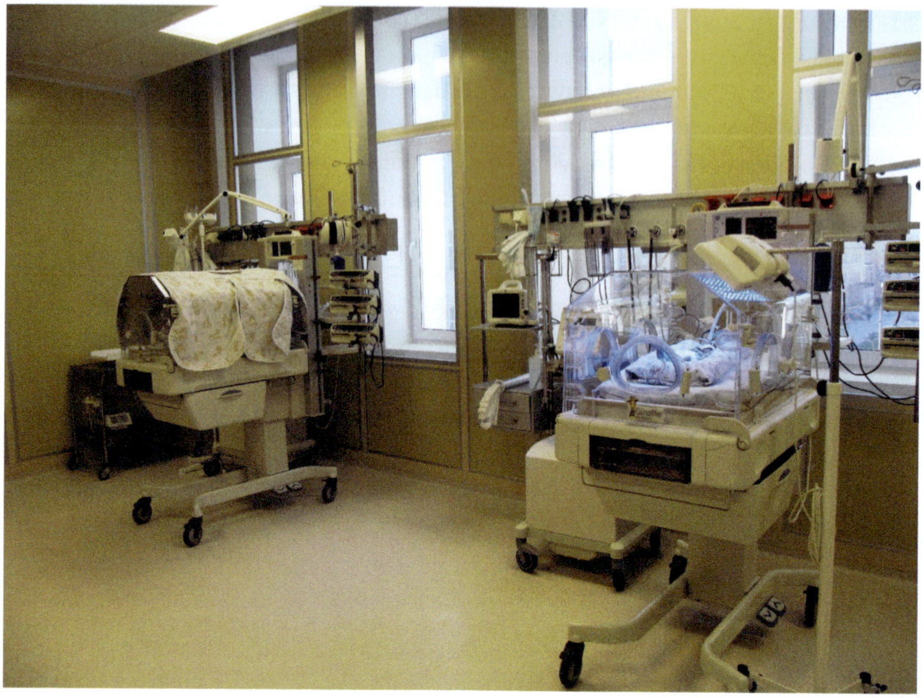

Figure 7.1 The neonatal intensive care environment

caregivers (Toivonen et al., 2020). To enable parents to be involved in their baby's care, many units are developing family support programmes to improve education and psychosocial support for parents (Waddington et al., 2021) within a family integrated care (FiCare) philosophy (Lee & O'Brien, 2018; see Chapter 6 for further information on FiCare).

Preterm infants may spend months in the NNU during a critically important period of brain development. Preterm infants experience multiple noxious stimuli such as toxic light and sound, social deprivation, and chemical exposure, all of which can have a negative impact on neurodevelopment. Optimising the neonatal environment could improve neurobehavioural outcomes for infants born preterm (Cheong et al., 2020). IFCDC is regarded as a neonatal care strategy that integrates the dynamics of evolving family systems with the biological, environmental, and psychological risks associated with preterm birth.

Recognising developmental theory and systematic behavioural assessment, the emphasis of IFCDC provides a more individualised and holistic approach, rather than the general introduction of developmentally supportive initiatives. Individualised assessment is necessary to understand the developmental agenda for the infant and enable care to be delivered contingently according to infant cues.

PRINCIPLES OF INFANT AND FAMILY-CENTRED DEVELOPMENTAL CARE

Developmental support programmes/interventions have been guided by different theoretical models and approaches have varied from single interventions to a collation of individualised developmentally focused care strategies aiming to minimise the negative effects of neonatal intensive care and to maximise infant and family outcomes (Burke, 2018). Representing this transformative shift in neonatal care, the core principles of IFCDC are:

- *Family engagement:* A partnership model which acknowledges the vital role families have in neonatal care, highlighting shared decision-making tailored to the individual needs and strengths of each family.
- *Developmentally supportive environment:* Prioritisation of providing a caregiving environment which is tailored to an infant's specific developmental needs. Key practices embedded within a developmentally supportive environment include managing external stimuli to reduce stress, encouraging skin-to-skin contact (Figure 7.2), and providing proper postural support and gentle touch. Interventions which enhance positive sensory experiences and reduce pain contribute to improved neurological and functional development.

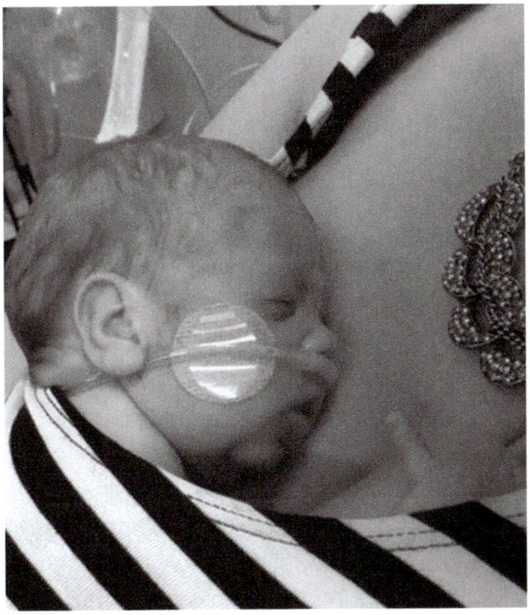

Figure 7.2 Skin-to-skin contact

- *Evidence-based practices*: Interventions should follow evidence-based guidelines and be aligned with the infant's developmental requirements. These include routines to support sleep, strategies to alleviate pain and stress, and strategies which support early feeding experiences.
- *Holistic care approach:* Acknowledging the interrelated medical, developmental, familial, and environmental influences on an infant's wellbeing, this approach promotes interventions that not only address physical health but also nurture emotional and psychological development, ensuring comprehensive care for both infants and their families.
- *Communication and behavioural understanding:* Clear and effective communication among healthcare professionals, infants, and families is a key component of IFCDC. Understanding an infant's behavioural signals and supporting parents in responding appropriately strengthens the parent-infant relationship and supports emotional wellbeing. This focus on behavioural interactions encourages responsive caregiving, which is vital for the development of secure attachment between infants and their parents (GFCNI, 2025).

FAMILY ENGAGEMENT

A key aspect of successfully implementing IFCDC is recognising the differing perspectives between families and healthcare professionals regarding the support provided. Studies indicate that while nurses often feel they offer adequate support, families frequently perceive it as lacking, underscoring the importance of reflective practices to better align care with family needs (Browne et al., 2020; Franck & O'Brien, 2023). Enhancing communication and family involvement fosters stronger collaboration and improves the emotional and psychological support available to families during critical care experiences (Franck et al., 2023).

The birth of an infant that requires admission to a NNU inevitably results in separation of the baby from their parents. The stress, uncertainty, and anxiety that many parents of preterm infants experience can significantly affect development of parent-child bond and parental mental health (Browne, 2021), having a detrimental impact on the successful establishment of the parenting role. The importance of early social interactions between infants and their parents, such as holding, touching, and eye contact, have been well researched in relation to attachment (Siva et al., 2025). There is a plethora of literature advocating the importance of involving mothers in caregiving activities with the aim of improving maternal-infant bonding, attachment, and outcomes (Pineda et al., 2018). There is also increasing information about the experiences of preterm infants' fathers during the NNU stay (Merritt et al., 2022). It is imperative that professionals offer enhanced support to fathers/partners to facilitate their involvement and participation during their newborn infant's admission to the NNU. This is crucial for achieving gender equality and fostering co-parenting. Additionally, it is important to acknowledge the diversity among parents and families. For instance, not all parents have biological ties to their newborn infants, and families may consist of one or multiple parents, as well as parents of the same or different genders. Professionals must approach each of these specific situations with sensitivity, fostering family involvement in the care of the newborn infant (Treyvaud et al., 2019).

With the recent adoption of FiCare, a comprehensive programme for parents of preterm infants (Broom et al., 2017), it is essential that developmental care is included as an interconnected component. These programmes demonstrate many benefits to both parents and infants (Moreno Sanz et al., 2025). Understanding infant behaviour allows parents to recognise their baby's individuality, adjust their expectations, and provide better support tailored to the infant. This involvement helps parents feel more empowered to make decisions about their baby's care.

DEVELOPMENTALLY SUPPORTIVE ENVIRONMENT

The hospital environment can be challenging for infants and their parents. Early brain development is influenced by genetics, but by the third trimester of pregnancy, sensory experiences also play a role. This makes hospitalisation a crucial period since these experiences can affect neurodevelopment through factors like synaptogenesis, synapse elimination, and epigenetics (Montirosso & Provenzi, 2015).

It is crucial to shield infants from harmful environmental stimuli and to facilitate their exposure to beneficial sensory experiences through their parents and other caregivers. Sensory interventions in the NNU should be tailored to the infants' needs and responses, aligning with their current developmental stage, and are optimally delivered through individualised programmes. Skin-to-skin contact remains the most effective strategy to address some of the sensory disruptions associated with preterm birth.

Creating a sensory-supportive environment is informed by an understanding of how the sensory systems develop in very preterm infants, as well as their heightened sensitivity and specific expectations of sensory input. A preterm infant's reactions to environmental stimuli can be observed through physiological, behavioural, and brain-level responses. The infant can easily become stressed, displayed by a variety of signals or cues (see Figures 7.3 and 7.4 and Table 7.1).

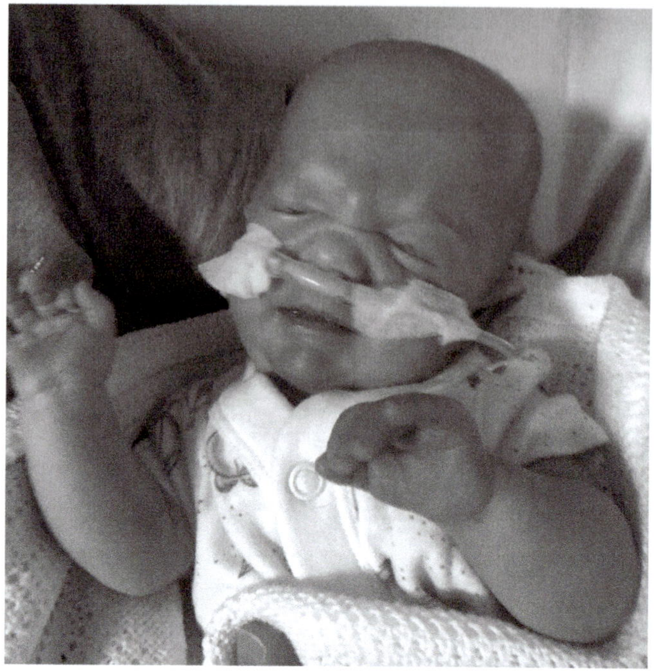

Figure 7.3 The stressed infant

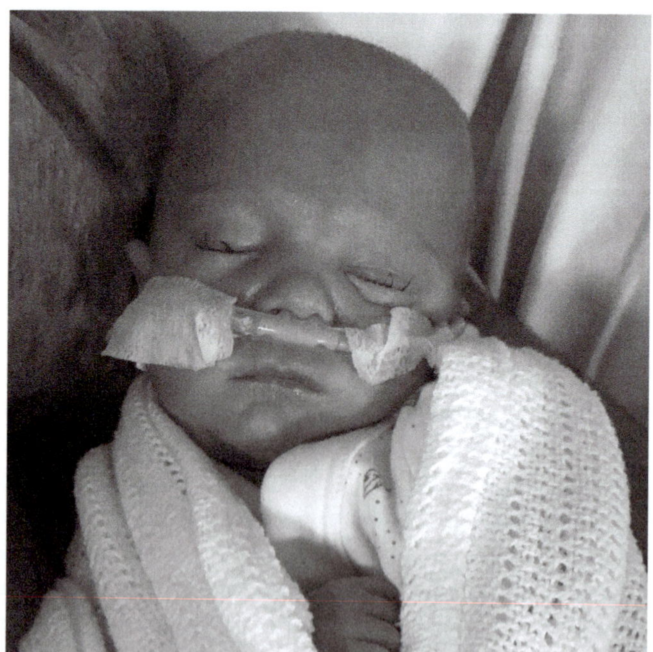

Figure 7.4 The calm infant

TABLE 7.1 STRESS AND STABILITY SIGNALS

Stress signals	*Stability and organisation signals*
Autonomic system	
Respiratory pause, tachypnoea, gagging, gasping, or sighing Colour, vascular, and visceral changes Tremor, twitch, or startle Posset, vomit, or hiccough Bowel strain Cough, sneeze, or yawn	Stable heart rate, respiratory rate, oxygenation, and colour Tolerance of enteral feeds
Motor system	
Hyperflexion; trunk, limbs, fists, feet, neck Protective manoeuvres; hand on face, salute, high guard arm position Frantic, diffuse activity Fixed, stereotypical postures	Smooth, well-modulated movements Relaxed postures and tone, with increasing flexion towards midline Mobility and efficient self-regulatory activity, e.g. ■ hand and foot clasping ■ hand-to-mouth activity, ■ grasping and handholding, ■ suck-searching, and sucking
State system	
Diffuse, oscillating sleep–wake state, whimper or high-pitched cry Strained or irritable fussiness or cry, lack of consolability Eye floating or staring, lack of facial expression, strained or panicked alertness Active averting	Clear, robust sleep states Clear, robust, rhythmic cry Ability to self-quiet or to be consoled Alert, intent, or animated facial expression Focused wide-eyed alertness

Understanding that the environment impacts experience-dependent brain organisation, various effective strategies have been developed to limit infants' exposure to harmful stimuli commonly found in hospital settings, such as painful procedures, excessive noise, strong odours from medical products, and constant bright lighting. These will be further described later in the chapter. Practices such as early skin-to-skin contact and **couplet care**, which ensures continuous proximity and prevents separation between the infant and mother, are designed to maintain close parent-infant interaction. This consistent and predictable multisensory engagement supports improved medical and developmental outcomes for preterm infants. Most of these strategies are included in well evaluated and validated developmental care programmes such as the neonatal individualised developmental care and assessment programme (NIDCAP) (Klein et al., 2021) and family nurture intervention (Woodward et al., 2025).

A HOLISTIC CARE APPROACH

The holistic care approach refers to a comprehensive and integrated model of care that addresses the entire spectrum of needs, medical, developmental, emotional, psychological, and environmental, of both the infant and their family. This approach recognises that an infant's health is deeply influenced by their environment and relationships, especially with their parents. Therefore, as care providers in the NNU, it is imperative that care is not limited to treating medical conditions but also supports the infant's neurological, sensory, and emotional development. Holistic care in IFCDC sees the infant not just as a patient, but as a developing human being embedded in a family, and it ensures that care supports the whole person and their relational context.

Communication and behavioural understanding

Healthcare providers in neonatal care often support parents who experience significant anxiety and fear. This emotional strain on healthcare professionals should be acknowledged and addressed within the neonatal unit environment (Browne, 2021). IFCDC is characterised as a collaborative partnership between parents and healthcare professionals, involving shared responsibility for the infant's care, open communication, cooperation, and joint decision-making. Open communication is essential for establishing a supportive connection between staff and parents, helping parents feel included, enhancing parent-infant attunement, and boosting parents' sense of control.

Preterm infants have the important capacity to communicate their needs and states through subtle behavioural and physiological cues. This unique repertoire of behaviours that caregivers can observe is a window for understanding the developing brain (Vittner & McGrath, 2019).

Well term newborns have stable autonomic and motor systems function and rapidly acquire distinct state system organisation. State refers to the level of consciousness displayed by the infant, which in turn, is determined by the level of arousal and the ability to respond to stimuli. Sleep and drowsy states predominate, but term infants can achieve quiet and active alert states as well as fussy, irritable, and lusty cry states.

Als (1982) was among the first to assert that preterm infants also had distinct behavioural patterns and that it was possible to assess and interpret them. These behaviours are grouped according to five physiological and behavioural subsystems of functioning and include an integrated set of autonomic (respirations, colour, tremors/startles), motor (tone, movement and postures), state (ranges of state and patterns of transitional states), and interaction attention (range and transition into and out of alertness) behaviours (Als, 1986). Preterm infants have immature systems organisation, and their behaviours are consequently more diffuse and less stable. These sub-systems are summarised below:

- The autonomic subsystem is responsible for respiratory, cardiovascular, and digestive functions. This system often needs support to maintain stability, especially when disturbed by handling, environment, pain, or illness. Stability in other subsystems relies on autonomic stability, forming the foundation for more complex developmental tasks.
- The motor system refers to a baby's muscle tone, posture, and movements. Preterm infants have less muscle bulk and power and an immature central nervous system, which can lead to less smooth and purposeful movements, and a flattened, extended posture.
- The state system refers to the ability to attain sleep and wake state. State regulation indicates the maturity of the central nervous system, the infant's interaction with their external surroundings, and their capacity to regulate and maintain internal stability. The pattern and organisation of these states are closely linked to brain development. Sleep and wake cycles start to develop around 26 to 28 weeks of gestation. Preterm infants tend to spend more time in light sleep or drowsy states and often struggle to reach deep sleep. Deep sleep and quiet alertness, when infants are more socially responsive, are rarely seen in NNU settings and typically require support through responsive handling and environmental adjustments.
- The attention-interactional system can be assessed when the infant is in an alert state by considering the infant's success in achieving a balance in the subsystems.

Understanding infant communication involves observing and interpreting infant behavioural cues. These behaviours fall into two categories: stress or avoidance signals, where the stimulation is beyond the infant's capacity to assimilate and approach, or stability signals, where the behaviours demonstrate organisation or self-regulatory activity (Table 7.1). Approach signals inform the observer of the infant's current stable functioning and point to the next level of developmental goals.

PRACTICE POINT

Behaviours should be assessed throughout handling activity, noting the context, infant responses, and environmental influences. A developmental review includes observing infant behaviour, assessing current functioning, and providing personalised recommendations to ensure stability in care. Broader factors like environmental modifications, staff and parent education, and institutional awareness also affect developmentally focused care, but systematic observation is crucial.

EVIDENCE-BASED PRACTICES IN DEVELOPMENTAL CARE

The IFCDC evidence base is built upon research demonstrating the benefits of developmentally supportive care practices for infants and families in NNUs. These practices have been shown to positively impact infant and family outcomes. Developmentally supportive care grounded in evidence emphasises implementing practices that promote healthy sleep, minimise pain and stress, and support early feeding, each tailored to meet the developmental needs of the infant. A model to approach the various elements of developmental care is put forward by Altimier and Phillips (2016; Figure 7.5) with some of these components explained in further detail thereafter and/or in other chapters.

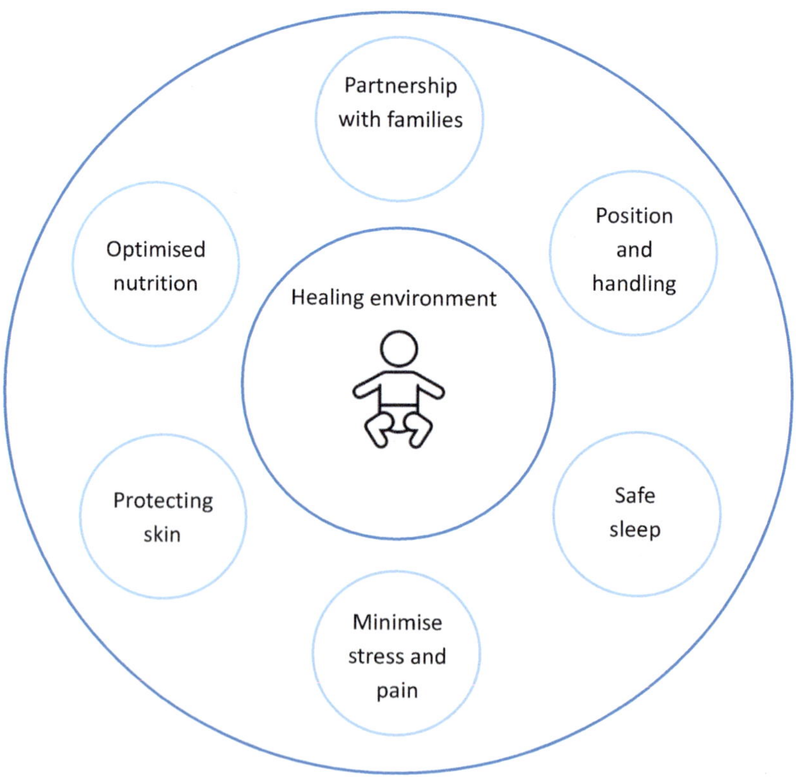

Figure 7.5 A model of Developmental care (Altimier & Phillips, 2016)

Protecting and promoting sleep

Both quantity and quality of sleep are essential to normal growth and development of preterm and term babies. Sleep plays an important role in preterm infants' illness recovery, brain development, and energy utilisation (Mahmoodi et al., 2016). Inpatients in the NNU are exposed to repeated environmental stimuli, causing frequent disruptions to the infant's sleep/wake cycles. With a recognition of the importance of sleep to the developing preterm infant, it is essential that health professionals providing care in the NNU environment incorporate developmentally supportive care strategies into their caregiving routine.

Sleep-state organisation refers to an infant's ability to move smoothly between sleep and wakefulness, and to regulate the transition between different levels of alertness. Active sleep is more commonly seen in earlier gestational ages, while the duration of quiet sleep increases as the infant matures. Sleep and arousal states are associated with physiological functions, including body temperature, breathing, heart rate, and digestion.

The vital role of sleep in conserving energy, promoting growth, and supporting healing for infants in the NNU is well recognised, and protecting infant sleep is commonly recommended as part of developmentally supportive care. An infant's sleep state and arousal level during routine care can affect how they respond to interventions and their readiness to feed (Neukamm et al., 2025). It is essential for neonatal nurses to receive targeted training on the importance of evaluating an infant's sleep and arousal levels before, during, and after care.

Strategies to reduce pain and stress

Extensive evidence confirms that both term and preterm infants experience pain and exhibit both behavioural and physiological pain responses (Walker, 2019). However, the assessment of pain and the application of both pharmacological and non-pharmacological pain management strategies differ widely across NICUs. Chapter 8 will explore infants' experience of and appropriate management for pain and stress in more detail.

Non-pharmacological approaches, such as skin-to-skin contact, have been proven effective in reducing both physiological and behavioural indicators of pain and stress (Zhao et al., 2022). Parents are particularly well suited to take part in these interventions; however, they are frequently excluded during painful or stressful procedures, despite their potential to positively influence the infant's experience during such interventions.

To effectively manage pain and stress in infants, care should be customised based on each baby's specific signals and reactions to interventions. Ensuring consistency in delivering individualised care can be supported through the use of standardised protocols, enabling all caregivers, both healthcare professionals and parents, to respond more uniformly to an infant's signs of pain or stress.

Supporting early feeding experiences

Education on the feeding process is essential and encompasses multiple aspects. A core principle of IFCDC is the need to understand and respond to an infant's cues. In terms of the neonatal environment and its impact on feeding development, in comparison to the gentle and predictable environment of the womb, the neonatal unit is a markedly different and overwhelming experience for infants. Bright lights, noxious smells, and necessary yet invasive medical interventions, such as endotracheal tube placement, continuous positive airway pressure masks, facial tape, and gastric tube placement, can be the infant's first tactile experiences outside the womb (Pados et al., 2025). This can contribute to sensory stress beyond the typical stress associated with the birth process itself, further impacting the infant's adaptation to life outside of the womb (Pineda et al., 2023). These early experiences are especially significant for the preterm infants who are born during a critical period of brain development, where early repeated experiences are shaping neural pathways and the subsequent architecture of the brain (Sarda et al., 2021). Any disruption, such as premature birth or maternal separation, can affect the development of these skills and has the potential to alter feeding experiences throughout childhood (Pados et al., 2021).

Feeding outcomes have been shown to improve with programmes that emphasise observing, interpreting, and reacting appropriately to infant behaviours (Ilahi et al., 2023). Feeding preterm infants or those with medical complexities requires a knowledgeable caregiver who can recognise and adapt to the baby's unique needs (Thoyre et al., 2016). Education should encompass the recognition of physiological stress signs in addition to motor and behavioural state stress indicators. Education and training on infant feeding for families, both within the NNU and after discharge, constitute standard care practices and have been shown to improve feeding outcomes. Chapter 19 will provide an in-depth exploration of supporting infant nutrition and early feeding experiences.

Supportive, cue based, co-regulated care following birth will support later infant-parent feeding confidence, connection, and positive experiences (Thomas et al., 2021). Long-term feeding difficulties, which are common among NNU graduates and often persist post-discharge and into the first two years of life, have been linked to these early sensory and neurodevelopmental experiences (Connell et al., 2023). With thanks to Chapter 19 authors (Murphy et al) for this section on the feeding context.

Managing the sensory environment

When a preterm infant is admitted to a NNU, the immaturity of their physiological systems makes this transition difficult and this environment can create a state of sensory overload in the baby. While there are several sources of stress, of particular concern are non-contingent or aversive handling events; noxious touch experiences, and the effect of sound and light on the sensory modalities of hearing and vision which are particularly immature in the preterm infant. The goal of nursing care then is to create a physical environment and approach to caregiving interventions that support the infant's physiological and neurodevelopmental needs.

There are recommendations for NNU design, including the structure, lighting, noise control, infection control, family space, and other considerations (O'Callaghan et al., 2019). In general, these suggest that there are many practical ways in which subdued calmness and appropriate caregiving commensurate with an infant's developmental maturation can be achieved without making structural changes.

AUDITORY ENVIRONMENT

Early auditory development involves the structural parts of the ears that develop in the first 20 weeks of gestation, and the neurosensory part of the auditory system that reaches the critical stage of development from 25 weeks' gestation to approximately 5–6 months post-term (Graven & Browne, 2008a). *In utero* sounds are muted through a fluid-filled environment. In contrast, on NNU infants are frequently exposed to noise that is often undesirable. Noise may cause apnoea, hypoxaemia, alternation in oxygen saturation, and increased oxygen consumption secondary to elevated heart and respiratory rates and may, therefore, decrease the amount of calories available for growth (Almadhoob & Ohlsson, 2020). The auditory experience is therefore very different, and greater care is needed to protect babies.

Current guidelines recommend that sound levels in the NNU should not exceed the maximum acceptable level of 45 decibels which is equivalent to a quiet library setting (Di Fiore et al., 2024). Optimising the acoustic environment in the NNU is vital; it must be quiet enough to prevent physiological instability yet provide optimal stimuli for cognitive and language development of preterm infants (Chow & Shellhaas, 2016). Maternal voice has been shown to promote weight gain, oral feeding skills, achieving better state regulation, and improved visual and auditory performance (Provenzi et al., 2018).

LIGHT ENVIRONMENT

In NNUs, lighting levels are variable with some units providing continuous high-intensity light and others reduced levels with diurnal patterning. Infants may also be exposed to additional amounts of light from their proximity to windows and the use of medical equipment and procedural lamps.

The visual system of the preterm infant is functionally and structurally incomplete and infants require dimness and sleep to support development (Graven &

Browne, 2008b). When *in utero*, the visual system is developing in the absence of light stimulation. Therefore, the bright lighting conditions in the NNU can provoke stress responses in the infant. Reduced lighting has been found to stabilise the baby's heart rate, respiratory rate, blood pressure, and motor activity. The lighting of clinical areas is an important environmental consideration. Practitioners need to balance the need for soft lighting to promote rest and sleep and support alertness with the need for close observation of the infant. While there are limits to the extent of environmental modification, it is possible to focus on the immediate cot space to reduce the adverse impacts of light exposure on vulnerable infants. Incubator covers can be used to absorb noise and attenuate lighting conditions. Lighting should be adjusted according to the infant's stage of development and strategies should be able to be individualised to accommodate the needs of the caregiver and the infant.

TOUCH

Being born prematurely or ill and requiring admission to a NNU unfortunately exposes infants to necessary but painful and stressful medical procedures. A recent review of observational studies on neonatal pain and stress found that newborns typically undergo a median of 16 procedures daily, with preterm infants experiencing more painful interventions than full term babies. Common procedures include heel lancing, suctioning, venipuncture, catheter insertion, and tape removal, while arterial line insertion and intubation are identified as the most painful (Siva et al., 2025). More robust infants often try to self-regulate through actions like grasping, sucking, and seeking boundaries, whereas more vulnerable infants lack the capacity to mobilise the resources necessary to stabilise and organise their behaviour. There is an association between painful experiences in preterm infants and adverse developmental outcomes, including cognitive and motor development (Pereira & Gaspardo, 2024). Chapter 8 has a detailed focus on pain and stress management in neonatal care.

POSITIVE TOUCH

Providing positive touch can be one of the most effective ways to offer comfort and pleasure to infants. This type of touch is carefully adapted for premature or fragile babies and is delivered based on each infant's individual behavioural and physiological responses (Royal College of Occupational Therapists, 2022). The ability of preterm infants to tolerate and gain benefits from positive touch is limited at earlier postmenstrual ages but improves as they mature; gentle human touch is generally well tolerated by infants between 27 and 32 weeks postmenstrual age.

The provision of skin-to-skin care (SSC) is one of the most well-recognised strategies for supporting parent and infant engagement in positive touch experiences. SSC describes the nappy-clad upright holding of the infant on the chest, providing maximum skin-to-skin contact between the baby and parent. SSC is recognised as a key component of developmentally supportive care because it creates a calm and soothing environment for both the infant and family, positions the infant to support physiological stability and motor development, and supports infant state regulation by aligning care with the infant's sleep-wake cycles.

ACTIVITIES

Explore the following reference for detailed information on the barriers and enablers to SSC in the neonatal unit

Cunningham et al. (2022). Neonatal kangaroo care – what we know and how we can improve its practice: An evidence review. *Journal of Neonatal Nursing*, *28*, 383–387.

Handling and positioning

CONTINGENT CARE

Infant stress resulting from aversive tactile caregiving can be lessened by implementing strategies that help stabilise the infant's condition and avoid overwhelming their ability to process experiences. Autonomic and motor stability can be enhanced through hands-on comfort holding; placing the baby in a concave nest with deep boundaries for postural support; and maintaining flexed, midline positions with proper head support during care activities. Using techniques that respond directly to the baby's signals of approach and avoidance increases the likelihood that the infant will tolerate the intervention. For the most vulnerable infants undergoing potentially stressful procedures, it may be necessary for two caregivers, one of whom may be the baby's parent, to work together: one to provide comfort and maintain the baby's flexed position, and the other to carry out the treatment or care. This method of handling can significantly improve the infant's physiological stability, and evaluating the outcomes of various handling approaches is valuable.

POSTURAL SUPPORT

The delivery of developmental care for infants in the NNU includes the use of individualised postural support strategies for infants. Brain development, along with fetal and newborn movements and posture, plays a key role in musculoskeletal development. In full term infants, the uterine environment in late pregnancy, combined with fetal brain development, promotes a naturally flexed, midline-oriented posture and movements. This midline position is essential for adequate brain development and for reaching future developmental milestones (GFCNI, 2025). In preterm infants these conditions are disrupted. Once born, the force of gravity encourages an extended posture, making it difficult for these infants, due to muscle weakness, to maintain a flexed, midline position. As a result, they often display uncoordinated movements and struggle with self-regulation (GFCNI, 2025).

Inadequate or incorrect positioning of preterm infants in the NNU can lead to physiological instability, behavioural disorganisation, and issues with soft-tissue integrity and postural alignment (Carneiro et al., 2024). Therefore, the goal of positioning in the NNU is to support infants in symmetrical postures in order to reduce infant stress and promote optimal musculoskeletal development (Wiley et al., 2020). Appropriate positioning (see Figures 7.6 and 7.7) promotes self-regulation and facilitates the infant's participation in normal sensorimotor experiences, such as bringing the hand to mouth and face (Skelton et al., 2023). This supportive positioning is intended to be a non-intrusive intervention that allows infants to develop adaptive responses comparable to those of full-term babies.

Key attributes of postural support identified in best practice guidelines (Sweeney & McElroy, 2020) include:

- Provide containment and a sense of security for a smoother adjustment to the extrauterine environment.
- Promote flexion to achieve postural and movement patterns that resemble those of healthy term infants.
- Optimise physiological stability and neurobehavioural organisation to enhance infant self-regulation.
- Maintain proper body alignment to prevent postural asymmetries and head shaping.
- Expose the infant to a variety of postures to prevent the development of fixed postural patterns.
- Maintain skin integrity and prevent skin breakdown.
- Maximise the infant's developmental potential and engagement in family-expected age-appropriate activities and interactions

Using positioning methods customised for each baby has been proven to enhance motor development, boost self-regulation, and help maintain stable breathing. It is important to emphasise that these positioning guidelines apply specifically to interventions for high-risk infants in the NNU. All infants must be transitioned to established safe sleep principles prior to their discharge home.

(a)

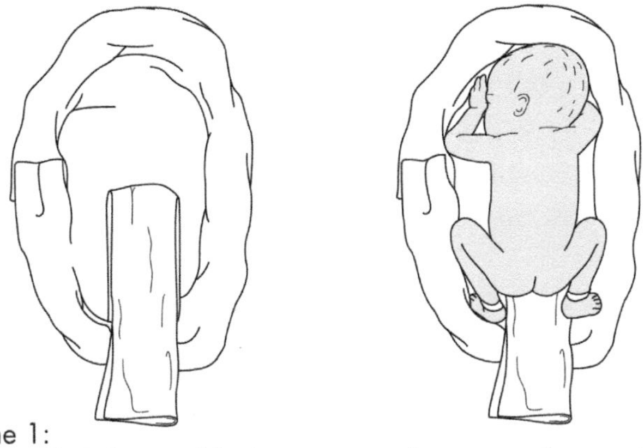

Prone 1:
Softly rolled sheet or blanket positioned in a complete circle. One smaller softly rolled sheet placed over the sheet circle and cover sheet, folded to support pelvic and thoracic lift. Arms and shoulders can be elevated to improve lung function, or fixed and tucked under the thorax. An additional cover may be needed to tuck under the nesting sheet. This serves to draw the nest closer into the infant, supporting flexed containment.

(b)

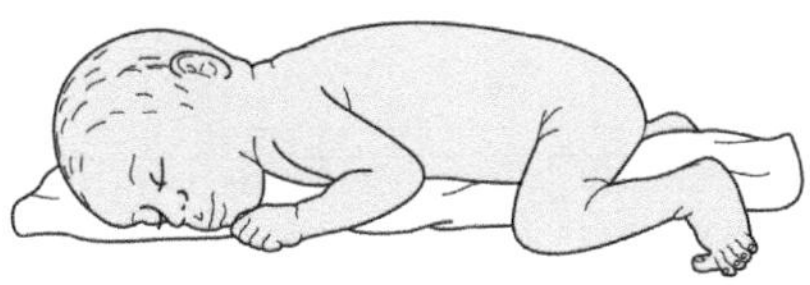

Prone 2:
Nappy roll length-wise under the body from head to hips. This may require additional rolls or blankets across the baby. The head can be supported at an oblique angle, if tolerated.

(c)

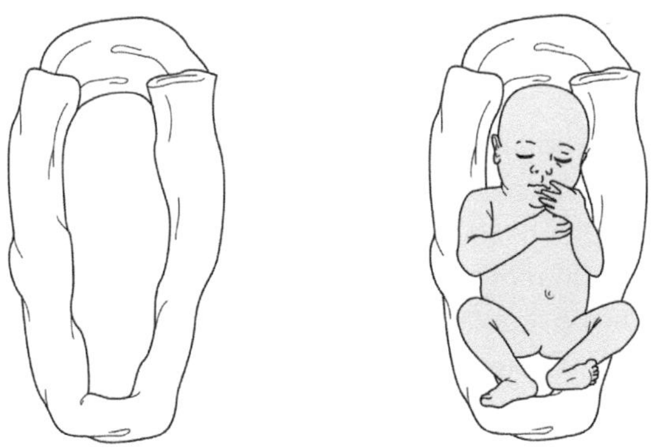

Supine 1:
Soft blanket or sheet rolled into a nest encourages flexion of lower limbs, brings shoulders forward and keeps the head in mid-line. If this continues round the contours of the head it may promote comfort. A small degree of neck flexion, if tolerated, can provide greater stability.

Figure 7.6 Postural support for infants in the NNU – prone and supine (adapted from Edinburgh Sick Children's NHS Trust, Maureen Grant, Superintendent Physiotherapist)

(d)

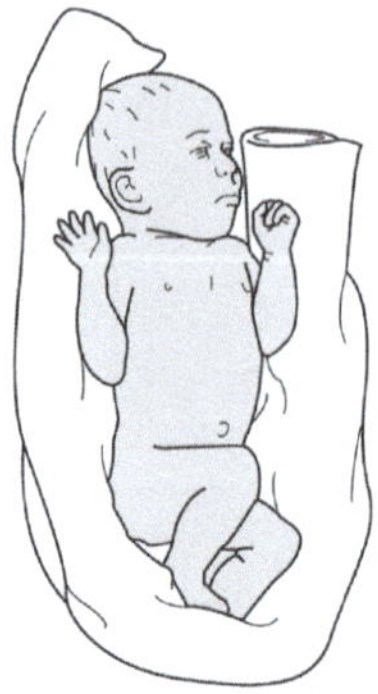

Supine 2:
Supine quarter turns can be utilised to vary position and reduce head flattening.

(e)

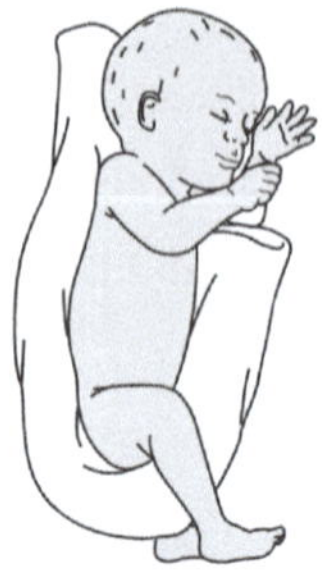

Side-lying:
One firmly rolled blanket in a 'U' shape. May need to be supported by tucked covers. Note the opportunity for tactile and visual stimulation in this position.

Figure 7.7 Postural support for infants in the NNU –supine and side-lying (adapted from Edinburgh Sick Children's NHS Trust, Maureen Grant, Superintendent Physiotherapist)

CRANIAL MOULDING

Premature infants in a Neonatal Intensive Care Unit (NICU) are at greater risk of developing **plagiocephaly** or an associated head deformity because of their malleable cranial bones and respiratory difficulties which may result limited positioning and/or prolonged supine positioning (Yang et al., 2019). Infants with head flattening tend to position themselves preferentially on the flattened side, which can lead to contractures of the neck muscles and **torticollis**.

Preventative measures such as developmentally appropriate positioning can minimise the risk of positional plagiocephaly, with a reduction in bilateral head flattening in infants who receive regular repositioning (Kubik et al., 2024). In addition to repositioning, many infants also benefit from a soft head boundary. When in supine postures, the head can be supported to enable occipital lying, the only position which aims to reduce the incidence and severity of head flattening. This can be achieved using a gel cushion. The use of neck rolls should be avoided as they may cause neck extension and thus, through damage, the delicate vessels at the back of the neck may alter cerebral blood flow.

PRONE POSITION

Prone positions have been demonstrated to improve ventilation and reduce the frequency of bradycardias and desaturations (Shepherd et al., 2020; Barka et al., 2025). It has also been demonstrated to improve sleep quality (Skelton et al., 2023). In prone postures, gravity has its greatest effect. The provision of postural support is imperative to enable the infant to maintain a flexed, midline-oriented position while in prone. Positional supports such as a prone positioner (clavicle to pubis) can be used to elevate the upper trunk to allow for shoulder and hip protraction and prevent over-rotation of the neck. Circumferential boundaries should also be used. As infants mature, prone positions are normally replaced in accordance with the recommendations for reducing the risk of sudden infant death syndrome by supine or side-lying postures.

SUPINE POSITION

Supine positions may be required for medical or surgical reasons; however, they have demonstrated disadvantages including increased stress responses, increased difficulty controlling movements, and incidence of reflux (Wiley et al., 2020; Skelton et al., 2023). Individualised postural support for infants nursed supine should consider the use of supportive boundaries (nests) to prevent shoulder retraction, promote hands to face/mouth, promote hip flexion and avoidance of excessive neck rotation.

SIDE-LYING POSITION

Side-lying postures can be positions of choice for comfort and support an infant's own efforts of self-regulation (Skelton et al., 2023). Side-lying promotes flexion and midline orientation that gravity supporting hand to face/mouth and minimising hip and shoulder rotation and **abduction**. Additional, left side-lying has been demonstrated to reduce **gastro-oesophageal reflux (GOR)** (Pados & Davitt, 2020).

In all positions, it is essential that boundaries are flexible to closely follow the contours of the body. Various commercial products are available for swaddling, **facilitated tucking**, nesting, and stabilising positions, but 'home-made' resources can be equally effective.

Overall for postural care, attention to detail is crucial to the dual goals of prevention of postural deformity and the facilitation of self-regulation and mobility. It is important that position changes are planned to incorporate a varied range of positions. It is also essential to assess the effectiveness of the intervention by ensuring that the infant tolerates the new position and that it supports both mobility and comfort.

THINK POINT

Consider the postural support provided to infants receiving care in your neonatal unit, including what type of aids are available and how they are used to support to individualise care for each infant in promoting flexion, midline orientation, and opportunities for self-regulation in all positions. Also consider how infant comfort and/or postural alignment is assessed to ensure that the postural support provided is meeting the infant's needs.

DEVELOPMENTAL MODELS OF CARE

Developmentally supportive care models are designed to shift neonatal care away from a traditional focus on tasks and procedures, toward an emphasis on caregiving processes and relationship-building, particularly by encouraging greater family involvement. This approach encompasses a variety of targeted interventions or structured programmes. While the specific components and methods of these programmes may vary, they typically share several core features, including:

- Recognising the infant's strengths and vulnerabilities and modifying caregiving approaches according to the infant's communication, medical history, and current medical status.
- Providing individualised care based on the strengths, needs, and availability of each infant and family.
- Recognising the essential nature of the family within the interprofessional team to provide developmental support for the baby.
- Providing environmental protection
- Enabling **neuroprotection** of the developing brain through individualised, sensitive caregiving.
- Incorporating infant mental health strategies.

(Jaeger & Browne, 2022)

As developmentally supportive care programmes have evolved, studies have been conducted to evaluate their effectiveness in enhancing the developmental outcomes of high-risk infants. While research results have shown some variability, evidence of potential advantages has led to the widespread adoption of this approach in many NNUs (Jaeger & Browne, 2022). To fully utilise developmental knowledge, it is essential to incorporate theoretical concepts and practical skills into the model of care. This will ensure that experienced practitioners convey their values to less experienced team members and developmental practice is regarded as an essential component of neonatal nursing care. In fact, factors such as mobility, sensory exposure, comfort, and communication needs are considered to be as important as physiological needs, and developmental considerations become fundamental to neonatal care.

The support of parent–infant relationships is perhaps the most important developmental intervention of all, as it is this relationship which will have the greatest impact on long-term developmental outcome. Developmental models of care must therefore place the emotional and educational needs of parents at the centre of practice. This means going beyond the practical caregiving approach and providing structured support for behavioural observation and contingent handling skills development. Parents should be encouraged to actively contribute to care planning decisions and be fully informed and supported as partners in care.

Chapter takeaways

- Developmental care is a neuroprotective care concept aimed at preventing long-term consequences associated with the environment of care, promoting the optimal organisation and neurodevelopment of preterm infants, as well as involving parents as partners in care.
- Developmentally supportive interventions have the potential to enhance the effectiveness of neonatal services by supporting traditional medical and nursing care.
- Neonatal nurses are the primary caregivers in the neonatal environment; they are in a key position to influence the environment of the developing neonate, as well as therapeutic interventions; however, the provision of an IFCDC approach is the responsibility of all members of the multi-professional neonatal care team.
- An understanding of developmental theory and knowledge of individualised behavioural assessment will serve to promote a creative approach to individualised holistic family-centred care which reflects the fundamental values and beliefs of neonatal nursing.

CASE STUDIES

CASE STUDY

Case study 1: Two-day old premature baby

Jacob is a 2-day-old baby boy born at 24 weeks' gestation. Following a traumatic delivery requiring resuscitation, he is fully ventilated within a humidified incubator and is also being monitored by ECG, pulse oximetry, and arterial line blood gas analysis. He also has an intravenous long line in situ for nutrition and drugs.

Q.1. First, consider the uterine environment: the consistent temperature, gravitational support and containment, attenuated light and sound,

CASE STUDY

and nutritional, hormonal, and psychological influences. Now consider the postnatal environment that Jacob was born into and his early care in the first few hours. How has this affected him and how would you manage the neonatal environment?

As someone who is looking after Jacob and his parents, you watch him for a while and note the following:

You note an infant in light sleep who, upon handling, immediately becomes hyperalert and agitated with extensor postures and 'panicked' facial expression. You have the additional problem of being unable to detect distinct states due to the infant's immature behaviours and the environment in which the infant is nursed.

Q.2. What do you notice about Jacob's behaviour?

Q.3. How would you explain this to the parents and how would you work with the parents to address the behaviours?

Q.4. What developmental care strategies could parents employ with your support, in this case, and why?

Case study 2: Three-week-old premature twin boys

Sebastian and Paulo are 3-week-old twins who were born at 25 weeks' gestation to Italian parents, visiting the UK on holiday. Sebastian has suffered a grade 2 intraventricular haemorrhage on his left side, but regardless of this, he has progressed well and has been taken off all forms of respiratory support, now just requiring some low flow oxygen in the special care unit. Paulo, however, has not progressed so well, had become septic, and was re-ventilated after being on high flow oxygen therapy, currently being nursed in the intensive care unit. He has been diagnosed with a grade 2 and 3 bleed intraventricular haemorrhage on the right and left sides respectively.

Q.1. How would you work with the parents to manage this situation?

Q.2. What strategies are required for both infants to optimise their well-being and prevent any longer-term development problems?

Q.3. What members of the neonatal multidisciplinary team should you involve to also work with the parents?

CASE STUDY

Case study 3: An eight-week-old premature baby on a developmental care programme

Baby Callum was born at 23 weeks and is now 8 weeks old. After a very unstable few weeks, he is starting to show progress in all areas but remains oxygen-dependent with difficulty tolerating his feeds. He has been reviewed by a developmental care specialist who is trained in NIDCAP. Along with the parents, they explain to you about the importance of observing the reactions of Callum in different environmental conditions. They also note the circumstances which support his efforts to quieten and relax or reach alertness. They observe his behaviour during periods of high activity and note the stress responses as well as comparing state system stability in relation to the environment of care.

Q.1. What do these observations and explanations mean to you and why are they important for the infant and family?
Q.2. How can you support the family during this current time in line with these types of observations?
Q.3. What interventions are required, working towards discharge home, to minimise adverse outcomes?

For suggested answer guides to the questions posed in these case studies, please refer to the web-based companion site specific to this chapter. See www.routledge.com/cw/petty

References

Almadhoob, A., & Ohlsson, A. (2020). Sound reduction management in the neonatal intensive care unit for preterm or very low birth weight infants. *Cochrane Database of Systematic Reviews*, *1*, Article CD010333. https://doi.org/10.1002/14651858.CD010333.pub3

Als, H. (1982). Toward a synactive theory of development: Promise for the assessment and support of infant individuality. *Infant Mental Health Journal*, *3*(4), 229–243.

Als, H. (1986). A synactive model of neonatal behavioural organisation: Framework for the assessment of neurobehavioural development in the premature infant and for support of parents in the intensive care environment. In J. K. Sweeney (Ed.), *The high-risk neonate: Developmental therapy perspectives* (pp. 3–53). The Haworth Press.

Altimier, L., & Phillips, R. (2016). The Neonatal Integrative Developmental Care Model: Advanced clinical applications of the seven core measures for neuroprotective family-centered developmental care. *Newborn and Infant Nursing Reviews*, *16*(4), 230–244. https://doi.org/10.1053/j.nainr.2016.09.030

Barka, K., Papachatzi, E., Fouzas, S., Dimitriou, G., & Dassios, T. (2025). Respiratory function in ventilated newborn infants nursed prone and supine. *Pediatric Pulmonology*, *60*(94), e71075.

Boland, R. A., Cheong, J. L. Y., & Doyle, L. W. (2021). Changes in long-term survival and neurodevelopmental disability in infants born extremely preterm in the post-surfactant era. *Seminars in Perinatology*, *45*(8), 151479.

Broom, M., Parsons, G., Carlisle, H., Kecskes, Z., Dowling, D., & Thibeau, S. (2017). Exploring parental and staff perceptions of the family-integrated care model. *Advances in Neonatal Care*, *17*(6), E12–E19.

Bröring, T., Oostrom, K. J., Lafeber, H. N., Jansma, E. P., & Oosterlaan, J. (2017). Sensory modulation in preterm children: Theoretical perspective and systematic review. *PLoS ONE*, *12*(2), e0170828.

Browne, J. V. (2021). Infant mental health in intensive care: Laying a foundation for social, emotional and mental health outcomes through regulation, relationships and reflection. *Journal of Neonatal Nursing*, *27*, 33–39.

Browne, J. V., Jaeger, C. B., Kenner, C., & on behalf of the Gravens Consensus Committee on Infant and Family Centered Developmental Care. (2020). Executive summary: Standards, competencies, and recommended best practices for infant- and family-centered developmental care in the intensive care unit. *Journal of Perinatology*, *40*(Suppl 1), 5–10. https://doi.org/10.1038/s41372-020-0767-1

Burke, S. (2018). Systematic review of developmental care interventions in the neonatal intensive care unit since 2006. *Journal of Child Health Care*, *22*(2), 269–286.

Carneiro, M. M. C., Ribeiro, S. N. S., Menegol, N. A., Okubo, R., Montemezzo, D., & Sanada, L. S. (2024). Nest positioning on motor development, sleep patterns, weight gain in preterm infants: Systematic review. *Pediatric Research*, *96*, 57–63. https://doi.org/10.1038/s41390-023-02972-w

Cheong, J. L. Y., Burnett, A. C., Treyvaud, K., & Spittle, A. J. (2020). Early environment and long-term outcomes of preterm infants. *Journal of Neural Transmission*, *127*, 1–8.

Chow, V. Y., & Shellhaas, R. A. (2016). Acoustic environment profile of the neonatal intensive care unit: High ambient noise and limited language exposure. *Journal of Neonatal Nursing*, *22*(4), 159–162.

Connell, A., Knudsen, K., Marginean, H., & Raddish, M. (2023). Associations between feeding and development in preterm infants in the NICU and throughout the first year of life. *Early Human Development*, *177*, 105719.

Cunningham, C., Patton, D., Moore, Z., O'Connor, T., Bux, D., & Nugent, L. (2022). Neonatal kangaroo care – What we know and how we can improve its practice: An evidence review. *Journal of Neonatal Nursing*, *28*(6), 383–387. https://doi.org/10.1016/j.jnn.2021.10.004

Di Fiore, J. M., Liu, G., Loparo, K. A., & Bearer, C. F. (2024). The effect of early postnatal auditory stimulation on outcomes in preterm infants. *Pediatic Research*, *96*, 1389–1396. https://doi.org/10.1038/s41390-024-03329-7

Dusing, S. C., Tripathi, T., Marcinowski, E. C., Thacker, L. R., Brown, L. F., & Hendricks-Muñoz, K. D. (2018). Supporting play exploration and early developmental intervention versus usual care to enhance development outcomes during the transition from the neonatal intensive care unit to home: A pilot randomized controlled trial. *BMC Pediatrics*, *18*(1), 46.

Franck, L. S., & O'Brien, K. (2023). Gravens by design: Family integrated care: An evidence-based and inclusive model for delivering on your NICU's commitment to family-centered care. *Neonatology Today*. https://neonatologytoday.org/archives/2023/06/1790/

Global Foundation for the Care of the Newborn Infants (GFCNI). (2025). *Infant-and family-centered developmental care*. Retrieved February 14, 2026, from https://www.gfcni.org/maternal-newborn-health/newborn-health/infant-and-family-centered-developmental-health

Graven, S. N., & Browne, J. V. (2008a). Auditory development in the fetus and infant. *Newborn and Infant Nursing Reviews*, *8*(4), 187–193.

Graven, S. N., & Browne, J. V. (2008b). Sensory development in the fetus, neonate, and infant: Introduction and overview. *Newborn and Infant Nursing Reviews*, *8*(4), 169–172.

Ilahi, Z., Capalongo, T., DiMeglio, A., Demissie, S., & Rahman, A. (2023). Impact of an infant-driven feeding initiative on feeding outcomes in the preterm neonate. *Advances in Neonatal Care*, *23*(3), 205–211.

Jaeger, C. B., & Browne, J. V. (2022). The science. In C. Kenner & C. K. J. McGrath (Eds.), *Developmental care of newborns and infants* (3rd ed.). National Association of Neonatal Nurses.

Klein, V., Zores-Koenig, C., Dillenseger, L., Langlet, C., Escande, B., Astruc, D., Le Ray, I., Kuhn, P., & Strasbourg NIDCAP Study Group. (2021). Changes of infant- and family-centered care practices administered to extremely preterm infants during implementation of the NIDCAP program. *Frontiers in Pediatrics*, *9*, 718813. https://doi.org/10.3389/fped.2021.718813

Kubik, A., Welton, J., Holmes, L., Struwe, L., & Gonzales, K. (2024). The PLAY bundle for head deformities: A NICU quality improvement project. *Journal of Neonatal Nursing*, *30*(3), 263–270. https://doi.org/10.1016/j.jnn.2023.10.006

Lee, S. K., & O'Brien, K. (2018). Family integrated care: Changing the NICU culture to improve whole-family health. *Journal of Neonatal Nursing*, *24*(1), 1–3.

Maatman, S. M. O., Bohlin, K., Lilliesköld, S., Garberg, H. T., Uitewaal-Poslawky, I., Kars, M. C., & Van den Hoogen, A. (2020). Factors influencing implementation of family-centered care in a neonatal intensive care unit. *Frontiers in Pediatrics*, *8*, 222.

Mahmoodi, N., Arbabisarjou, A., Rezaeipoor, M., & Mofrad, Z. P. (2016). Nurses' awareness of preterm neonates' sleep in the NICU. *Global Journal of Health Science*, *8*(6), 226–233.

Merritt, L., Maxwell, J., & Urbanosky, C. (2022). The needs of NICU fathers in their own words: A qualitative descriptive study. *Advances in Neonatal Care*, *22*(3), E94–E101. https://doi.org/10.1097/ANC.0000000000000934

Montirosso, R., & Provenzi, L. (2015). Implications of epigenetics and stress regulation on research and developmental care of preterm infants. *Journal of Obstetric, Gynecological and Neonatal Nursing JOGNN*, *44*(2), 174–182.

Moreno Sanz, B., Alferink, M. T., O'Brien, K., & Franck, L. S. (2025). Family integrated care: State of the art and future perspectives. *Acta Paediatrica*, *114*(4), 710–730.

Neukamm, A. C., Quante, M., Poets, C. F., Shellhaas, R. A., & Neonatal Sleep Talks (NEST) Group. (2025). The impact of sleep in high-risk infants. *Pediatric Research*. https://doi.org/10.1038/s41390-025-04049-2

Nourah Alsadaan, N., Ramadan, O. M. E., Alqahtani, M., Shaban, M., Nadia Bassuoni Elsharkawy, N. B., Enas Mahrous Abdelaziz, E. M., & Ali, S. I. (2023). Impacts of integrating family-centered care and development care principles on neonatal neurodevelopmental outcomes among high-risk neonates. *Children*, *10*(11), 1751.

O'Callaghan, N., Dee, A., & Philip, R. K. (2019). Evidence-based design for neonatal units: A systematic review. *Matern Health, Neonatol and Perinatol*, *5*, 6. https://doi.org/10.1186/s40748-019-0101-0

Pados, B. F., Briceno, G., Feaster, V., & Chiu, M. (2025). Prevalence of parent-reported problematic eating behaviours and skills at 8–24 months of age in infants born at less than 34 weeks gestation. *American Journal of Speech-Language Pathology*, *34*(2), 535–546.

Pados, B. F., & Davitt, E. S. (2020). Pathophysiology of gastroesophageal reflux disease in infants and nonpharmacologic strategies for symptom management. *Nursing for Women's Health*, *24*(2), 101–114. https://doi.org/10.1016/j.nwh.2020.01.005

Pados, B. F., Hill, R. R., Yamasaki, J. T., Litt, J. S., & Lee, C. S. (2021). Prevalence of problematic feeding in young children born prematurely: A meta-analysis. *BMC Pediatrics*, *21*(1), 110. https://doi.org/10.1186/s12887-021-02574-7

Pereira, F. L., & Gaspardo, C. M. (2024). Neonatal pain and developmental outcomes in children born preterm: An updated systematic review. *Psychology & Neuroscience*, *17*(1), 1–15. https://doi.org/10.1037/pne0000332

Pineda, R., Bender, J., Hall, B., Shabosky, L., Annecca, A., & Smith, J. (2018). Parent participation in the neonatal intensive care unit: Predictors and relationships to neurobehaviour and developmental outcomes. *Early Human Development*, *117*, 32–38.

Pineda, R., Kellner, P., Ibrahim, C., Sense Advisory Team Working Group, & Smith, J. (2023). Supporting and enhancing NICU sensory experiences (Sense), 2nd edition: An update on developmentally appropriate interventions for preterm infants. *Children*, *10*(6), 961. https://doi.org/10.3390/children10060961

Provenzi, L., Broso, S., & Montirosso, R. (2018). Do mothers sound good? A systematic review of the effects of maternal voice exposure on preterm infants' development. *Neuroscience & Biobehavioural Reviews*, *88*, 42–50. https://doi.org/10.1016/j.neubiorev.2018.03.009.

Royal College of Occupational Therapists. (2022). *Occupational therapy in neonatal services and early intervention: Practice guideline* (2nd ed.). RCOT. https://www.rcot.co.uk/practice-resources/rcot- publications/downloads/neonatal-services

Sarda, S. P., Sarri, G., & Siffel, C. (2021). Global prevalence of long-term neurodevelopmental impairment following extremely preterm birth: A systematic literature review. *Journal of International Medical Research*, *49*(7), 03000605211028026.

Shepherd, K. L., Yiallourou, S. R., Odoi, A., Yeomans, E., Willis, S., Horne, R. S. C., & Wong, F. Y. (2020). When does prone sleeping improve cardiorespiratory status in preterm infants in the NICU?, *Sleep*, *43*(4), zsz256. https://doi.org/10.1093/sleep/zsz256

Siva, N., Nayak, R., & Ghosh, D. (2025). Pain and pain-related stress in high-risk neonates at NICU – a narrative review. *Journal of Neonatal Nursing*, *31*(3), 101675. https://doi.org/10.1016/j.jnn.2025.101675

Skelton, H., Psaila, K., Schmied, V., & Foster, J. (2023). Systematic review of the effects of positioning on nonautonomic outcomes in preterm infants. *Journal of Obstetric, Gynecologic & Neonatal Nursing*, *52*(1), 9–20. https://doi.org/10.1016/j.jogn.2022.09.007

Sweeney, J., & McElroy, J. (2020). *IFCDC: Recommendations for best practice for positioning and touch*. NICU Recommended Standards. University of Notre Dame. Retrieved June 16, 2025, from https://nicudesign.nd.edu/nicu-care-standards/ifcdc-recommendations-for-best-practice-for-positioning-and-touch/

Thomas, T., Goodman, R., Jacob, A., & Grabher, D. (2021). Implementation of cue-based feeding to improve preterm infant feeding outcomes and promote parents' involvement. *Journal of Obstetric, Gynecologic & Neonatal Nursing*, *50*(3), 328–339.

Thoyre, S. M., Hubbard, C., Park, J., Pridham, K., & McKechnie, A. (2016). Implementing co-regulated feeding with mothers of preterm infants. *American Journal of Maternal/Child Nursing*, *41*(4), 204–211.

Toivonen, M., Lehtonen, L., Löyttyniemi, E., Ahlqvist-Björkroth, S., & Axelin, A. (2020). Close Collaboration with Parents intervention improves family-centered care in different neonatal unit contexts: A pre-post study. *Pediatric Research*, *88*(3), 421–428.

Treyvaud, K., Spittle, A., Anderson, P. J., & O'Brien, K. (2019). A multi-layered approach is needed in the NICU to support parents after the preterm birth of their infant. *Early Human Development*, *139*, 104838.

Vittner, D., & McGrath, J. M. (2019). Behavioural assessment. In E. P. Tappero & M. E. Honeyfield (Eds.), *Physical assessment of the newborn: A comprehensive approach to the art of physical examination* (6th ed.). Springer Publishing Company.

Waddington, C., van Veenendaal, N. R., O'Brien, K., Patel, N., & International Steering Committee for Family Integrated Care. (2021). Family integrated care: Supporting parents as primary caregivers in the neonatal intensive care unit. *Pediatric Investigations*, *5*(2), 148–154.

Walker, S. M. (2019). Long-term effects of neonatal pain. *Seminars in Fetal and Neonatal Medicine*, *24*(4), 101005. https://doi.org/10.1016/j.siny.2019.04.005

Wiley, F., Raphael, R., & Ghanouni, P. (2020). NICU positioning strategies to reduce stress in preterm infants: A scoping review. *Early Child Development and Care*, *191*(15), 2333–2350. https://doi.org/10.1080/03004430.2019.1707815

Woodward, L. J., Ludwig, R. J., Gong, A., Myers, M. M., & Welch, M. G. (2025). Family Nurture Intervention and mother-preterm infant autonomic emotional connection in the neonatal intensive care unit: A review. *Acta Paediatrica*, *114*(4), 760–771. https://doi.org/10.1111/apa.17456

Yang, W., Chen, J., Shen, W. Wang, C., Wu, Z., Chang, Q., Li, W., Lv, K., Pan, Q., Li, H., Ha, D., & Zhang, Y (2019). Prevalence of positional skull deformities in 530 premature infants with a corrected age of up to 6 months: A multicenter study. *BMC Pediatrics*, *19*(1), 520. https://doi.org/10.1186/s12887-019-1864-1

Zhao, Y., Dong, Y., & Cao, J. (2022). Kangaroo Care for relieving neonatal pain caused by invasive procedures: A systematic review and meta-analysis. *Computational Intelligence and Neuroscience*, *2022*(1), 2577158. https://doi.org/10.1155/2022/2577158

8 MANAGEMENT OF PAIN AND STRESS IN THE NEONATAL UNIT

Jenni Jones

CONTENTS

DOI: 10.4324/9781003591405-11

GUIDANCE ON HOW TO ENHANCE PERSONAL LEARNING FROM THIS CHAPTER

Key points covered in this chapter

- The pathophysiology and long-term effects of pain in neonates
- Neonatal pain assessment tools and management strategies
- Parental perception of pain in the neonatal unit

Reflection

Reading through the chapter, you are encouraged to engage with the key points and related literature in an enquiring way. Ask these questions:

- Why is the recognition and management of neonatal stress and pain so important?
- What is the wider impact of stress and pain in the neonatal unit? Consider short- and long-term outcomes and how it may affect families.
- What measures for pain management are in place in your work environment? Do you need to address this?

Implications for nursing care

- Finally: How will this chapter enable you to holistically assess and manage pain and stress experienced by the infants in your care? Consider the implications of what you learn for your nursing practice relating to this area.

INTRODUCTION AND BACKGROUND

Sick and premature neonates admitted to neonatal intensive care units (NICUs) are exposed to an average of 14 painful procedures per day (Williams & Lascelles, 2020), with most procedures inflicting mild-moderate to severe pain (Laudiano-Dray et al., 2020). Contrary to earlier beliefs, research over the past three decades has demonstrated that due to the immaturity of their nervous system, neonates experience a hypersensitivity to painful stimuli (Perry et al., 2018). In addition, research has revealed that prolonged and/or repeated exposure to pain during early neonatal life has both short- and long-term detrimental effects and adversely affects physiological, neurological, psychosocial, and behavioural development of infants (Williams & Lascelles, 2020).

The effective prevention and management of neonatal pain is therefore of crucial importance. Moreover, access to pain management within the healthcare setting is globally perceived as a fundamental human right (Brennan et al., 2019), and healthcare professionals (HCPs) have a moral and ethical obligation to assess and manage the pain of all infants in their care (Ilhan et al., 2020).

Nurses prevail on the front line in ensuring that neonates and their families receive the best care for managing painful interventions. Despite an overwhelming volume of research, an evidence-practice gap for the assessment and management of pain in neonates persists (Zhao et al., 2022).

DEVELOPMENT OF PAIN PATHWAYS

Pain pathways consist of a network that communicates unpleasant sensations of noxious stimuli throughout the body. At birth, neonates have a developing and incomplete myelinated nervous system; however, all the components of the nociceptive (pain) pathways are present. Thus, a newborn infant's nervous system is fully capable of transmitting, perceiving, responding to, and remembering noxious stimuli even though it is not yet fully developed.

Nociception (the detection of noxious stimuli) occurs when harmful impulses are transferred to the spinal cord through thinly myelinated and unmyelinated nerve fibres (see Figure 8.1).

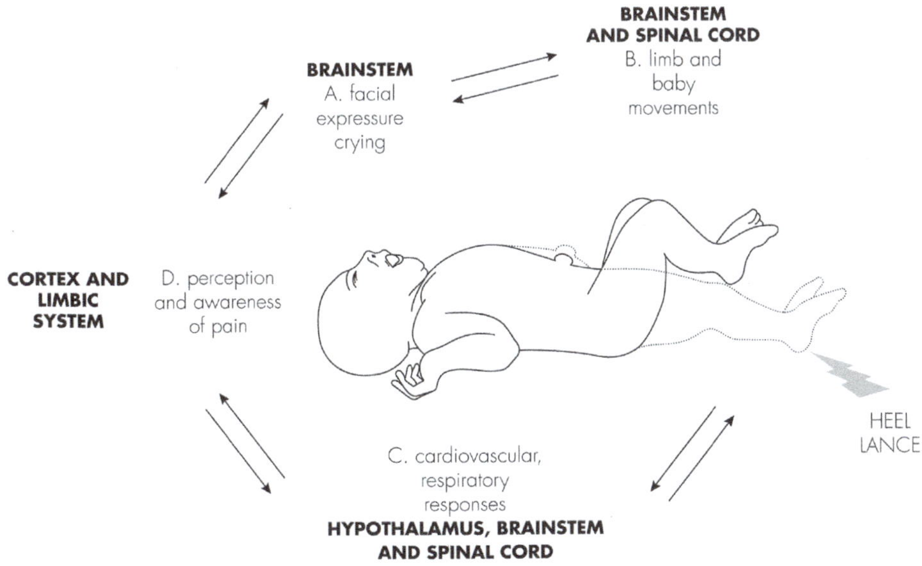

Figure 8.1 Pain pathways in the neonate (adapted from Slater et al., 2007, with permission from Elsevier)

Three key aspects of sensory processing in the spinal cord underlie responses to pain in the neonate. First, an infant's spinal sensory nerve cells are more excitable than an adult's. This makes their spinal reflex response to a harmful stimulus much greater and more prolonged. Second, individual sensory nerve cells in neonates have a much larger area of skin, or receptive fields, than in adults. This means reflex responses can be triggered from a larger body area. Receptive fields combine to form a 'map' or image of our body surface in our brain and enable us to locate a stimulus in a particular part of our body. In neonates, the larger receptive fields result in a less precise or 'smeared' body map, where the newborn responds less selectively and produces the same reflex to a light touch (Tucker et al., 2023).

PAIN AND STRESS

The terms 'neonatal pain' and 'neonatal stress' are often used interchangeably. Stress responses can be specific to a particular source or non-specific and more generalised. Stress is not necessarily painful, and in the preterm infant, a stress response may be elicited by routine procedures such as a nappy change, as well as environmental factors including excess light and noise. On the other hand, pain caused by skin-breaking or invasive procedures is always stressful. Figure 8.2 outlines the context of pain or stress when assessing pain in neonates.

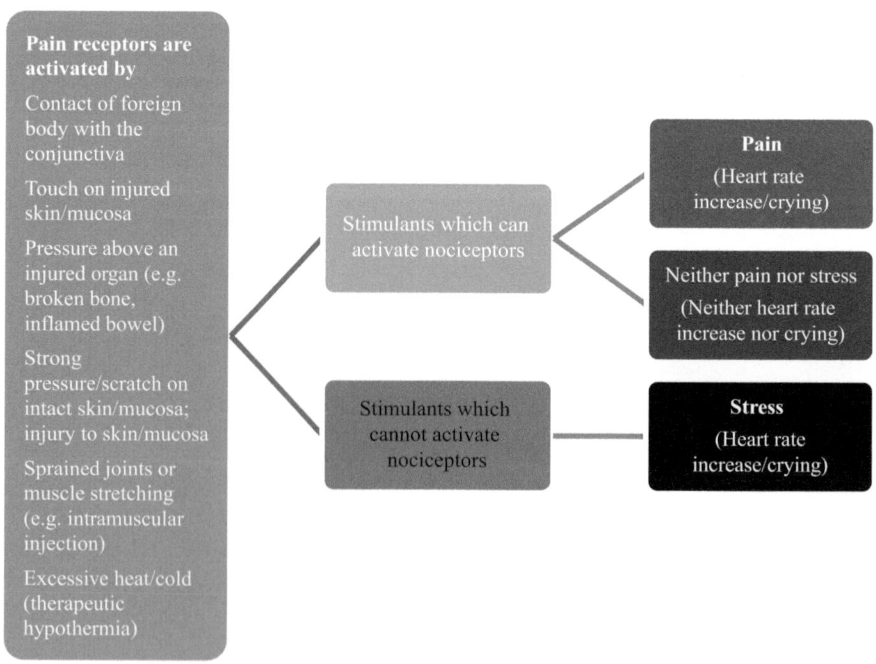

Figure 8.2 Contextual assessment of pain (adapted from Bellieni et al., 2015)

Both pain and stress lead to an immediate disturbance of vital signs, including an increase in heart rate as well as mean arterial pressure, and a drop in oxygen saturation levels in both term and preterm infants (Agrawal & Samayam, 2025). Furthermore, exposure to either pain or stress during the neonatal period results in the same adverse impact on long-term developmental outcomes (British Association of Perinatal Medicine (BAPM), 2025; Siva et al., 2025).

EARLY PAIN EXPERIENCES AND LONG-TERM OUTCOMES

During their stay on the neonatal unit (NNU), infants experience a plethora of painful procedures, including heel-lancing, venepuncture, and endotracheal tube suctioning. Frequently, pain is experienced as an acute event which has an immediate onset and a clearly defined end point, usually once the procedure it is associated with comes to a conclusion. On other occasions, infants may experience prolonged or chronic pain, lasting longer and persisting despite treatment attempts, and which may cause changes in the nervous system, including increased sensitivity to pain and a pain response from normally non-painful stimuli (Ilhan et al., 2022).

The **plasticity** of the developing brain contributes to its vulnerability to the stressors that cause long-term developmental changes, ultimately leading to adverse neurological outcomes. A multitude of studies have highlighted the detrimental impact of early pain experience upon physiological, neurological, psychosocial, and behavioural development of infants, in particular those born preterm (Williams & Lascelles, 2020; van Dokkum et al., 2021). Boggini et al. (2021) found that cumulative experiences of procedural pain in preterm infants was associated with a reduction of both white and grey matter volume at school age, while Pavlyshyn et al. (2024) reported a reduction in interpersonal, communication and problem-solving abilities in preterm infants exposed to pain and stressful experiences during early life when followed up at 24–30 months corrected gestational age (GA). Psychosocial impairment, including increased anxiety, depression and internalisation of negative behaviours is associated with early exposure to painful procedures (William & Lascelles, 2020), as is an increased risk of developing autism in later life (Cook et al., 2023).

The message for the neonatal nurse is that being aware of the consequences of pain, no matter how harmless it may appear, is to know that it has the potential to cause harm. Modifications of practice to meet the individualised needs of each infant should be part of every nurse's practice.

FAMILY INVOLVEMENT IN PAIN MANAGEMENT

Parents of infants in the NNU may worry that their baby is experiencing pain, and this concern will undoubtedly contribute to increased parental stress. Frequently, parents have a strong desire to be present during painful procedures and to play an active part in mitigating their baby's pain (Ullsten et al., 2021). Parental involvement in pain management strategies can significantly reduce neonatal pain (Eissler et al., 2022), and recognising parents as part of the healthcare team positively correlates with a multitude of improved short and long-term outcomes for the infant, including improved growth, reduced supplemental oxygen requirement, improved infection rates, and shorter duration of hospital stay (Waddington et al., 2021; BAPM, 2025). Despite this, a theory-practice gap persists, as in clinical practice methods of pain management involving parents frequently remain underused (Ullsten et al., 2024). Whilst nurses may be reluctant to involve parents in pain management in order to protect their mental health and for fear of causing additional stress during an already traumatic time, parents themselves can feel empowered when involved in the assessment and management of their baby's pain. Assigning them an active role in the process and encouraging them to embrace their role as primary caregiver can allow parents to regain a sense of control, thereby improving their mental wellbeing.

With support, parents can become actively involved in all aspects of pain management. They are often ideally placed to participate in pain assessment due to their consistent presence at the cot side and their sensitivity to subtle changes in their baby's condition. Furthermore, they can play an active role in delivering non-pharmacological pain management interventions. Skin-to-skin kangaroo care, non-nutritive sucking at the breast or pacifier, and facilitated tucking delivered by parents have been shown to be effective methods to reduce pain expression during painful procedures (Eissler et al., 2022). Other parent-delivered strategies may include massage, singing, swaddling, or a combination of a number of interventions (Ullsten et al., 2021), and in order to give parents the opportunity to deliver these it is crucial to schedule non-urgent procedures for times when they are likely to be present at the cot-side.

Parents may feel anxious about participating in their baby's pain management due to a perceived lack of knowledge and skills or for fear of getting in the way or appearing demanding. Good communication from the healthcare team is paramount when supporting parents to take on an active role in infant pain management, as is revisiting the subject on a regular basis due to the fact that parents' feelings towards participating in comforting their baby during painful procedures may change over time.

Box 8.1 contains suggestions for a parent-information brochure about the support parents can offer their baby to mitigate the effects of pain and stress. Table 8.1 lists the important discussion points to be covered when talking to parents about painful procedures.

BOX 8.1 EXAMPLE OF A PARENT INFORMATION BROCHURE ABOUT SUPPORTING THEIR BABY DURING A PAINFUL PROCEDURE

Observing your baby for signs of pain

Over the coming days, you will get to know your baby and start to recognise when they are uncomfortable, stressed, or in pain. Signs that your baby is experiencing discomfort can include crying, yawning, grimacing, or placing a hand in front of their face. For some babies, especially those born prematurely, it is difficult to show that they are experiencing pain. But it will become easier for you to spot the signs once you have had the chance to get to know them a bit better. You may also see a change in your baby's heart rate, a drop in their oxygen levels, or pauses in their breathing when he or she is uncomfortable.

You can support your baby by alerting the healthcare team of any signs that he or she is unhappy.

Being present during procedures

Holding your baby during a procedure can be comforting for him or her. However, some parents feel that this is too uncomfortable for them to do. If for any reason you are not able to be there, the nursing staff will comfort and support your baby instead.

How to comfort your baby

If a procedure is required that is likely to cause your baby pain, there are many ways in which you can comfort him or her. If you are breastfeeding, you can give your baby a breastfeed a couple of minutes before the procedure, and you may even be able to carry on feeding while it is ongoing. During some procedures, you may be able to have your baby skin-to-skin so they can be soothed by your touch and smell. Where this is not practical, the nursing staff can show you other ways to hold, comfort, and support your baby.

TABLE 8.1 TALKING TO PARENTS ABOUT PAINFUL PROCEDURES (ADAPTED FROM BLISS UK)

WHAT is going to happen	Explain the procedure in simple terms. Acknowledge if it is likely to cause pain/discomfort to their baby. Try to avoid terms that are likely to influence their decision such as 'you don't want to see this.'
WHY it is needed	Give the rationale and expected outcome using simple language.
HOW parents can be involved	Explain how parents can support their baby if they wish to, and explain what the benefits of parental touch are. Show them ways in which they can comfort their baby before and during the procedure.
WHEN it is expected to happen	Ensure that parents know the timing of any procedures to enable them to be present, if they want to be.
Questions?	Give the opportunity to ask questions and communicate their thoughts, feelings, and preferences.

THINK POINT

Think of the last time you had to perform a painful procedure on a baby. Were the parents present? Did they take part in supporting their baby? If not, why? What else could you have done to empower them to take on an active role during the event?

ASSESSMENT OF NEONATAL PAIN

The neonatal nurse plays a crucial role in the assessment of pain, which should form part of routine observations. However, nurses can find the assessment of neonatal pain challenging, as neonatal pain signals are frequently complex, subtle, or lacking altogether, particularly in sedated, premature, and severely ill infants. Consequently, neonatal pain often remains underassessed by nursing staff (Carlsen Misic et al., 2021). Table 8.2 provides an overview of common behavioural and physiological pain signals in neonates.

Furthermore, standardised pain assessment tools remain underused in neonatal nursing care (Mala et al., 2021). This may be due to lack of integration of pain scoring

TABLE 8.2 NEONATAL PAIN AND STRESS SIGNALS

Category	*Description*
Behavioural Signs	
Alertness	- Hyper alertness, in particular during prolonged pain - Prolonged time to self-soothe and return to rest - Reduced sleep quality
Body	- Yawning - Hiccupping - Finger and toe splaying - Back arching - Limb withdrawal away from painful stimulus, usually in term infants - Term/Strong infants: Increased muscle tension of all four limbs - Preterm and sick infants: Flaccidness
Crying	- Term/Well infants: Crying which intensifies with longer duration of painful stimulus - Preterm/Sick infants: Weak moaning, or vocal reaction may be absent altogether
Facial Activity, grimacing	- Most commonly observed facial expressions: * Brow bulge * Squeezed eyes * Distinct furrows from the nose to the corners of the mouth * Tense and stretched mouth and tongue * Raised cheeks
Physiological Signs	
Heart Rate and Heart Rate Variability (HRV)	- Term/Well infants: Increased heart rate, increased blood pressure, and red skin colour - Preterm/Sick infants: Heart rate may increase or decrease, bradycardias are possible - Pain, in particular prolonged, reduces HRV
Respiration Rate	- Term/Well infants: Tachypnoea due to fight-or-flight response - Preterm infants: Decreased respiration rate, apnoea may be observed
Oxygen Saturation	- Changes in oxygen saturation following pain-associated changes in respiration and heart rate - Saturations may increase or decrease, depending on context
Cortisol	- Increased levels following painful procedures or surgery

Adapted from Campbell-Yeo et al. (2022).

charts into routine clinical practice, or because the prevailing lack of a universal pain assessment chart that is suitable to be utilised for all neonates. At present, there are over 35 pain assessment instruments available for use in the NNU; however, none can be recommended as gold standard, as different tools are suitable for different patients (Arabiat et al., 2023). The nurse must therefore choose a pain scoring tool depending on gestational age, type of painful stimulus and the infant's environment. Some tools available also score level of sedation, thereby rendering them suitable for the assessment of ventilated or post-operative infants receiving regular analgesia or continuous opiate infusions. In the United Kingdom (UK), guidance on the selection of a suitable pain scoring tool has recently been published (BAPM, 2025).

Utilising a pain scoring tool can enable the assessment of the level of pain, open up the dialogue between clinicians and lead to joint decisions in the management of an infant's pain or discomfort. Any pain assessment tool used to guide clinical practice must be reliable and validated; however, due to conflicting, often contradictory evidence, this can be difficult to achieve (Giordano et al., 2019; Arabiat et al., 2023).

Table 8.3 describes some of the assessment tools in current use.

ACTIVITY

Think about the pain assessment tool used on your unit. Do you think it is suitable for the babies in your care? Consider the different tools listed in Table 8.3. Might one of these be better at assessing pain in the babies you look after?

TABLE 8.3 OVERVIEW OF PAIN ASSESSMENT TOOLS

Tool	*Measured Variables*	*Type of pain*	*Population*	
APN (Acute Pain in Neonates) (Carbajal et al., 1997)	Facial expression, crying, limb movement	Procedural/ Acute	Preterm neonates Term neonates	One of the pain assessment tools recommended by the American Academy of Paediatrics. Potential high risk of bias
BIIP Behavioural Indicators of Infant Pain (Holsti & Grunau, 2007)	Sleep/wake states, five facial actions and two hand actions.	Procedural/ acute	Preterm neonates Term neonates	Reliability, moderate concurrent validity with a multidimensional pain scale (NIPS)

TABLE 8.3 (CONT.)

Tool	*Measured Variables*	*Type of pain*	*Population*	
CHIPPS (Children's and Infants' Post-operative Pain Scale) (Büttner & Finke, 2000)	Facial expressions, crying, leg and trunk posture, degree of restlessness	Post-op	Preterm neonates Term neonates	Reliability, validity, clinical utility with low to moderate risk of bias
COMFORT (van Dijk et al., 2005)	Movement, calmness, facial tension, alertness, respiration rate, muscle tone, heart rate, blood pressure.	Prolonged Procedural/ acute Sedation	Preterm neonates Term neonates	Reliability, validity, clinical utility with low risk of bias, includes assessment of sedation
COMFORT B (Caljouw et al., 2007)	Alertness, agitation, respiratory effort, movement, muscle tone, facial expressions	Prolonged Procedural/ acute Ventilated Sedation	Preterm neonates Term neonates	Reliability, validity, clinical utility with low risk of bias, includes assessment of sedation
COMFORTneo* (Meesters et al., 2023)	Alertness, calmness/agitation, respiratory response, crying, body movement, facial tension, and muscle tone	Prolonged	Preterm neonates	Reliability and validity, correlates well with other pain scales
EDIN (Échelle Douleur Inconfort Nouveau-Né, Neonatal Pain and Discomfort Scale) (Debillon et al., 2001)	Facial movements, sleep-wake pattern, consolability, limb movements, interaction with caregivers	Prolonged	Preterm neonates	High degree of validity with low risk of bias
EVENDOL (Evaluation Enfant Douleur/Child Pain Assessment) (Fournier-Charrière et al., 2012)	Facial expressions, crying, posture and movement, interaction with environment	Procedural/ acute	Term neonates	High degree of validity with low risk of bias

TABLE 8.3 (CONT.)

Tool	*Measured Variables*	*Type of pain*	*Population*	
FLACC (Face, Legs, Activity, Cry and Consolability) (Merkel et al., 1997)	Facial expressions, limb movement cry and consolability, activity	Procedural/ acute Post-op	Term neonates	High degree of interrater reliability but lack of evidence for content validity
N-PASS* (Neonatal Pain, Agitation and Sedation Scale) (Hummel et al., 2007)	Crying, irritability, behavioural state, facial expression, extremity tone, vital signs	Prolonged Procedural/ acute Sedation	Preterm neonates Term neonates	High degree of reliability and validity, includes sedation end of scale
NFCS (Neonatal Facial Coding System) (Peters et al., 2003)	Facial expressions, eyes squeezed, bulging brow, open lips, taut tongue, and deepening of nasolabial folds	Prolonged Procedural/ acute	Preterm neonates Term neonates	Reliability, validity, clinical utility, high degree of sensitivity to analgesia
NIPS* (Neonatal Infant Pain Score) (Lawrence et al., 1993)	Facial expression, crying, breathing patterns, arm and leg movements, arousal	Procedural/ acute	Preterm neonates Term neonates	Reliability, validity
PAT (Pain Assessment Tool) (Spence et al., 2005)	Physiological, behavioural, nurse's, perception	Post-operative Ventilated	Preterm neonates Term neonates	Reliability and validity, comfort measures part of use, clinical utility
PIPP-R* (Premature Infant Pain Profile – Revised) Gibbins et al., 2014)	Heart rate, oxygen saturation, facial actions; takes state and gestational age into account	Prolonged Procedural/ acute	Preterm neonates Term neonates	Reliability, validity, clinical utility well established

* recommended tools in the BAPM framework (2025)
Collated from Giordano et al. (2019) and Arabiat et al. (2023)

MANAGEMENT OF PAIN, STRESS, AND DISCOMFORT

Comfort/non-pharmacological interventions

The first line of pain management is to ensure basic comfort measures are instituted. These include positioning the infant in a non-stressful way and ensuring there are boundaries in-situ to assist in self-regulation as a method of relieving stress, the use of a pacifier to encourage non-nutritive sucking, and ensuring the nappy is dry and comfortable. Modification of environmental factors to ensure lights are dimmed, and the noise and activity kept to a minimum, can further promote wellbeing and decrease the likelihood of a stress response.

To protect the neurodevelopment of preterm and sick term infants and to provide best practice in neonatal intensive care, emphasis has been put on humane neonatal care, individualised developmentally supportive care, and family integrated care (Soleimani et al., 2020); these are discussed in detail in Chapters 6 and 7. There are many non-pharmacological interventions that can be implemented either singularly or in conjunction with each other, many of which have been shown to be effective in reducing neonatal pain without the risk of causing adverse reactions (Shen et al., 2022), and consequently, the initial focus should be on utilising these to address neonatal pain. Box 8.2 lists the most common non-pharmacological strategies, as well as the actions and evidence for reducing pain and/or stress during acute pain interventions. Figure 8.3 depicts a suggested non-pharmacological approach to the management of procedural pain.

BOX 8.2 NON-PHARMACOLOGICAL PAIN MANAGEMENT STRATEGIES IN NEONATAL CARE

Non-nutritive sucking

- Sucking on a pacifier, finger, or empty breast for a purpose other than nutritional
- Reduces physiological and behavioural response to pain
- Reduces pain reactivity
- Improves immediate pain regulation
- Low-certainty evidence due to limitations and potential risk for bias in existing studies (Pillai et al., 2023)

Breastfeeding

- Reduces crying time
- Reduces physiological and behavioural response to pain, reflected in

overall lower pain scoring on NIPS, NFCS, and APN pain assessment tools
- Moderate-certainty evidence due to some limitations and potential risk for bias in existing studies (Shah et al., 2023)

Breastmilk administration

- **Buccal** administration of small amounts of expressed breastmilk
- Reduces crying time
- Reduces physiological and behavioural response to pain, reflected in overall lower pain scoring on NFCS and APN pain assessment tools
- Moderate certainty evidence due to some limitations and potential risk for bias in existing studies (Shah et al., 2023)

Sucrose therapy

- Buccal administration of oral sucrose
- May reduce crying time
- May reduce physiological and behavioural response to pain, reflected in overall lower pain scoring on PIPP pain assessment tool
- Low-certainty evidence due to limitations, potential risk for bias in existing studies and lack of homogeneity of existing studies (Yamada et al., 2023)

Swaddling

- Prevention of excess movement of limbs by tightly wrapping the infant to stimulate **proprioceptive** system
- Reduces pain reactivity in term infants
- Improves immediate pain regulation in term and preterm infants
- Low-certainty evidence due to limitations and potential risk for bias in existing studies (Pillai et al., 2023)

Facilitated tucking

- The infant is placed in a midline position and the legs, arms, torso, or head are gently cradled (see Figure 8.4)
- Reduces pain reactivity
- Improves immediate pain regulation
- Reduces crying time
- Low to very low-certainty evidence due to limitations and high risk for bias in existing studies (Pillai et al., 2023)

Kangaroo care

- Placing the infant onto the parent's chest, usually as skin-to-skin contact, to stimulate proprioceptive system
- Reduced pain intensity
- Reduced physiological and behavioural response to pain, reflected in overall lower pain scoring on PIPP pain assessment tool
- Low risk of bias in most studies, but high heterogeneity in existing studies (Sharma & Ruikar, 2022)

Touch/Massage

- Gentle touch to provide tactile and **kinaesthetic** stimuli
- Modulates behaviour to pain response
- Reduces pain reactivity
- Improves immediate pain regulation
- Reduces crying time
- Low to very low-certainty evidence due to limitations and high risk for bias in existing studies (Pillai et al., 2023)

Auditory

- Exposing the infant to soothing sounds, including maternal voice recordings and white noise
- Affects descending pain modulation mechanism
- Improves immediate pain regulation
- Reduces crying time
- Low to very low-certainty evidence due to limitations and high risk for bias in existing studies (Pillai et al., 2023)

Pharmacological interventions

Pharmacological agents may be required to alleviate pain in hospitalised neonates who are subjected to numerous invasive procedures, or during the post-operative period. There is considerable clinical and experimental evidence to support the practice of providing adequate analgesia for newborns undergoing invasive medical, surgical, diagnostic, or therapeutic procedures, or who develop conditions associated with considerable pain, such as necrotising enterocolitis.

Figure 8.5 depicts a suggestion of escalating analgesia in neonates. It is recommended that all NNUs have a plan for the use of analgesia, and this

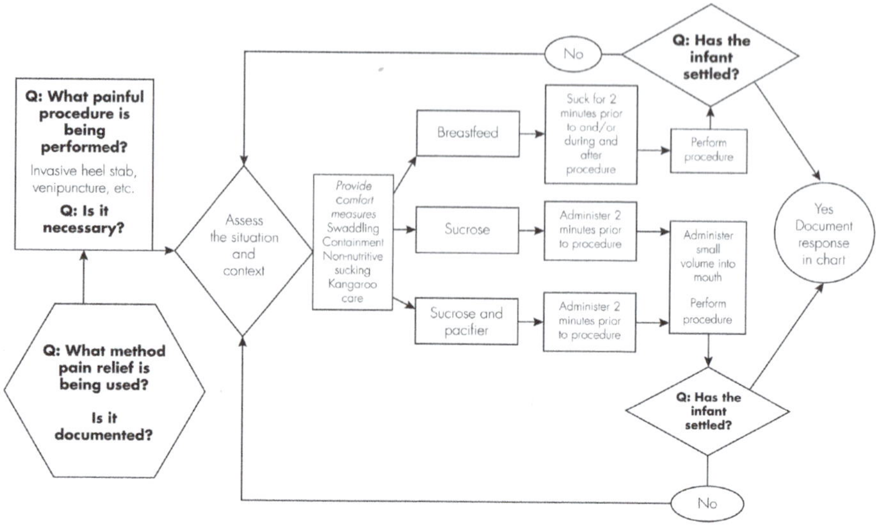

Figure 8.3 An approach to procedural pain

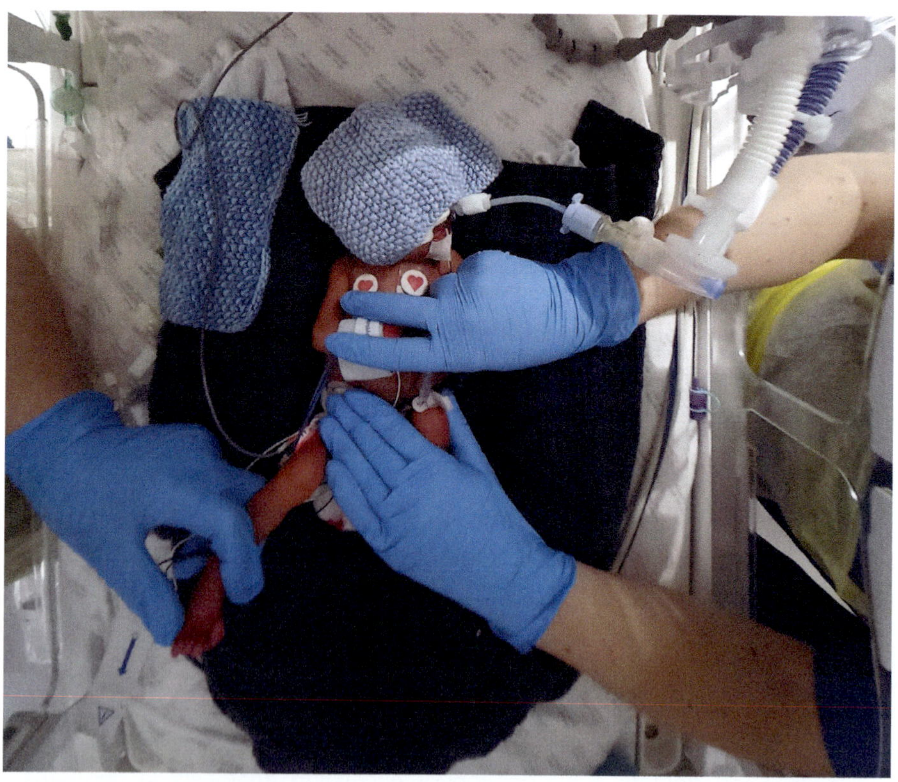

Figure 8.4 Facilitated tucking during a procedure

should include regular identification and assessment of pain. Uncertainty regarding the long-term impact of neonatal opioid administration on long-term neurodevelopmental outcomes persists (Bellù et al., 2021), although more recently the BAPM framework for the management of neonatal pain discourages the routine infusion of opioid analgesics in ventilated preterm infants. In general, careful consideration of potential risks versus benefits must precede the administration of any pharmacological agent to this vulnerable patient group (BAPM, 2025). Fundamentally, as indicated in Figure 8.5, the aim should be the prevention of unnecessary pain, followed by a stepwise approach to pharmacological pain management. Pharmacological agents used in the NNU are described in Box 8.3.

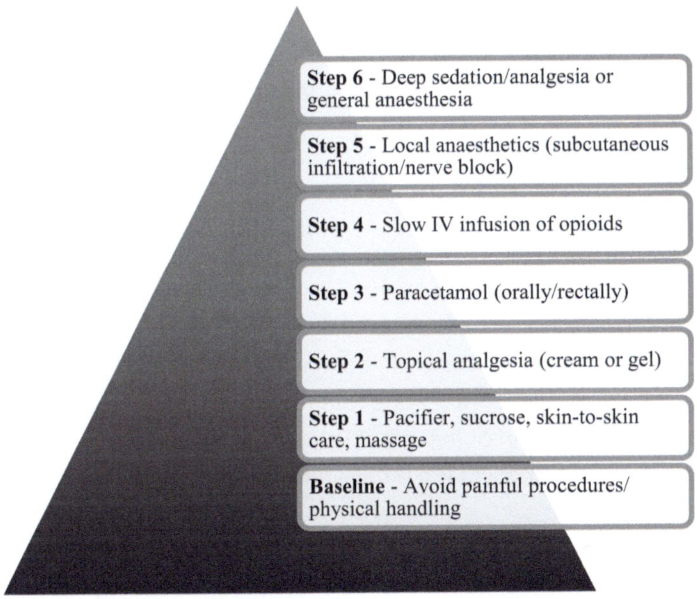

Figure 8.5 Stepwise approach to neonatal analgesia (adapted from Witt et al., 2016; BAPM, 2025)

BOX 8.3 PHARMACOLOGICAL INTERVENTIONS FOR PAIN MANAGEMENT IN THE NNU

Opioids

- The gold standard for relief of moderate to severe pain in neonates
- Morphine and fentanyl are the most commonly used and most widely studied opioids in neonates (Kinoshita et al., 2021; BAPM, 2025)

- Potential adverse effects of opioids include urinary retention, the slowing of gastric and intestinal motility, and feeding intolerance
- Some evidence of possible long-term adverse neurological effects (Szatkowski et al., 2023)
- Prolonged use may lead to opioid dependence and tolerance

Morphine

- Has a long half-life (6 to 14 hours in preterm, 2 to 11 hours in term infants)
- Side effects include marked respiratory depression, bradycardia, and hypotension
- Can be administered as bolus dose or via continuous intravenous infusion
- Tolerance may develop after prolonged use (3–4 days in preterm infants)
- Slow weaning is recommended

Fentanyl

- A potent synthetic opioid
- It penetrates the central nervous system (CNS) rapidly and the serum half-life is 1 to 15 hours
- Rapid bolus administration or continuous intravenous infusion may cause chest wall rigidity, urine retention, and laryngospasm; therefore, careful monitoring of the infant is imperative
- Infusions of fentanyl for >5 days have shown significant withdrawal symptoms.

Paracetamol

- Infants who receive intravenous paracetamol as primary analgesic after major surgery require significantly less morphine than those who receive a continuous morphine infusion (Zeilmaker-Roest et al., 2024)
- Prolonged administration of paracetamol (>72h) is not associated with liver injury or metabolic changes (Haslund-Krog et al., 2023)
- Caution is warranted, as safety data on the prolonged administration of paracetamol in very preterm infants remains sparse

Epidural analgesia

- Used for pain relief following neonatal surgery
- Popular method for delivery of post-operative analgesia, as it lacks the side effects associated with opioids, including respiratory depression and reduced gut motility
- The commonest drugs are bupivacaine, lidocaine, and ropivacaine

Local wound analgesia

- The wound catheter is placed during surgery to provide post-operative pain relief via a continuous infusion of local anaesthetic
- Infrequently used in neonates
- Lack of evidence for effectiveness and potential side effects in neonates (Jyoti et al., 2024)

Topical agents

- Topical local anaesthetics can be used for venepuncture pain
- Topical local anaesthetics alone are insufficient for heel lance pain
- When using a topical local anaesthetic, it must be applied correctly, and sufficient time allowed for it to become effective
- EMLA contains lidocaine 2.5% and prilocaine 2.5%, which can produce local anaesthesia when applied to intact skin as a cream. It is applied to the centre of the area to be anaesthetised and covered with an occlusive dressing. Cream and dressing are removed after a maximum of 60 minutes
- A rare side effect of EMLA cream is methaemoglobinaemia, an increase in haemoglobin lacking the capacity to bind and carry oxygen molecules, resulting in hypoxaemia and hypoxia
- Not recommended for use in infants <37 weeks gestation due to the increased risk of methaemoglobinaemia

Sweet-tasting oral solutions

- Oral sucrose administration likely reduces pain response in examination for retinopathy of prematurity as well as during heel-lancing (Yamada et al., 2023)

CLINICAL PRACTICE

Clinical guidelines

Despite the evidence available, neonatal pain frequently remains poorly assessed and under-treated in NNUs across the world (Mitello et al., 2021; Treiman-Kiveste et al., 2021) and evidence of poor knowledge regarding neonatal pain management prevails (Kassab et al., 2021; Popowicz et al., 2021). Even in settings where knowledge is adequate, a knowledge-practice gap persists (Santos et al., 2021).

In response, position statements and clinical practice recommendations for pain assessment in the nonverbal patient have been developed and issued in many countries by professional groups, project teams, and individual institutions (Harris et al., 2016). Subsequently, many organisations have released both national and international standards in order to translate these into practical guidelines designed to act as a template for local policy makers (American Academy of Pediatrics Committee on Fetus and Newborn and Section on Anesthesiology and Pain Medicine, 2016; Oude-Reimer et al., 2018), including the recent BAPM framework for the management of neonatal pain in the UK (BAPM, 2025).

Guidelines are a useful way of putting the evidence for pain assessment and management into practice. However, existing neonatal pain management guidelines can be vague in their recommendations and are not always based on best available evidence (Campbell et al., 2025). Furthermore, the existence of neonatal pain assessment and management guidelines does not always translate into their application in practice (Carlsen Misic et al., 2021). It is the responsibility of practicing clinicians to be aware of the guidelines supporting their own practice and to adhere to these recommendations. Part of the nurse's role is advocacy for best practice by ensuring guidelines are in place and used to inform practice. Effectiveness of practice is measured by way of clinical audits monitoring whether pain management is individualised, and practice based on evidence.

Caregiver attitude to infant pain assessment and management

Nurses generally have a positive attitude towards neonatal pain assessment and management (Carlsen Misic et al., 2021); however, this does not automatically translate into practice. Strong interprofessional collaboration between different HCPs can result in an increased application of neonatal pain management guidelines (Ulmer et al., 2022) and it has been suggested that increased interdisciplinary cooperation enhances care delivery and improves patient outcomes (McLaney et al., 2022). This is a challenging task which requires both support on an organisational level as well as from individual HCPs, who must play an active part in fostering a culture of collaboration and teamwork (Schot et al., 2019). In addition, recognising parents as part of the healthcare team positively correlates with improved short- and long-term outcomes for the infant (Waddington et al., 2021).

Fear of inadvertently causing an adverse drug reaction or negatively impact long-term neurological outcomes may present a barrier to pain management; however, most non-pharmacological strategies are safe to use and can be effective in addressing neonatal pain and discomfort (Shen et al., 2022).

PRACTICE POINT

Many nurses feel that they are able to assess neonatal pain without the use of a pain assessment tool (De Clifford Faugère et al., 2022). However, behavioural markers of neonatal pain are subject to bias and vary depending on an infant's gestational age and ability to express pain or the degree of their illness or paralysis.

Pain scores can act as a common language and facilitate interprofessional discussions about the need for pain management. When implementing pain assessment tools in practice, careful selection of the most appropriate one for the clinical setting is therefore warranted. In addition, the different ways neonates of varying gestational ages and clinical conditions express pain may necessitate the implementation of more than one pain scale within the same clinical setting, in order to allow for the assessment of all types of patients as well as all types of pain (Eriksson & Campbell-Yeo, 2019).

Lack of resources, in particular staff shortages, has previously been identified as a barrier to neonatal pain management (Mala et al., 2021). Many pharmacological and non-pharmacological pain management strategies require participation of more than one person, often in the form of another HCP, and adequate staffing is therefore a necessary prerequisite for successful and consistent neonatal pain management.

ACTIVITY

Consider the attitude towards neonatal pain management in your area of work. Is it a priority? If not, why? What barriers to effective pain management in your own clinical practice can you identify, and what could you do to overcome these?

Ethical aspects of neonatal pain

Nurses, like all healthcare professionals, have a moral and ethical obligation to limit the neonate's exposure to pain wherever possible, as is reflected in the principles of beneficence and non-maleficence, two of the four ethical principles which govern professional decision-making (Varkey, 2021), and which require HCPs to promote their patients' wellbeing and to protect them from preventable harm. Therefore, pain assessment and management can raise ethical issues for neonatal professionals with the infant's best interests being of primary concern. When neonates are subjected to painful procedures, it can be argued that this is not in the infant's best interest (see Chapter 11) to withhold pain relief. If pain relief is withheld on the assumption that the medicine may be harmful to the infant, then this raises the issue of the boundaries of preserving life and health. The ethical issues associated with the treatment for neonatal pain are complex. The long-term consequences of continued exposure to pain experienced by neonates are unknown. Therefore, the focus for this dilemma should be to try and reduce exposure to pain. Consideration of each potentially painful procedure needs to be a priority for each caregiver. The number of painful procedures carried out in the NNU needs to be reduced, and the indiscriminate use of routine procedures without a clear rationale reviewed by the multidisciplinary team.

Chapter takeaways

- Neonatal nurses can help alleviate pain and suffering through careful assessment and ensuring appropriate interventions are provided.
- By understanding the mechanisms of neonatal pain pathways, nurses are able to demonstrate effective assessment skills, which in turn contribute to best practice.
- Despite a large amount of evidence regarding painful procedures and effective pain management, clinical practice is still variable and not always in keeping with this evidence.
- Nurses with an awareness of pain in the newborn will be empowered to provide interventions to ensure that neonates in NNU will receive adequate relief not only from procedural pain but also from chronic pain associated with ventilation and surgery, as well as exposure to stress.
- Most parents want to be able to actively support their baby during painful procedures, and empowering them to do so not only positively impacts their own mental health but also significantly reduces neonatal pain and improves both short and long-term outcomes for the baby.

CASE STUDY

CASE STUDIES

Case study 1: Managing neonatal stress

Naomi has been in the NNU for four weeks now. She was delivered by caesarean section at 28 weeks' gestation because her mother went into labour with ruptured membranes. Naomi was on mechanical ventilation for two weeks and is now on non-invasive respiratory support (CPAP). She is receiving small volumes of expressed breastmilk via her gastric tube. You have been assigned to care for Naomi on your shift.

Q.1. On receiving handover from your colleague, how would you determine if Naomi is comfortable?

Q.2. What signs of stress would you be looking for when you are undertaking care activities for Naomi?

Q.3. How might you determine if Naomi has been experiencing stressful events either on the past shift or during your shift?

Q.4. What are some of the detrimental effects of stress for neonates in the NNU?

Case study 2: Undertaking pain assessment in a preterm neonate

Angus was born at 34 weeks'gestation and he is now 5 days of age. On his mother's antenatal ultrasound scan he was diagnosed with a congenital heart defect. He had surgery on the second day of life for a narrowing of his aortic arch. He was ventilated in the post-operative period for 3 days and was receiving a fentanyl infusion for his pain. On the medical ward round, the team asked for the rate of his fentanyl infusion to be reduced in preparation for extubation.

Q.1. How would you assess Angus' readiness for a reduction in his analgesia?

Q.2. You have been asked what the trends in his pain score are prior to reducing the analgesia. Using a suitable pain assessment scale, check the algorithm to gauge the scores that would be suitable for weaning the analgesia.

Q.3. You have been assigned a new staff member to work with you in caring for Angus. As part of your mentorship, you decide to teach them about how to assess a baby's pain. What do you need to consider in explaining how to assess a baby's pain using a pain scale?

CASE STUDY

Case study 3: Management of pain in the NNU

Malik is a 26-week gestation infant weighing 875 grams. He was born by emergency caesarean section following maternal antepartum haemorrhage. His mother did not receive antenatal corticosteroids. He was born in fair condition and was intubated and given surfactant immediately after delivery. Following stabilisation, he was transferred to the NNU, where he continued to require mechanical ventilation. Umbilical arterial and venous lines were sited for monitoring and intravenous therapy and medication.

Q.1. Does Malik need any pain relief given that he is so premature? What is the rationale for your answer?
Q.2. Which drugs could be used in this situation?
Q.3. Are there any non-pharmacological strategies you could employ to keep Malik comfortable?
Q.4. How would you assess whether the pain-relieving strategies were effective?
Q.5. Can you think of any pharmacological interventions appropriate for procedural pain?

For suggested answer guides to the questions posed in these case studies, please refer to the web-based companion site specific to this chapter. See www.routledge.com/cw/petty

References

Agrawal, P., & Samayam, P. (2025). View of variations in physiological responses to painful stimuli in preterm and term neonates: An observational study. *International Journal of Contemporary Pediatrics*, *12*(1), 89–93.

American Academy of Pediatrics Committee on Fetus and Newborn and Section on Anesthesiology and Pain Medicine. (2016). Prevention and management of procedural pain in the neonate: An update. *Pediatrics*, *137*(2), 1–13.

Arabiat, D., Mörelius, E., Hoti, K., & Hughes, J. (2023). Pain assessment tools for use in infants: A meta-review. *BMC Pediatrics*, *23*(1), 1–22.

Bellieni, C. V., Tei, M., & Buonocore, G. (2015). Should we assess pain in newborn infants using a scoring system or just a detection method? *Acta Paediatrica*, *104*(3), 221–224.

Bellù, R., Romantsik, O., Nava, C., de Waal, K. A., Zanini, R., & Bruschettini, M. (2021). Opioids for newborn infants receiving mechanical ventilation. *Cochrane Database of Systematic Reviews*, *2021*(3), CD013732.

BLISS UK. *A quick guide to parents' involvement in their baby's care and procedures*. https://www.bliss.org.uk/parents/in-hospital/being-involved-in-your-babys-care-and-procedures/quick-guide-to-involvement-in-babys-procedures

Boggini, T., Pozzoli, S., Schiavolin, P., Erario, R., Mosca, F., Brambilla, P., & Fumagalli, M. (2021). Cumulative procedural pain and brain development in very preterm infants: A systematic review of clinical and preclinical studies. *Neuroscience & Biobehavioral Reviews*, *123*, 320–336.

Brennan, F., Lohman, D., & Gwyther, L. (2019). Access to pain management as a human right. *American Journal of Public Health*, *109*(1), 61–65.

British Association of Perinatal Medicine. (2025). *Management of neonatal pain. A framework for practice*. BAPM. Retrieved March 4, 2026, from https://hubble-live-assets.s3.eu-west-1.amazonaws.com/bapm/file_asset/file/3857/Management_of_Neonatal_Pain_Nov_25.pdf

Büttner, W., & Finke, W. (2000). Analysis of behavioural and physiological parameters for the assessment of postoperative analgesic demand in newborns, infants and young children: A comprehensive report on seven consecutive studies. *Pediatric Anesthesia*, *10*(3), 303–318.

Caljouw, M. A. A., Kloos, M. A. C., Olivier, M. Y., Heemskerk, I. W., Pison, W. C. R., Stigter, G. D., & Verhoef, A.-M. J. H. (2007). Measurement of pain in premature infants with a gestational age between 28 to 37 weeks: Validation of the adapted COMFORT scale. *Journal of Neonatal Nursing*, *13*(1), 13–18.

Campbell, N., Adair, P., Doherty, N., McCormack, D., & Walsh, A. (2025). A systematic review of clinical practice guidelines for the assessment and management of pain in neonates. *Journal of Neonatal Nursing*, *31*(2), 1–6.

Campbell-Yeo, M., Eriksson, M., & Benoit, B. (2022). Assessment and management of pain in preterm infants: A practice update. *Children*, *9*(2), 1–18.

Carbajal, R., Paupe, A., Hoenn, E., Lenclen, R., & Olivier-Martin, M. (1997). APN: A behavioral acute pain rating scale for neonates. *Archives De Pédiatrie*, *4*(7), 623–628.

Carlsen Misic, M., Andersen, R. D., Strand, S., Eriksson, M., & Olsson, E. (2021). Nurses' perception, knowledge, and use of neonatal pain assessment. *Paediatric and Neonatal Pain*, *3*(2), 59–65.

Cook, K. M., De Asis-Cruz, J., Kim, J.-H., Basu, S. K., Andescavage, N., Murnick, J., Spoehr, E., Liggett, M., Du, J., & Limperopoulos, C. (2023). Experience of early-life pain in premature infants is associated with atypical cerebellar development and later neurodevelopmental deficits. *BMC Medicine*, *21*(1), 1–15.

Debillon, T., Zupan, V., Ravault, N., Magny, J.-F., & Dehan, M. (2001). Development and initial validation of the EDIN scale, a new tool for assessing prolonged pain in preterm infants. *Archives of Disease in Childhood – Fetal and Neonatal Edition*, *85*(1), F36–F41.

De Clifford Faugère, G., Aita, M., Feeley, N., & Colson, S. (2022). Nurses' perception of preterm infants' pain and the factors of their pain assessment and management. *Journal of Perinatal & Neonatal Nursing*, *36*(3), 312–326.

Eissler, A., Zwakhalen, S., Stoffel, L., & Hahn, S. (2022). Systematic review of the effectiveness of involving parents during painful interventions for their preterm infants. *Journal of Obstetric, Gynecologic & Neonatal Nursing*, *51*(1), 6–15.

Eriksson, M., & Campbell-Yeo, M. (2019). Assessment of pain in newborn infants. *Seminars in Fetal and Neonatal Medicine*, *24*(4), 1–7.

Fournier-Charrière, E., Tourniaire, B., Carbajal, R., Cimerman, P., Lassauge, F., Ricard, C., Reiter, F., Turquin, P., Lombart, B., Letierce, A., & Falissard, B. (2012). EVENDOL, a new behavioral pain scale for children ages 0 to 7 years in the emergency department: Design and validation. *PAIN*, *153*(8), 1573–1582.

Gibbins, S., Stevens, B. J., Yamada, J., Dionne, K., Campbell-Yeo, M., Lee, G., Caddell, K., Johnston, C., & Taddio, A. (2014). Validation of the premature infant pain profile-revised (PIPP-R). *Early Human Development*, *90*(4), 189–193.

Giordano, V., Edobor, J., Deindl, P., Wildner, B., Goeral, K., Steinbauer, P., Werther, T., Berger, A., & Olischar, M. (2019). Pain and sedation scales for neonatal and pediatric patients in a preverbal stage of development. *JAMA Pediatrics*, *173*(12), 1186–1197.

Harris, J., Ramelet, A.-S., van Dijk, M., Pokorna, P., Wielenga, J., Tume, L., Tibboel, D., & Ista, E. (2016). Clinical recommendations for pain, sedation, withdrawal and delirium assessment in critically ill infants and children: An ESPNIC position statement for healthcare professional'. *Intensive Care Medicine*, *42*(6), 972–986.

Haslund-Krog, S., Barry, J. M., Birnbaum, A. K., Dalhoff, K., Henriksen, T. B., Charul Avachat, C., Poulsen, S., Christensen, U., Remmel, R. P., Wilkins, D., & Holst, H. (2023). Pharmacokinetics and safety of prolonged paracetamol treatment in neonates: An interventional cohort study. *British Journal of Clinical Pharmacology*, *89*(11), 3421–3431.

Holsti, L., & Grunau, R. E. (2007). Initial validation of the Behavioral Indicators of Infant Pain (BIIP). *Pain*, *132*(3), 264–272.

Hummel, P., Puchalski, M., Creech, S. D., & Weiss, M. G. (2007). Clinical reliability and validity of the N-PASS: Neonatal pain, agitation and sedation scale with prolonged pain. *Journal of Perinatology*, *28*(1), 55–60.

Ilhan, E., Pacey, V., Brown, L., Spence, K., Ganzewinkel, C. van, Riddell, R. P., Campbell-Yeo, M., Stevens, B. J., Eriksson, M., Shah, V., Anand, K. J. S., Bellieni, C., Daly, M., Johnston, C., & Hush, J. (2022). What is the definition of acute episodic and chronic pain in critically ill neonates and infants? A global, four-stage consensus and validation study. *BMJ Open*, *12*(3), 1–9.

Ilhan, E., Pacey, V., Brown, L., Spence, K., Gray, K., Rowland, J. E., White, K., & Hush, J. M. (2020). Neonates as intrinsically worthy recipients of pain management in neonatal intensive care. *Medicine, Health Care and Philosophy*, *24*(1), 65–72.

Jyoti, J., Sloukova, E., Spence, K., Webb, A., Shun, A., & Popat, H. (2024). Continuous local anaesthetic wound infusion in infants undergoing thoracic or abdominal surgery: A systematic review. *Journal of Pediatric Surgery Open*, *8*, 1–8.

Kassab, M., Joseph, R., Alhammad, N., & Mohammad, K. I. (2021). Oral sucrose for neonatal pain: Perception of Jordanian nurses. *Neonatal Network*, *40*(1), 25–30.

Kinoshita, M., Olsson, E., Borys, F., & Bruschettini, M. (2021). Opioids for procedural pain in neonates. *Cochrane Database of Systematic Reviews*, *12*, CD015056.

Laudiano-Dray, M. P., Pillai Riddell, R., Jones, L., Iyer, R., Whitehead, K., Fitzgerald, M., Fabrizi, L., & Meek, J. (2020). Quantification of neonatal procedural pain severity: A platform for estimating total pain burden in individual infants. *Pain*, *161*(6), 1270–1277.

Lawrence, J., Alcock, D., McGrath, P., Kay, J., MacMurray, S. B., & Dulberg, C. (1993). The development of a tool to assess neonatal pain. *Neonatal Network*, *12*(6), 59–66.

Mala, O., Forster, E. M., & Kain, V. J. (2021). Neonatal nurse and midwife competence regarding pain management in neonates. *Advances in Neonatal Care*, *2*(22), E34–E42.

McLaney, E., Morassaei, S., Hughes, L., Davies, R., Campbell, M., & Di Prospero, L. (2022). A framework for interprofessional team collaboration in a hospital setting: Advancing team competencies and behaviours. *Healthcare Management Forum*, *35*(2), 112–117.

Meesters, N. J., Dilles, T., van Rosmalen, J., van den Bosch, G. E., Simons, S. H. P., & van Dijk, M. (2023, May). COMFORTneo scale: A reliable and valid instrument to measure prolonged pain in neonates? *Journal of Perinatology*, *43*(5), 595–600. https://doi.org/10.1038/s41372-023-01628-1

Merkel, S. I., Voepel-Lewis, T., Shayevitz, J. R., & Malviya, S. (1997). The FLACC: A behavioral scale for scoring postoperative pain in young children. *Journal of Pediatric Nursing*, *23*(3), 293–297.

Mitello, L., Marucci, A. R., Salvatore, S., Sii Onesto, A., Baglio, G., & Latina, R. (2021). Predictors of nurses' attitudes and knowledge towards pain management in Italy. A cross-sectional study in the hospital settings. *Applied Nursing Research*, *62*, 1–6.

Oude-Reimer, M., Frauenfelder, O., Binter, J., Cámba, F., Ceccatelli, M., Hankes-Drielsma, I., Jørgensen, E., & Silva, E. (2018). *European standards of care for newborn health: Support during painful procedures and pain assessment.* European Standards of Care for Newborn Health.

Pavlyshyn, H., Sarapuk, I., & Kozak, K. (2024). The relationship between neonatal stress in preterm infants and developmental outcomes at the corrected age of 24–30 months. *Frontiers in Psychology, 15*, 1–13.

Perry, M., Tan, Z., Chen, J., Weidig, T., Xu, W., & Cong, X. S. (2018). Neonatal pain. *Critical Care Nursing Clinics of North America, 30*(4), 549–561.

Peters, J. W. B., Koot, H. M., Grunau, R. E., de Boer, J., van Druenen, M. J., Tibboel, D., & Duivenvoorden, H. J. (2003). Neonatal facial coding system for assessing postoperative pain in infants: Item reduction is valid and feasible. *The Clinical Journal of Pain, 19*(6), 353–363.

Pillai, R. R., Bucsea, O., Shiff, I., Chow, C., Gennis, H. G., Badovinac, S., DiLorenzo-Klas, M., Racine, N. M., Kohut, S. A., Lisi, D., Turcotte, K., Stevens, B., & Uman, L. S. (2023). Non-pharmacological management of infant and young child procedural pain. *The Cochrane Library, 6*, CD006275.

Popowicz, H., Mędrzycka-Dąbrowska, W., Kwiecień-Jaguś, K., & Kamedulska, A. (2021). Knowledge and practices in neonatal pain management of nurses employed in hospitals with different levels of referral – multicenter study. *Healthcare, 9*(48), 1–15.

Santos, C. S., De Almeida Soares, J., Azevedo Pinheiro, J., & Dos Santos Queiroz, M. (2021). Perception of the nursing team about pain evaluation in premature newborns. *Revista de Enfermagem e Atenção à Saúde, 10*(2), 1–17.

Schot, E., Tummers, L., & Noordegraaf, M. (2019). Working on working together: A systematic review on how healthcare professionals contribute to interprofessional collaboration. *Journal of Interprofessional Care, 34*(3), 1–11.

Shah, P. S., Torgalkar, R., & Shah, V. (2023). Breastfeeding or breast milk for procedural pain in neonates. *The Cochrane Library, 8*, CD004950.

Sharma, H., & Ruikar, M. (2022). Kangaroo mother care (KMC) for procedural pain in infants: A meta-analysis from the current evidence of randomized control trials and cross-over trials. *Journal of Family Medicine and Primary Care, 11*(4), 1250–1256.

Shen, Q., Huang, Z., Leng, H., Luo, X., & Zheng, X. (2022). Efficacy and safety of non-pharmacological interventions for neonatal pain: An overview of systematic reviews. *BMJ Open, 12*(9), 1–8.

Siva, N., Nayak, R., & Ghosh, D. (2025). Pain and pain-related stress in high-risk neonates at NICU – A narrative review. *Journal of Neonatal Nursing, 31*(3), 1–7.

Slater, R., Fitzgerald, M., & Meek, J. (2007). Can cortical responses following noxious stimulation inform us about pain processing in neonates? *Seminars in Perinatology, 31*(5), 298–302.

Soleimani, F., Azari, N., Ghiasvand, H., Shahrokhi, A., Rahmani, N., & Fatollahierad, S. (2020). Do NICU developmental care improve cognitive and motor outcomes for preterm infants? A systematic review and meta-analysis. *BMC Pediatrics, 20*(1), 1–16.

Spence, K., Gillies, D., Harrison, D., Johnston, L., & Nagy, S. (2005). A reliable pain assessment tool for clinical assessment in the neonatal intensive care unit. *Journal of Obstetric, Gynecologic & Neonatal Nursing, 34*(1), 80–86.

Szatkowski, L., Sharkey, D., Budge, H., & Ojha, S. (2023). Association between opioid use during mechanical ventilation in preterm infants and evidence of brain injury: A propensity score-matched cohort study. *The Lancet, 65*, 1–9.

Treiman-Kiveste, A., Pölkki, T., Kalda, R., & Kangasniemi, M. (2021). Nurses' perceptions of infants' procedural pain assessment and alleviation with non-pharmacological methods in Estonia. *Journal of Pediatric Nursing, 62*, 156–163.

Tucker, M. H., Tiwari, P., & Carter, B. S. (2023). The physiology, assessment, and treatment of neonatal pain. *Seminars in Fetal and Neonatal Medicine*, *28*(4), 101465–101465.

Ullsten, A., Andreasson, M., & Eriksson, M. (2021). State of the art in parent-delivered pain-relieving interventions in neonatal care: A scoping review. *Frontiers in Pediatrics*, *9*, 1–19.

Ullsten, A., Campbell-Yeo, M., & Eriksson, M. (2024). Parent-led neonatal pain management – a narrative review and update of research and practice. *Frontiers in Pain Research*, *5*(16), 1–9.

Ulmer, M., Martakis, K., Scholten, N., & Kuntz, L. (2022). Existence and perceived application of pain management protocols in German neonatal intensive care units. *Paediatric and Neonatal Pain*, *118*(4), E992–E1000.

van Dijk, M., Peters, J. W. B., van Deventer, P., & Tibboel, D. (2005). The COMFORT Behavior Scale: A tool for assessing pain and sedation in infants. *The American Journal of Nursing*, *105*(1), 33–36.

van Dokkum, N. H., de Kroon, M. L. A., Reijneveld, S. A., & Bos, A. F. (2021). Neonatal stress, health, and development in preterms: A systematic review. *Pediatrics*, *148*(4), 1–13.

Varkey, B. (2021). Principles of clinical ethics and their application to practice. *Medical Principles and Practice*, *30*(1), 17–28.

Waddington, C., Veenendaal, N. R., O'Brien, K., & Patel, N. (2021). Family integrated care: Supporting parents as primary caregivers in the neonatal intensive care unit. *Pediatric Investigation*, *5*(2), 148–154.

Williams, M. D., & Lascelles, B. D. X. (2020). Early neonatal pain – a review of clinical and experimental implications on painful conditions later in life. *Frontiers in Pediatrics*, *8*(30), 1–18.

Witt, N., Coynor, S., Edwards, C., & Bradshaw, H. (2016). A guide to pain assessment and management in the neonate. *Current Emergency and Hospital Medicine Reports*, *1*(4), 1–10.

Yamada, J., Bueno, M., Santos, L., Haliburton, S., Campbell-Yeo, M., & Stevens, B. (2023). Sucrose analgesia for heel-lance procedures in neonates. *The Cochrane Library*, *8*, CD014806.

Zeilmaker-Roest, G., de Vries-Rink, C., van Rosmalen, J., van Dijk, M., de Wildt, S. N., Knibbe, C. A. J., Koomen, E., Jansen, N. J. G., Kneyber, M. C. J., Maebe, S., Van den Berghe, G., Haghedooren, R., Vlasselaers, D., Bogers, A. J. J. C., Tibboel, D., & Wildschut, E. D. (2024). Intermittent intravenous paracetamol versus continuous morphine in infants undergoing cardiothoracic surgery: A multi-center randomized controlled trial. *Critical Care*, *28*(1), 143–153.

Zhao, T., Starkweather, A. R., Matson, A., Lainwala, S., Xu, W., & Cong, X. (2022). Nurses' experiences of caring for preterm infants in pain: A meta-ethnography. *International Journal of Nursing Sciences*, *9*(4), 533–541.

9 NEONATAL PALLIATIVE CARE: RECOGNISING UNCERTAINTY AND ENHANCING THE FAMILY EXPERIENCE

Alex Mancini and Jo Bennett

CONTENTS

DOI: 10.4324/9781003591405-12

GUIDANCE ON HOW TO ENHANCE PERSONAL LEARNING FROM THIS CHAPTER

Key points covered in this chapter

- Acknowledging the changing landscape of neonatal palliative care and the implications for practice ensuring consistent and equitable care for babies and their families.
- The background of neonatal palliative care, highlighting the importance of recognising uncertainty aligned with national guidance and frameworks.
- Highlighting the very specialised support the workforce requires, which must be tailored to individual needs, including access to high-quality education and training and equipping the workforce with fundamental skills and knowledge.
- The concept that neonatal palliative care is 'everyone's business' and is inclusive of all members of the healthcare team across acute and community teams.
- Examples of good practice which may be adapted to various care settings.

Reflection

Reading through this chapter, you are encouraged to engage with the key points and related literature in an enquiring way. Ask yourself these questions:

- Why is perinatal/neonatal palliative care considered 'everyone's business'?
- Think of how you might apply the three key approaches to recognising uncertainty and the need for palliative care during the daily ward round?
- Why is it important for parents and the wider family to be given information and choices which may influence care planning?
- Which specialities within the multidisciplinary team (within your organisation and externally) are important to be involved in palliative care planning?

Implications for nursing care

This chapter should increase your understanding of the principles of perinatal/neonatal palliative care and how they can be incorporated into routine neonatal care.

Consider how you might change your current practice, the way you communicate and share information might influence the impact of consistent high-quality care for each baby and family you care for?

INTRODUCTION AND BACKGROUND

Across the United Kingdom (UK), recent advances in technology and perinatal care have made survival amongst the most vulnerable babies more commonplace. With advancements in medical care, the prevalence of complex **life-limiting conditions** (LLCs) in children has increased over the last two decades (Smith et al., 2023). The need for **palliative care** for children under the age of one should be seen as a priority given that they have the highest prevalence of LLC and mortality rates. LLC account for the majority of child deaths: 54 % (5,134 of 9,517) were in children with LLCs, with 58 % occurring under one year of age. An estimated 12,123 babies admitted to the neonatal unit (NNU) across England and Wales over a 6-year period had palliative care needs. This equates to around 2,000 babies per year (around 2% of total admissions; Harnden et al., 2023). Fraser et al. (2021) previously described a significant increase in prevalence of babies and older children surviving with life-limiting and life-threatening conditions, with the largest increase in babies under the age of 1 year. Deaths associated with LLC were disproportionately higher among children from socioeconomically deprived areas and Asian ethnic background (National Child Mortality Database (NCMD), 2025). The Office for National Statistics (ONS, 2025) reported that approximately 4,000 infant deaths occur annually in the UK, many on NNUs, and between 2019 and 2022, there were 2,991 recorded child deaths of infants under 1 year, who also had a LLC or perinatal/neonatal event (NCMD, 2025).

In 2024, the British Association of Perinatal Medicine (BAPM) in partnership with the Association of Paediatric Palliative Medicine (APPM) developed a national framework 'Recognising Uncertainty: An Integrated Framework for Palliative Care in Perinatal Medicine' focusing on a shift and modification in language and approach to neonatal palliative care emphasising that

> "palliative care is not synonymous with end of life care, but rather represents an active and total approach to care which can be delivered from the point of diagnosis and alongside treatments directed at survival. It includes symptom management and parallel planning, but also empowering parents to be involved in the care of their baby and in decisions"
>
> (BAPM, 2024, p. 3)

This current framework focuses on recognising the uncertain future and uncertain path many babies and their families are faced with, rather than a list of specific conditions, as was referred to previously.

> Palliative care is very much 'everyone's business' and can and should be delivered by existing perinatal teams with support from community and specialist services where required. Many of the elements of palliative care overlap with elements of family integrated care and are very familiar to perinatal teams.
>
> (BAPM, 2024)

TERMINOLOGY AND LANGUAGE USED IN NEONATAL PALLIATIVE CARE

Historically there have been misconceptions and unhelpful narratives around neonatal palliative care. Recently there has been significant work nationally (HEARD, 2023) in changing the narrative and highlighting the value of palliative care for babies and their families. The focus is on reframing the language positively, such as using words like collaboration, connection, partnership, embracing, comprehensive, simple pleasures, moments of happiness, 'firsts,' and experiences rather than presenting hopelessness, struggle, unthinkable, and tragedy. It is acknowledged that there may be different terms used to describe neonatal palliative care or used alongside the term. Table 9.1 explains some terminology which may be used.

TABLE 9.1 TERMINOLOGY RELATING TO PALLIATIVE CARE

Palliative Care	Refers to an active approach to the care of neonates and their families with life-limiting conditions from the time of diagnosis through to death and bereavement. It embraces physical, emotional, social, and spiritual needs and focuses on the enhancement of quality of life, and support for the patient's family (Together for Short Lives (TFSL), 2018). Palliative care is not the same as end-of-life care, though it includes such care as appropriate. In other words, it is an umbrella term that includes all elements of supportive care and end of life care. This includes many babies who are not receiving end of life care, those for whom the outcome is not certain, and some who may recover fully and live a normal lifespan. Palliative care will often be provided alongside and in addition to elements of routine survival focused care (sometimes misleadingly called 'active treatment'). Palliative care should be 'integrated' in that it involves general elements provided by the same neonatal and perinatal care teams who provide other elements of care, together with (in some cases, and as required) the support of specialist palliative care teams.

TABLE 9.1 (Cont.)

End of Life Care	'End of life care' refers to the care of a patient in the dying phase, including symptom management, decision-making about appropriate treatments, and family support.
Supportive Care	'Supportive care' is sometimes used to refer to an approach to care which aims to support patients and families to live as well as possible by providing high quality pain and symptom control alongside practical and psychological support (Hui et al., 2013; Together for Short Lives, 2018). Supportive care is provided for patients in the setting of uncertain outcome, for example patients who may recover but also are at risk of dying. Many families and healthcare providers are comfortable referring to this as 'palliative care,' while others find the term 'supportive care' more accessible or preferable.
Comfort Care	This term has been used to imply that active care or resuscitation will not be initiated. However, following clinical consensus and many discussions this term has been deemed to be confusing for parents and healthcare teams alike. It is suggested that the term 'palliative care' is used with a clear explanation of what it means.

Adapted from (BAPM, 2024)

THINK POINTS

- Think about what the terms palliative care, supportive care, comfort care, end of life care, and bereavement care mean to you.
- Where have you heard these terms used?
- Do they have different meanings to you?

RECOGNISING BABIES AND THEIR FAMILIES WHO MAY BENEFIT FROM PALLIATIVE CARE

It is important to recognise which babies and their families may benefit from a palliative care approach at the earliest opportunity, so that clear discussions with parents and the healthcare team can start planning a comprehensive care plan inclusive of all key multi professionals and relevant specialties. Figure 9.1 helps explore three ways of approaching this.

The Diagnostic Approach: there may be a diagnosis antenatally or post-natally, where there is uncertainty regarding the baby's survival, or the baby may have a health condition which is considered life-limiting. There may also be some situations where a baby with palliative care needs who survives the neonatal period, may be discharged from the NNU and continues living at home in the community.

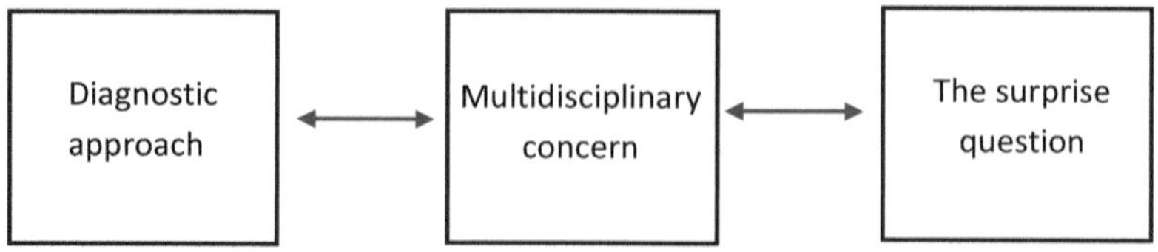

Figure 9.1 Three ways to recognise babies who may benefit from palliative care (adapted from BAPM, 2024)

Multidisciplinary Concern: this is where there may be concerns from the parents and within the multidisciplinary team regarding a baby's uncertain future in the absence of a confirmed diagnosis. It may be helpful to discuss these concerns together with the parents and the multidisciplinary team caring for the baby at the earliest opportunity. This situation and the level of uncertainty may encourage additional discussions. Further guidance for parents exists in a parent information booklet developed by Together for Short Lives and Bliss (2024).

The Surprise Question: this approach is used widely with older children, and teams may incorporate this within regular multidisciplinary meetings. Suggested prompts may be 'would you be surprised if this baby died in the short or longer term.' If the answer is 'no,' that may suggest exploring a palliative approach to care with involvement of specialist paediatric palliative care where they exist.

THINK POINTS

- Think of a neonate whom you have cared for with whom it might have been helpful to use the above approaches to identification and care planning.
- Would using these three tools have changed the plan of care?
- In retrospect, do you think some neonates you have cared for might have had an improved plan of care?
- Having read the BAPM framework (2024), do you think you may change your practice?

Some NNUs have developed regular integrated meetings where the focus is on the identification of babies and their families who will benefit from a palliative care approach and further discussions will be needed.

KEY PRINCIPLES OF NEONATAL PALLIATIVE CARE

Many of the key principles of palliative care align with the core principles of family integrated care (FiCare), in particular partnership with families being central to all discussions, decision-making, and the development of care plans and pathways for their babies. The acknowledgement of uncertainty for the future of their baby is paramount and will require sensitive and advanced communication skills, focusing on understanding their baby's clinical condition, what matters most to them, and consideration of their hopes and fears. Compassionate inclusive communication with parents from the very beginning of their baby's experience all the way through the neonatal journey is paramount in ensuring robust partnership in care. The most up-to-date information available must be shared with parents at the earliest opportunity regarding choices and the possibilities and opportunities available to include planning of their baby's care (see Table 9.2).

Addressing diverse cultural needs of families

Increasing cultural diversity has led to greater numbers of families whose first language differs to that of the healthcare team, resulting in situations where an interpreter may help facilitate communication and translate important discussions between the healthcare team and the family. It is important to acknowledge that in some cultures there may be preferences from the family regarding a male or female interpreter wherever possible. It is also advisable to spend some time with the interpreter before the meeting to discuss key issues, give warning to challenging information being shared, and how this will be conveyed sensitively to the family. Attention must also be paid to differences in cultural and religious beliefs around death and dying. After the meeting it is also good practice to spend some time to debrief with the interpreter (Prentice et al., 2014).

A whole team approach with shared responsibility, collaboration with relevant teams and robust pathways are essential to providing consistent, high-quality care. No one professional group can provide the comprehensive care required, but different specialities are fundamental in working towards a shared goal for personalised care. These interdisciplinary teams across the continuum of care may include fetal medicine, obstetrics, maternity, neonatal, specialist paediatric palliative care, children's hospices, and community teams.

CARE PLANNING IN NEONATAL PALLIATIVE CARE

Parallel planning is the heart of neonatal palliative care. Through honest, clear conversations with parents at the earliest opportunity, various possible scenarios and several different plans may be considered.

Advance Care Planning (ACP): Discussing with the family what the future may look like and what choices are available to them and helping them explore their priorities and goals is a dynamic process occurring as a series of discussions evolving over a period of time rather than just one meeting or conversation (Downie et al., 2020). It may be appropriate to have these conversations for an unborn baby or baby for whom death is a possible outcome, recognising the uncertainty of their future. Wherever possible, there should be continuity in the professionals involved, so the family do not need to repeat information and can build a rapport and relationship.

In all planning, it is key that the family's wishes are central and parents are included as partners in care. Research has shown that language barriers are an important consideration in providing equitable palliative and bereavement care (Clancy et al., 2024). Therefore, different modes of communication may be considered; the use of an interpreter, written information or access to websites with accessibility and language options may help in ensuring all parents are able to be fully informed and involved throughout. Cultural humility and cultural curiosity are fundamental within routine neonatal care and neonatal palliative care incorporated into all care planning and every interaction with parents and the wider family.

Table 9.2 and Figure 9.2 illustrate the key elements of individualised palliative care planning, which overlap with FiCare principles (see Chapter 6).

TABLE 9.2 KEY ELEMENTS OF PERINATAL PALLIATIVE CARE (ADAPTED FROM BAPM, 2024)

	To consider and include

Recognise babies with an uncertain future	■ Three approaches to identification:
	  ■ Diagnostic approach: antenatally or postnatally diagnosed with a LLC or an uncertain future
	  ■ Multidisciplinary concern and family perspective: encourage to share concerns as a useful starting point for conversations and planning
	  ■ The surprise question (see page 228) to prompt further discussion

Communicating with families	Once a baby has been recognised as having the potential to benefit from palliative care, it is important that this is shared with parents and other members of the healthcare team at the earliest opportunity. This involves acknowledging uncertainty and will require honest, compassionate, and often repeated conversations including details of what parents understand regarding their baby's clinical needs and prognosis. In particular discussions should include what is important to them and what their priorities are regarding choices of care. Conversations must include using the most appropriate strategies for each family, ensuring a personalised approach, by not making assumptions or stereotyping. These include: ■ Creating a safe space ■ Being culturally curious and sensitive, recognising and respecting differences ■ Culturally sensitive and inclusive language

TABLE 9.2 (Cont.)

	To consider and include
	■ Using clear and concise language which is mirrored when there is the necessity of engaging an interpreter ■ Curiosity regarding culture, traditions, and beliefs. Respectfully explore traditions and beliefs and how these may be supported ■ Active listening; listening to hear and not to respond ■ Being attentive to non-verbal cues ■ Considering multiple approaches to communicating information, including visuals, large text ■ Authenticity and honesty, especially where there are unknowns or uncertainty Some key questions you might consider asking parents (adapted from Mancini et al., 2020) ■ Tell me about your baby ■ What is your understanding of your baby's illness? ■ What are your hopes and priorities for your baby? ■ What are your fears for him/her? ■ Where do you get your strength to cope?
Holistic family support	■ Consider the needs of siblings and the wider family ■ Think about who else might be helpful to involve in providing support (local hospice, specialist palliative care team, psychology, community support, social care charity) ■ Cultural support within own network of family and friends ■ Financial, social, and practical support
Supporting parents to feel empowered	■ What are the priorities for the family at that point in time ■ Flexibility around key goals ■ Celebrating everyday joys, feeding, cuddles, developmental milestones ■ Every moment is a memory
Parallel planning	■ Discuss parallel plans with parents, preparing for a range of possible outcomes or scenarios and plan for them ■ Consider developing an advance care plan together ■ Consider referral to specialist palliative care teams/local children's hospices
Symptom management	■ Consider developing a symptom management plan with specialist palliative care teams
Grief and bereavement care after loss	■ Parents' experience of loss and anticipatory grief ■ Ensure parents are involved in the care of their baby after death as much or as little as they wish ■ Explore if they would like to take their baby home or to a local children's hospice for continuing care after death ■ Identify a named point of contact for ongoing bereavement support

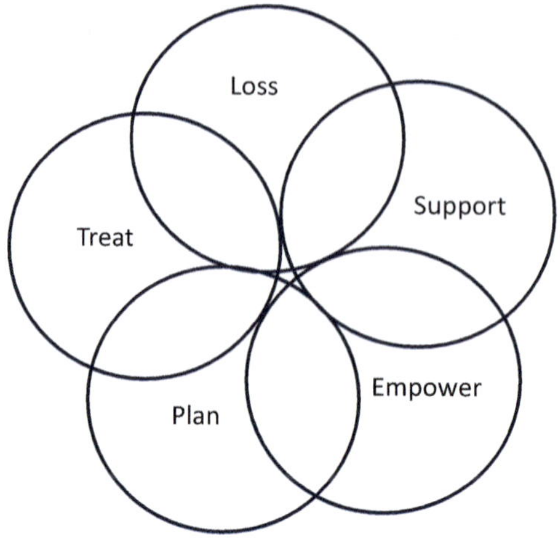

Figure 9.2 Key elements of neonatal palliative care (adapted from BAPM, 2024)

PRACTICE POINTS

- In relation to a baby that you have cared for with palliative care needs, apply the five key elements (support, empower, plan, treat, and loss).
- Consider and discuss how you might approach planning of care and which communication approach might be helpful when discussing uncertainty of the baby's future with the parents.
- Does the place you currently work in have a toolkit or guidance document to support care planning?

HOLISTIC FAMILY SUPPORT

When planning a palliative care pathway for a baby, support for the family needs to be considered just as much as for the infant's ongoing medical and nursing needs. The use of an ACP is a helpful tool for discussions and documentation of the family's wishes and priorities. This may involve support from maternity in case of an antenatal diagnosis of a LLC.

All families require an individualised and personalised approach to care for their baby and support for themselves, including these who may require a tailored approach taking into account the bespoke nature of their needs. This might involve families who consider themselves to be neurodivergent, part of the LGBTQ+ community, travellers, or migrant families. Communication with parents must be non-judgemental and respectful and not based on assumptions.

The 'Caring for Your Baby When the Future Is Uncertain' booklet (Together for Short Lives and Bliss, 2024) provides information about the nature of palliative care as well as support and choices available to them. It can act as a supportive tool for conversations on the NNU. The family's needs or wishes may change as their baby's condition changes, particularly where there is uncertainty over prognosis, so that professionals need to be open to adaptations in any palliative care plan. Involvement of other services such as the children's palliative care or children's hospice teams can support with offering information and options to families to help them in how their needs and wishes can be met. There is evidence that having children's palliative care professionals embedded within the NNU positively influences how effectively parents are able to access hospice support (Tatterton et al., 2023).

The neonatal team should inform the family's local primary care team to ensure continuity of support. Health visitors provide universal services for all children under school age, including those with LLCs. Social and practical needs should be assessed on an individual basis; some babies with complex needs, such as those requiring long-term ventilation, may need social care or family support services during transition from hospital to home. Other families may require practical assistance, for example with sibling care or transport. Charitable organisations, such as the Rainbow Trust Children's Charity, may also be able to offer additional support.

ACTIVITY

Can you list the services and charities available in your local area or nationally which may be able to offer support to families? This could be for practical support for the family or peer support through linking with others whose baby has a similar diagnosis.

CHOICES IN LOCATION OF CARE

For some infants with a very limited life expectancy or an uncertain prognosis, their entire palliative care journey may take place in hospital, either on the delivery suite or within the NNU. However, choices can still be offered to the family:

- Who would they like to be present alongside them?
- Is birth at home or in the children's hospice possible?
- Would they like to have a naming ceremony for their baby?
- Would they like to be in a family room (if on the NNU)?
- Would they like to go home with their baby for continuing care or after the death of their baby?
- Would they like to transfer to a local children's hospice with their baby for continuing care?

If a family choose to take their baby's body home after death, some preparation may be considered in advance for keeping baby's body cool with cooling technologies, e.g. portable air conditioning unit, cooling pads (Techni Ice), a CuddleCot, or cooling sheets. In the absence of cooling technologies, guidance around keeping the room cool, opening windows, and turning off heating appliances can be provided. The absence of access to cooling technologies should not be a barrier to taking their baby home. Other choices include using a temperature-controlled bedroom within a children's hospice (cool bedroom).

When there is an antenatal diagnosis of a LLC, or significant uncertainty about a neonate's prognosis, such as in cases of extreme prematurity at 22–23 weeks' gestation, every effort should be made to offer parents a delivery-room cuddle. This provides an opportunity for parents to hold their baby while alive and reduces the risk that death occurs before this can take place (Clarke, 2017). Where there is more time, additional options for place of care may be explored. For families receiving care on a tertiary neonatal intensive care unit that is not their booking hospital, **repatriation** to the family's local NNU may be possible. Families may also wish to consider transfer to a children's hospice or, where appropriate, discharge home.

For babies whose palliative care needs continue for months or years, care at home can be supported by a children's community nursing team, a community paediatrician, and/or a children's palliative care team, with respite care available through the local children's hospice. Even when life expectancy is limited to days or weeks, home-based end-of-life care may still be an option if appropriate community services are available. This aligns with National Institute for Health and Care Excellence (2016) quality standards, which recommend 24-hour access to children's nursing care and specialist paediatric palliative care advice for end-of-life care at home. However, these services are not yet available in all areas of the UK.

DISCHARGE PLANNING

General considerations for discharge from the NNU and the role of neonatal outreach services are outlined in Chapter 3. While many of these principles also apply to infants discharged on a palliative care pathway, several additional points require attention.

As discussed previously, an ACP is a comprehensive document outlining the family's wishes for the ongoing care of their baby, including plans for end-of-life care. A symptom management plan may also be required to address current symptoms and anticipate probable future symptoms (Maynard, 2020). This should prioritise non-pharmacological strategies before progressing to pharmacological interventions. Important supportive measures such as skin-to-skin contact and non-nutritive sucking can be highly effective and are opportunities for parents to take a leading role (Together for Short Lives, 2020). Pain assessment should continue seamlessly after discharge, using the same validated tools employed on the NNU. Ongoing support may be provided by the neonatal outreach team, children's community nursing team, or the local children's hospice. Pharmacological guidance should follow the APPM Formulary (APPM, 2024).

A discharge planning meeting (see Table 9.3) involving the family, neonatal, and relevant community professionals is essential, whether the baby is transitioning home or to a children's hospice for ongoing care.

TABLE 9.3 DISCHARGE PLANNING IN THE CONTEXT OF NEONATAL PALLIATIVE CARE

Medicines	Alongside a symptom management plan, any medicines required will need to be prescribed and ordered in advance of discharge.
Equipment	If any equipment is required e.g. oxygen or suction, this will need to be ordered in advance and parents taught how to use it.
Nursing Care Plan	The nursing needs for the baby, how much input will be required from neonatal outreach or children's community nurse services, need to be established. This may include consideration for home oxygen, a feeding plan, and symptom management.
Escalation	Contacts for parents in case of deterioration at home.
Readmission	Possibility of readmission, familiarising parents with the appropriate children's ward in the hospital.
Financial Support	If longer-term palliative care is anticipated, parents may be entitled to disability living allowance. Parents should be informed of this.
Language	If English is not the family's first language, ensure an interpreter is in attendance at the meeting and arrangements are made for interpreter provision for ongoing care.
Vulnerable Families	For vulnerable or migrant families, social care support may be required.
End of Life Care	If being transferred home for end-of-life care, ensure ambulance service and primary healthcare professionals are aware.
Compassionate Extubation	If transferring to home or hospice for compassionate extubation, the family will need to be prepared for how this may happen and what to expect.
Care after Death	Preparation for end-of-life care and care of the baby's body after death may be required, depending on prognosis. This will include whom to contact when they die and providing cooling equipment at home if family wish to keep baby at home with them afterwards.

All comprehensive plans should be clearly documented and shared with relevant teams in a timely manner. Care plans may change frequently either following discussions with parents or in response to changes in the baby's clinical condition and needs.

SPECIFIC ASPECTS OF PALLIATIVE CARE

Caring for families with twins and multiple births

There may be situations in a twin or multiple pregnancy where one or more infants have been diagnosed with a life-limiting condition and are not expected to survive the pregnancy or birth. Compassionate consideration must be given to parents faced with the devastating position of balancing the experience of loss and death at the same time as new life, and processing the complexity of emotions attached. Parents have relayed that the loss of 'special status' associated with having twins was particularly painful. A purple butterfly symbol to recognise twin status has been developed as part of a large study undertaken with parents. The symbol is placed on or at the cotside, and parents are offered the opportunity to write the name of the twin or baby who died onto it.

Parents have suggested the key points below to help teams caring for families who have twins or multiple births

- Recognise twin status
- Acknowledge the bereavement
- Provide emotional support
- Provide appropriate information
- Provide continuity
- Offer memory making – suggest photos of the babies together with parents and other siblings if possible
- Handle cot occupancy sensitively on the NNU
- Prepare parents for discharge from hospital

For further information and resources, please access the Neonatal Butterfly Project (see companion website for link).

Delivery room cuddle or birthday cuddle

UNICEF, along with the World Health Organization (WHO), established the Baby-Friendly Hospital Initiative, which highlights that kangaroo care (skin to skin) improves chances of survival for preterm or low birthweight babies when started immediately after birth. It also supports parents in bonding with their baby, reduces stress and anxiety, and helps parents feel more confident about looking after their premature baby. This key element of FiCare care is also known as 'delivery room cuddles' or 'birthday cuddles' and is even more poignant if parents have this opportunity when their baby's future is uncertain. Whilst the benefits of delivery room cuddles are well documented for the baby and their parents, it must be acknowledged that not all NNUs offer this as a standard of routine care. Many studies have supported this as a safe and feasible concept; however, it requires time, planning, and robust collaboration across specialties (Clarke et al., 2021).

Breast care choices after loss

Discussions around breast care after loss help to create a holistic, parent-centred approach to bereavement care on the NNU. The BAPM Lactation After Loss framework (2022) emphasises the importance of offering families clear, compassionate information about their choices, recognising that every response to loss is unique. Whilst some families wish to supress lactation to minimise discomfort and emotional distress, a growing number of families find comfort in donating milk through initiatives such as the Memory Milk Gift (see companion website for information) which provides a meaningful way to honour their baby whilst helping families who have a baby receiving neonatal care. Safe guidance on managing lactation, whether suppression, expression, or donation, must be delivered with compassion (Oreg, 2019). By acknowledging the emotional significance of breast care, health care professionals can support parents to feel empowered and respected in their shared decision-making at a particularly vulnerable time (Atherton & Savage, 2022). Some key points to consider when discussing choices with parents are below.

- When discussing lactation suppression, always offer the option of milk donation.
- Take the time to discuss the potential benefits of donation to the donor and recipients.
- Have literature available for the family to take away.
- Pre-screen the family to determine whether the milk will be used for donation or research.
- Gain a signed consent form.
- Speak to the milk bank about the most appropriate way to take blood samples for serological testing (bearing in mind that some families will not want to return to hospital).
- Pass the referral to the milk bank.

Non-tangible memories and meaning making

It is important to create space and time for parents to reflect on their baby, and to support them in building meaningful family experiences, where every interaction, however small, may become a cherished memory. Providing opportunities to celebrate everyday moments, acknowledge milestones, and share experiences as a family is vital. Tools such as the *Baby Steps* Journey Cards, developed by the Kent, Surrey & Sussex and Thames Valley & Wessex Neonatal Networks (see companion website), can help families recognise and record these significant moments.

Creating opportunities to be together as a family are essential elements of neonatal palliative care when a baby's future is uncertain. Every moment together is treasured and of utmost importance and value, as reflected on in a poignant and moving personal account of baby loss by Norwood (2021). Examples of how babies and their families can have opportunities together which form part of their memories and can help them find meaning include creative therapies, a form of psychotherapy, that uses expressive techniques, such as art, music, and dance, to help people process emotions and improve their mental and physical wellbeing. An example of this within neonatal palliative care is music therapy which can support the parent-infant relationship, enhancing psychological support for both parents and neonatal staff (Jane et al., 2025).

Fresh air therapy and access to nature

It may be possible for the baby and their family to access outdoor spaces within the hospital grounds. Access to nature and natural environments plays a direct and indirect role in health and wellbeing (WHO, 2021) including physiological, cognitive, and psychological benefits, with growing emphasis to see these benefits integrated into inpatient spaces (Edwards et al., 2023; Carroll et al., 2024). The inclusion of natural environments in neonatal palliative care reflects a broader culture shift toward holistic, personalised care, one that honours the emotional, psychological, and spiritual dimensions of end-of-life experiences.

Tantam et al. (2025) describe the benefits and growing culture change across NNUs in offering fresh air therapy to families and their babies when their future is uncertain. They explored the role of access to nature spaces for neonatal palliative care, offering families a chance to experience connection, calm, and dignity beyond the confines of the clinical environment. The integration of outdoor spaces within healthcare settings provides opportunity for parents to engage in everyday acts of parenting such as holding their child in natural light and sharing quiet moments with siblings nearby, which can be profoundly affirming during emotionally complex times (Downing et al., 2014). These experiences help reinforce parental identity and support the psychological processing of grief (Wilkinson et al., 2025).

From a clinical perspective, fresh air therapy also contributes to staff wellbeing. Neonatal professionals often face high emotional demands, with studies reporting significant rates of burnout and post-traumatic stress symptoms (Ravaldi et al., 2023; Butcher et al., 2024). Access to restorative environments, such as hospital gardens, has been shown to reduce emotional fatigue and improve coping strategies, offering a protective buffer against the psychological toll of intensive care work (Cordoza et al., 2018). These spaces not only benefit families but also foster a more supportive and sustainable work environment for healthcare teams.

SELF-AWARENESS AND WELLBEING FOR THE HEALTHCARE TEAM

It is essential that healthcare professionals caring for babies and their families are appropriately trained and have continuing learning opportunities to improve and optimise the care they provide. The neonatal workforce must be equipped with the relevant skills, knowledge, and capabilities to provide consistent high-quality neonatal palliative care. It is well recognised that the impact on individual healthcare professionals can be far reaching, with consideration to the dual demands of clinical excellence and compassionate caregiving (Box 9.1). The National Neonatal Palliative Care Programme provides core e-Learning modules alongside regular virtual training sessions freely accessible to all healthcare and social care teams nationally (see web-based companion for link).

BOX 9.1 THE IMPACT OF PALLIATIVE CARE ON NEONATAL PROFESSIONALS

Providing compassionate care, while beneficial for patient outcomes, can come at a personal cost to nurses and midwives. The emotional labour inherent in healthcare roles increases the risk of burnout and compassion fatigue when work demands are high and support is lacking (Kinman et al., 2020)

Alongside essential tailored training and education enhancing knowledge and confidence, it is paramount that individuals have self-awareness and give consideration to their own wellbeing as well as that of the whole team. It is important to make space and time to reflect on experiences of providing care and the interactions with families receiving it. There are many ways this can be facilitated which include reflection and reflective practice.

ACTIVITY

Consider and reflect on a time when you have been allocated or asked to support the care of a baby with an uncertain future, including supporting their parents.

Using the Model of Reflection for Children's Palliative care by McNeilly et al. (2022), below are some questions for reflection which have been adapted from the model:

Family story

What is the issue for discussion?

Contextual factors

Were there any cultural, spiritual, ethical, legal, social, or political issues?

The event

Who was involved? What went well? What did not go well? How did you feel? What was the emotional impact on you?

Personal factors

How was the event influenced by: Your personal and professional values? Your current knowledge (empirical and experiential) or gaps in your knowledge base, taking account of your scope practice?

Considering the above factors

What have you learned? Has this altered your initial perspective on the situation? Does anything need to change?

Was there an action plan put in place?

Other approaches to support neonatal care staff.

- Debrief – this can be immediately following a traumatic episode in the workplace, sometimes known as a 'hot debrief,' or at a scheduled time later on ('cold debrief'). The aim of a debrief is to give all staff involved the chance to discuss what happened and how a similar situation might be managed in the future. It is not a space for appointing criticism or blame.

- Peer support – offered by colleagues within the team or outside your organisation. This may be formal or informal.
- Restorative clinical supervision with a professional nurse advocate – this can be on a one-to-one or group basis. It gives practitioners the chance to reflect, assimilate, and possibly look at a quality improvement project which has been found to have many beneficial effects for staff as well as enhancing patient care.
- Joining a neonatal palliative care specialist interest group, either locally, regionally, or nationally, can offer another avenue for support through sharing of best practice and knowledge in a safe forum.
- Online wellbeing resources for healthcare professionals.

ACTIVITY

Identify what is on offer where you work to support staff when caring for a patient who dies or after a traumatic event in the workplace. Have you accessed any of these? What did you find beneficial? If you have not accessed any of these services, explore what is available and think about what would best suit your needs.

A GLOBAL PERSPECTIVE

The WHO defines palliative care for children, including babies as

> "the active total care of the child's body, mind and spirit and also involves giving support to the family. It begins when illness is diagnosed, and continues regardless of whether or not a baby or child receives treatment directed at the disease."
>
> (WHO, 2023, para. 1)

Annually in the UK, 60,000 babies are born prematurely and admitted to NNUs. Globally, 15 million babies are born prematurely and remain the leading cause of neonatal death and lifelong complex health needs with an uncertain future, often requiring palliative care. Whilst this chapter focuses on care delivery in the UK, it is important to acknowledge that across Europe and further afield, there are many examples of good practice in neonatal palliative care. Despite different levels of development and resources available, the goals and key principles remain the same: high-quality consistent and equitable neonatal palliative care for all babies who have an uncertain future and enhanced support for their parents and wider family.

All healthcare teams aim at improving the quality of life for babies and their families, whilst supporting individualised and very personal priorities for each family. Diverse cultures, beliefs, faiths, and spiritual focus will invariably influence the choices each family make in partnership with health and social care teams. With advancements in technology and accessibility, digital platforms, information sharing of guidelines and experiences have become commonplace. Internationally and collectively, professionals are able to share learning opportunities and improve the care for infants and their families.

Chapter takeaways

- Neonatal palliative care is an integrated, active approach that begins at diagnosis and continues alongside survival-focused treatment. It prioritises recognising uncertainty early and providing consistent, equitable care across all settings. Family-centred communication and shared decision-making are central throughout.
- Identifying babies who may benefit from palliative care requires multiple approaches, including diagnostic indicators, multidisciplinary concern, and the 'surprise question.' Early recognition enables timely discussions and personalised planning. These approaches help ensure families receive coordinated and compassionate support.
- Communication with families must be compassionate, honest, and culturally sensitive. Creating a safe environment, avoiding assumptions, and adapting communication to each family's needs are essential. Interpreters and multi-modal communication tools support inclusive, equitable care.
- Parallel planning and advance care planning are key components of neonatal palliative care. They help families understand possible scenarios and explore their priorities and goals. Plans are dynamic and should be revisited as a baby's condition evolves.
- Holistic family support includes emotional, cultural, social and practical needs for the whole family, recognising that parents, siblings, and extended family may each need tailored support. Children's hospice teams, community services, and charities play vital roles. Embedding paediatric palliative care specialists in NNUs improves access to hospice support.
- Families should be offered meaningful choices regarding the location of care, including hospital, home, or hospice. Even when life expectancy is short, options such as delivery-room cuddles, home-based end-of-life care, or transitional hospice care can enhance family experience. These choices must be supported by clear planning and appropriate community services.
- Discharge planning for babies on a palliative pathway requires rigorous multidisciplinary coordination. Plans must address medicines, equipment,

symptom management, escalation, and ongoing community support. Clear communication and documentation ensure safe, seamless care across settings.

- Staff wellbeing and reflective practice are essential for sustaining high-quality neonatal palliative care. Healthcare professionals must have access to training, debriefing, supervision, and peer support to help manage the emotional demands of this work. A supported workforce is better equipped to provide compassionate, consistent care to families.

CASE STUDIES

CASE STUDY

Case study 1: Antenatal diagnosis of a life-limiting condition

Immy and Steve are parents to three children; Jack who is 10 years old, Reggie who is 5 years, and Maya who is 3. Immy is pregnant with their fourth child, a girl whom they are calling Ruby. The initial screening test at 12 weeks indicated a higher chance of Edwards syndrome or Patau syndrome. Patau syndrome was then confirmed on amniocentesis. They chose to continue with their pregnancy. At the 20 week scan they were informed that Ruby measured small, with her head appearing microcephalic, and there were concerns with her heart and kidneys. Fetal medicine referred to neonatology, and following their 24-week appointment, a neonatologist and specialist neonatal palliative care nurse meet with Immy and Steve to begin discussions on options for care for Ruby following birth.

Q1. After introducing themselves to Immy and Steve, how should the neonatologist and specialist neonatal palliative care nurse begin the conversation with them?

Q2. What options might they offer to Immy and Steve, considering the potential for Ruby to die *in utero* or at birth or to survive delivery and receive palliative care?

Q3. What other services might they discuss with them?

Immy and Steve decide that they would like to move to a children's hospice with Ruby and their older children if Ruby survives birth. At 37^{+3} weeks' gestation Immy goes into labour, and at 1:30am Ruby is born alive. She is small but breathing by herself and is kept warm with skin-to-skin cuddles with her

CASE STUDY

parents. The transport team are going to take Ruby and Immy in the ambulance to the local children's hospice in the morning.

Q4. Until transfer, what care needs would you need to consider for Ruby?
Q5. What information would you need to ensure is handed over to the hospice team?

Case study 2: Palliative care on a level 2 NNU

Yasmin was the fourth baby for Davi and Nita and was born at 36 weeks' gestation in good condition following an uneventful pregnancy. At birth, she only required minimal intervention with facial oxygen. She was reviewed on the postnatal ward for increased work of breathing, and soft dysmorphic features were noted. She stayed on the NNU due to increasing oxygen requirements and deteriorated, requiring intubation.

Yasmin was also noted to have a fracture to her femur, hypotonia, limited movement, and minimal respiratory effort.

Davi and Nita were consanguineous with a family history of infant loss due to spinal muscular atrophy (type 1); Yasmin has two older brothers, 6 and 8 years old, who were unaffected by the condition.

Yasmin was reviewed by the geneticist, who confirmed it was likely the same condition.

Parents expressed a wish to stay in their local NNU so that they were close to home and the environment was familiar.

There was a full multidisciplinary discussion with the tertiary centre and the family. It was considered that in the best interest of the family, the baby was to remain on the local unit for ongoing palliative care and support for the other children.

Q1. What key aspects need to be considered when supporting the parents, siblings, and wider family?
Q2. Consider how the parents Davi and Nita felt when Yasmin was noted to need intubation along with complications following an uneventful pregnancy. How might you support them during this time on the NNU, and whilst waiting for results from investigations?
Q3. Choices for the family: consider how you might be involved in discussions regarding the planning for Yasmin's care. Which other healthcare professionals might be included and why?
Q4. What support do you think the team might need?

CASE STUDY

Case study 3: Palliative care on a level 3 NNU with twin girls

Sophia and Peter had a history of 6 years of IVF treatment before this twin pregnancy with two girls. The 12 week scan showed Twin 2, Lisa, was not growing well, with some abnormalities detected. Twin 1, Sarah, was unaffected and growing well, but the decision was made to deliver early at 29 weeks to increase the chance of Twin 1 being born in reasonable condition. Lisa and Sarah were born by caesarean section at 29 weeks' gestation.

Twin 1, Sarah, was born in good condition at 1350g requiring ventilatory support and transferred to NNU. Twin 2, Lisa, was born in poor condition at 850g and remained with Mum and Dad on the postnatal ward to cuddle and for palliative care.

Twin 2, Lisa, lived for 2 hours.

Twin 1, Sarah, continued to have care on the NNU and was discharged at 38 weeks corrected gestation. Sophia and Peter spent as much time as possible on the NNU with their surviving twin, Sarah. During this time, they also planned Lisa's funeral.

Q1. What key aspects need to be considered when supporting the parents and wider family at the time of antenatal appointment, at the time of birth, and after birth?

Q2. Consider how the parents might feel when their twin daughters are born and how you can best support them. How might you continue to support the parents throughout their neonatal journey?

Q3. Consider choices available for the parents when they are spending time with their daughter Lisa on the postnatal ward following her birth and providing palliative care. What do you need to consider about the location, privacy, cultural needs, and emotional/psychological needs.

Q4. What support do you think the team might need?

For suggested answer guides to the questions posed in these case studies, please refer to the web-based companion site specific to this chapter. See www.routledge.com/cw/petty

References

Association of Paediatric Palliative Care Medicine. (2024). *Formulary* (6th ed.). APPM.

Atherton, L., & Savage, E. (2022, March). The Memory Milk Gift Initiative: Donation after loss. *Infant*, *18*(2). https://www.infantjournal.co.uk/journal_article.html?id=7281

British Association of Perinatal Medicine. (2022). *Lactation and loss: Management of lactation following the death of a baby*. https://www.bapm.org/resources/lactation-and-loss-management-of-lactation-following-the-death-of-a-baby

British Association of Perinatal Medicine. (2024). *Recognising uncertainty: An integrated framework for palliative care in perinatal medicine.* https://www.bapm.org/resources/palliative-care-in-perinatal-medicine-framework

Butcher, I., Morrison, R., Balogun, O., Duncan, H., St Louis, K., Webb, S., & Shaw, R. (2024). Burnout and coping strategies in pediatric and neonatal intensive care staff. *Clinical Practice in Pediatric Psychology*, *12*(1), 16–30.

Carroll, C., Higgs, J., McCray, S., Utter, J. (2024). Implementation and impact of health care gardens: A systematic scoping review. *Journal of Integrative and Complementary Medicine*, *30*(5), 431–449.

Clancy, M., Thomas, F., Redman, H., Fowke Doyle, H., & Gasiorowski, E. (2024). Informing culturally sensitive neonatal palliative care: Focus on communication. *Infant*, *20*(6).

Clarke, P. (2017). Family-centred care right from birth: The irreplaceable birthday cuddle. *Acta Paediatrica*, *106*, 1534–1539.

Clarke, P., Allen, E., Atuona, S., & Cawley, P. (2021). Delivery room cuddles for extremely preterm babies and parents: Concept, practice, safety, parental feedback. *Acta Paediatrica*, *110*(5), 1439–1449.

Cordoza, M., Ulrich, R. S., Manulik, B. J., Gardiner, S. K., Fitzpatrick, P. S., Hazen, T. M., Mirka, A., & Perkins, R. S. (2018). Impact of nurses taking daily work breaks in a hospital garden on burnout. *American Journal of Critical Care*, *27*(6), 508–512.

Downie, J., Kerr-Elliott, T., & Criag, F. (2020). Advance care planning (Chap. 13). In A. Mancini, J. Price & T. Kerr-Elliott (Eds.), *Neonatal palliative care for nurses*. Springer.

Downing, J., Marston, J., & Fleming, E. (2014). Children's palliative care: Considerations for a physical therapeutic environment. *Journal of Palliative Care*, *30*(2), 116–124.

Edwards, N., Dunn, S., Barach, P., & Vaughan, L. (2023). The Wolfson Prize: Designing the hospital of the future. *Future Healthcare Journal*, *10*(1), 27–30. https://doi.org/10.7861/fhj.2022-0105

Fraser, L. K., Gibson-Smith, D., Jarvis, S., Norman, P., & Parslow, R. C. (2021). Estimating the current and future prevalence of life-limiting conditions in children in England. *Palliative Medicine*, *35*(9), 1641–1651.

Harnden, F., Lanoue, J., Modi, N., Uthaya, S. N., & Battersby, C., UK National Collaborative (2023). Data-driven approach to understanding neonatal palliative care needs in England and Wales: A population-based study 2015–2020. *Archives of Disease in Childhood – Fetal and Neonatal Edition*, *108*(5), 540–544

HEARD. (2023). *How to talk about children's palliative care.* https://heard.org.uk/wp-content/uploads/2023/01/Heard_How-to-talk-about-childrens-Palliative-Care_draft_v2.pdf

Hui, D., De La Cruz, M., Mori, M., Parsons, H. A., Kwon, J. H., Torres-Vigil, I., Kim, S. H., Dev, R., Hutchins, R., Liem, C., Kang, D. H., & Bruera, E. (2013). Concepts and definitions for 'supportive care,' 'best supportive care,' 'palliative care,' and 'hospice care' in the published literature, dictionaries, and textbooks. *Supportive Care in Cancer*, *21*(3), 659–685. https://doi.org/10.1007/s00520-012-1564-

Jane, K., Hayns-Worthington, R., Gallagher, K., Livermore, P., Shoemark, H., & Robert, G. (2025). Supporting continuing bonds for parents with infants with uncertain futures on neonatal units in the United Kingdom: Co-designing a culturally sensitive music therapy intervention. *Frontiers in Psychiatry*, *16*, 1633878. https://doi.org/10.3389/fpsyt.2025.1633878

Kinman, G., Teoh, K., & Harris, A. (2020). *The mental health & wellbeing of nurses and midwives in the UK.* https://www.som.org.uk/sites/som.org.uk/files/The_Mental_Health_and_Wellbeing_of_Nurses_and_Midwives_in_the_United_Kingdom.pdf

Mancini, A., Price, J., & Kerr-Elliott, T. (2020). *Neonatal palliative care for nurses*. Springer.

Maynard, L. (2020). Fundamental principles of effective symptom management in neonatal palliative care (Chap. 16). In A. Mancini, J. Price & T. Kerr-Elliott (Eds.), *Neonatal palliative care for nurses*. Springer.

McNeilly, P., McCloskey, S., Peacock, V., & Price, J. E. (2022). Reflecting on palliative care for children, young people and their families: A revised model. *International Journal of Palliative Nursing, 28*(10), 482–490. https://doi.org/10.12968/ijpn.2022.28.10.482

National Child Mortality Database (NCMD). (2025, July). *Infants, children, and young people with life-limiting conditions. Learning from child death reviews on palliative and end of life care provision.* National Child Mortality Database Programme Thematic Report.

National Institute for Health and Care Excellence (NICE). (2016). *End of life care for infants, children and young people.* Quality Standard QS160.

Norwood, T. (2021). Something good enough. *The Lancet, 398*(10318), 2305–2306.

Office for National Statistics (ONS). (2025). *Child and infant mortality in England and Wales: 2023.* Office for National Statistics. https://www.ons.gov.u

Oreg, A. (2019). Milk Donation after losing one's baby: Adopting a donor identity as a means of coping with loss. *Social Science & Medicine, 238,* 112519.

Prentice, J., Nelson, A., Baillie, J., Osborn, H., & Noble, S. (2014). Don't blame the middleman. *The Royal Society of Medicine, 107*(7), 271–276.

Ravaldi, C., Mosconi, L., Mannetti, L., Checconi, M., Bonaiuti, R., Ricca, V., Mosca, F., Dani, C., & Vannacci, A. (2023). Post-traumatic stress symptoms and burnout in healthcare professionals working in neonatal intensive care units: Results from the STRONG study. *Front Psychiatry, 14,* 1050236.

Smith, L. K., van Blankenstein, E., Fox, G., Seaton, S. E., Martinez-Jimenez, M., Petrou, S., Battersby, C., & MBRRACE-UK Perinatal Surveillance Group. (2023). Effect of national guidance on survival for babies born at 22 weeks' gestation in England and Wales: Population-based cohort study. *BMJ Medicine, 2*(1), e000579.

Tantam, K., Philipps, M., Rogers, C., Clarke, R, Keeling, D. (2025). End of life care in a fresh air space – a case report. *Journal of Neonatal Nursing, 31,* 101726.

Tatterton, M., Fisher, M., Storton, H., Mcshane, Z., & Walker, C. (2023). Holding families in uncertainty: A framework analysis of the role and impact of children's hospices in the provision of perinatal palliative care. *Illness, Crisis & Loss, 33*(1), 152–171.

Together for Short Lives. (2018). *A guide to children's palliative care: Supporting babies, children and young people with life-limiting and life-threatening conditions and their families* (4th ed.). Together for Short Lives. https://www.togetherforshortlives.org.u

Together for Short Lives. (2020). *Perinatal pathway for babies with palliative care needs.* Together for Short Lives. https://www.togetherforshortlives.org.u

Together for Short Lives and Bliss. (2024). *Caring for your baby when the future is uncertain.* Retrieved November 2025, from https://www.bliss.org.uk/news/2024/bliss-and-together-for-short-lives-launch-new-information-for-families-whose-babys-future-is-uncertain

Wilkinson, D., Bertaud, S., Mancini, A., & Murdoch, E. (2025). Recognising uncertainty: An integrated framework for palliative care in perinatal medicine. *Archives of Disease in Childhood – Fetal and Neonatal Edition, 110*(3), 236–244.

World Health Organization (WHO). (2021). *Green and blue spaces and mental health: New evidence and perspectives for action.* https://www.who.int/europe/publications/i/item/9789289055666

World Health Organization (WHO). (2023). *Palliative care for children.* https://www.who.int/europe/news-room/fact-sheets/item/palliative-care-for-children

10 NEONATAL BEREAVEMENT CARE

Jo Cookson

CONTENTS

DOI: 10.4324/9781003591405-13

GUIDANCE ON HOW TO ENHANCE PERSONAL LEARNING FROM THIS CHAPTER

Key points covered in this chapter

- Definitions of bereavement, mourning, and grief, and the nature of the grieving process.
- How to care for families experiencing a bereavement on the NNU.
- The wider impact of the perinatal death of a baby.

Reflection

Reading through the chapter, you are encouraged to engage with the key points and related literature in an enquiring way. Ask these questions:

- What emotional responses and behaviours might be exhibited by bereaved parents, and how can healthcare professionals provide appropriate and compassionate support in response?
- How can bereavement care be delivered in a manner that is sensitive to the parents' individual needs and preferences, with the intention of fostering positive and meaningful recollection of their experience in the future?
- What key considerations should be considered in relation to the extended family, and what strategies can be implemented to ensure continued support for parents following discharge after the death of their baby?

Implications for neonatal practice

- Finally: this chapter aims to enhance your understanding of perinatal death and inform the provision of compassionate, individualised care for affected families. Reflecting on this knowledge, how might your approach to care be influenced or transformed as a result?

INTRODUCTION AND BACKGROUND

Globally, neonatal mortality remains a significant challenge, with approximately 2.3 million newborns dying in 2023, accounting for nearly half of all deaths in children under 5. The highest neonatal mortality rates are found in lower income countries such as sub-Saharan Africa and southern Asia, where access to quality maternal and newborn care is often limited (World Health Organization, 2024; UNICEF, 2025). The death of a neonate is relatively uncommon in higher income countries as mortality rates have declined dramatically over the course of the twentieth century. However, due to extreme prematurity, congenital anomalies, or other complex medical issues, some babies are unable to survive despite medical interventions. Quality of life issues are also integrated into decision-making where potentially medical interventions may be withdrawn or withheld if they are not deemed to be in the infant' best interests.

Experiencing the death of a baby is a profound and often unexpected loss that generates significant emotional turmoil for parents, triggering a complex grieving process. Perinatal and neonatal death must be acknowledged as a unique form of loss, often eliciting an intense emotional response that affects many dimensions of parents' lives, including their emotional, physical, financial, spiritual, and social wellbeing. This deeply personal experience also profoundly impacts healthcare professionals (HCPs), highlighting the need for both compassionate care and the implementation of best practices. The quality of care provided during pregnancy, birth, and following a neonate's death is especially critical, as parents will always remember how they were treated during this time. It can influence their short- and long-term wellbeing, their ability to care for others, and their future interactions with health services. This chapter highlights the unique nature of grief associated with neonatal death, addressing the individual needs of families and emphasising the importance of consistent, compassionate bereavement care. It also explores how effective and sensitive communication can enhance the support provided to bereaved families, ultimately improving their experience during one of the most challenging times in their lives.

BEREAVEMENT, MOURNING, AND GRIEF

Terms such as bereavement, mourning, and grief are often used interchangeably, but understanding their distinct differences is crucial. It is important to recognise that loss and grief may not be solely associated with the death of a baby. These feelings can arise when reality diverges from expected futures. Many parents of preterm and sick neonates experience a sense of loss and grief, even if their baby survives. Often, there is a feeling of lost opportunity, particularly when long-term morbidity issues arise despite avoiding mortality (Steele & Mancini, 2013).

Bereavement

Bereavement is an objective condition, denoting the state of having experienced the death of a significant other. In neonatal settings, parents may question whether the death of their baby, particularly in cases where the neonate was their only child, renders them no longer parents in a social or cultural sense. This perceived loss of parental identity can exacerbate the emotional impact of their grief, as it may be experienced as a form of disenfranchised loss, whereby the legitimacy of their grief is minimised or unacknowledged by society. Parental bereavement following neonatal death presents a distinct form of grief, shaped by the limited duration of the parent-infant relationship. The brief time spent with the baby often results in a scarcity of tangible memories, which can complicate the grieving process (Currie et al., 2018).

Mourning

Mourning refers to the outward expression of grief following a death and is often shaped by cultural and societal norms. Across diverse ethnic populations, structured rituals, such as wearing designated clothing, abstaining from regular activities, or engaging in symbolic behaviours, serve to acknowledge and communicate the experience of loss. In the context of the United Kingdom (UK), mourning can be particularly complex for parents who have experienced neonatal death, as their grief may not be fully recognised or validated by others. The societal tendency to underestimate the depth of this loss can lead to feelings of isolation, further complicating the mourning process and impeding emotional recovery.

Grief

Grief is a multifaceted biological and psychological response to death, which can present through a range of physical, emotional, behavioural, and psychosocial manifestations. HCPs working within neonatal units (NNUs) must be attuned to the diverse and individualised expressions of grief encountered among bereaved parents. Although the experience of loss is a universal human phenomenon, its outward expression is deeply influenced by cultural, religious, and personal values. While some cultural frameworks emphasise emotional restraint and stoicism, others encourage open verbal expression or seek solitude and privacy during bereavement. It is therefore imperative that health professionals adopt a culturally sensitive, non-judgmental approach, ensuring that care remains responsive to the values, beliefs, and preferences of the grieving family.

MODELS OF GRIEF AND LOSS

The grieving process has been the studied intensely, with early theoretical models frequently emphasising stage-based frameworks. One of the most influential of these is Kübler-Ross's (2014) model, which identifies emotional responses such as denial, confusion, anger, bargaining, depression, and acceptance. However, it is essential for HCPs to recognise that grief is a highly individualised experience with various ethnic, cultural, and religious nuances; not all individuals will encounter each stage, nor will they necessarily progress through them in a linear or sequential manner. While such models can offer a useful lens for understanding the emotional landscape of bereavement, they should not be applied rigidly or prescriptively in clinical practice.

More recent theorists have emphasised the social and cultural context of bereavement and grief, leading to the dual process model (Stroebe & Schut, 2010; see Figure 10.1). This model acknowledges the individuality of the grief response and the journey through grief. It suggests that bereaved parents often oscillate between confrontation and avoidance rather than experiencing grief as a linear series of stages. This oscillation involves moving between passive and active styles of grief without a set timeline. Bereaved individuals may fluctuate between confronting their grief and engaging in everyday tasks or seeking distractions from their intense emotions.

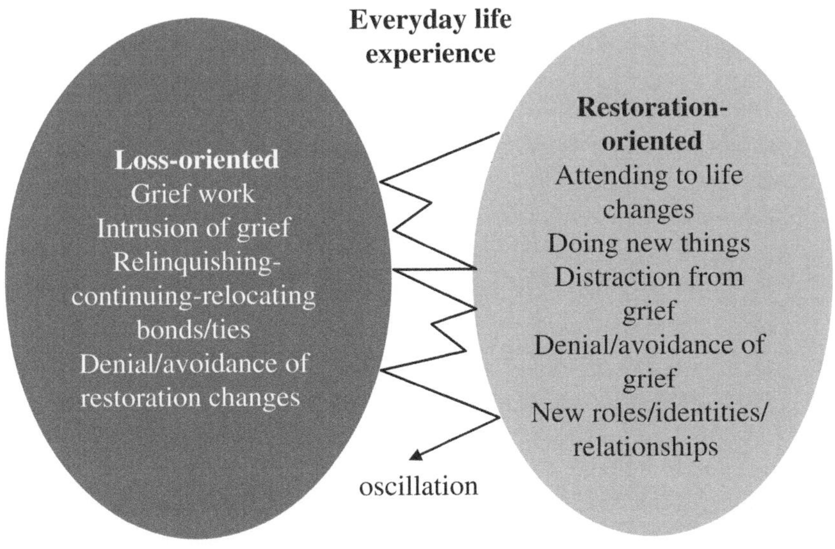

Figure 10.1 A dual process model of coping with loss (adapted from Stroebe & Schut, 2010)

RESPONDING TO LOSS

Grief is widely recognised as a dynamic and emotionally labile process, often characterised by fluctuations in intensity and expression over time (Worden, 2018). For some parents, the death of their baby may represent their first encounter with death, leaving them unprepared for the complex emotional upheaval that follows. It is crucial for HCPs to sensitively communicate that grief is an inherently individual experience, encompassing a broad spectrum of emotional and physiological responses. Acknowledging this variability can help validate parents' experiences and support their coping mechanisms during an intensely vulnerable period (see Box 10.1). It is important to acknowledge and communicate to parents that grief is a deeply personal and individualised process, with no singular or universally 'right' way to experience or express it. Nevertheless, empirical evidence indicates that bereaved parents often benefit from receiving information about the diverse emotional responses commonly associated with grief (Lakhani et al., 2024). Providing such information can aid in normalising their experiences, offering reassurance that their emotional reactions, however varied, are valid and shared by others who have endured similar losses. This approach can foster a sense of connection and support, mitigating feelings of isolation during the grieving process

BOX 10.1 A MOTHER'S REFLECTION ON THE COMPLEX NATURE OF GRIEF IN THE PERINATAL PERIOD

Bereaved parents, no matter how long ago our loss, we carry on, we might smile and we might laugh and we might be genuinely happy – but what we never, ever do – is forget. You can help us make our memories rich and meaningful. I wish I had photographs of my son naked. It might seem strange but years later, I feel guilty as his mother that I never saw him properly. I know he was in poor condition, so the nurse very kindly wrapped him up and took him away to dress him. She meant well, but I regret not dressing him myself, I would have been so proud of myself for doing that. I could have really been a Mum to him in those brief moments, and photographs that took me back to that special time would have been amazing!

Mother of Rowan

> **Reflection point**
>
> Consider how this bereaved mother's story will affect your own professional practice? Think of how you could adapt practice in your own clinical area to improve the memories of bereaved parents.

Conventional models of grief typically suggest that it concludes after a set timeframe. However, it is now understood that those who are bereaved often maintain an ongoing connection with the deceased, who continues to hold a place in their lives. This perspective is especially significant for grieving parents, as it helps them to rebuild their relationship in a way that keeps their deceased baby as an enduring part of the family. This concept links closely with Tonkin's model of grief, known as Growing Around Grief, which suggests that grief does not necessarily diminish over time; instead, life grows around the grief. Initially, grief may permeate every aspect of a person's life. Over time, rather than shrinking, the individual's life expands, allowing them to experience new things and create new parts of their life while still carrying the grief (Tonkin, 1996).

DEATH IN THE NEONATAL UNIT – PROVIDING HOLISTIC AND INCLUSIVE CARE

After the death of a neonate, it is essential that parents and families receive holistic care that is attuned to their unique needs. HCPs should adopt a person-centred approach, ensuring they listen carefully to the parents' wishes. Parents should be given the time and space to express their individual needs, supported and guided by compassionate professionals. Recognising and respecting the parents' personal, cultural, spiritual, and religious values is crucial in providing meaningful and sensitive care (Brooten et al., 2016). A holistic approach to care should be adopted by the wider healthcare teams involved in the family's care. This necessitates clear communication and cooperation between teams, with appropriate referrals to relevant organisations for ongoing support. Collaboration with maternity services is particularly crucial, so parents are well supported during the immediate postnatal period (see Box 10.2).

BOX 10.2 THE IMPORTANCE OF COMMUNICATION BETWEEN NEONATAL AND MATERNITY SERVICES

While my husband had left to arrange overnight accommodation at the hospital, I asked the doctor if I should express milk, as the midwives had suggested I should do so. I was told, 'Let's see if he survives first.' These words were like a bullet through my heart. The doctor was shocked I didn't know how serious his condition was, but all day we had been told he was stable and not given the full details, even the midwives that had been with us were shocked by this news.

Mother of Isaac

CULTURAL ELEMENTS OF LOSS

While it is important for professionals to understand how parents' personal, cultural, spiritual, and religious beliefs may shape their choices, it is equally vital that they avoid making assumptions (Sadeghi et al., 2016). Professionals should not presume to know parents' wishes based on factors such as socioeconomic status, religion, or personal circumstances. Although these aspects may influence decisions around funerals and post-mortem consent, they do not necessarily determine them. Those supporting parents must adopt a non-judgemental, attentive approach, ensuring that parents feel heard and respected.

COMMUNICATION

HCPs play a critical role in supporting parents through the profound trauma of perinatal death. The intensity of grief reactions often displayed by bereaved parents can evoke discomfort among healthcare providers, who may fear saying the wrong thing or inadvertently exacerbating the parents' emotional distress. Such fears frequently become barriers to providing compassionate and effective care. However, trauma-informed practice emphasises the importance of presence, validation, and emotional safety in navigating these difficult encounters (Berry et al., 2023). Recognising and normalising the parents' emotional responses is fundamental to fostering an environment conducive to healing.

A core principle of effective communication in this situation is active and intentional listening, which involves offering undivided attention and demonstrating empathy. This approach grants parents the meaningful experience of being truly heard in their grief, providing them with the space to share their narrative, explore complex emotions, and identify what matters most in their journey. By adopting this communication strategy, healthcare professionals will not only be acknowledging the depth of parental suffering but also support the gradual restoration of agency and control. It is essential to acknowledge that neither the death of a neonate nor the profound grief it evokes can be 'fixed.' Trauma-informed care reframes the role of healthcare providers from that of problem-solvers to facilitators of a safe, respectful space where parents can openly express their sorrow and their enduring love for their baby. This approach prioritises emotional safety, empowerment, and collaboration, allowing parents to engage with their grief at their own pace while feeling supported and validated (Berry et al., 2023).

ACTIVITY

Take a look at these resources and consider how they inform your nursing care:

- Child Bereavement UK. *Faiths, beliefs, cultures and communities.* https://www.childbereavementuk.org/pages/faqs/category/faiths-beliefs-cultures-and-communities Consider the diverse perspectives on neonatal bereavement care.
- Stillbirth and Neonatal Death Society (SANDS) Professionals page. https://www.sands.org.uk/professionals Consider how to apply your care to improve the quality of care offered during pregnancy and in the event of a neonate dying.

Verbal communication

The use of carefully considered language is critical when communicating with parents following the death of a neonate. Empirical evidence suggests that bereaved families place a high value on receiving clear, honest, and direct information about their baby's condition, even when such communication involves the disclosure of distressing or life-limiting news (SANDS, 2022). However, shortcomings in communication training among HCPs can lead to the delivery of information in ways that parents may perceive as impersonal or insensitive (Lakhani et al., 2024). To enhance communication effectiveness and emotional support, professionals should prioritise the use of plain, comprehensible language and minimise reliance on medical jargon. Additionally, adopting the terminology and language preferred by parents, including the use of the baby's given name, demonstrates respect, empathy, and a family-centred approach to care. Furthermore, it is crucial to acknowledge that the delivery of traumatic information can significantly impair cognitive processing and memory retention. Consequently, healthcare professionals may need to repeat key information multiple times, perhaps rephrasing it to aid understanding. Parents should be actively encouraged to ask questions and seek clarification regarding aspects they find difficult to comprehend. Consistent access to knowledgeable staff between formal discussions is also essential, as it provides opportunities for parents to have their concerns addressed in a timely and supportive manner.

Parents generally value healthcare providers who convey the gravity of the information with appropriate empathy and seriousness. Maintaining honesty, including transparency about uncertainties, and recognising the emotional toll such conversations have on parents, are critical components of compassionate care. Ultimately, the provision of sensitive, therapeutic communication constitutes a cornerstone of high-quality bereavement support (Currie et al., 2018).

Nonverbal communication

Nonverbal communication plays a pivotal role in all interpersonal interactions and must be carefully considered in clinical contexts. Elements such as posture, facial expressions, gestures, physical proximity, and vocal tone convey significant meaning, often independent of spoken language. In situations involving bereaved parents, these nonverbal cues can be particularly salient; such individuals are often acutely attuned to subtle communicative signals and may detect distressing information even before it is verbally disclosed (Siassakos et al., 2018). In these emotionally charged circumstances, parents tend to rely on intuition, frequently anticipating the nature of bad news. This anticipatory anxiety can heighten emotional distress and erode trust in the HCP responsible for their infant's care (SANDS, 2016).

Cultural sensitivity is essential when interpreting nonverbal communication, as norms regarding facial expressions, eye contact, and other behaviours vary significantly across cultures. HCPs must therefore avoid making assumptions based solely on nonverbal indicators. In cases where English is not the parents' first language, the use of trained interpreters should be considered a standard component of care. Interpreters not only facilitate accurate transmission of medical information but can also bridge cultural divides, helping both staff and parents navigate potential misunderstandings and foster mutual comprehension. HCPs should ensure that interpreters are made aware of the sensitive nature of the information they will be conveying and that they receive appropriate support after the communication has taken place

Box 10.3 summarises important aspects of communication in bereavement.

BOX 10.3 COMMUNICATION WITH BEREAVED PARENTS

- All communication with parents experiencing a pregnancy loss or the death of a baby must be empathic, sensitive, non-judgemental, and parent-led.
- Use warm, open body language by sitting near parents, facing them, making eye contact, and using touch if appropriate.
- Communicate with honesty while remaining as sensitive as possible. Showing genuine emotion is acceptable; however, care must be taken to ensure that parents do not feel responsible for managing the professional's emotional response.
- Professionals should maintain their natural empathic approach, avoiding extremes of being overly detached or overly demonstrative.
- Parents may experience shock or significant distress, which can impair their ability to process information or think clearly. Staff should communicate in a calm, clear manner using straightforward language, and parents should be encouraged to ask questions at any time.
- Be aware that cultural norms or individual circumstances may influence a parent's readiness to ask questions, request clarification, or express their needs and preferences.

Adapted from SANDS National Care Bereavement Pathway (2022)

CARING FOR THE DYING BABY

Parents who have experienced neonatal death consistently emphasise the importance of having their role and identity as a parent acknowledged and respected as well as ensuring they are enabled to function as a parent while being an advocate for their baby (Redshaw et al., 2021). Neonates who die within the NNU often do so following a period of intensive medical intervention. During this time, parents are frequently confronted with the emotionally distressing experience of seeing their baby surrounded by complex life-support equipment, situated within a highly technological environment, and physically separated by the barriers of an incubator. Such experiences can understandably lead to emotional detachment or physical withdrawal, as parents begin to process the anticipated loss of their child (Hindmarch, 2018). It is essential that HCPs acknowledge and understand these responses and actively engage in compassionate, sensitive strategies to support and encourage parental involvement in their baby's care, even during this profoundly difficult time.

Actively involving parents in the care of their baby, in accordance with the principles of family integrated care (FiCare), supports the development of parental confidence and emotional connection, even in the context of critical illness or impending death (British Association of Perinatal Medicine (BAPM), 2021). Facilitating participation in caregiving tasks, such as feeding, bathing, and dressing, and enabling physical contact with the baby where appropriate, are integral to affirming the parental role and supporting psychological wellbeing. Such active engagement has been shown to mitigate the profound feelings of guilt that parents may otherwise experience following their baby's death (SANDS, 2022). Furthermore, careful attention must be given to the physical and emotional environment at the time of death, as outlined by the National Bereavement Care Pathway (2022), which emphasises the importance of compassionate and family-centred end-of-life care practices. These considerations have also been explored in Chapter 9, where salient points for creating a supportive environment are identified.

An individualised and sensitive approach to the care provided during the immediate period surrounding a neonate's death is essential. Parental preferences at this time can vary considerably; while some parents may wish for solitude with their baby before, during, or after death, others may derive comfort from the presence of HCPs who can offer emotional support and answer any emerging questions. Similarly, while some parents may choose to hold their baby as they die, others may not find solace in doing so. The practice of offering parents the opportunity to see and hold their baby after death has become routine in many NNUs, yet it remains important to recognise that this is not universally beneficial. Encouraging parents to hold their baby under the presumption that it will facilitate grieving may be counterproductive and risks placing undue emotional pressure on them.

HCPs must adopt a compassionate and non-directive approach, presenting the available options clearly while following the expressed wishes of the parents. These discussions should be approached with sensitivity, as parents in acute distress may feel compelled to comply with suggestions that are perceived as clinical recommendations rather than optional choices (SANDS, 2022).

Spiritual and religious considerations

Some bereaved parents may find solace in participating in spiritual or religious ceremonies to honour and commemorate their child's life. However, it is imperative that HCPs refrain from making assumptions regarding the desirability or cultural appropriateness of such practices. Rather, these options should be presented with sensitivity and cultural humility, ensuring that parents are supported to make informed decisions that reflect their individual beliefs and values (Lakhani et al.,

2024). Following the death of a neonate, specific cultural or religious traditions may influence the care of the deceased baby, including stipulations about who may handle the body and the prescribed procedures for washing and dressing. Parents, particularly those experiencing neonatal death for the first time, may feel uncertain about the rituals associated with their cultural or faith traditions and may therefore look to healthcare staff for guidance.

In such situations, it is crucial that practitioners are equipped to provide informed, culturally sensitive support. Establishing and maintaining relationships with a range of faith leaders and community representatives enables healthcare teams to offer appropriate advice and facilitate desired rituals in accordance with family wishes. Proactive engagement with diverse cultural and religious communities prior to such events ensures that NNUs are prepared to deliver holistic and respectful care that honours the cultural values of all families.

THINK POINT

Can you think of an example of a neonate that has died on the NNU? How were the family cared for? If you have not yet observed a neonatal death, what do you think are the important areas to prepare yourself for this aspect of care? Finally, also consider how this chapter aligns closely with Chapter 9 on palliative care and Chapter 11 on ethical considerations in neonatal care.

Memory making

Perinatal death presents profound emotional and psychological challenges for bereaved parents. While many parents have formed an attachment to their baby, the brevity of the baby's life often results in an absence of tangible memories that can be shared with others, potentially complicating the grieving process (SANDS, 2022). In this context, the role of the HCP in sensitively facilitating opportunities for memory-making becomes crucial. Compassionate encouragement to engage in physical closeness, such as talking to, gently touching, or holding their baby, including the option of skin-to-skin contact, can provide parents with cherished moments that offer comfort in the future. Moreover, supporting parents to create keepsakes, photographs, or videos enables families to establish concrete memories that may be shared within their wider social networks, reinforcing the recognition of the child's life and significance.

To support this process, many NNUs now collaborate with specialist charities such as 4Louis and SANDS, which provide memory boxes containing items

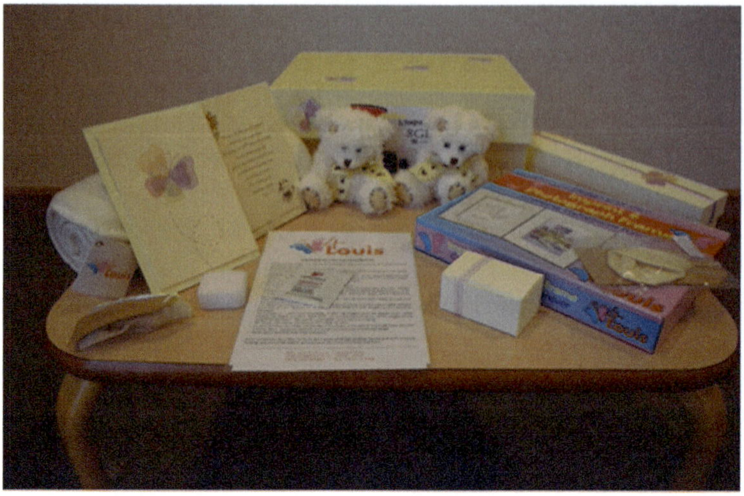

Figure 10.2 Louis memory box

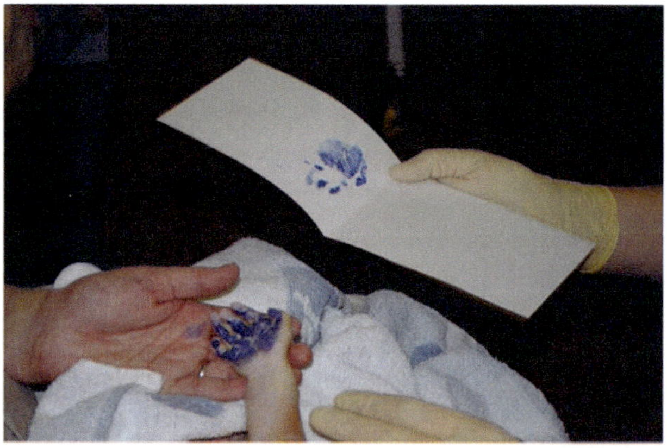

Figure 10.3 Memory-making

designed to preserve mementoes of the baby's life (see Figures 10.2 and 10.3). These resources not only offer a dedicated space for keepsakes (see Box 10.4) but also play a vital role in acknowledging the child's existence and supporting parental grief. The integration of such initiatives aligns with the National Bereavement Care Pathway, which advocates for offering meaningful memory-making opportunities as an essential component of high-quality, compassionate bereavement support (SANDS, 2022).

Tangible mementoes connected to the baby will help to confirm their existence and provide comfort to the parents in the long term (see Box 10.5).

BOX 10.4 KEEPSAKES

- Hand- and footprints
- Lock of hair
- Clay models of the baby's hands or feet if possible
- A record of baby's weight and length
- Clinical items used when caring for the baby
- Any blankets or toys used by the baby
- Baby's cord clamp
- Identification bracelet
- Cot card
- Photographs

BOX 10.5 THE IMPORTANCE OF MEMORY BOXES

> *When we made the decision to turn his life support off, we realised that he didn't have a teddy. I made the decision to buy him one but had no idea where I could get one from. I asked the staff member who told me not to worry and that she would sort it; she came back a short time later with a memory box which included a change of clothes and two teddy bears. This meant that the last few precious moments could be spent with our baby.*
>
> Father of Isaac

Where appropriate, parents should be offered support in considering the transfer of their baby's care to a specialist children's hospice. Hospices provide a less clinical and more family-centred environment, allowing parents unrestricted time to be with their baby in a setting that fosters intimacy and emotional connection. This transition can also alleviate some of the pressures faced by clinical staff within busy NNUs, where time and resources to support bereaved families are often limited. Please see Chapter 9 for more details on palliative care planning.

It is essential that HCPs present choices to bereaved parents with the clear assurance that their preferences will be respected wherever possible. Parents should also be informed that their decisions are not necessarily final; for example, while some may initially decline the opportunity to hold their deceased baby, they may later wish to do so. HCPs must remain sensitive to such evolving preferences and provide compassionate support throughout this process (SANDS, 2022).

Furthermore, it is imperative that professionals possess a sound understanding of the physiological changes that occur after death and communicate this sensitively to parents, as unanticipated changes in the neonate's appearance may contribute to additional distress. Environmental factors, such as elevated ambient temperatures, can accelerate such changes. Where feasible, access to a cold cot should be facilitated, as this enables families to maximise the time spent with their baby in a dignified and respectful manner (BAPM, 2024). It is suggested that the use of a cooling facility can reduce the immediate distress experienced by parents in the early stages of bereavement by allowing the deceased baby to remain in a familiar environment, thereby affording parents greater control over the timing of final separation (Hackett et al., 2022). While there are no formal legal requirements mandating specific documentation for the transfer of the baby's body home, it is considered best practice to provide a letter of confirmation to accompany the family, helping to prevent potential misunderstandings or difficulties (SANDS, 2022).

Photographs

Photography can serve as a meaningful means for families to remember their baby, though it is crucial to recognise that cultural factors may influence whether this is perceived as acceptable. For many parents, photographs offer a tangible connection to their child, providing a visual testament to the existence of their baby. Specialised bereavement photography courses are being developed for healthcare providers to ensure that sensitive and enduring images are captured with the utmost care (see Figure 10.4 for an example). Additionally, it is important to consider the potential impact on other family members, particularly siblings, who may find comfort in having photographs taken with the baby. Families should never feel coerced into taking photographs; however, HCPs should gently inform them that many parents have expressed regret over not capturing more memories

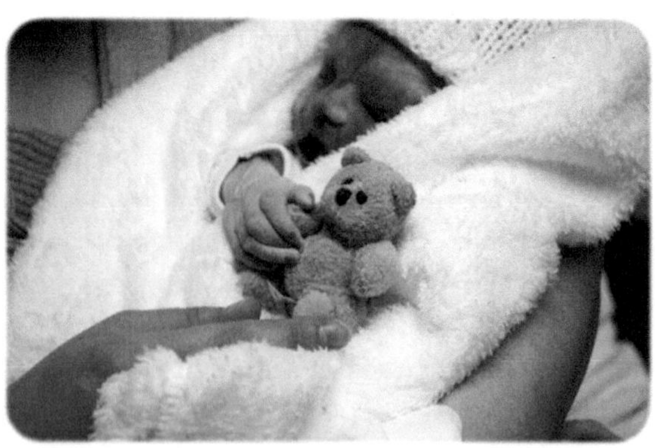

Figure 10.4 Minimising the presence of invasive medical devices

or being dissatisfied with the quality and quantity of photographs taken (Blood & Cacciatore, 2014).

POSTNATAL CARE FOLLOWING A LOSS

The psychological impact of stillbirth and neonatal death on parents is both profound and enduring. Social support is a critical factor in promoting biopsychosocial wellbeing in the aftermath of such life-altering experiences (Cacciatore et al., 2021). However, the distinct and often paradoxical nature of perinatal death frequently results in inadequate social support, with many parents reporting feelings of isolation and emotional disconnection. Interactions with family, friends, and colleagues are often perceived as insensitive or invalidating, compounding the sense of grief and marginalisation (Berry et al., 2023). Connecting parents to a supportive community becomes a priority as well as educating parents on the importance of being connected to a strong support network should be coupled with information on what resources are available to ensure parents are both informed and empowered during their bereavement journey. In accordance with recommendations from BAPM, it is essential that families have access to specialist psychological and mental health support both during their time on the NNU and following discharge (BAPM, 2021). This recommendation is further supported by National Health Service (NHS) England (2021), which advocates for the integration of clinical psychologists within multidisciplinary teams to ensure the delivery of high-quality, psychologically informed care throughout the perinatal period.

It is imperative that all mothers who experience neonatal death are provided with comprehensive, evidence-based lactation support as an integral component of bereavement care. This should involve collaboration with the local infant feeding team to ensure that mothers receive expert guidance and support. Care provision should include anticipatory counselling regarding lactation suppression, helping mothers make informed decisions about managing their milk production in the context of loss (Noble-Carr et al., 2023). Additionally, the option of milk donation should be sensitively discussed as a potential avenue for some mothers, recognising that for certain individuals, donating expressed breastmilk may provide a meaningful and purposeful action amidst bereavement (BAPM, 2022). Proactive, compassionate support in this area can play a vital role in addressing both the physical and emotional aspects of lactation following perinatal loss.

MULTIPLE PREGNANCIES

When one neonate in a multiple birth is facing imminent death, the situation becomes particularly complex and emotionally fraught. Parental needs may be especially complex, particularly when outcomes for each baby differ. Parents may express distinct preferences regarding their involvement with each baby, necessitating an individualised and compassionate approach by HCPs. It is essential that parents are encouraged to spend time with both their surviving baby and the one who is unlikely to survive. In such cases, it is critical that both infants be held and photographed together, allowing families to create memories that reflect the entirety of their experience. HCPs, while providing the standard bereavement support, must also recognise and address the conflicting emotions of joy and grief that parents may experience during this difficult time (SANDS, 2022).

FATHERS AND SAME-SEX PARTNERS

The emotional impact of perinatal death on fathers and partners is often insufficiently recognised or acknowledged in clinical practice. Additionally, societal pressures and the expectation to return to work may compel partners to suppress their grief, thereby reintegrating into everyday life without fully processing the death.

Neonatal death creates a distinct form of grief that affects both parents equally and simultaneously. Therefore, parents should be guided in understanding the complexity of this shared grieving process, fostering mutual respect and acceptance of each other's emotional responses. Additionally, couples must recognise the challenges of supporting one another while navigating their individual grief. HCPs play a crucial role in encouraging parents to engage in open communication and to seek specialist counselling if needed, thereby promoting emotional wellbeing during this difficult time.

EXTENDED FAMILY

Where a decision has been made to reorientate a baby's care to a palliative care pathway, it is important to actively consider the involvement of siblings, as their inclusion can be integral to the family's grieving process. Parents may require sensitive guidance and support from HCPs on how best to facilitate sibling engagement within the constraints of the NNU setting. The quality of communication siblings experience during this time will significantly impact their ability to cope with the evolving circumstances. Historically, it was believed that children would not be affected by illness and death if they were not directly involved or informed; however, this assumption has been disproven. The psychological risks associated with withholding information from children are now acknowledged and recognised to lead to maladaptive thinking and behavioural issues later in life (D'Alton et al., 2022). Resources, such as those provided by Child Bereavement UK, offer valuable guidance to help parents engage in age-appropriate and

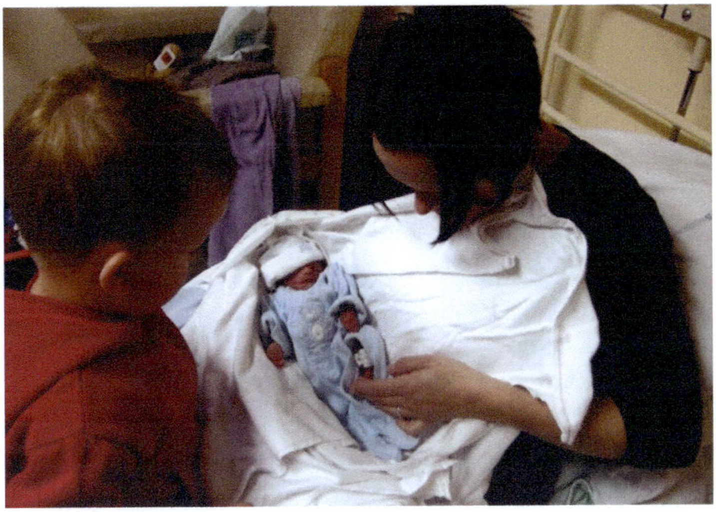

Figure 10.5 Involving siblings in bereavement care

sensitive conversations with their children, supporting their emotional wellbeing during this challenging time.

Parents should be encouraged to involve other family members, if they choose to do so, in the process of grieving and memory making. In addition to addressing the needs of siblings (see Figure 10.5), it is essential to consider the emotional needs of grandparents and other close relatives, who may wish to have the opportunity to see and hold the baby. Such interactions can be instrumental in fostering their own grieving process and can strengthen their capacity to support the parents in the long term, particularly when they, too, have meaningful memories to share. To facilitate this, it is important that visiting restrictions be lifted, where possible, to ensure that the diverse needs of the family are appropriately addressed during this sensitive time.

CHALLENGING ISSUES TO CONSIDER

Perinatal autopsy

All parents who experience the death of their baby should be offered the option of a post-mortem examination, as part of comprehensive care and to support understanding of the circumstances surrounding the death. In England, Wales, and Northern Ireland, this practice is regulated by the Human Tissue Act 2004 and overseen by the Human Tissue Authority (HTA). HCPs require specific training to engage in these sensitive conversations effectively and empathetically.

While discussions regarding post-mortem examinations are typically led by medical staff, it is imperative that nursing and midwifery teams are equally prepared to provide accurate information and respond to parental queries. Such discussions can become particularly challenging when parents who both hold parental responsibility have conflicting views regarding the consent for a post-mortem examination. In these instances, it is essential that NNU staff possess a clear understanding of the relevant legal frameworks to navigate these complex situations appropriately (see Box 10.6).

BOX 10.6 CONSENT FOR POST-MORTEM EXAMINATION

> *Where there is a conflict between those accorded equal ranking, this should be discussed sensitively with all parties, whilst explaining clearly that so far as the Human Tissue Act is concerned, the consent of one of those ranked equally in the hierarchy is sufficient for the procedure to go ahead. This does not mean that the consent of one person must be acted on, and a decision not to proceed may be made on the basis of the emotional impact that this would have on family and friends.*
>
> (HTA, 2023, p. 10)

Organ donation

Newborn organ donation is still relatively uncommon practice within the UK. Cases across the general population continues to rise; however, this has not been replicated in the neonatal population. Often a paternalistic approach to bereavement care results in professionals not discussing the option of organ donation as part of palliative care conversations, believing it may cause more emotional distress for the family. Chapter 11 details the ethical implications of organ donation.

To assist in improving current neonatal donation rates, a strategic plan has been released to develop a framework which will embed organ donation as a routine end-of-life choice for all families facing the death of their child, where organ donation may be possible (NHS Blood and Transplant, 2019). It is crucial that, where neonatal organ donation is being considered, any initial discussions involve the transplant team (BAPM, 2024). This should include notifying the specialist nurse in organ donation (SNOD). All NHS Trusts will have a SNOD who will not only be able to offer advice to professionals regarding the suitability of organ donation in individual cases, but will also, where possible, attend as preliminary discussions with parents are raised. This topic needs to be broached with parents at a suitable time, in a sensitive manner, with appropriate professionals involved. As well as being trained to open the discussion sensitively, they will be able to support and guide clinical staff through the process and will ensure parents are given all information relating to the end-of-life care, post-mortem examination, and how memory-making will be facilitated.

Parents should be reassured that their decision regarding organ donation, whether to proceed or decline, will in no way influence the standard or quality of care provided to their baby. In instances where parents choose not to consider organ donation, their wishes must be fully respected without pressure or judgment. The option of organ donation represents a significant development in bereavement care, as some families have found solace in the knowledge that, through their loss, others may benefit. For these parents, the ability to contribute to the lives of others has provided a sense of meaning and comfort during an otherwise devastating experience.

SUPPORT AND TRAINING FOR PROFESSIONALS

Both the beginning and end of life profoundly affect those involved, and the meaning attributed to these events is often shaped by social and cultural constructs. Accordingly, the emotional and psychological impact on HCPs who support families through neonatal death warrants careful consideration. Although there is an expanding body of literature outlining best practices for providing effective care to bereaved families within NNUs, considerably less attention has been given to the grief and emotional toll experienced by healthcare providers themselves (Levick et al., 2017). Members of the multidisciplinary team who are involved must recognise and address the personal impact that the death of a newborn can have on their emotional wellbeing. The dual responsibility of providing end of life care for the baby while simultaneously supporting the grieving family can generate intense emotional strain and moral distress.

Acknowledging the emotional burden associated with such care should be embedded within the culture of NNUs (BAPM, 2021). However, support for staff is often informal and inconsistent, with limited opportunities for professionals to develop structured strategies for managing grief and emotional fatigue. Establishing accessible and ongoing clinical supervision, where staff are encouraged to reflect on and discuss their experiences, may serve to mitigate some of the psychological distress frequently reported by those working in this challenging field.

PRACTICE POINT

Consider both the practical and emotional aspects of nursing that are essential for quality practice in this sensitive area of care. List them for future reference given that neonatal bereavement is a relatively uncommon area of practice. Practical care might include necessary procedures to follow in the event of a neonatal death and advice for the family. Emotional care might be, for example, the provision of support from religious figures as applicable to faith and culture and other bereavement support sources.

Chapter takeaways

- The complexity of bereavement care can evoke considerable anxiety among members of the neonatal team and in such emotionally charged circumstances, it is crucial to anchor care in the core principles of supportive practice, effective communication, and an individualised approach.
- As parents will carry the memories formed during this profoundly difficult time for the rest of their lives, the way these experiences are shaped is of critical importance; therefore, sensitive communication by the neonatal team is imperative.
- To minimise psychological trauma and facilitate emotional recovery, the principles of safety, autonomy, and empowerment must be prioritised by culturally sensitive, inclusive, and compassionate care.
- A commitment to upholding parental autonomy through collaborative decision-making processes is vital, rather than imposing predetermined choices to ensure that bereavement care tailored to the unique needs and values of each family.

CASE STUDY

CASE STUDIES

First, looking back at Boxes 10.1 and 10.2, consider how these bereaved mothers' stories will affect your own professional practice. Think of how you could adapt practice in your own clinical area to improve the memories of bereaved parents.

Case study 1: Organ donation

Dale and Chloe have given birth to a daughter, Ellie, at 39 weeks' gestation. Chloe presented to the maternity services with a heavy vaginal bleed and was immediately taken for an unplanned caesarean section because of placental abruption. Ellie was born in poor condition, and no heart rate was noted at birth. She had advanced resuscitation by the attending neonatal team including intubation, cardiac compressions, and resuscitation drugs. A heart rate was first heard at 10 minutes of age. Ellie fulfilled the criteria for therapeutic hypothermia. After a period of 3 days of cooling, she remained neurologically compromised and did not demonstrate any spontaneous respiratory effort. On examination, she had fixed dilated pupils and absent gag and deep tendon reflexes.

Magnetic resonance imaging (MRI) was undertaken on day 5 and demonstrated extensive changes in the white matter and basal ganglia, suggestive of severe hypoxic-ischaemic brain damage. The neonatal team agree that further intensive care is futile and are considering re-orienting Ellie's care to palliation. Throughout Ellie's stay on the NNU, Dale and Chloe have been made aware of how critical her status was and have 'prepared themselves for the worst' prior to her MRI. Once the results are discussed with the parents, they express a wish to donate Ellie's organs following her death.

Q.1. Would Ellie be eligible for organ donation?
Q.2. How would the family be supported and prepared through this whole situation and who would be involved?
Q.3. What resources and support services could be provided for the parents?

Case study 2: Planning holistic bereavement care

Ammar was born at 24 weeks and doing well initially but sadly deteriorated with fulminant necrotising enterocolitis at 10 days of age. He is too unstable for an operation, and within a few hours it becomes evident that Ammar will not survive for much longer. His parents, Fatima and Jamil, have two other children, Saba, aged 7, and Sameer, aged 4 years. The family practice the Muslim faith and raise their children in accordance with it.

Q.1. What are your immediate considerations with regard to planning Ammar's care around his death?
Q.2. Given that Jamil and Fatima are practicing Muslims, how would you address religious aspects as part of the family's bereavement care?
Q.3. Which points would you like to discuss with Fatima and Jamil regarding their other children?

For suggested answer guides to the questions posed in these case studies, please refer to the web-based companion site specific to this chapter. See www.routledge.com/cw/petty

References

Berry, S. N., Winsor, T., & Huene, L. (2023). A proposed framework for perinatal loss trauma informed care. *Journal of Neonatal Nursing*, *29*(6), 916–921.

Blood, C., & Cacciatore, J. (2014). Best practice in bereavement photography after perinatal death: Qualitative analysis with 104 parents. *BMC Psychology*, *2*(1), 15.

British Association of Perinatal Medicine. (2021). *Family integrated care. A framework for practice.* https://www.bapm.org/resources/ficare-framework-for-practice

British Association of Perinatal Medicine. (2022). *Lactation and loss: Management of lactation following the death of a baby.* https://www.bapm.org/resources/lactation-and-loss-management-of-lactation-following-the-death-of-a-baby.

British Association of Perinatal Medicine. (2024). *Recognising uncertainty: An integrated framework in perinatal medicine.* https://www.bapm.org/resources/palliative-care-in-perinatal-medicine-framework

Brooten, D., Youngblut, J. M., Charles, D., Roche, R., Hidalgo, I., & Malkawi, F. (2016). Death rituals reported by white, black, and hispanic parents following the icu death of an infant or child. *Journal of Pediatric Nursing*, *31*(2), 132–140.

Cacciatore, J., Thieleman, K., Fretts, R., & Jackson, L. B. (2021). What is good grief support? Exploring the actors and actions in social support after traumatic grief. *PLoS ONE*, *16*(5), e0252324–e0252324.

Currie, E. R., Christian, B. J., Hinds, P. S., Perna, S. J., Robinson, C., Day, S., Bakitas, M., & Meneses, K. (2018). Life after loss: Parent bereavement and coping experiences after infant death in the neonatal intensive care unit. *Death Studies*, 1–10.

D'Alton, S. V., Ridings, L., Williams, C., & Phillips, S. (2022). The bereavement experiences of children following sibling death: An integrative review. *Journal of Pediatric Nursing*, *66*, e82–e99.

Hackett, J., Heavey, E., & Beresford, B. (2022). 'It was like an airbag, it cushioned the blow': A multi-site qualitative study of bereaved parents' experiences of using cooling facilities. *Palliative Medicine*, *36*(2), 365–374.

Hindmarch, C. (2018). *On the death of a child* (3rd ed.). CRC Press.

Human Tissue Authority (HTA). (2023). *Code A: Guiding principles and the fundamental principle of consent.* Human Tissue Authority.

Kübler-Ross, E. (2014). *On death and dying* (Reprint ed.). Routledge.

Lakhani, J., Mack, C., Kunyk, D., Kung, J., & Van Manen, M. (2024). Considerations for practice in supporting parental bereavement in the neonatal intensive care unit – A systematic review. *Journal of Palliative Care*, *39*(2), 138–160.

Levick, J., Fannon, J., Bodemann, J., & Munch, S. (2017). NICU bereavement care and follow-up support for families and staff. *Advances in Neonatal Care*, *17*(6), 451–460.

NHS Blood and Transplant. (2019). *Paediatric and neonatal deceased donation. A strategic plan.* NHS Blood and Transplant. www.odt.nhs.uk/odt-structures-and-standards/key-strategies/paediatric-and-neonatal-donation-strategy/

NHS England. (2021). *Supporting mental healthcare in a maternity and neonatal setting.* https://www.england.nhs.uk/wp-content/uploads/2021/08/B0233-Health-in-Maternity-and-Neonatal-Settings-including-Neonatal-Loss-July-2021.pdf

Noble-Carr, D., Carroll, K., Copland, S., & Waldby, C. (2023). Providing lactation care following stillbirth, neonatal and infant death: Learning from bereaved parents. *Breastfeeding Medicine*, *18*(4), 254–264.

Redshaw, M., Henderson, J., & Bevan, C. (2021). 'This is time we'll never get back': A qualitative study of mothers' experiences of care associated with neonatal death. *BMJ Open*, *11*(9), e05083.

Sadeghi, N., Hasanpour, M., Heidarzadeh, M., Alamolhoda, A., & Waldman, E. (2016). Spiritual needs of families with bereavement and loss of an infant in neonatal intensive care unit: A qualitative study. *Journal of Pain and Symptom Management*, *52*(1), 35–42.

Siassakos, D., Jackson, S., Gleeson, K., Chebsey, C., Ellis, A., Storey, C., Heazell, A., Draycott, T., Winter, C., Hillman, J., Cox, R., Lewis, J., & Davey, L. (2018). All bereaved parents are entitled to good care after stillbirth: A mixed-methods multicentre study (INSIGHT). *BJOG: An International Journal of Obstetrics and Gynaecology*, *125*(2), 160–170. https://doi.org/10.1111/1471-0528.14765

Steele, P., & Mancini, A. (2013). The neonatal experience–loss and grief without a bereavement. *Infant*, *9*(3), 92–93.

Stillbirth and Neonatal Death Society (SANDS). (2016). *Pregnancy loss and the death of a baby: Guidelines for professionals* (4th ed.).

Stillbirth and Neonatal Death Society. (2022). *National bereavement care pathway: Neonatal death*. https://www.nbcpathway.org.uk/wp-content/uploads/2024/03/NBCP-Neonatal-July-2022.pdf

Stroebe, M., & Schut, H. (2010). The dual process model of coping with bereavement: A decade on. *OMEGA-Journal of Death and Dying*, *61*(4), 273–289.

Tonkin, L. (1996). Growing around grief – another way of looking at grief and recovery. *Bereavement Care*, *15*(1), 10.

UNICEF. (2025). *Neonatal mortality*. https://data.unicef.org/topic/child-survival/neonatal-mortality/

Worden, J. W. (2018). *Grief counseling and grief therapy: A handbook for the mental health practitioner* (5th ed.). Springer Publishing Company.

World Health Organization. (2024). *Newborn mortality*. https://www.who.int/news-room/fact-sheets/detail/newborn-mortality

11 LEGAL AND ETHICAL ISSUES IN NEONATAL PRACTICE

Debra Nicholson and Katherine Noble

CONTENTS

DOI: 10.4324/9781003591405-14

GUIDANCE ON HOW TO ENHANCE PERSONAL LEARNING FROM THIS CHAPTER

Key points covered in this chapter

- Legal considerations in neonatal care: fetal and neonatal rights, viability limits, consent, organ and tissue donation, and duty of care.
- Application of ethical principles guided by the infant's best interests.
- Decision-making in the neonatal unit, including conflict management, legal-ethical application, and responses to moral distress

Reflection

Reading through the chapter, you are encouraged to engage with the key points and related literature in an enquiring way. By the end of this chapter, you will be able to:

- Describe the nurse's role in legal and ethical issues within neonatal care.
- Explain legal and ethical principles guiding practice.
- Understand fetal rights in relation to peri-viability and viability thresholds.
- Discuss decision-making around withdrawing care, applying the best interests principle, and managing conflict.
- Recognise moral distress and how nurses can continue to support families in difficult situations.

Implications for nursing care

This chapter emphasises the nurse's central role in bioethical discussions and decisions in neonatal care. In partnership with parents and the multidisciplinary team (MDT), nurses must recognise ethical challenges and act within legal, professional, and ethical frameworks to address them (Nursing and Midwifery Council (NMC), 2024).

INTRODUCTION AND BACKGROUND

In the past four decades, advances in medical technology and clinical care have led to major improvements in neonatal care, and the limit of viability has shifted toward lower gestations, meaning that extremely premature and very ill neonates have better chances of survival and making a good recovery. However, surviving very premature neonates have been shown to have more prematurity-associated complications and long-term neurodevelopmental deficits compared with more mature infants (Kornhauser Cerar & Lucovnik, 2023). It is difficult to predict which neonates will survive, with or without future disabilities, or which may not survive. This means that families and health professionals sometimes must make complex and emotionally demanding decisions about an infant's treatment and care (Nuffield Council on Bioethics, 2014; Green et al., 2017). An understanding therefore of these complexities is essential for the multidisciplinary team to make sense of situations that present legal and/or ethical dilemmas. Although ethical dilemmas occur across all specialties, they are particularly common in modern neonatal practice.

THE NURSE'S ROLE IN LEGAL AND ETHICAL ISSUES IN THE NEONATAL UNIT

Nurses should have knowledge and skills to practice safe acts in line with regulations that will ultimately guide and influence them to provide holistic, ethical, and compassionate care; this is the essence of good nursing practice for the best interests of the neonatal population and their families (Al-Breiki, 2017). It is essential that nurses be able to recognise legal and ethical challenges and practise in line with national guidance and frameworks. Neonatal nurses are in a unique position to be advocates for the babies and families they care for as they understand the beliefs and values of families including the individualised wishes they may have within their ethnic, cultural, and religious backgrounds. Cultural competence is vital in line with respecting the cultural, ethnic, and socioeconomic diversity of all families in the neonatal unit (NNU) and ensuring their best interests are upheld. In line with this, culturally inclusive care should be considered and implemented by the whole MDT and nurses as a key player in the team should continue to work towards greater cultural competence to ensure families' diverse and holistic needs are met (Hendson et al., 2015; Heitzler, 2017).

LEGAL PRINCIPLES

Understanding of a clear concept of law is necessary in clinical decision-making as it affects almost everything we do and can be defined as a rule enacted and recognised as commanding or forbidding certain actions, or a body of such rules (Griffith & Tengnah, 2023). Rules can both guide and serve as standards for behaviour. But all rules, whether they are legal, moral, ethical, or social, have the same basic characteristics: they set standards of how things ought or ought not to be and lay down a standard of behaviour which must be complied with if the rule affects us (Hendrick, 2000).

For nurses, the NMC Code of Conduct (2024) represents an extended statement of the accountability of registered practitioners. It revolves around four key themes: prioritise people, practice effectively, preserve safety, and promote professionalism and trust. Within medicine, guidance on appropriate conduct is contained in the Good Medical Practice document (General Medical Council (GMC), 2024), which covers much the same as the NMC but endeavours to be more specific to medical professionals. The codes represent best available guidance for practitioners upon what is expected of them as a bare minimum. It is important to note that these codes impose a higher standard upon practitioners than the law actually demands (Avery, 2017). Nurses therefore should be aware of relevant legislation, health and social care policies, and their professional code in order that they can apply them to their practice.

Knowledge of specific legal principles and laws relevant to neonatology is essential. Table 11.1 outlines some key legal principles that should be understood by nurses and the MDT to protect themselves, the infant, and the family at a vulnerable time.

FETAL RIGHTS, PERSONHOOD, PERI-VIABILITY, AND AGE OF VIABILITY

The discussion about the age of fetal **viability** involves two quite separate issues. One is the increase in survival rates for babies born extremely prematurely; the second is abortion which, based on current United Kingdom (UK) legislation, the Abortion Act, 1973 allows for termination up to 24 weeks gestation (Buka, 2020). Under English law, fetuses have no independent legal status. Once born, babies have the same rights to life as other people (Nuffield Council on Bioethics, 2014). The law's main concern with gestational age (GA) lies in the concept of viability. This is not only a matter of UK jurisprudence; viability is universally regarded as an important milestone (Laurie et al., 2016).

There are varied positions on when a fetus is afforded the status of personhood. These positions have foundations in law, morality, religion and biomedical science. In some instances, the fetus is considered a person from the point of conception, but there are many thresholds during embryonic development that differing perspectives consider attainment of moral status. For many, however, birth is a highly significant moment in the fetus becoming a person with full moral status. The Nuffield Council could not reach a unanimous conclusion as to the point in time at which moral status should be afforded to the fetus; however, they regard the moment of birth, which is straightforward to identify and usually

TABLE 11.1 LEGAL PRINCIPLES IN NEONATAL CARE

Legal Issue	*Application to Neonatal Care*
Safeguarding/ Child Protection	Safeguarding and child protection in neonatal settings involves nurses proactively preventing harm and responding to incidents. Working in collaboration with various agencies, ensuring a coordinated response to safeguarding concerns. It also involves addressing the needs of the family and supporting those utilising family integrated plans of care. There are many policies and guidelines in place and nurses should be familiar with their own unit procedures.
Minimising Risk and Litigation	To protect vulnerable neonates, neonatal care practices should be delivered with safety as a central consideration, with appropriate governance processes in place, following the service and quality standards expected (British Association of Perinatal Medicine (BAPM), 2022).
Accountability	Neonatal nurses are morally, ethically, and legally accountable for their nursing judgements and actions and must comply with the NMC Code of Conduct (NMC, 2024).
Consent	It is a legal and ethical requirement to gain informed, valid consent before examining and initiating any investigation and treatment for any patient. Consent for neonatal care should involve provision of clear information and the building of trust between health professionals and parents to facilitate shared decision-making (BAPM, 2019a).
Confidentiality	A nurse has a duty of confidentiality to all those who are receiving care, including neonates and their family (NMC, 2024).
Duty of Care	Duty of care is a legal and ethical obligation for nurses to ensure the safety and wellbeing of those they support, acting in their best interest and preventing harm.
Parental responsibility	This refers to the legal rights and responsibilities of the parents, it is distinct from legal parentage and is defined by the Children Act (1989) as 'all the rights, duties, powers and responsibilities and authority which by law a parent of a child has in relation to the child and [their] property' (Children Act, 1989, Section 3(1)). Neonatal nurses need to have awareness of this and how it might apply to their practice when dealing with parents.

represents a significant threshold in potential viability, as the significant point of transition not just for legal judgments about preserving life but also for moral ones (Nuffield Council on Bioethics, 2014). In neonatal care, personhood is not the only consideration regarding moral, legal, and ethical thinking. Age of viability is tremendously relevant to determine whether life of the fetus is sustainable. Peri-viability is defined as the stage of fetal maturity with a marginal chance of extra-uterine survival (Gkiougki et al., 2021), and the time window between 22 and 26 weeks of GA is considered the peri-viability period, which can often be a 'grey zone' for clinical and ethical decision-making. There is a widespread consensus that 22 weeks of gestation is the lowest threshold of human viability (Sayeed, 2014; Janvier et al., 2017), limited by the physiological development of the lungs, as it is during the period of 22 to 24 weeks that the basic structure of the area of the lung where gaseous exchange occurs is formed and vascularised (Glass et al., 2015) and surfactant production begins; both are paramount to enable life.

The ethical principles that formed the basis of earlier guidelines have not changed but advances in perinatal care have led to steadily improving outcomes for babies admitted to UK NNUs, particularly at the lowest GAs (BAPM, 2019b). A key ethical consideration for decisions about instigating life sustaining treatment for an extremely preterm baby is the baby's prognosis and the risk of an acceptable (or unacceptable) outcome if active management is undertaken. BAPM (2019b) developed a consensus for risk categories that professionals can refer to during discussions with parents (see Box 11.1). There is no objective way of defining a risk as 'extremely high' versus 'high,' and families differ in the outcome that they regard as unacceptably poor. Thus, risk assessment may need to be modified in the light of parents' knowledge, views, and values.

From a legal perspective it is clear that international human rights law deems human rights to apply prior to birth, but by reducing the 'normal' limit for abortion to 24 weeks, UK law seems to recognise that a fetus has acquired some additional human rights at this stage of its gestation that it did not have prior to this (British Medical Association, 2007).

BOX 11.1 CONSENSUS OF THE WORKING GROUP IN REGARD TO RISK CATEGORIES FOR THE PURPOSES OF THE BAPM FRAMEWORK (2019B)

Extremely high risk: The Working Group considered that neonates with a >90% chance of either dying or surviving with severe impairment if active care is instigated would fit into this category. For example, this would include:

Neonates at 22+0–22+6 weeks of gestation with unfavourable risk factors

Some neonates at 23+0–23+6 weeks of gestation with unfavourable risk factors, including severe fetal growth restriction (rarely) Neonates at >24+0 weeks of gestation with significant unfavourable risk factors, including severe fetal growth restriction

High risk: The Working Group considered that neonates with a 50–90% chance of either dying or surviving with severe impairment if active care is instituted would fit into this category. For example, this would include:

Neonates at 22+0–23+6 weeks of gestation with favourable risk factors
Neonates >24+0 weeks of gestation with unfavourable risk factors and/or co-morbidities

Moderate risk: The Working Group considered that neonates with a <50% chance of either dying or surviving with severe impairment if active care is instituted would fit into this category. For example, this would include:

Most neonates >24+0 weeks of gestation
Some neonates at 23+0–23+6 weeks of gestation with favourable risk factors

THINK POINTS

A baby is born at 22+2 weeks gestation following spontaneous preterm labour. There was limited antenatal counselling due to the rapid delivery. The infant requires resuscitation at birth and is admitted to the NNU. Early imaging suggests a high risk of severe neurodevelopmental impairment. Parents request 'everything possible' be done.

- What clinical and ethical factors do you think should inform decisions at the limits of viability?
- How do you think survival statistics and long term outcomes should be presented to parents?
- What role do you think the nurse plays in supporting the infant's best interests and the parental wishes?

ETHICAL PRINCIPLES

Although a preterm neonate is one born before 37 weeks, there is a wide variation in that group, from extremely preterm to late preterm (Paterson & Redpath, 2013). Advances in this area have been remarkable, leading to a substantial reduction in mortality. Nevertheless, ethical questions remain, about resources, about whether the outcomes for some neonates are too burdensome, about criteria and authority for decision-making, and on stress and burnout for adults involved, both professionals and parents. Of these, the most challenging is the issue of over-burdensome outcomes of treatment to achieve survival. Parents too may feel 'overwhelmed by the demands of having to care for a preterm infant while at the same time coming to terms with a pregnancy that did not meet their expectations' (Paterson & Redpath, 2013, p. 19). Where a neonate appears to have poor prognosis, it may be argued that it is best either not to begin or to withdraw treatment. The difficulty of a decision to act is that, while resuscitation may be successful, the result may be a survivor with severe neurodisability, and this is not even to mention the resource implications of such a decision (Laurie et al., 2016).

Neonatal ethical standards seem to have lagged behind delivery of neonatal intensive care. Potential reasons for this include: agreement of how to manage care varies among nurses, allied health professionals and families, all who have different values, beliefs, and priorities; advances in neonatal technology have determined that those caring for neonates have not been afforded with sufficient training and time to resolve difficult end-of-life dilemmas; both of these factors therefore contribute to an overall lack of capability of providers to discuss ethical care (Pasarón, 2013). In these frequently uncertain circumstances, decision-making may be influenced by the consequences of quality of life and the possibility of severe disability, which undoubtedly raises ethical questions. However, extending an individual's lifespan frequently implies a compromised quality of life, while the medical field continues to advance and push the limits of healthcare treatment possibilities (Wilkinson, 2009; Tosello, 2016).

Gillon (1994) was one of the pioneers in adapting and applying ethics to healthcare. This arose in the form of bioethical principles in the UK. This focused on Principlism (the four principles) which includes **beneficence, non-maleficence, autonomy**, and **justice.** In implementing treatment decisions healthcare professionals may look to a framework and should be informed by their professional codes of conduct for guidance based on a framework of moral norms (Buka, 2020). These four principles can provide a useful framework for discussing ethical dilemmas. However, these principles conflict with each other, and it is conceivable that the principles cannot capture cultural differences, so that guidance may miss things that are important for some. These principles are closely related to the Seedhouse Grid (Freegard, 2007), and this puts ethics at the centre of decision-making in complex situations (Buka, 2020). Application of the Seedhouse Grid (Seedhouse, 1998; Figure 11.1) aims to improve a multidisciplinary and partnership approach; it allows for application of ethical principles as well as duty of candour and openness. It is a tool which can enhance deliberation and throw light into unseen corners, suggesting new avenues of thought. Each of the principles will be discussed next.

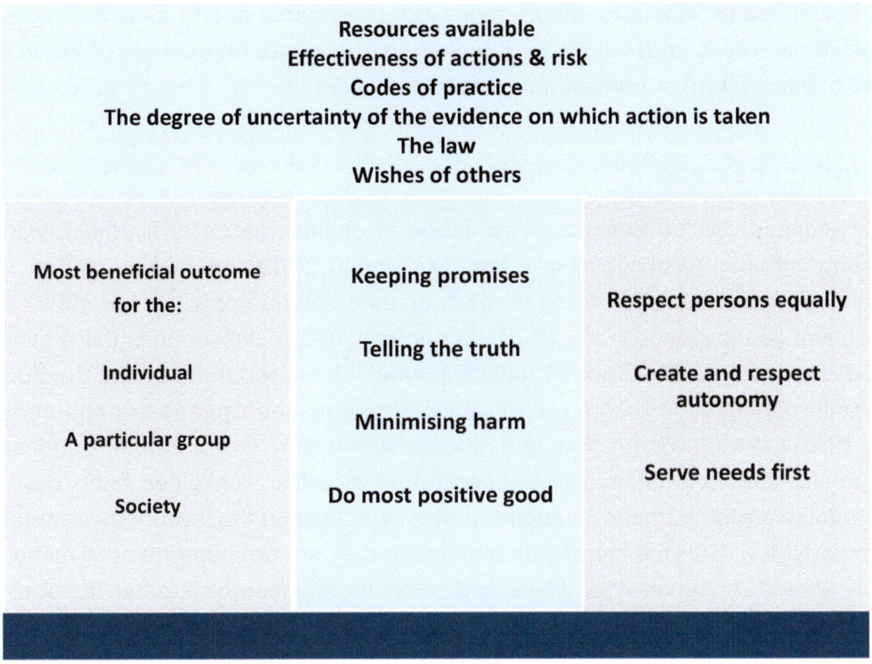

Figure 11.1 Seedhouse Grid (adapted from Seedhouse, 1998)

Autonomy

When considering making decisions within neonatal care, it is important to remember the neonate is not an autonomous being. To be considered autonomous, it is widely thought that a person must be able to perceive themselves as a rational individual who has the capacity to make informed choices through un-coerced decisions. Where the patient is considered incompetent or non-autonomous, decisions are made by a proxy or surrogate decision-maker. This would usually be the baby's parents; under the terms of the Mental Capacity Act (2005), they must be presumed to be competent to do so unless otherwise proven. In some cases, the courts will be forced to act in the capacity of surrogate decision-maker to ensure the rights of the neonate are protected and care is delivered considering their best interest (Wilkinson, 2006). The decision-making process within neonatal care is unique in nature, as it considers an infant who has never been autonomous, and the natural focus of neonatal care tends to be the baby's interests opposed to their rights (Spence, 2000). The best interest standard is disputed in this principle and is meant to be protective of a person unable to make decisions of their own by transferring the assessment of risks and benefits of treatment options and their alternatives to a surrogate. The neonate's parents may not be best placed to make decisions in isolation as they may not possess the appropriate knowledge or perspective to do so. It is the responsibility of healthcare providers to ensure that every reasonable effort has been made to enable parents to understand the information presented. An example of this is the use of interpreters or relevant communication aids.

Beneficence and non-maleficence

Beneficence can be defined as an action of charity, mercy, or kindness with a strong intention to do good to others (Kinsinger, 2009), so relating to benevolence. Beneficence also strives to reach an outcome that provides benefit for the recipient (Baumrucker et al., 2008). In contrast, non-maleficence is the principle of doing no harm. The Code is very clear when identifying that fulfilling the duties of both principles is a core responsibility for all nurses. Nurses are and should be held accountable for their practice, ensuring they are competent and safe professionals. Ignorance is not accepted as a justification when harm occurs, as nurses are duty bound to ensure that they act within the level of their competence (NMC, 2024). If faced with a situation they are not competent to manage, they should recognise their limits and refer the situation to another member of the team. Harm incidents that occur within clinical practice are usually caused by human error or **iatrogenesis**, harm caused by initiating treatment/care. When such incidents occur, the practitioners involved are assessed using the Bolam principle, in which they are measured by the standard of practice deemed acceptable and reasonable by a responsible group of practitioners from the same specialty (Tingle & Cribb, 2013). This ensures a fair and just review of the incident as to whether it was avoidable and managed appropriately.

As principles, non-maleficence and beneficence are usually in tension with one another, primarily because beneficence considers burden versus benefit of treatment within the best interest standard, whereas non-maleficence could be considered as continuing futile treatment by not causing death. It is important to acknowledge that the purpose of intensive care is not to prolong life with futile treatment but to restore the health of the person (Stone, 2018). From this perspective, continuation of futile intensive care could even be considered a technological form of harm, as it is not going to achieve the desired outcome (Wyatt, 2009). It is difficult to balance these two principles when applying them to specific dilemmas in neonatal intensive care such as withholding and withdrawing life-sustaining treatment, again highlighting the need for a pragmatic approach when approaching ethical principles in isolation.

Justice

The fourth ethical principle, justice, refers to ensuring each person is given what they are due. It can be considered in terms of fairness, equality, need, or any other criterion that is material to the justice decision. In healthcare, justice often focuses on equitable access to care resource allocation and protection of the patient's rights. It would therefore seem obvious that the cost of neonatal care, while just for the patients that receive it, may not be considered so in a struggling healthcare economy. When resources are already limited, it could be considered unjust to fund an expensive area of healthcare when this funding could be used elsewhere for patients that may have better outcomes and survival rates. Pasarón (2013) objects to this perspective, highlighting that there is insufficient data to support these claims. There are no easy answers as to how justice can be truly implemented within an imperfect society (Beauchamp & Childress, 2013). The application of ethics and moral decision-making to practice is not just about life and death decisions or the provision of resources on a national scale. It is present in everyday life, and neonatal nurses, as autonomous practitioners, should be encouraged to develop their awareness of the subject. When in context, it is easy to determine how these ethical considerations can be seen in everyday practice. An example of this is allocating nursing staff to infants, when considering the needs of the neonates is matched against the skills of the nurses and the overall needs of the unit. This can be seen as an unconscious use of the ethical principles to ensure that care is provided safely and effectively.

PRACTICE POINT

Parents are often asked to consent to numerous invasive interventions and procedures within hours of the birth of a preterm or sick newborn who requires admission to the NNU. Consider the following situation: a baby is admitted to NNU and consent is obtained from one parent recovering from a general anaesthetic following a caesarean section and the other parent who is clearly overwhelmed by the ongoing situation. Questions later arise about how much information the parents understood.

How do you think parental autonomy can be respected when decision-making capacity is affected by stress and trauma?

WITHHOLDING AND WITHDRAWING TREATMENT

Due to the advancements in both perinatal and neonatal care, there are more frequent instances where infants of borderline viability are resuscitated at birth. These situations call for medical and nursing teams in collaboration with parents to make some very difficult decisions regarding withholding or withdrawing life-sustaining treatments (BAPM, 2019b). Professionals should not only be fully aware of the ethical and legal issues but also about how to manage such difficult decisions to the satisfaction of parents, the judiciary, and the public (Avery, 2017). There are also instances where infants have been born and developed past the age of viability but have conditions that are incompatible with life, such as congenital abnormalities, for example, anencephaly or Trisomy 18 (Edwards syndrome). In other situations, on-going treatment has become futile and continuing to provide care is no longer considered to be in the best interest of the baby; examples of this are infants that have received therapeutic hypothermia, and when the treatment is completed, they have no cerebral function present. In these situations, it is imperative that all the ethical and legal considerations have been addressed to ensure the most appropriate outcome. Health professionals are duty bound to act in the best interest of the baby and should use all available guidance to do so. Internationally, the literature appears to advocate a shared decision-making approach, in which staff (members of medical and nursing teams in the UK) and parents work collaboratively to recognise the infant's best interests. The guidance provided by the Royal College for Paediatrics and Child Health (RCPCH, 2014); which has foundations in UK law and strives for best ethical practice, agrees that parental agreement is essential when considering withholding or withdrawing treatment for neonates (Larcher et al., 2015). The dynamics of complex decision-making between all parties will be explored further later in this chapter. The RCPCH provides an essential framework that echoes the voice of law, and although it is a clinical guideline, it assumes much of the same language as a legal ruling (Bhatia, 2015). It is common and accepted practice to withdraw life-sustaining treatment where parents and the neonatal MDT believe that the distress caused by such intervention outweighs the benefits.

CONFLICT

No matter how clear the guidelines for making critical care decisions, health professionals and parents will sometimes disagree. All staff working with children and young people encounter parental concerns about treatment plans from time to time. Experience teaches us that disagreements in healthcare can usually be managed by a process of shared decision-making with active early involvement of parents and whenever possible with the child/young person. The importance of honest and open communication with families as early as possible cannot be understated. In most cases, resolution can be achieved by careful listening and understanding and where possible early involvement of mediation services (Linney et al., 2019).

Potential areas of conflict include uncertain gestational age, rapid birth without time for counselling, baby born in unexpectedly good/poor condition, parents request second opinion, and threatened birth before 22+0 weeks gestation. Miscommunication is a frequent occurrence and may in part arise from providers' insufficient or inadequate knowledge of outcomes of extremely low birthweight infants (Papadimitriou et al., 2019). In addition, the decision-making process around critically ill neonates begins during the pregnancy and involves a wide range of people, including maternity, obstetrics, neonatal, and possibly surgeons; the greater the number of people involved in decision-making, the greater the number of values and beliefs that are reflected, leading to conflicts (Sakai et al., 2024). Box 11.2 looks at potential strategies for dealing with some areas of conflict.

The number of court cases relating to neonatal medicine seems to be increasing; however, involving the courts can be a very stressful experience for the child's family as well as the professionals, and it is a costly process (Nuffield Council on Bioethics, 2014). Conflict is damaging, stressful, and emotionally challenging for all involved. Taking the correct steps early may prevent early disagreements reaching conflict. Regardless of the presence of conflict in all situations the legal and ethical basis for decisions is that the best interest of the child is paramount (Linney et al., 2019), and this will be discussed next.

BOX 11.2 ADDRESSING ETHICAL CONFLICT

Challenges & Conflicts	*Strategies*
Conflict within the family	Give honest, timely information. Involve key members of the family and/or religious leaders in accordance with the beliefs and values of the family.
Conflict between parents and the neonatal MDT	Regular meetings with the MDT. Involvement of the family in the shared decision-making process.
Communication challenges and barriers	Consider language/information need barriers and ensure both written and verbal communication is in line with cultural background and first language of the family.
Parents with limited competence to make decisions (due to age, capacity, illness)	Involvement of supportive services, family support workers, psychological support, social workers, family advocates.

> **THINK POINT**
>
> - The MDT believes ongoing treatment for an infant with a life-limiting congenital condition is causing unnecessary suffering and may not be in the infant's best interests. However, the parents insist on continuation of full intensive care citing religious beliefs and tensions rise during meetings between the parents and MDT.
> - How do you think conflict between parents and the MDT should be managed ethically and compassionately?

DECISION-MAKING AND THE 'BEST INTERESTS' STANDARD

When an infant is admitted to an NNU, parents are faced with many challenges, and the number and complexity of decisions faced by parents will vary between families (Fairhurst & Long, 2020). Nonetheless, parents may be asked to sanction proposed interventions based on medical 'best interests' (Vasu, 2017). The principle of 'best interests' is central to medical practice and UK law. It states that in all matters affecting any child, his or her best interest should be the paramount consideration. Parents, doctors, and others involved in the decision-making process may have different ideas about what is in the best interest of the baby (Nuffield Council on Bioethics, 2014).

Under the best interest standard, a surrogate decision-maker must determine the highest net benefit among the available options. Best interest judgements are meant to focus attention entirely on the value of life for the person who must live it (Beauchamp & Childress, 2013).

Perinatal care for very preterm gestations must always be tailored to the individual and led by senior midwives, obstetricians, and neonatologists. Parents should be involved in discussions regarding perinatal care, and their goals and expectations should be examined honestly, compassionately, and realistically. Decisions should be made in collaboration with parents, using the best available evidence about the baby's prognosis and keeping the baby's best interests in mind (BAPM, 2019a).

Parents are generally considered to have the moral authority to make decisions in their child's best interests in all circumstances of life; they are best placed to know what is in the interests of their child because they share a special bond that begins during pregnancy and develops over time. Doctors have a responsibility to promote the best interest of the neonate and will be able to give a prediction of the outcome based on knowledge and experience. Other people such as family members, religious advisors, or healthcare specialists may contribute, and nurses are often well placed to provide additional insights into the best interest of both the child and family (Nuffield Council on Bioethics, 2014).

The 'best interest' principle has its foundation in the Children Act 1989. The overriding principle of this is that the neonate's or child's welfare and best interests must be of the highest regard in all decisions concerning their upbringing. The way the 'best interest' of the very premature neonate is determined needs to keep time with the evolving importance of shared decision-making and family integrated care (Jefferies et al., 2012). This evolution requires that the very concept of 'best interest,' as well as the modalities to clinically determine it, be transformed to transcend the traditional basis in the principles of bioethics and the definition of ethical dilemmas as 'conflicts between principles.' However, there is no single, unequivocal definition of the 'best interest' of a seriously compromised neonate (Daboval & Shidler, 2014). The GMC (2018) states that authoritative clinical guidance must be used to determine what treatment may be in a neonate's best interests. The RCPCH (2014) describes five situations in which it is considered ethical, legal and in the child's best interest to withhold life-sustaining treatment, one of which is the 'no chance' situation. This situation is described as 'such severe disease that life-sustaining treatment simply delays death without significant alleviation of suffering' (RCPCH, 2014, p. 10).

Although clinical practices are evolving toward shared decision-making, it has been claimed that some medical professionals believe they provide the 'best' answers in the quest for the best interest of sick neonates, not recognising the fact that the interpretation of research data predicting prognosis may vary even among themselves (Haward et al., 2011, 2017). Thus, a collaborative approach is paramount, meaning that all persons with relevant advocacy for the baby, having considered long- and short-term issues, partake in the decision-making process (Kohsman, 2016).

THINK POINT

An infant born at 23+4 weeks initially responds well to intensive care but later develops sepsis and is identified to have an evolving intraventricular haemorrhage. Prognosis is uncertain, with a risk of severe disability. Parents ask if continuing intensive care is in their baby's best interest.

- How do you think 'best interests' should be defined in this situation?
- Do you think uncertainty can be acknowledged without removing hope?
- Whose perspectives do you think should be considered in best interest decision-making?

MORAL DISTRESS

Although it has been accepted that moral distress is common among healthcare professionals, it is unclear how common it is in the NNU (Thorne et al., 2018). According to Prentice et al. (2018), 76% of healthcare professionals believe that providing care for extremely ill infants necessitates moral distress. While every complicated circumstance can cause moral distress, the most frequent ones in the NNU are conflicts regarding care plans, medical utility and futility, end-of-life care, and peri-viability (Field et al., 2016). Burton et al. (2020) describe moral distress in nurses caring for critically ill neonates as the result of patient care situations in which there is a mismatch or incongruence between the behaviour expected of nurses and their personal values/beliefs. In other words, it centres on organisational policies and practices that prevent nurses from acting in ways they believe are morally right.

The entire healthcare team, the patient, and the family are all impacted by moral distress, which spans all healthcare professions. A careful and customised approach to patient care is necessary due to the wide range of situations that can result in moral distress. It is critical to recognise that moral distress will vary in intensity among team members. The understanding of moral distress as a phenomenon, its influence on the care given, and assisting professionals in recognising its existence are of utmost importance. Burnout and job dissatisfaction can be avoided by promoting an environment that values transparency, moral sincerity, and assistance for those in need (Mills & Cortezzo, 2020).

THINK POINT

Reflect on the signs of moral distress, the organisational factors that may contribute to moral distress and how nurses can be supported if experiencing ethical conflict.

TISSUE AND ORGAN DONATION

A particularly rare and sensitive aspect of neonatal end of life care, which requires further exploration, is that of neonatal organ donation (see also Chapter 10). Although neonates have the potential to donate tissues and/or organs to other neonates, children, and even adults, it is unknown whether during these situations, the option of neonatal donation is being discussed with specialist organ donation teams and families where appropriate (Ali et al., 2025). Despite the existence of guidelines and strategies to support its implementation, neonatal organ donation remains rare in the UK (RCPCH, 2015; National Health Service (NHS) Blood and Transplant, 2021). Although some cases of neonatal transplantation have been reported in the literature, the use of neonatal organs and tissues is limited (Bluhme et al., 2023). Neonatal organ and tissue donation represent a desire to make an altruistic gift and can play a key role in the care and support provided to families around the time of a neonate's death. Indeed, many families who have made the decision to donate organs and tissues of their deceased neonate say it brought them solace and comfort which can be vital to families' healing processes and should be supported wherever possible.

Legal and ethical questions that must be addressed require an adherence to a variety of laws, regulations, and ethical principles. The donation of organs and tissues from neonates for transplantation has been a relatively infrequent occurrence, with donation of organs and tissues for research being even less common, primarily because family members who receive a prenatal diagnosis of a lethal anomaly or experience the death of a neonate are not routinely offered information about research donation, but social media, blogs, and websites have increasingly connected parents who have received a diagnosis of a lethal anomaly, which may increase parental awareness. Moreover, neonatal donation of organs and tissues for research is proving increasingly important in a variety of areas including neural tube defects, treating vision impairment, diabetes, and organ system development (Anderson et al., 2020).

However, it is important that families are provided with a realistic expectation if considering organ and tissue donation, as there are several legal and ethical barriers to negotiate, not all areas are able to offer the service, and the baby may not be a suitable donor.

FAMILY INTEGRATED PRINCIPLES OF INCLUSIVE, ETHICAL CARE

This chapter has touched on the nurse's position as a vital member of the neonatal MDT. Nonetheless, it is worthwhile to make a few further observations regarding the nursing context before concluding the chapter. Nurses must be able to identify ethical and legal dilemmas and follow national frameworks and guidelines when practicing. Being advocates for the infants and families they look after puts neonatal nurses in a special position. They are aware of the values and beliefs of families, as well as any unique desires that members of their ethnic, cultural, and religious backgrounds may have. Some parents may find the NNU environment daunting due to its complexity and the attachment between the parents and baby, which is essential for stability and psychological development, may be disrupted (Adama et al., 2022). The many challenges that NNU babies and their parents must overcome may negatively affect the establishment of the best possible relationship, which may have long-term effects on the mental health and development of both the parents and the infant. Therefore, nurses are in a privileged position to guide and support these families (Givrad et al., 2021).

Chapter takeaways

- Professional codes of conduct provide guidance on topics such as safeguarding, accountability, consent, confidentiality, duty of care, and parental responsibility.
- The four ethical principles are autonomy (usually affecting parents in neonatal cases); beneficence (aim to do good); non-maleficence (do no harm); and justice. These should be central to treatment decisions, alongside the best interest standard, which has the baby's welfare at heart.
- Fetuses have no independent legal status until birth. Advances in neonatal care have resulted in improved survival at lower gestations, but prognosis is often uncertain, creating ethical and legal dilemmas. BAPM provides a framework to aid decision-making for babies expected to be born at the edge of viability (22–26 weeks GA), which includes three risk categories ranging from moderate to extremely high.
- Conflict may arise from uncertainty, miscommunication, or cultural factors. Enabling shared decision-making with a baby's family in the context of family integrated care can preclude disagreements.
- Organ and tissue donation is as yet rare practice in neonatal care, but should be explored where possible, as it is associated with benefits such as comfort to bereaved families, improving the span or quality of life of the recipient of a transplant, and furthering research.
- Moral distress is common on the NNU, particularly around end-of-life care, or those where prolonging of life appears futile. Openness and team support are important to reduce burnout.
- The neonatal nurse provides safe, compassionate, and ethical care, and advocacy for neonates and their families, with cultural competence and inclusivity.

CASE STUDY

CASE STUDIES

For all cases, consider the following ethical themes

- Best interests and proportionality: Choose treatments that offer meaningful benefit relative to burden; both withholding and withdrawing may be appropriate when burdens outweigh benefits.
- Shared decision-making: Parents are central partners; ensure clear, compassionate counselling and documented plans (BAPM's emphasis on agreeing and documenting is key).
- Borderline of viability: At 22 weeks, use individualised risk assessment and senior led counselling; some babies may be considered for active care, but palliative care remains appropriate for many.
- Transparency and process: Where disagreement persists, Nuffield recommends structured processes (second opinions, ethics input) and a focus on communication quality.

Case study 1: Birth at the threshold of viability (22+1 weeks)

A 19-year old woman has presented to her booking labour ward at a district general hospital (DGH) with rupture of the membranes at 21+6 weeks' gestation. This is her first pregnancy. She has so far not received any antenatal corticosteroids or magnesium sulphate. The fetal weight is estimated at 470 grams, fetal heart rate shows good variability. The baby is in breech presentation.

The nearest tertiary NICU is 90 minutes away.

The father, who is anxious but engaged, is present, but there is otherwise limited social support for the couple.

Q.1. Applying a risk-based approach, how would you support the parents in a decision between active (survival-focused) vs palliative (comfort-focused) perinatal plans?

Q.2. What is the difference between withholding vs withdrawing life-sustaining treatment?

Q.3. How would you make best-interest judgments and involve the parents at the borderline of viability?

Q.4. Consider how the neonatal team could present prognosis without extinguishing hope?

CASE STUDY

Case study 2: Long-term NNU infant with complex respiratory morbidity: palliative care integration

Ibrahim was born at 24+4 weeks at a tertiary hospital. After a complicated postnatal course, he is now 5 months corrected age. He has severe bronchopulmonary dysplasia with tracheostomy and ventilator dependence, recurrent ventilator-associated infections, severe growth failure, evolving pulmonary hypertension, abnormal neuroimaging, and repeated desaturations requiring high FiO_2 and sedation. Parents express exhaustion: 'We don't want him to suffer.'

Q.1. Can you recognise triggers for palliative care alongside disease-directed care in long-stay NNU infants? How would you approach parallel planning?

Q.2. Consider how you would structure a best-interests meeting that revisits goals as the trajectory clarifies, distinguishing proportionate benefit vs ongoing burdens?

Q.3. What symptom management bundle would you implement (dyspnoea, agitation, secretion burden), and how do you communicate that palliative care can be concurrent, not 'giving up'? (Consistent with Nuffield's recommendation for high-quality palliative options and family support)

Q.4. How will you document treatment ceilings and ensure continuity across out-of-hours and transport? (BAPM highlights documenting and communicating a clear management plan)

Case study 3: Re-orientation of care for an infant >6 months in NNU without ongoing long-term paediatric facilities

Abdallah is a 7-month chronological age infant born at 23+1 weeks. He is cared for at his local level 2 NNU. Abdallah has severe multisystem morbidity, profound neurodevelopmental impairment, gastrostomy dependence, ventilator dependence with frequent apnoea/bradycardia events, stage 3 retinopathy treated, and repeated sepsis. The regional long-term paediatric complex care unit has no capacity for the foreseeable future.

The MDT is split on whether to continue full intensive support. However, Abdallah's family are devout Muslims and have expressed the wish to continue care under all circumstances.

Q.1. How would you navigate the complexity of re-orienting care when a child is beyond the neonatal period, balancing best interests, resource realities, and service configuration, without compromising ethical duties to the child and family?

Q.2. Consider Abdallah's case using the BAPM risk/benefit and documentation approach to structure decision-making even when infants are older than the perinatal window. What does it say about ethical principles, risk-based assessment, parental partnership, and making clear plans.

Q.3. What constitutes a fair, transparent process for recommending palliative redirection when the MDT is divided?

Q.4. How will you plan location of end-of-life care (NNU vs hospice vs home) given the lack of long-term paediatric beds?

Q.5. Consider how you can be supportive of familial religious beliefs and the family's position to continue treatment at all costs?

For suggested answer guides to the questions posed in these case studies, please refer to the web-based companion site specific to this chapter. See www.routledge.com/cw/petty

CASE STUDY

References

Adama, E. A., Adua, E., Bayes, S., & Mörelius, E. (2022). Support needs of parents in neonatal intensive care unit: An integrative review. *Journal of Clinical Nursing*, *31*(5–6), 532–547.

Al-Breiki, M. (2017). What influence nurses practice more: Law or ethics. *JOJ Nurse Healthcare*, *5*(3), 103.

Ali, F., Chant, K., Scales, A., Sellwood, M., & Gallagher, K. (2025). An exploration of neonatal staff knowledge and attitudes towards neonatal organ donation. *Journal of Neonatal Nursing*, *31*(2), 101589.

Anderson, M., Youngner, S., Smith, R. D., Nandyal, R. R., Orlowski, J. P., Jessie Hill, B., & Barsman, S. G. (2020). Neonatal organ and tissue donation for research: Options following death by natural causes. *Cell and Tissue Banking*, *21*, 289–302.

Avery, G. (2017). *Law and ethics in nursing and healthcare: An introduction* (2nd ed.). Sage Publications.

Baumrucker, S. J., Sheldon, J. E., Stolick, M., Morris, G. M., VandeKieft, G., & Harrington, D. (2008). The ethical concept of "best interest". *American Journal of Hospice and Palliative Medicine*, *25*(1), 56–62.

Beauchamp, T. L., & Childress, J. F. (2013). *Principles of biomedical ethics* (7th ed.). Oxford University Press.

Bhatia, N. (2015). *Critically impaired infants and end of life decision making: Resource allocation and difficult decisions*. Routledge.

Bluhme, E., Henckel, E., & Jorns, C. (2023). Potential of neonatal organ donation and outcome after transplantation. *Pediatric Transplantation*, *27*(3), e14486.

British Association of Perinatal Medicine. (2019a). *Enhancing shared decision making in neonatal care. A BAPM framework for practice*. British Association for Perinatal Medicine. Retrieved November 11, 25, from https://www.bapm.org/resources/158-enhancing-shared-decision-making-in-neonatal-care

British Association of Perinatal Medicine. (2019b). *Perinatal management at less than 27 weeks' gestation. A framework for practice*. British Association of Perinatal Medicine. Retrieved November 11, 2025, from https://www.bapm.org/resources/80-perinatal-management-of-extreme-preterm-birth-before-27-weeks-of-gestation-2019

British Association of Perinatal Medicine. (2022). *Service and quality standards for provision of neonatal care in the UK*. British Association for Perinatal Medicine. Retrieved November 11, 2025, from https://www.bapm.org/resources/service-and-quality-standards-for-provision-of-neonatal-care-in-the-uk

British Medical Association. (2007). *The law and ethics of abortion*. British Medical Association.

Buka, P. (2020). *Essential law and ethics in nursing: Patients, rights and decision-making*. Routledge.

Burton, M., Caswell, H., Porter, C., Mott, S., & DeGrazia, M. (2020). Moral distress: Defined and described by neonatal and pediatric critical care nurses in a quaternary care free-standing pediatric hospital. *Dimensions of Critical Care Nursing*, *39*(2), 101–109.

Children Act 1989, s. 3. Retrieved September 2, 2025 from https://www.legislation.gov.uk/ukpga/1989/41/contents/enacted

Daboval, T., & Shidler, S. (2014). Ethical framework for shared decision making in the neonatal intensive care unit: Communicative ethics. *Paediatrics & Child Health*, *19*(6), 302–304.

Fairhurst, N., & Long, T. (2020). Parental involvement in decision-making in the neonatal intensive care unit: A review of the International evidence. *Paediatrics & Child Health*, *30*(4), 119–123.

Field, D., Deeming, J., & Smith, L. K. (2016). Moral distress: An inevitable part of neonatal and paediatric intensive care? *Archives of Disease in Childhood*, *101*(8), 686–687.

Freegard, H. (Ed.). (2007). *Ethical practice for health professionals*. Thomson Learning.

General Medical Council. (2018). *Ethical guidance*. General Medical Council.

General Medical Council. (2024). *Good medical practice*. www.gmc-uk.org/professional-standards/the-professional-standards/good-medical-practice

Gillon, R. (1994). Medical ethics: Four principles plus attention to scope. *BMJ*, *309*(6948), 184.

Givrad, S., Hartzell, G., & Scala, M. (2021). Promoting infant mental health in the neonatal intensive care unit (NICU): A review of nurturing factors and interventions for NICU infant-parent relationships. *Early Human Development*, *154*, 105281. https://doi.org/10.1016/j.earlhumdev.2020.105281.

Gkiougki, E., Chatziioannidis, I., Pouliakis, A., & Iacovidou, N. (2021). Periviable birth: A review of ethical considerations. *Hippokratia*, *25*(1), 1.

Glass, H. C., Costarino, A. T., Stayer, S. A., Brett, C. M., Cladis, F., & Davis, P. J. (2015). Outcomes for extremely premature infants. *Anesthesia and Analgesia*, *120*(6), 1337–1351.

Green, J., Darbyshire, P., Adams, A., & Jackson, D. (2017). Quality versus quantity: The complexities of quality of life determinations for neonatal nurses. *Nursing Ethics*, *24*(7), 802–820.

Griffith, R., & Tengnah, C. A. (2023). *Law and professional issues in nursing* (6th ed.). SAGE Publications.

Haward, M. F., Gaucher, N., Payot, A., Robson, K., & Janvier, A. (2017). Personalized decision making: Practical recommendations for antenatal counselling for fragile neonates. *Clinics in Perinatology*, *44(2)*, 429–445.

Haward, M. F., Kirshenbaum, N. W., & Campbell, D. E. (2011). Care at the edge of viability: Medical and ethical issues. *Clinics in Perinatology*, *38*(3), 471–492.

Heitzler, E. T. (2017). Cultural competence of obstetric and neonatal nurses. *Journal of Obstetric, Gynecologic & Neonatal Nursing*, *46*(3), 423–433.

Hendrick, J. (2000). *Law and ethics in nursing and health care*. Nelson Thornes.

Hendson, L., Reis, M. D., & Nicholas, D. B. (2015). Health care providers' perspectives of providing culturally competent care in the NICU. *Journal of Obstetric, Gynecologic & Neonatal Nursing*, *44*(1), 17–27.

Janvier, A., Prentice, T., & Lantos, J. (2017). Blowing the whistle: Moral distress and advocacy for preterm infants and their families. *Acta Paediatrica*, *106*(6), 853–854.

Jefferies, A. L., Kirpalani, H. M., Canadian Paediatric Society, & Fetus and Newborn Committee. (2012). Counselling and management for anticipated extremely preterm birth. *Paediatrics & Child Health*, *17*(8), 443–443.

Kinsinger, F. S. (2009). Beneficence and the professional's moral imperative. *Journal of Chiropractic Humanities*, *16*(1), 44–46.

Kohsman, M. G. (2016). Ethical considerations for perinatal toxicology screening. *Neonatal Network*, *35*(5), 268–276.

Kornhauser Cerar, L., & Lucovnik, M. (2023). Ethical dilemmas in neonatal care at the limit of viability. *Children*, *10*(5), 784.

Larcher, V., Craig, F., Bhogal, K., Wilkinson, D., & Brierley, J. (2015). Making decisions to limit treatment in life-limiting and life-threatening conditions in children: A framework for practice. *Archives of Disease in Childhood*, *100*(Suppl 2), s1–s23.

Laurie, G. T., Harmon, S. H. E., & Porter, G. (2016). *Law and medical ethics* (10th ed.). Oxford University Press.

Linney, M., Hain, R. D., Wilkinson, D., Fortune, P. M., Barclay, S., Larcher, V., Fitzgerald, J., & Arkell, E. (2019). Achieving consensus advice for paediatricians and other health professionals: On prevention, recognition and management of conflict in paediatric practice. *Archives of Disease in Childhood*, *104*(5), 413–416.

Mental Capacity Act. (2005). www.legislation.gov.uk/ukpga/2005/9

Mills, M., & Cortezzo, D. E. (2020). Moral distress in the neonatal intensive care unit: What is it, why it happens, and how we can address it. *Frontiers in Pediatrics*, *8*, 581.

NHS Blood and Transplant. (2021). *Paediatric care*. Retrieved March 2025, from https://www.odt.nhs.uk/deceased-donation/best-practice-guidance/paediatric-care/

Nuffield Council on Bioethics. (2014). *Critical care decisions in fetal and neonatal medicine: Ethical issues. A guide to the report*. Nuffield Council on Bioethics.

Nursing and Midwifery Council (NMC). (2024). *Professional standards of practice and behaviour for nurses, midwives and nursing associates*. NMC. www.nmc.org.uk/standards/code/

Papadimitriou, V., Tosello, B., & Pfister, R. (2019). Effect of written outcome information on attitude of perinatal healthcare professionals at the limit of viability: A randomized study. *BMC Medical Ethics*, *20*, 1–8.

Pasarón, R. (2013). Neonatal bioethical perspectives: Practice considerations. *Neonatal Network*, *32*(3), 184–192.

Paterson, L., & Redpath, I. (2013). Preterm infant care. *Nursing Standard*, *27*(49), 19–21.

Prentice, T. M., Gillam, L., Davis, P. G., & Janvier, A. (2018). Always a burden? Healthcare providers' perspectives on moral distress. *Archives of Disease in Childhood-Fetal and Neonatal Edition*, *103*(5), F441–F445.

Royal College of Paediatrics and Child Health. (2014). *Making decisions to limit treatment in life limiting and life-threatening conditions in children: A framework for practice*. Royal College of Paediatrics and Child Health.

Royal College of Paediatrics and Child Health. (2015). *The diagnosis of death by neurological criteria in infants, children and adolescents*. Royal College of Paediatrics and Child Health.

Sakai, M., Tanaka, K., Nagata, K., & Ichinoyama, R. (2024). Moral distress in the neonatal intensive care unit experienced by nurses caring for critically Ill neonates: A phenomenological study. *Journal of Advanced Nursing*, *81*(7), 4160–4171. https://doi.org/10.1111/jan.16625

Sayeed, S. A. (2014). Peri-viable birth: Legal considerations. *Seminars in Perinatology*, *38*(1), 52–55.

Seedhouse, D. (1998). *Ethics: The heart of health care* (2nd ed.). John Wiley & Sons.

Spence, K. (2000). The best interest principle as a standard for decision making in the care of neonates. *Journal of Advanced Nursing*, *31*(6), 1286–1292.

Stone, E. G. (2018). Evidence-based medicine and bioethics: Implications for health care organizations, clinicians, and patients. *The Permanente Journal*, *22*, 18–30.

Thorne, S., Konikoff, L., Brown, H., & Albersheim, S. (2018). Navigating the dangerous terrain of moral distress: Understanding response patterns in the NICU. *Qualitative Health Research*, *28*(5), 683–701.

Tingle, J., & Cribb, A. (Eds.). (2013). *Nursing law and ethics* (3rd ed.). John Wiley & Sons.

Tosello, B. (2016). Perinatal palliative care in France: Who? Why? How?. *Archives de Pediatrie: Organe Officiel de la Societe Francaise de Pediatrie*, *23*(9), 983–989.

Vasu, V. (2017). Pilot evaluation of parental and professional views regarding consent in neonatal medicine by telephone interviews and questionnaires. *BMJ Paediatrics Open*, *1*(1).

Wilkinson, D. (2006). Is it in the best interests of an intellectually disabled infant to die? *Journal of Medical Ethics*, *32*(*8*), 454–459.

Wilkinson, D. (2009). The window of opportunity: Decision theory and the timing of prognostic tests for newborn infants. *Bioethics*, *23*(9), 503–514.

Wyatt, J. S. (2009). *Matters of life and death* (2nd ed.). InterVarsity Press.

PART 3

CLINICAL ASPECTS OF NEONATAL CARE

DOI: 10.4324/9781003591405-15

12 TRANSITION TO EXTRAUTERINE LIFE

Delivery room and early care practices

Sarah Fitchett

CONTENTS

DOI: 10.4324/9781003591405-16

GUIDANCE ON HOW TO ENHANCE PERSONAL LEARNING FROM THIS CHAPTER

Key points covered in this chapter

- Preparation for caring for the newborn infant in the first hour of life, including antenatal and perinatal considerations.
- Principles of neonatal resuscitation and the newborn life support algorithm.
- Care considerations after successful resuscitation.

Reflection

Reading through the chapter, you are encouraged to engage with the key points and related literature in an enquiring way. Ask these questions:

- How can you ensure perinatal optimisation is considered for every preterm birth?
- How can you improve outcomes by optimising care in the first hour?
- Would you feel confident and competent to participate in neonatal resuscitation, and are you familiar with the algorithm?
- How can you support families in caring for their baby after he or she has required resuscitation at birth?

Implications for nursing care

Finally: this chapter should facilitate your understanding of how early neonatal care for the newborn is structured and organised. Consider how you can contribute towards antenatal and perinatal optimisation in your own neonatal unit in your own country.

How might you be able to contribute to the implementation and quality improvement of this care requirement if this is not standardised practice already?

INTRODUCTION AND BACKGROUND

Most newborns adapt well to extrauterine life. Up to 85% of babies at birth breathe spontaneously and approximately 10% respond following drying, stimulation, and effective airway opening manoeuvres (Madar et al., 2021). Therefore, 5% will require respiratory support using positive pressure with varied intubation rates from 0.4–2%, less than 0.3% receiving chest compressions and only 0.05% requiring adrenaline (Fawke et al., 2025b). These numbers suggest that most newborns will respond to good airway and respiratory management but that a small proportion will go on to require further interventions.

In the context of neonatal clinical care specifically, the need for stabilisation at birth is a relatively frequent occurrence. The first hour of life in newborns that require intervention, who are compromised and/or born prematurely, is a critical time when tailored care must be aimed at supporting the transition to extrauterine life. Neonatal nurses, as either the lead practitioner or a key team member, are often involved in the resuscitation and stabilisation of high-risk newborns in the delivery room and subsequently in their care on the neonatal unit (NNU). In order to comply with the Code (Nursing and Midwifery Council (NMC), 2018), it is imperative that they deliver care based upon best evidence and practice available and that associated knowledge and skills are kept up to date.

This chapter examines the literature currently available with regard to effective practices in the early care of the newborn baby requiring neonatal care, starting with a discussion of the first 60 minutes of postnatal life known as the 'the golden hour' (Sharma, 2017) or '1st hour of care' and then moving onto to discuss resuscitation of the newborn in line with current evidence-based practice. Care relating to antenatal and perinatal periods specifically is covered in Chapter 2.

THE GOLDEN HOUR

The transition and adaptation from **intrauterine** (fetal) to **extrauterine** (neonatal) life is required for all infants, and this commences in the first minutes following birth in the delivery room, supported through the interventions that are implemented as part of the **'golden hour'** (Bellingham & Warren, 2025). The concept of the golden hour incorporates high-quality, timely, and efficient evidence-based interventions and standardisation of care for term and preterm neonates in the first 60 minutes of postnatal life, which can improve short and long-term outcomes. It reinforces the philosophy of communication and collaboration ensuring a standardised approach by all healthcare professionals involved (Fathi et al., 2018). The golden hour interventions (see Box 12.1) include neonatal resuscitation, post-resuscitation care, transportation of the sick newborn to the NNU, respiratory and cardiovascular support, and initial care in the nursery environment. Amuji et al. (2025) outline key areas of the golden hour, namely, resuscitation, thermoregulation, rapid treatment of sepsis, timely parenteral nutrition administration, euglycaemia, and completed admission within 60 minutes of delivery. Every minute of life following birth is critical to the overall survival and the potential morbidities of the neonate (Verklan, 2018). Acknowledging that neonates can experience issues similar to adult trauma patients will facilitate the application of trauma principles within the NNU, enabling staff to address the components of the golden hour (Doak & Waskosky, 2022). Studies evaluating the golden hour concept in preterm neonates demonstrated a reduction in detrimental short-term outcomes such as hypothermia and hypoglycaemia and subsequently the decrease in intraventricular haemorrhage (IVH), bronchopulmonary dysplasia (BPD), and retinopathy of prematurity (ROP) when a policy, guideline, or protocol is followed (Sharma, 2017; Sheng et al., 2024).

BOX 12.1 COMPONENTS OF THE GOLDEN HOUR

- Attendance at delivery and team role assignment
- Supporting the respiratory system; preventing hypoxia
- Resuscitation
- Prevention of hypothermia/temperature maintenance
- Optimal cord management
- Support to cardiovascular system
- Early nutritional care
- Prevention of hypoglycaemia
- Initiation of breastfeeding
- Infection prevention
- Starting of therapeutic hypothermia for perinatal hypoxia-ischaemia
- Laboratory investigations
- Monitoring/record keeping
- Communication with family

(adapted from Sharma, 2017; Lamary et al., 2023; Bellingham & Warren, 2025)

The first four areas from this list of care interventions (1: attendance at delivery, 2: supporting the respiratory system, 3: resuscitation, 4: prevention of hypothermia/temperature maintenance) will now be discussed. Further detail about these important topics along with the remaining topics are covered in the relevant chapters elsewhere in the book.

ATTENDANCE AT DELIVERY AND TEAM ROLE ASSIGNMENT

Decisions about resuscitation should be made by an experienced neonatologist or paediatrician to whom this responsibility has been designated in accordance with current Resuscitation Council UK (RCUK) guidance or country-specific guidance as applicable to elsewhere in the world. Experienced neonatal practitioners need to be present at delivery and ensure that introductions have been made to the parents with explanations as to their presence (local guidelines may vary depending on the team availability). The team should be aware of and confirm any treatment plans agreed with parents during antenatal counselling, also ensuring familiarity with obstetric history. A significant amount of preparation is required not only for the pending delivery but the baby's care during the first hour of life. In neonatal resuscitation, clear team role assignment is crucial for effective and timely intervention and the team attending the birth of an extremely high-risk neonate should decide on a team leader and allocate roles prior to the delivery of the baby (British Association of Perinatal Medicine (BAPM), 2019; see Table 12.1). This role allocation can avoid confusion over interventions, thus

TABLE 12.1 CORE TEAM ROLE ASSIGNMENT AT RESUSCITATION

Team leader	■ Oversees the entire resuscitation process. ■ Assigns roles, ensures communication, and makes critical decisions. ■ Often a senior clinician or neonatologist.
Airway management	■ Responsible for positioning the baby, opening the airway, initiating inflation breaths. ■ Undertaking airway manoeuvres and use of airway adjuncts. ■ Removal of any obstruction using suction under direct vision if needed. ■ Delivering ventilation breaths. ■ May also perform intubation if required.
Chest compressions	■ Begins chest compressions if the heart rate (HR) remains below 60 beats per minute (bpm) despite adequate inflation or ventilation breaths. ■ Coordinates with the person managing the airway to ensure synchronised compressions and ventilations.
Record keeper/ scribe	■ Documents all actions, times, and responses during the resuscitation. ■ Vital for post-event review and legal documentation.

TABLE 12.1 (Cont.)

Thermoregulation/ temperature management	■ Monitoring temperature and ensuring a thermoneutral zone with/without adjuncts – polyethylene bag/wrap, thermal chemical mattress.
Supporting roles	■ May include ANNPs, neonatal nurses, or doctors who help with equipment setup, attachment of the saturation probe, umbilical access, and post-resuscitation care. ■ In some trusts there may be equipment technicians checking, preparing, and setting up equipment ready for the team.

streamlining the process of resuscitation. A pre-brief checklist may be beneficial, as well as professionals present confirming their responsibilities prior to the resuscitation. A 'hands-off' leadership role at resuscitation allows an objective view of events to occur.

Best practices include:

- *Pre-resuscitation briefing*: Assign roles before delivery if risk factors are known.
- *Equipment checklists*: Ensure all necessary equipment items are available and functioning.
- *Closed-loop communication*: Confirm instructions are heard and understood.
- *Post-resuscitation debriefing*: Review performance and outcomes to improve future care.

SUPPORTING THE RESPIRATORY SYSTEM: PREVENTING HYPOXIA

Hypoxia before, during, or after birth is an important cause of neonatal mortality and morbidity (Seikku et al., 2016; Turner et al., 2020). Hypoxia is defined as a condition in which an extreme decrease in the concentration of oxygen in the body leads to loss of consciousness or death. In the perinatal period, this hypoxia with concurrent **hypercapnia** and acidosis leading to circulatory compromise is usually secondary to impaired placental gas exchange (Thompson et al., 2015; Fawke et al., 2025a). Early detection is essential to minimise any potential irreparable damage. Assessment of hypoxia at the moment of birth is undertaken by cord blood gas analysis, where blood is sampled from the umbilical artery and umbilical vein and analysed on a blood gas analyser.

Hypoxia is the stimulus for the onset of breathing at birth, therefore relative oxygen depletion is part of the normal process of labour, with the healthy fetus being equipped with several protective mechanisms to prevent hypoxic damage to vital organs. The high affinity for oxygen of fetal haemoglobin supports the delivery of oxygen to the tissues. This mechanism allows oxygen extraction at tissue level to increase by almost 100% during **hypoxaemic** events, delaying hypoxic damage. The fetal HR is a major determinant of cardiac output. It is four times greater than that of an adult per kilogram body weight, as it is the combined output of right and left ventricles, with 50% of the output directed to the placenta). The combination of these mechanisms allows a wide safety margin of adequate oxygen delivery during labour.

In short-duration hypoxaemic events, the HR of the mature fetus will fall, but myocardial contractility is increased, and cardiac output is maintained due to an associated increase in arterial blood pressure. This autoregulatory process is modulated at cellular level via metabolic feedback regulation of the calibre of the arterioles and capillary sphincters. The heart and brain are efficient at **autoregulation** and can maintain their blood flow over a wide range of perfusion pressures and oxygen contents. Hypoxaemic events of this type are intermittent during labour, and the ability of the fetus to quickly redistribute oxygenated blood is very important.

When there is no stress, the fetal and newborn heart is working at close to capacity merely to satisfy normal demands of tissues and growth; therefore, any increased output requirement to satisfy suboptimal tissue oxygen demand cannot be sustained for long and myocardial contractility will fail. So, while the fetus can make circulatory adjustments to compensate for the rigours of labour, under severe conditions these adaptive mechanisms will be overwhelmed, the shunting of blood towards vital organs and cerebral oxygen delivery will reduce, as blood pressure and cardiac output fall.

The ability of an organ to maintain **aerobic** metabolism is dependent on the amount of energy needed to maintain functional activity, the amount of oxygen delivered to the tissue and the amount of oxygen extracted by the tissue. The variation in response during labour is related to maturity, with immature fetal tissue being generally more robust. The smaller body mass to placental size gives a larger oxygen reserve to the premature fetus. As ventricular pressure falls there is a corresponding decrease in cerebral blood flow (CBF). During severe **asphyxia**, CBF is directed to the brain stem rather than the cerebrum, which increases the likelihood of damage to the cerebrum and cortex. When organ blood flow and oxygen delivery are severely compromised, increased tissue extraction of oxygen will not be able to compensate fully for the decrease in oxygen delivery.

Hypoxia is the most common cause of perinatally acquired severe brain injury in the full-term infant (Thompson et al., 2015; Turner et al., 2020). Practitioners working within the field of neonatal care need to be able to ameliorate its potentially devastating effects by prompt and skilled resuscitation. This is true also in management of the preterm infant who, if neglected in the first few minutes of life, is more likely to succumb to hypoxic and thermal stresses that will undoubtedly adversely affect that infant's outcome.

THINK POINT

Consider a delivery and admission that you have attended; did your preparation, stabilisation, and admission processes align to the golden hour's key considerations and principles? If not, which areas were not possible or an option and how might this be remedied for future experiences?

Many preterm neonates can be stabilised with non-invasive ventilation such as continuous positive airway pressure (CPAP). This mode of support maintains the functional residual capacity (FRC) of the lung and eases the work of breathing in the delivery room within the first 15 minutes of life, thus reducing the need for intubation for the spontaneously breathing neonate (Martherus et al., 2019; National Institute for Health and Care Excellence (NICE), 2019). If required, it is possible to administer surfactant using less invasive techniques. These will be discussed in more detail in Chapter 14.

RESUSCITATION

The aims of resuscitation are to establish and maintain a clear airway by ventilation and oxygenation, ensure effective circulation, correct acidosis, prevent hypothermia, hypoglycaemia, and haemorrhage. Successful resuscitation requires the coordinated efforts of a professional team. Infants who require resuscitation at birth fall into two broad categories: those who have undergone a period of hypoxic stress *in utero* and those who are prone to hypoxaemia in the immediate postnatal period due to inadequate pulmonary development, airway obstruction, or congenital malformations. Significant hypoxia will lead to irreparable hypoxic tissue damage, so anticipation of the need for resuscitation prior to delivery is crucial.

It is important to have an appreciation for the events that may lead to acute hypoxia. An interruption to placental oxygen supply causes the fetus to make breathing attempts. If these fail to inflate the lungs with air, the baby loses consciousness. A continuation of hypoxia of the respiratory centre within the brain results in the cessation of breathing, usually within two to three minutes; this is termed **primary apnoea**. After the baby has been in a state of primary apnoea for 1 to 2 minutes, the result is a period of gasping, which is followed by **terminal apnoea**. If no intervention occurs at this point, the baby will die.

Anticipation

The likelihood of neonatal resuscitation is increased by certain several known maternal, fetal, and intrapartum factors. These include maternal conditions, such as pre-eclampsia, maternal infection/chorioamnionitis, substance misuse in pregnancy or maternal sedation, fetal abnormality, intrauterine growth restriction, antepartum or intrapartum haemorrhage, prolonged rupture of membranes, fetal compromise indicated by decelerations of the HR or meconium-stained amniotic fluid, preterm labour, induction of labour, prolonged labour, instrumental and operative delivery, and obstetric emergencies such as a **cord prolapse** or shoulder dystocia. However, unexpected situations where resuscitation is required will also arise. Therefore, on arriving in the delivery room, details with regard to the gestation of the infant and any known problems should be elicited prior to the baby being born. If time permits, a more detailed history can be taken, but the above will enable a plan to be formulated quickly as to whether the infant may need intervention or whether more help may be needed in the case of multiple births.

Preparation of environment and equipment

Preparation prior to the birth is the key to success. Before every delivery, the room should routinely be prepared as a warm, draught-free environment so heat loss is minimised. The working condition of any equipment should be checked and prepared, so that everything that may be required is close to hand. Practitioners should check there is adequate equipment supply on each Resuscitaire® or in the resuscitation trolley, if twins, triplets, or higher multiples are being expected. The use of a pre-resuscitation check list can make the process of equipment checking quick and easy and helps avoid safety incidents.

Equipment preparedness is essential and while it may appear obvious that equipment is checked, and be sufficient for the task in hand, failure of this simple procedure has been previously implicated in a proportion of neonatal deaths reported annually in the UK (National Patient Safety Agency (NPSA), 2010) and the implementation of safety equipment checklists has been recommended in low resource settings to improve overall equipment preparedness (Hassen et al., 2024). Equipment for resuscitation may vary depending on the place of birth, e.g. community or hospital setting, yet all staff must be familiar with what is available for use, including the decontamination procedure following equipment use (Box 12.2).

The RCUK also provide guidance on what should be the minimum equipment for newborn resuscitation and the support of transition of infants at

BOX 12.2 BASIC RESUSCITATION EQUIPMENT REQUIRED IN HOSPITAL

- Radiant warmer – flat surface, heat source, light source, timer/clock
- Stethoscope
- Warm towels
- Suction unit with tubing, yankauer and various sizes of suction catheters
- Blended air/oxygen supply with flow regulation and adjustable pressures
- Pulse oximetry
- T-piece system, e.g. Neopuff
- Self-inflating bag
- Assorted face mask sizes
- Supraglottic/laryngeal mask airway (LMA) size 1, lubricant gel sachets and a 5mL syringe for cuffed LMAs
- Laryngoscope with a size 1 blade
- Polyethylene bags/wraps for preterm babies (e.g. Neohelp™ bags).

Delivery rooms should have equipment available for more advanced resuscitation:

- Laryngoscope handles (disposable options are now available)
- Various blades (disposable options are now available)
- Endotracheal tubes (ETT) – various sizes and introducers
- ETT fixation equipment according to local procedures
- End-tidal CO_2 detectors
- Resuscitation drugs
- Syringes, needles
- Umbilical artery catheter (UAC)/umbilical venous catheter (UVC) insertion pack
- Intraosseous needle
- Nasogastric tube and fixation source
- Surfactant administration/instillation kit.

birth in the pre-hospital setting (Fawke et al., 2025b). It is paramount to ensure that all professionals conform to the use of correct personal protective equipment which should be readily available and worn to protect the baby and the attending practitioner.

The ABC (D and E) of resuscitation

The RCUK suggests the use of an algorithm which incorporates an ABCD approach to neonatal resuscitation, based on continuous assessment of the baby (see Figure 12.1). As this forms the basis for education of midwives, nurses and

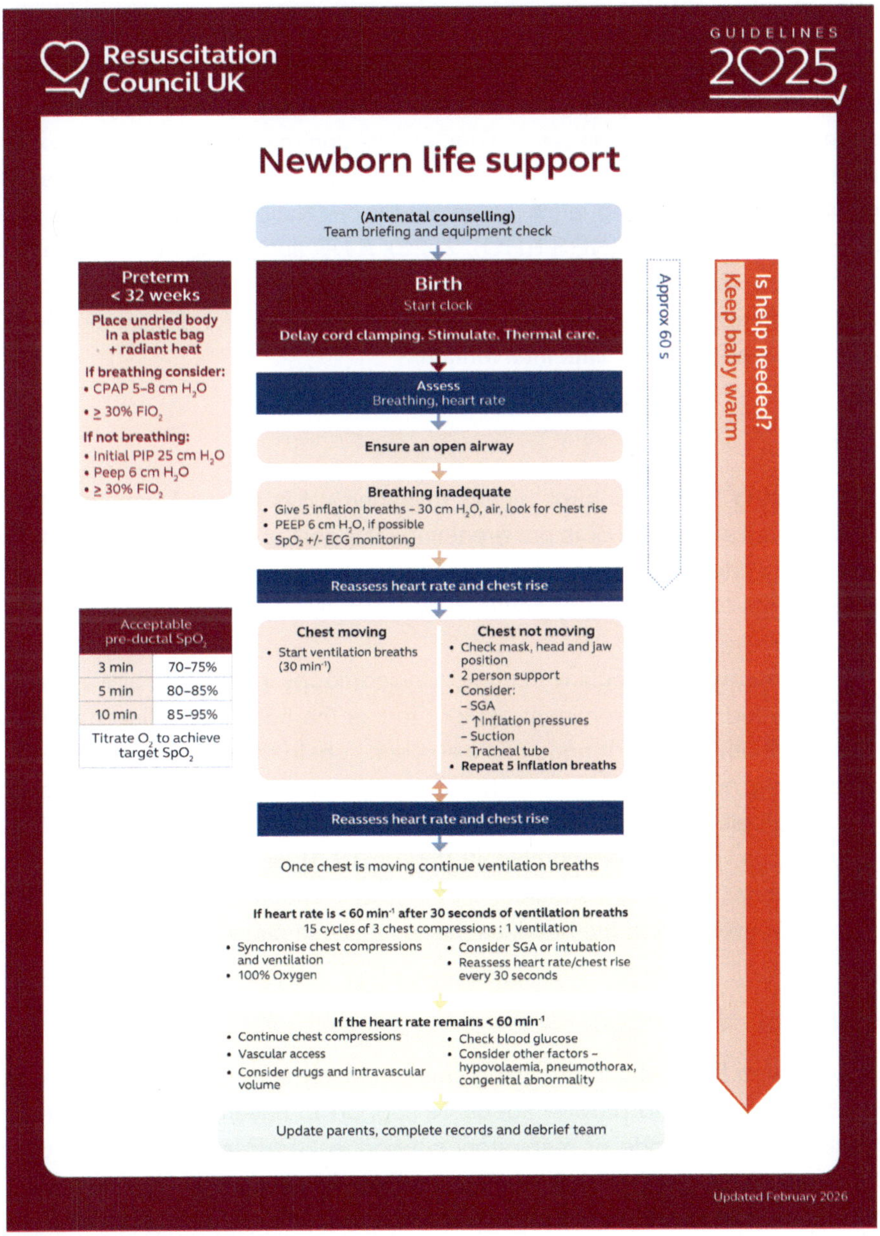

Figure 12.1 The NLS algorithm

medical staff during neonatal life support (NLS) courses, aiming to standardise the approach to resuscitation at birth, neonatal nurses should be familiar with this. Each aspect of the algorithm will be discussed in the following sections.

Assessment at birth

Every baby should be assessed immediately once they are born. At birth, newborn assessment focuses on evaluating HR, respiration, tone, response to stimulation, and appearance using the Apgar score (see Chapter 4). Appearance is no longer judged by overall skin colour, as this can mask hypoxia or cyanosis in babies with darker skin tones; instead, the healthcare team should assess the colour of the lips and tongue for central perfusion (National Health Service Race and Health Observatory (NHS RHO), 2023). A HR above 100 beats per minute, a strong cry, active limb flexion, and a prompt response to stimulation indicate good adaptation, while absent respirations, poor tone, weak reflexes, or slow HR signal the need for immediate intervention.

Airway

After ensuring thermal control, airway management is the next consideration if the infant has a slow HR or is not breathing. The goal of providing support to the respiratory system is to help in the smooth transition of the gas exchanging organ from placenta to lung. The key points in successful airway management are:

- *Open airway* Particularly in compromised/floppy infants, the airway can be occluded as the prominent occiput forces the head into a flexed position. The relatively large tongue can also cause obstruction.
- *Head in neutral position* This should provide an open airway by counteracting the problems described above. Neutral head position (see Figure 12.2) can be achieved by a simple chin lift (Figure 12.3), or by placing a 2-cm-thick roll under the baby's shoulder. With either manoeuvre, care must be taken not to over-extend the head, as this in itself can cause airway obstruction.

Breathing

In the preterm baby who is breathing spontaneously after birth without intervention there is a need to provide adequate support to ensure effective breathing, and the preferred mode of respiratory support is CPAP, a non-invasive means of support either by face mask or nasal prongs. This intervention will reduce the work of breathing and aims to prevent alveolar collapse during expiration.

The spontaneously gasping infant who has central cyanosis and/or a HR around 100 bpm is likely to respond quickly to airway opening and minimal

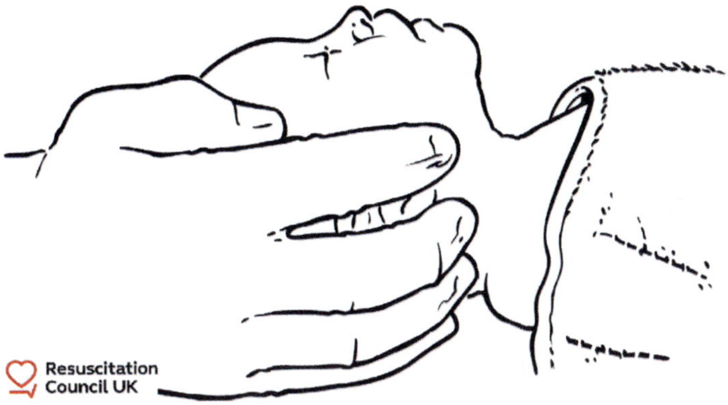

Figure 12.2 Neutral head position

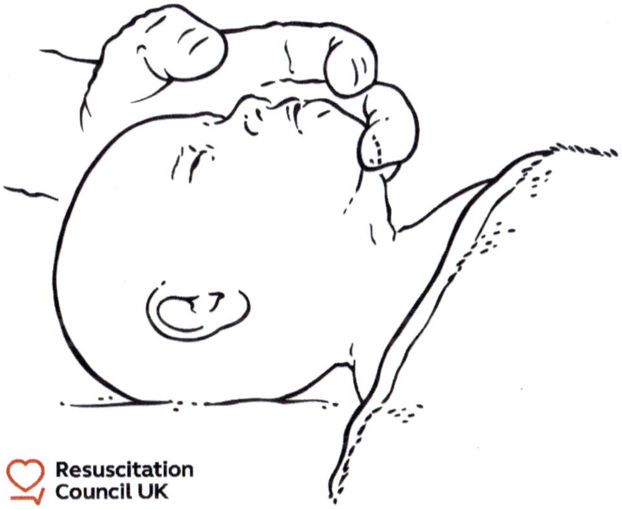

Figure 12.3 Chin lift of the newborn airway

resuscitative measures such as facial oxygen. Apnoea, pallor, or a HR less than 100 bpm indicate the necessity for positive pressure ventilation (PPV) via a mask. When an infant is born in less-than-optimal condition, it is resuscitation that mimics the adaptation to extrauterine life. A healthy baby born in good condition can clear approximately 100mL of lung fluid spontaneously within minutes of birth. It is this airway-liquid clearance and lung aeration, which allows for the establishment of FRC and the delivery of tidal volumes, which are essential for gaseous exchange. Table 12.2 explores the key aspects of 'breathing' during neonatal resuscitation.

Face mask With both the T-piece and self-inflating bag, an appropriate-sized mask is required, which should by applied by rolling from the chin to fit over

TABLE 12.2 THE 'B' OF NEONATAL RESUSCITATION

Equipment checks	■ Safety check of a 500mL self-inflating bag-valve mask system *or* ■ (preferably) a T-piece resuscitator ■ Peak Inspiratory Pressure (PIP) set at maximum pressures of **30cmH_2O for the term baby** and **25cmH_2O for the preterm baby** ■ Positive end-expiratory Pressure (PEEP) set at 5cmH_2O ■ Gas blender set to **air (21%) for term babies** or **30% for preterm babies <32 weeks' gestation** ■ Selection of mask sizes
5 inflation breaths	■ Give 5 inflation breaths, sustained for 2–3 seconds each ■ Observe for chest wall movement (the chest may not rise with the first few inflation breaths as the fluid is being moved out from the lungs, but it should be seen of the fourth or fifth inflation breath if the technique is correct and the airway is open ■ Reassess the HR
Ventilation breaths	Ventilation breaths are delivered at a rate of 30 breaths per minute if ■ Chest wall movement was observed during inflation breaths ■ The HR has improved but the baby remains apnoeic/is still breathing irregularly ■ The HR remains slow, but chest wall movement was seen during inflation breaths. Continue to observe for consistent chest wall movement and reassess the baby after 30 seconds

(Adapted from Fawke et al., 2025b)

the nose and mouth (Figure 12.4), without occluding the orbital ridges. When applying the face mask, an effective seal must be created; to ensure this, it is useful to remember the '3 Ps':

- *Position* To obtain a good seal, the mask should be aligned, then rolled on from the cleft of the chin to the bridge of the nose.
- *Pressure* Applying gentle, well-balanced pressure to the non-deformable top portion of the mask with thumb and forefinger held in a 'C' shape aids in achieving a good seal without leaks.
- *Pull* The remaining three fingers are placed to form an 'E' on the jaw line with the ring finger on the angle of the jaw. Drawing the mandibular ridge upwards lifts the jaw into the mask, thus applying a single-handed jaw thrust.

Troubleshooting If no chest wall movement is observed during PPV, the most likely reason is the absence of an open airway. Thus, the first steps should be

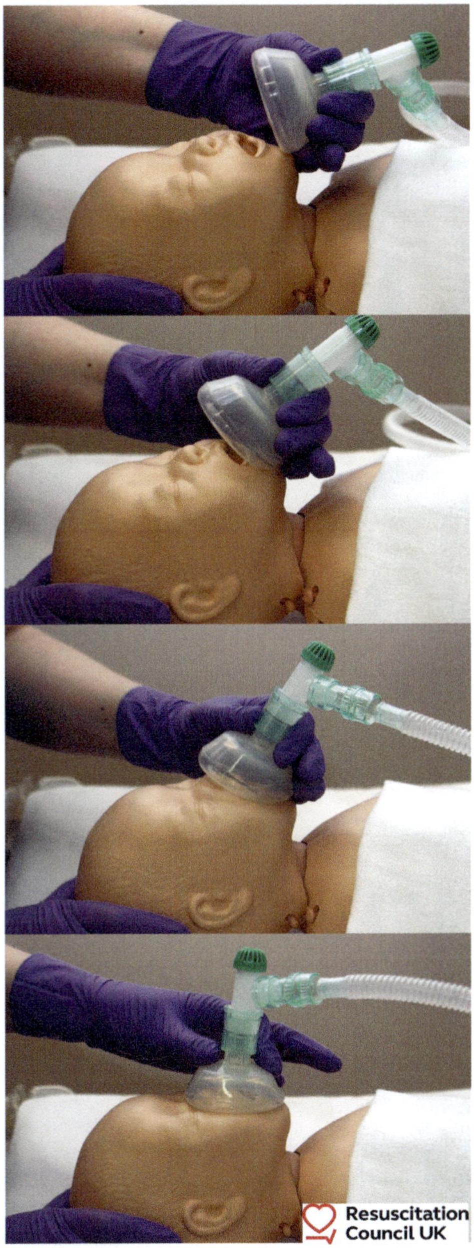

Figure 12.4 Applying the face mask

to revisit the fundamental basics, such as head positioning and mask fit, with an attempt to repeat inflation breaths. If there is only one person available at this stage, they should ensure the airway is in neutral position (Figure 12.2) and should support and lift the jaw to achieve this (Figure 12.5). The baby's condition

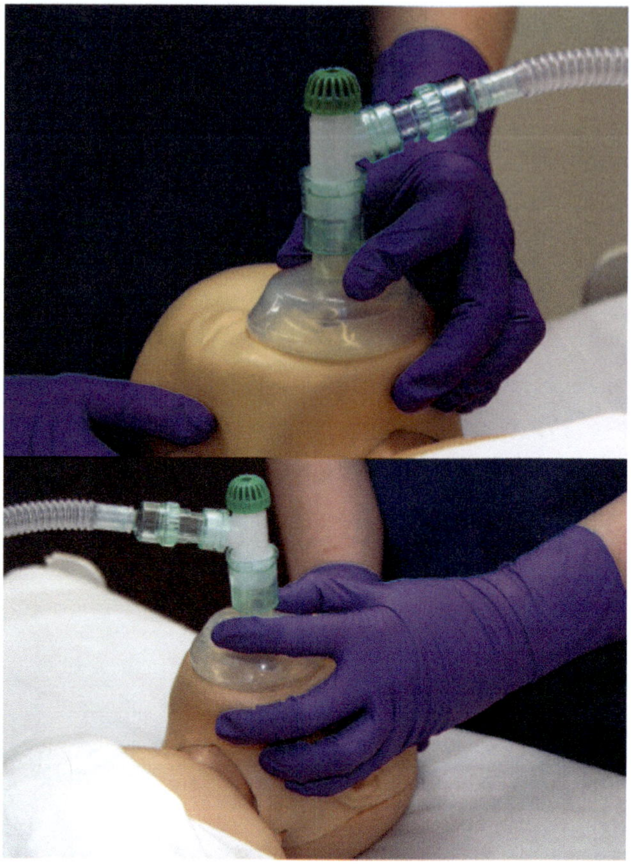

Figure 12.5 Applying one-person jaw support

will not change, and resuscitation cannot progress until an airway is established and chest wall movement is seen.

There are, however, two other airway manoeuvres that can be used if this is not successful:

- *Two-person jaw thrust* A jaw thrust will lift the tongue out of the oropharynx and open the airway. The first person applies the jaw thrust and maintains a good seal with the mask, while five inflation breaths are delivered by the second person (Figure 12.6).
- *Laryngeal mask/Supraglottic airway* Use of a 'size 1' LMA or supraglottic airway (e.g. i-gel) in a baby over 2000g will allow for the creation of a seal around the glottic opening and promotes a more direct flow of gases to the trachea. Insertion of the LMA (Figure 12.7)/i-gel (Figure 12.8) should be under direct vision with the aid of a laryngoscope to depress the tongue and optimise mouth opening. A water-soluble gel will be required for lubrication

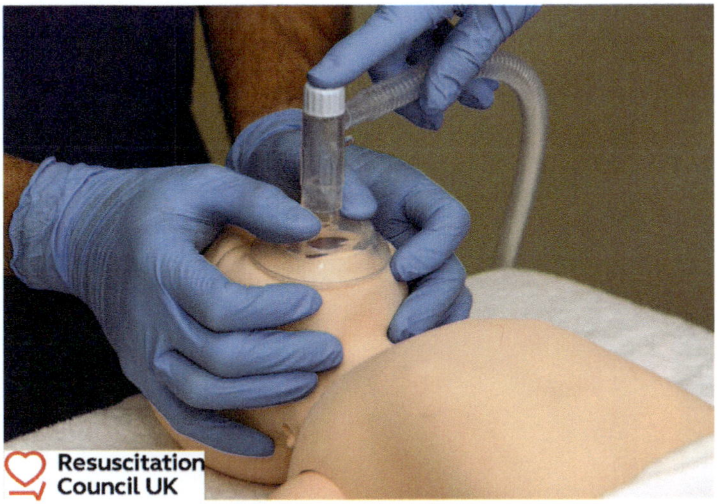

Figure 12.6 Two-person jaw thrust

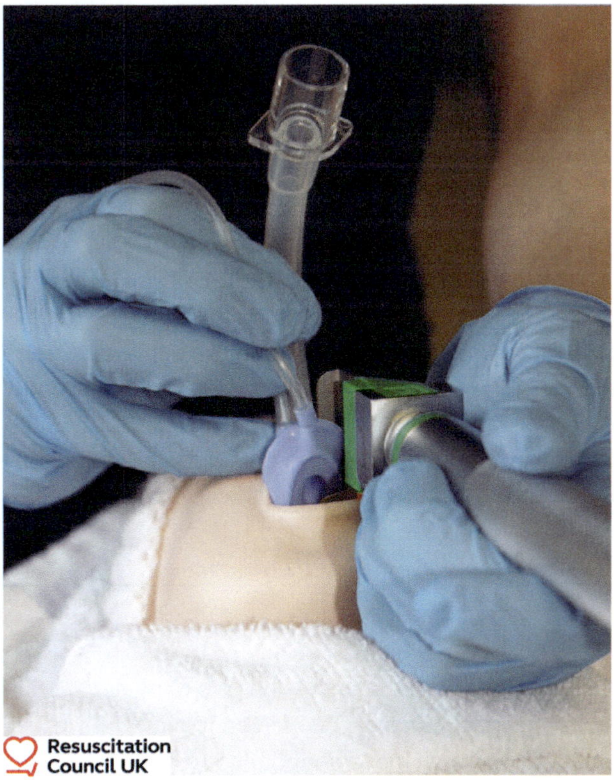

Figure 12.7 Insertion of a laryngeal mask airway

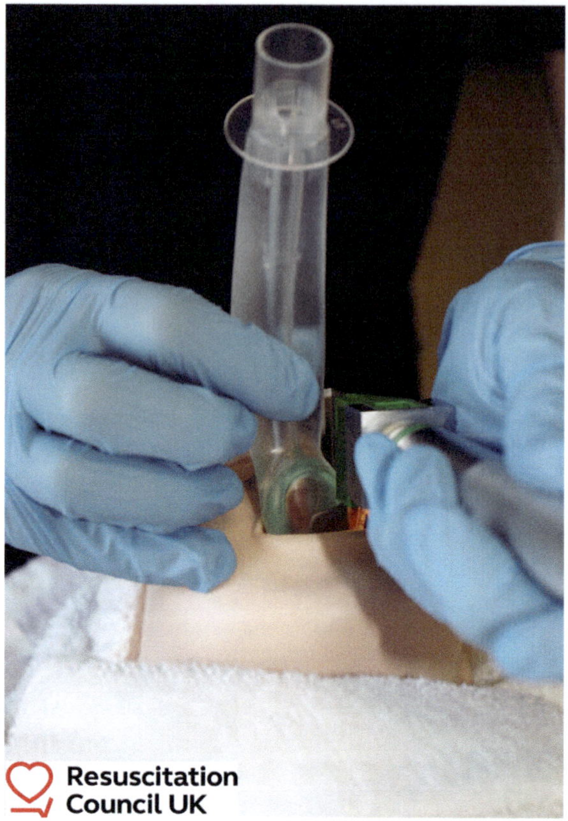

Figure 12.8 Insertion of an i-gel

of the LMA/i-gel. Prior to insertion of the LMA/i-gel, inspect the mouth and oropharynx for any particulate matter that may need removing by suction under direct vision. Suction should never be performed blindly or stimulate the **posterior** larynx or pharynx as this may induce **adduction** of the vocal cords or a profound vagal bradycardia. LMAs use an inflatable cuff to create the seal and can be secured like tracheal tubes, whereas the i-gel moulds to the airway to create a seal when it is warmed by the surrounding tissue and does not have the securing option.

PRACTICE POINT

- After any airway-opening manoeuvre, give 5 inflation breaths if the chest wall has not previously been seen to move.
- Observe for chest wall movement during PPV.
- Reassess the baby's HR after you have repeated your inflation breaths.

Most infants will respond favourably to mask ventilation, but a proportion will require endotracheal intubation, due to extreme prematurity, severe asphyxia, altered anatomy, or poor response to PPV. If this is anticipated or found to be required, a practitioner skilled in endotracheal intubation should be in attendance as unsuccessful intubation attempts are counterproductive and make subsequent attempts more difficult (Fawke et al., 2025a, 2025b).

Positive end-expiratory pressure The application of **positive end-expiratory pressure** (PEEP) at resuscitation may have several benefits for the premature infant. It is thought to optimise alveolar expansion, improve lung volumes, conserve and prolong the effectiveness of surfactant, and reduce oxygen requirements. Additionally, the application of PEEP reduces apnoea incidences in preterm infants with RDS and attenuates the potential damaging effects of high inspiratory pressures. If the use of a **bag-valve mask** (BVM) system is required due to the absence of a T-piece or gas supply, practitioners need to be aware that this does not provide PEEP.

Oxygen Current evidence available suggests that resuscitation should be commenced in air for babies > 32 weeks' gestation. Any preterm baby below 32 weeks' gestation should commence with 30% oxygen. In all gestations, oxygen titration should then be considered in response to pre-ductal pulse oximetry readings whilst avoiding bradycardia and the extremes of hypoxia and hyperoxia (Madar et al., 2021). High oxygen concentrations, leading to oxygen toxicity, can damage hypoxic cells and tissues. This is caused by the production of **free radicals** and antioxidants and contributes to brain injury in the baby who has suffered a hypoxic-ischaemic event. The antioxidant defence system develops towards the end of pregnancy and neutralises free radicals and antioxidants. Due to this system not being established, preterm babies below 30 weeks' gestation are at greater risk from oxidative stress and the inflammatory cycle. This can damage the heart, lungs, brain and kidneys, contributing to the pathogenesis of morbidities such as ROP, BPD, necrotising enterocolitis, and patent ductus arteriosus in the premature population (Falsaperla et al., 2020).

Hyperoxia reduces CBF in both term and preterm infants. Persistent cerebral vasoconstriction when high oxygen levels are used may make the brain more susceptible to hypoxic episodes or **ischaemia**, which may increase the risk of cerebral damage in the newborn period, delay the onset of spontaneous respirations, and increase the risk of short-term mortality. In the term hypoxic population, high oxygen concentrations may also be damaging due to hypoxic reperfusion injury. Research suggests that restoration of blood supply containing a high concentration of oxygen is more detrimental than restoration of the circulation alone, as it appears to create radical oxygen metabolites that lead to further pathological changes.

While the prevention of hypoxia must remain a high priority during neonatal resuscitation, the indiscriminate use of oxygen needs careful consideration in order to prevent potential long-term adverse sequelae. Pulse oximetry at birth provides real-time measurement of arterial haemoglobin saturations (SpO_2) during neonatal

TABLE 12.3 ACCEPTABLE PRE-DUCTAL SPO_2

3 minutes	70–75%
5 minutes	80–85%
10 minutes	85–95%

adapted from Dawson 2010 and Wolfsberger 2024 (cited by Fawke et al., 2025a, 2025b)

stabilisation and resuscitation. This allows practitioners to adjust oxygen delivery based on **pre-ductal** pulse oximetry level and hence cerebral oxygen saturations are also recorded. Accuracy may be affected if cardiac output and perfusion of the infant are very poor. Acceptable pre-ductal saturations can be seen in Table 12.3.

Circulation

The HR should be assessed by auscultation over the apex beat using a stethoscope. Palpation of the apex or the umbilical stump is not recommended, as it has been found that slow pulsation does not always accurately reflect the true HR. More recently, electrocardiography has been advocated as a quick and accurate way of determining HR in the delivery room (Dawson et al., 2018). The most frequent cause of an inadequate HR is ineffective lung inflation and ventilation, and once this is established, most HRs will increase. See Box 12.3.

BOX 12.3 THE 'C' OF NEWBORN RESUSCITATION

- The HR remains <60bpm after 5 inflation breaths (chest wall movement seen).
- Give 30 seconds of ventilation breaths (rate of 30 breaths per minute).
- Reassess the HR.
- If still no improvement, start chest compressions at a ratio of 3:1 (3 compressions: 1 breath) and increase oxygen to 100%.
- Consider intubation if not already been undertaken.

The aim of cardiac compressions is to re-establish effective heart pumping by moving oxygenated blood from the pulmonary veins to the coronary arteries. There are two options; however, the optimal and recommended method is chest encircling (Figure 12.9) as the 2 finger method (Figure 12.10), does not always consistently achieve the correct depth. As breaths are being delivered, ensure that the chest is inflating with each breath. At this stage, it is appropriate to increase the oxygen concentration to 100%. Help should have been requested, and if it has not already been applied, a pulse oximeter will be beneficial in assessing how effective the process is. The quality of compressions cannot be overemphasised;

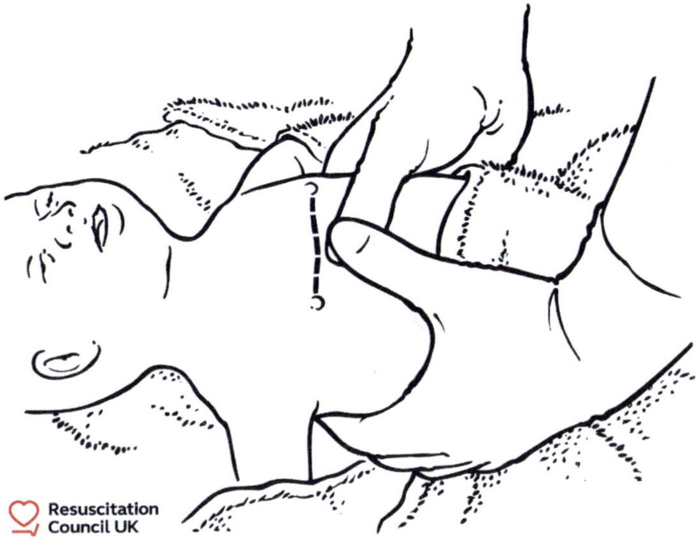

Figure 12.9 Chest compressions – encircling technique

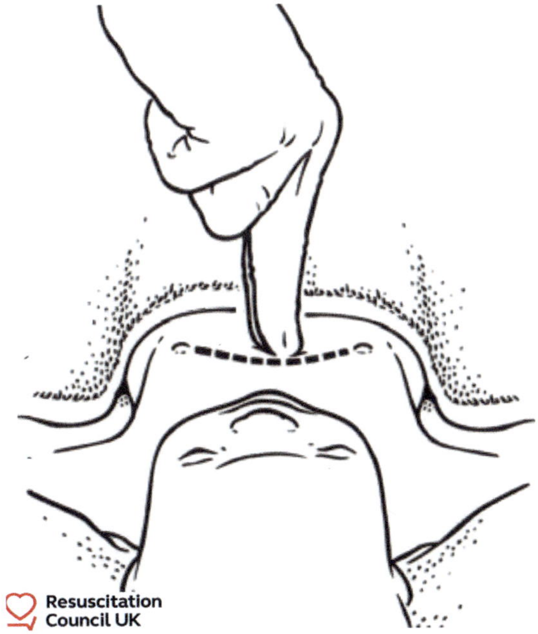

Figure 12.10 Chest compressions – two-finger technique

too rapid a rate will not allow for the recoil phase of the chest compressions, which will hinder its effectiveness. The 3:1 ratio will give 120 cycles per minute, for example, 90 cardiac compressions to 30 breaths (Box 12.3). Reassessment should take place every 30 seconds. Once the infant's HR is above 60bpm and rising, chest compressions can be discontinued. It is a continued increase that demonstrates improvement and a HR over 120 bpm that indicates stable HR. Ventilation breaths need to continue until spontaneous respiration occurs; reassess the HR every 30 seconds to ensure it remains above 100 bpm.

Resuscitation drugs

Neonatal cardiopulmonary resuscitation (CPR) in the delivery room is rare: only a small number of babies need chest compressions (0.3%), and even fewer, about 1 in 2,000 (0.05%), require adrenaline (Fawke et al., 2025a). In the unlikely event that the infant's HR is still not improving, remaining below 60bpm, or is not detectable despite adequate ventilation and good-quality compressions, drug therapy (see Table 12.4) needs to be considered. Drugs are not a first-line agent in neonatal resuscitation.

The administration of drugs needs to be achieved as close as possible to the heart, so best via an umbilical venous catheter (UVC). Administration into a peripheral vein is unlikely to reach the heart in the event of complete circulatory arrest, even

TABLE 12.4 DRUGS IN NEONATAL RESUSCITATION

Drug	*Dose*	*Mechanism of action*
Adrenaline (epinephrine)	0.2mL/kg of 1:10,000 Repeat doses are administered every 4 mins if HR remains <60 bpm.	■ Endogenous catecholamine with α- and β-adrenergic effects ■ α-mediated vasoconstriction results in improved coronary perfusion pressure and myocardial blood flow ■ Administration is intravenous (IV) or intraosseous (IO); consider endotracheal instillation if no other available access ■ Risk of arrhythmias when multiple doses administered
Glucose	2.5mL/kg of 10%	■ Intracardiac glycogen stores are likely to become depleted during acidosis ■ Glucose may be helpful where there has been no response to adrenaline and sodium bicarbonate ■ Administration is IV or IO
Volume	10mL/kg 0.9% sodium chloride or O negative blood	■ To correct hypovolaemia where this is suspected as the underlying cause for perinatal compromise ■ Avoid excessive volume replacement ■ Administration is IV or IO

(adapted from Fawke et al., 2025a, 2025b)

with effective ventilation and chest compressions. Umbilical catheterisation is also quicker and easier in a baby that is peripherally poorly perfused. An alternative route is the intraosseous route. After the administration of each drug a small flush, usually of 0.9% sodium chloride, must be given. The continuation of good-quality ventilation and cardiac compressions is imperative; drugs will otherwise not be effective.

When to stop resuscitation

Current guidance is to continue resuscitation for at least 20 minutes. The available literature does not establish exactly when resuscitation should be discontinued or a universally applicable resuscitation duration that accurately predicts poor outcomes; however, in the absence of the return of spontaneous circulation (ROSC) in neonates following 10–20 minutes of intensive resuscitation, there are close links to elevated mortality rates and a substantial risk of severe neurodevelopmental impairment among survivors (Foglia et al., 2020).

It is paramount that everybody with a responsibility of attending high-risk deliveries have an awareness of their local NNU/maternity unit guidance in relation to this. What is known is that the decision should be made in the best interest of the baby. After 10 minutes of resuscitation where the HR remains undetectable, the person leading the situation (ideally a consultant neonatologist or paediatrician) should consider the effectiveness and invite all other team members to suggest or contribute to further treatment options. Everybody involved should participate in the discussions whether resuscitation ought to be continued. This process should also include conversations with the obstetric team and a review of the obstetric history, and at this point the parents also need to be spoken to about potential plans to cease resuscitative measures.

Following 20 minutes duration of resuscitation it is reasonable to consider discontinuation if there has been no ROSC despite the implementation of the recommended stages of resuscitation and there has been the exclusion of all reversible causes which would require prolonged resuscitation measures. If the clinical decision is made to discontinue resuscitation, there needs to be ethical justification for stopping. This will need to be that a poor outcome is highly likely, a high risk of mortality, and that survival will be with severe disability. Parents' views are critical to the decision-making process, especially in marginally viable gestation neonates.

Meconium-stained amniotic fluid

Antenatal or intrapartum meconium release is referred to as meconium staining of amniotic fluid (MSAF). This is an important sign of deteriorating fetal wellbeing and adverse outcomes in terms of morbidity and mortality (Desai et al., 2017). Risk factors for the *in utero* passage of meconium includes post-maturity (>41 weeks' gestational age), small size for gestation, and conditions that compromise fetal wellbeing, such as placental insufficiency and cord compression (Gallo et al., 2023). Continuous fetal HR monitoring is recommended where there is evidence of MSAF, to detect possible fetal compromise in case this indicates acute or chronic hypoxia. MSAF is present in approximately 13% of all live births and reported rates documented are between 7 and 22%. It has been demonstrated to be as high as 23–52% at 42 weeks' gestation (Kashikar et al., 2021). Preterm births are not frequently associated with MSAF. The majority of neonates born with MSAF are healthy, but in about 2–10% meconium aspiration syndrome develops, presenting with severe respiratory compromise (Desai et al., 2017).

Witnessed resuscitation at birth

Newborn resuscitation is a unique parental experience where parents are facing the possibility of the death of their child. Evidence within the literature demonstrates that presence during resuscitation of adults and children is often preferred by families and can be beneficial. Studies indicate that parental presence during resuscitation enabled bonding, allowed them to comfort their child through touch, and in addition supported their adjustment to the loss of their child (McLean et al., 2016; Walker & Gavin, 2019). Parental presence during resuscitation aligns to family integrated care (FiCare) principles and the enabling of trauma-informed care delivery. Thus, by involving parents, teams are recognising the critical role of parents in their babies care during resuscitation, which subsequently provides reassurance that all possible interventions are being undertaken, empowers them to make appropriate treatment decisions whilst ultimately supporting a more realistic understanding of the resuscitation efforts, and the circumstances surrounding their child's death. The RCUK, along with the European Resuscitation Council (ERC) and the International Liaison Committee on Resuscitation (ILCOR), support parental presence during resuscitation (RCUK, 2023).

ACTIVITY

Reflect on the pros and cons of allowing parents to be present during the procedure of resuscitation. Do you think it is beneficial for parents?

Do you think that parents are provided with sufficient support and information during the resuscitation?

Consider whether nurses have the appropriate knowledge and training to support parents during the resuscitation of their child. How could this be improved?

Does your hospital have a policy or guidance on allowing parents to witness their child's resuscitation? If not, how would the case of parents wishing to do so be addressed?

Communication with parents

Communicating with the parents is a vital aspect of neonatal care and should always be a priority of care and not an afterthought. Clinicians should ensure that the parents understand about their baby's health at the time of delivery, during, and after resuscitation. Complete, direct, and honest individualised information from nurses and health professionals is paramount for enabling the parents to be partners in their baby's care, which is the central principle of FiCare. Wherever possible, the parents should be spoken to together regarding what is likely to happen following the delivery (for example, immediate transfer of the infant to the resuscitation area), so that they are aware of the situation and prepared as to why these interventions may be necessary. This is not always possible when a baby is born unexpectedly compromised. Neonatal resuscitation events are unique in that there are usually other persons in the immediate vicinity who are not directly (practically) involved with the situation. Where resuscitation has been necessary, it may be appropriate to involve the NNU psychologists with a referral for support of the parents to process the events witnessed.

Record keeping

Accurate, factual, and contemporaneous record keeping of the resuscitation and documentation of interventions undertaken during the golden hour alongside their timing is essential (Box 12.4). It allows the team to review this and identify a potential need for improvement. Having one member of the team allocated and solely dedicated to recording the events and interventions as they occur during resuscitation facilitates accurate and contemporaneous documentation. Prior to leaving the delivery room for transfer to the NNU, identification of the baby must be established in the form of name bands (NICE, 2021).

BOX 12.4 POINTS TO DOCUMENT FOLLOWING BIRTH

- Team members present during the resuscitation
- Antenatal and perinatal optimisation
- Duration of optimal cord management
- Apgar score
- Interventions required during resuscitation including oxygen concentrations
- Time respirations were established
- Birthweight
- Axillary temperature at time of admission to the NNU

- Timing of surfactant administration
- Time of umbilical catheterisation
- Time of commencement of ventilation or non-invasive respiratory support
- Time of commencement of therapeutic hypothermia
- Time of administration of first feed
- Time of commencement of intravenous fluids and parenteral nutrition
- Time of administration of the first dose of antibiotics
- Complications secondary to any neonatal procedure
- Size and depth of endotracheal tube (ETT), umbilical catheters, and depth of feeding tube fixation.

Post-resuscitation care

Continuing observation is necessary for any infant who has required resuscitation and has any need for ongoing support. This includes HR, oxygen saturations, and temperature. Determined on an individual basis, this may include cord gases, placental histology, screening for infection, and cardiovascular and respiratory management including the correction of any hypoglycaemia and/or metabolic acidosis. The main aim of post-resuscitation care is the early identification of the unwell or deteriorating neonate, as timely recognition will ensure appropriate referral, diagnosis and management.

ACTIVITY

Read BAPM (2023) *NEWTT 2 – Deterioration of the Newborn. A Framework for Practice.*

Explore what tools are used on your maternity unit for postnatal observations of the neonate. Reflect upon how this will be beneficial to familiarise yourself with the documentation and to understand the scores that might trigger a review and a subsequent admission to the NNU.

The signs and symptoms of a deteriorating neonate can be either obvious or initially non-specific. Nurses and midwives must have the required knowledge to recognise any deviations from the norm or the normal for each individual baby. Tools exist to assist healthcare professionals to identify signs and symptoms of deterioration. One such tool is the Newborn Early Warning Track and Trigger (NEWTT2) tool (BAPM, 2023). This incorporates parental concern to emphasise the value of family perspectives alongside input from the wider multidisciplinary team. This aligns with findings and recommendations from recent national maternity investigations, which highlight the importance of family involvement in clinical decision-making and safety monitoring. Any concerns with observations made should be escalated to the appropriate personnel utilising the frameworks recommendations for the score achieved. Utilising a recognised tool is a good indicator of physiological trends and a sensitive indicator of any abnormal physiology. Identifying problems prompts earlier review in those babies that are showing deterioration and using a standardised escalation system can aid in reducing sudden collapse or unexpected death. Infants who have required resuscitation or are preterm and meet the criteria for admission to the NNU will need to be transferred safely from the delivery room. During the transfer they will need to have their temperature maintained, airway secured and have HR and oxygen saturations monitored throughout. Occasionally, IV access is gained prior to moving. Transfer to the NNU will need a coordinated approach and should be undertaken either on a Resuscitaire® or in a transport incubator, depending on the unit's available equipment and location in relation to the delivery room.

Resuscitation training, education, and debrief

The presence of a practitioner experienced in neonatal resuscitation is crucial at high-risk deliveries. It is therefore essential that skills and competence are maintained, and refresher sessions are attended to ensure there is no deterioration in psychomotor skills following training. Three months after an educational session has been attended, skills have been shown to deteriorate (Hundscheid et al., 2021). Simulation-based training is the gold standard in both graduate and postgraduate education. When skills are acquired within a simulated setting, they are transferable into the clinical environment, with a resultant improvement in patient outcomes. Simulation should not replace exposure and experience of real-time clinical practice, but utilising this expansion of resuscitation training and dedicated airway management training can ensure that exposure to skills continues despite reduced bedside practice opportunities.

Practitioners involved in the resuscitation should also be included in a 'hot debrief' process at the earliest possible opportunity – the same shift where possible. Ensuring compassionate, non-judgemental, and supportive discussions take place, NNU psychologists may be involved in the provision of psychological first aid following events such as resuscitation.

PREVENTION OF HYPOTHERMIA/TEMPERATURE MAINTENANCE

Hypothermia remains a worldwide problem, especially for small infants and those born preterm. Effective thermal management is crucial to successful extrauterine transition. Definitions of thermal imbalances as well as interventions in the delivery room are covered in detail in Chapter 13.

Chapter takeaways

- Management in the perinatal and early postnatal period including the first hour of care can directly affect long-term outcomes, necessitating a careful, structured approach.
- Anticipation of the need for resuscitation is essential, and this should enable good preparation prior to delivery.
- Practitioners attending high-risk deliveries need to be familiar with the fundamental principles of neonatal resuscitation and be skilled in delivering this, for which ongoing training is required.
- Supporting and communicating with parents is an essential part of caring for the whole family. Post-resuscitation care needs to include conversations with the parents, discussions, and a debrief related to the perinatal events, confirming their understanding.
- Post-resuscitation care and the implementation of safety measures for the newborn infant are essential, this may include NNU admission or close observation in TC or on the postnatal ward. The midwife and neonatal nurse's role in this is central, ensuring that the needs of both parents and baby are met during this crucial time.

CASE STUDY

CASE STUDIES

Case study 1: Birth of an extremely preterm baby

Maya was born to Jo via spontaneous vaginal delivery at 24+3 weeks gestation. Jo is a primigravida and experienced spontaneous early onset of labour. There is no significant medical or antenatal history. Sam is her partner.

Q1. How would you prepare the equipment and environment prior to the birth of Maya?

Q2. Which members of the multidisciplinary team need to be present for Maya's delivery?

C A S E S T U D Y

Q3. How best can you prepare Sam and Jo for Maya's birth?
Q4. Explain how you would use the Apgar score to assess Maya's condition at birth.
Q5. Discuss the care for Maya in relation to the components of the golden hour.

Case study 2: Term baby compromised at delivery

Patience and Frank are Nigerian parents. Patience gave birth to their first baby, Ronni, in the delivery suite with a prolonged, difficult second stage of labour. When Ronni was born his HR was slow, he had reduced tone, and after stimulation he grimaced and gasped but made no further attempts to breathe.

Q1. What are the initial actions that you would take?
Q2. How would you assess Ronni for hypoxia or cyanosis?
Q3. What airway opening manoeuvres can be used to ensure Ronni's chest moves while giving inflation breaths?
Q4. What are your responsibilities in relation to Ronni's parents witnessing the resuscitation of their baby?

For suggested answer guides to the questions posed in these case studies, please refer to the web-based companion site specific to this chapter. See www.routledge.com/cw/petty

References

Amuji, N., Appaji Rao, S., Yemmethimmanahalli, N. P., Gautham, S. K., Steven, S., & Bada, S. C. (2025). Improving the quality of care for preterm infants in the golden hour. *BMJ Open Quality*, *14*, e002277. https://doi.org/10.1136/bmjoq-2023-0022

Bellingham, T., & Warren, I. (2025). The not-so-golden hour: A case study. *Journal of Neonatal Nursing*, *31*(3), 101662.

British Association of Perinatal Medicine (BAPM). (2019). *Perinatal management of extreme preterm birth before 27 weeks of gestation. A BAPM framework for practice*. https://www.bapm.org/resources/80-perinatal-management-of-extreme-preterm-birth-before-27-weeks-of-gestation-2019

British Association of Perinatal Medicine (BAPM). (2023). *NEWTT 2 – deterioration of the newborn. A framework for practice*. Retrieved April 14, 2025, from https://www.bapm.org/resources/deterioration-of-the-newborn-newtt-2-a-framework-for-practice

Dawson, J. A., Schmölzer, G. M., & Wyllie, J. (2018). Monitoring HR in the delivery room. *Seminars in Fetal and Neonatal Medicine*, *23*(5), 327–332. Retrieved August 18, 2025, from https://doi.org/10.1016/j.siny.2018.07.001

Desai, D., Maitra, N., & Patel, P. (2017). Fetal HR patterns in patients with thick meconium staining of amniotic fluid and its association with perinatal outcome. *International Journal of Reproduction, Contraception, Obstetrics and Gynecology*, *6*(3), 1030–1035.

Doak, A., & Waskosky, A. (2022). Golden hour education, standardization, and team dynamics: A literature review. *Neonatal Network*, *41*(5), 281–288. https://doi.org/10.1891/NN-2021-0005

Falsaperla, R., Lombardo, F., Filosco, F., Romano, C., Saporito, M. A. N., Puglisi, F., Piro, E., Ruggieri, M., & Pavone, P. (2020). Oxidative stress in preterm infants: Overview of current evidence and future prospects. *Pharmaceuticals (Basel, Switzerland)*, *13*(7), 145. Retrieved August 18, 2025, from https://doi.org/10.3390/ph13070145

Fathi, O., Bapat, R., Shepher, G., & Logan, J. W. (2018). Golden hour: An approach to postnatal stabilization and improving outcomes. *Neonatal Medicine*. IntechOpen. Retrieved August 18, 2025, from http://doi.org/10.5772/intechopen.82810

Fawke, J., Alexander-Elborough, E., Benson-Clarke, A., Bradfield, M., Cusack, J., Hamilton-Bower, I., Madar, J., Monnelly, V., Reeves, N., Tinnion, R., Wood, T., & Wyllie, J. (Eds.). (2025a). *Newborn life support* (6th ed.). Resuscitation Council UK (RCUK).

Fawke, J., Monnelly, V., Madar, J., Main, C., Tinnion, R., Wallace, F., Yates, J., Wyllie, J., Wood, T., & Benson Clarke, A. (2025b). *Newborn resuscitation and support of transition of infants at birth Guidelines*. Resuscitation Council UK. Retrieved February 22, 2026, from https://www.resus.org.uk/professional-library/2025-resuscitation-guidelines/newborn-resuscitation-and-support-transition-infants-birth

Foglia, E. E., Weiner, G., de Almeida, M. F. B., Wyllie, J., Wyckoff, M. H., Rabi, Y., Guinsburg, R., & International Liaison Committee on Resuscitation Neonatal Life Support Task Force. (2020). Duration of resuscitation at birth, mortality, and neurodevelopment: A systematic review. *Pediatrics*, *146*(3), e20201449. Retrieved March 24, 2025, from https://doi.org/10.1542/peds.2020-1449

Gallo, D. M., Romero, R., Bosco, M., Gotsch, F., Jaiman, S., Jung, E., Suksai, M., Ramón, Y., Cajal, C. L., Yoon, B. H., & Chaiworapongsa, T. (2023). Meconium-stained amniotic fluid. *American Journal of Obstetrics and Gynecology*, *228*(5S), S1158–S1178. https://doi.org/10.1016/j.ajog.2022.11.1283

Hassen, A. E., Agegnehu, A. F., Temesgen, M. M., Admassie, B. M., Abebe, T. A., & Admass, B. A. (2024). Equipment preparedness for neonatal resuscitation in neonatal intensive care unit in resource limited setting: Cross-sectional study. *Annals of Medicine and Surgery)*, *86*(4), 1915–1919. https://doi.org/10.1097/MS9.0000000000001801

Hundscheid, T., Bruinenberg, J., Dudink, J., de Jonge, R., & Hogeveen, M. (2021). Performing newborn life support in advance of neonatal advanced life support course-back to basics? *European Journal of Pediatrics*, *180*(5), 1647–1651. https://doi.org/10.1007/s00431-020-03917-9

Kashikar, S., Kotpalliwar, M. K., & Uttarwar, P. R. (2021). Meconium-stained liquor and its impact on maternal and neonatal outcome. *International Journal of Reproduction, Contraception, Obstetrics and Gynecology*, *10*(4), 1629–1636. https://doi.org/10.18203/2320-1770.ijrcog20211149

Lamary, M., Bertoni, C. B., Schwabenbauer, K., & Ibrahim, J. (2023). Neonatal golden hour: A review of current best practices and available evidence. *Current Opinion in Pediatrics*, *35*(2), 209–217.

Madar, J., Roehr, C. C., Ainsworth, S., Ersdal, H., Morley, C., Rüdiger, M., Skåre, C., Szczapa, T., te Pas, A., Trevisanuto, D., Urlesberger, B., Wilkinson, D., & Wyllie, J. P. (2021). European resuscitation council guidelines 2021: Newborn resuscitation and support of transition of infants at birth. *Resuscitation*, *161*, 291–326.

Martherus, T., Oberthuer, A., Dekker, J., Hooper, S. B., McGillick, E. V., Kribs, A., & Te Pas, A. B. (2019). Supporting breathing of preterm infants at birth: A narrative review. *Archives of Disease in Childhood. Fetal and Neonatal Edition*, *104*(1), F102–F107. Retrieved June 16, 2025, from https://doi.org/10.1136/archdischild-2018-314898

McLean, J., Gill, F., & Shields, L. (2016). Family presence during resuscitation in a paediatric hospital: Health professionals' confidence and perceptions. *Journal of Clinical Nursing*, *25*(7–8), 1045–1052. Retrieved June 16, 2025, from https://pubmed.ncbi.nlm.nih.gov/26923310/

National Institute for Health and Care Excellence (NICE). (2019). *Specialist neonatal respiratory care for babies born preterm* (NG 124). https://www.nice.org.uk/guidance/ng124/chapter/Recommendations

National Institute for Health and Care Excellence (NICE). (2021). *Postnatal care (NG194)*. Retrieved February 22, 2026, from https://www.nice.org.uk/guidance/ng194/chapter/recommendations

National Patient Safety Agency. (2010). *Neonatal resuscitation – Signal*. National Patient Safety Agency.

NHS Health and Race Observatory. (2023). *Review of neonatal assessment and practice in Black, Asian and minority ethnic newborns: Exploring the Apgar score, the detection of cyanosis, and jaundice*. National Health Service.

Nursing and Midwifery Council (NMC). (2018). *The code: Professional standards of practice and behaviour for nurses, midwives and nursing associates*. Retrieved February 22, 2026, from https://www.nmc.org.uk/globalassets/sitedocuments/nmc-publications/nmc-code.pdf

Resuscitation Council UK (RCUK). (2023). *Presence of family members at the clinical emergency of children and babies*. Retrieved February 22, 2026, from https://www.resus.org.uk/library/publications/publication-presence-family-members-clinical-emergency

Seikku, L., Gissler, M., Andersson, S., Rahkonen, P., Stefanovic, V., Tikkanen, M., Paavonen, J., & Rahkonen, L. (2016). Asphyxia, neurologic morbidity, and perinatal mortality in early-term and postterm birth. *Pediatrics*, e20153334. https://doi.org/10.1542/peds.2015-3334

Sharma, D. (2017). Golden hour of neonatal life: Need of the hour. *Maternal Health, Neonatology and Perinatology*, *3*(1), 16.

Sheng, L., Zhong, G., Xing, R., Yan, X., Cui, H., & Yu, Z. (2024). Quality improvement in the golden hour for premature infants: A scoping review. *BMC Pediatrics*, *24*, 88. https://doi.org/10.1186/s12887-024-04558-9

Thompson, L., Crimmins, S., Telugu, B., & Turan, S. (2015). Intrauterine hypoxia: Clinical consequences and therapeutic perspectives. *Research and Reports in Neonatology*, *5*, 79–89. https://doi.org/10.2147/RRN.S57990

Turner, J. M., Mitchell, M. D., & Kumar, S. S. (2020). The physiology of intrapartum fetal compromise at term. *American Journal of Obstetrics and Gynecology*, *222*(1), 17–26.

Verklan, T. (2018). The golden hour for high-risk neonates. *International Journal of Childbirth Education*, *33*(1), 13–21. https://search.ebscohost.com/login.aspx?direct=true&AuthType=shib,cookie,ip,url,uid&db=cin20&AN=127211605&site=ehost-live

Walker, W., & Gavin, C. (2019). Family presence during resuscitation: A narrative review of the practices and views of critical care nurses. *Intensive Crit Care Nurs*, *53*, 15–22. https://pubmed.ncbi.nlm.nih.gov/31053336/

13 THERMAL CARE OF THE NEONATE

Tracey Jones and Cassie Swire

CONTENTS

DOI: 10.4324/9781003591405-17

GUIDANCE ON HOW TO ENHANCE PERSONAL LEARNING FROM THIS CHAPTER

Key points covered in this chapter

- The physiological basis of neonatal thermoregulation, including mechanisms of heat loss and heat gain.
- Thermal instability and its consequences.
- Thermal assessment and management in the neonatal unit.

Reflection

Reading through the chapter, you are encouraged to engage with the key points and related literature in an enquiring way. Ask these questions:

- Have you encountered neonates presenting with hypothermia or hyperthermia, and what potential adverse outcomes were associated with these conditions?
- What symptoms did these infants present with?
- How were the neonates managed?

Implications for nursing care

- This chapter will support your understanding of best practices in neonatal thermal care. You are encouraged to reflect on how the knowledge gained may influence and enhance your clinical decision-making and nursing practice in this area.

INTRODUCTION AND BACKGROUND

Thermal care of the neonate is a vital aspect of neonatal nursing worldwide, specifically for vulnerable preterm or low birthweight neonates (World Health Organization, 2017). In England, the National Neonatal Audit Programme (NNAP) monitors neonatal admission temperatures as a key indicator of quality and patient safety. In 2024, 77.6% of neonatal admissions with gestational ages (GA) less than 34 weeks were within the recommended temperature range, a 1.1% increase from the previous year (NNAP, 2025). However, 20% of those most vulnerable neonates remained outside of the recommended temperature range. Admission temperatures are regarded not only as indicators of quality but also as predictors of outcomes (Madar et al., 2021). Comparable challenges have been reported internationally, and the importance of managing neonatal temperature regulation has been recognised in recent studies (Ferede et al., 2025; Yip et al., 2017; Frazer et al., 2018).

This chapter will examine the key challenges associated with maintaining effective thermal care in neonates, highlighting the physiological vulnerabilities that place certain newborns at greater risk of temperature instability. It will explore evidence-based strategies and best practices to support neonatal thermoregulation, with a focus on both prevention and early intervention to reduce the risk of hypothermia and associated complications.

During the transition from intrauterine to extrauterine life, the neonate must achieve independent thermal stability to maintain normothermia. The most widely cited definition of normothermia in the neonate originates from the WHO's Thermal Protection of the Newborn (WHO, 1997), which defines normothermia as a temperature range of 36.5°C to 37.5°C (see Table 13.1). Maintaining normothermia is crucial for maintaining physiological stability, which enables homeostasis and optimal metabolic function. Conserving energy for growth and immune function, rather than heat production, supports optimal development. This is an essential transition for any neonate, but specifically the preterm and very low birthweight (VLBW) neonatal populations, who have an increased risk of **hypothermia**.

TABLE 13.1 DEFINITIONS IN NEONATAL THERMOREGULATION

Thermoneutral zone	Where the neonate's temperature is maintained with minimal metabolic activity and energy expenditure. Also called neutral thermal environment (NTE)
Cold stress	The physiological response following exposure to an environment outside the thermoneutral zone.
Hypothermia	■ Mild (36.0°C–36.4°C) ■ Moderate (35.9°C–32.0°C) ■ Severe (<32.0°C)
Hyperthermia	■ >38.0°C

(WHO, 1997; British Association of Perinatal Medicine (BAPM), 2019; Dunne et al., 2024)

Internationally, hypothermia is a significant contributory factor in the high mortality rate related to preterm birth (McCall et al., 2018). Hypothermia is defined by Dang et al. (2023) as a temperature <36.5°C. The prevention of hypothermia and associated morbidity and mortality is a fundamental component of neonatal nursing care. Thermal management of the neonate can be a cost-effective intervention to reduce neonatal morbidity and mortality and improve long-term health, particularly in resource-limited settings.

PHYSIOLOGY OF THERMOREGULATION IN THE NEONATE

To maintain normothermia, it is important to understand how heat loss occurs and to implement strategies that reduce it. Newborns lose heat through four main mechanisms: evaporation, conduction, convection, and radiation. All of these processes are affected by the temperature of the surrounding environment. Evidence suggests that the optimal delivery room temperature is between 23°C and 25°C (British Association of Perinatal Medicine (BAPM), 2019; Dunne et al., 2024). Maintaining a warm ambient temperature helps minimise heat loss in several ways: it reduces **convection**, where heat is lost to cooler surrounding air; limits **radiation**, where heat is transferred to nearby cooler surfaces without direct contact; and decreases **conduction**, the direct transfer of heat to cooler objects (McCall et al., 2018). In addition, drying and wrapping term neonates, polyethylene wrapping use at birth, and incubator humidity for premature neonates, all prevent heat loss via **evaporation**, where heat is lost through evaporative water loss when wet skin is exposed to the cooler environmental temperatures.

Following birth, a neonate's temperature can decrease by between 0.1°C and 0.3°C per minute, unless management strategies are initiated (Lubkowska et al., 2020). Failure to so may lead to hypothermia, which is associated with adverse outcomes (Solvang et al., 2025). This evidence emphasises the importance of optimum thermal care immediately post-delivery, affecting both short-term and long-term outcomes. The term neonate already has a large surface area-to-body weight ratio and a thin layer of insulating fat, both of which increase heat loss (van de Kamp & Daanen, 2025), and these factors are further compromised as GA or birthweight decreases. Together with environmental factors in the birthing setting, this can result in significant heat loss during the crucial post-birth period.

Several innate mechanisms aid thermal stability in the immediate postnatal period. The term gestation neonate has a layer of subcutaneous fat, which provides insulation, to prevent heat loss. For heat production, a neonate relies on a process of **non-shivering thermogenesis** (Figure 13.1), which is stimulated by **brown adipose tissue** (BAT) during periods of hypothermia. Once the skin

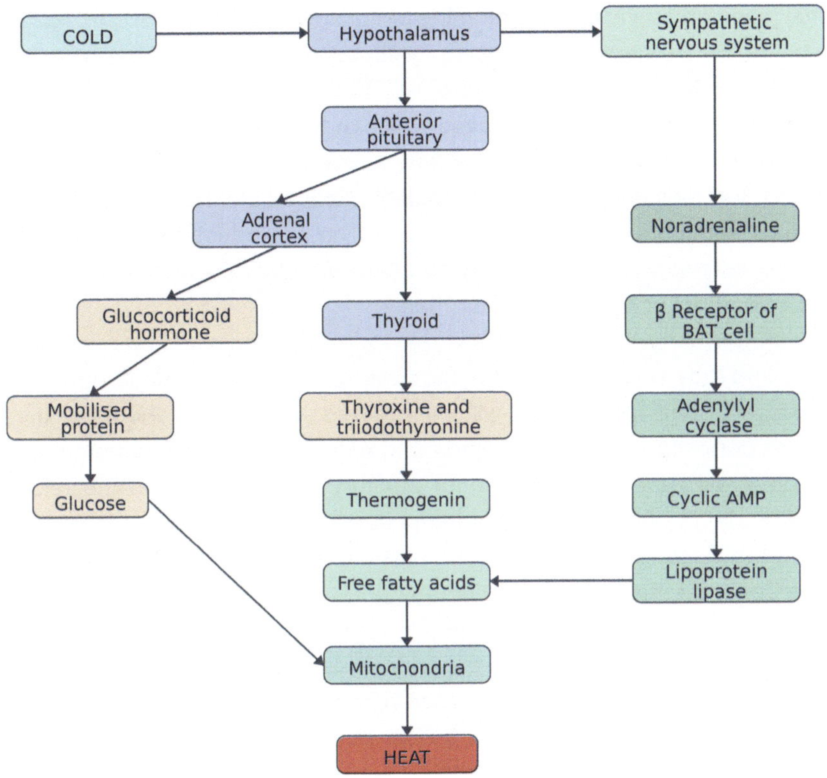

Figure 13.1 Mechanisms of non-shivering thermogenesis

temperature falls between 35°C and 36°C, non-shivering thermogenesis is initiated. Peripheral vasoconstriction of blood vessels directs blood flow to the core organs, which, in the term neonate, are well insulated with brown adipose tissue. The sympathetic release of noradrenaline initiates a process of BAT breakdown, of which heat production is a byproduct. The blood redirected through peripheral vasoconstriction is warmed by the heat produced and subsequently circulated (Kyokan et al., 2023).

This **thermogenic** process is triggered by three main factors: cutaneous cooling, increased oxygenation, and separation from the placenta. The rise in blood oxygen content and circulation is essential for activating this system. Additionally, the act of severing the umbilical cord plays a critical role in optimising the onset of non-shivering thermogenesis (McGregor, 2025). This process involves the metabolic activity of BAT. Importantly, the hypothalamus and other thermoreceptors in the body react to cold stimuli by causing vasoconstriction of the cutaneous blood vessels via the sympathetic nervous system (though this is limited) and increase the metabolic rate by releasing noradrenaline from the adrenal gland and thyroxine from the thyroid gland (Osilla et al., 2025). Noradrenaline binds to β_1-receptors increasing cyclic adenosine monophosphate (cAMP) by releasing **adenosine triphosphate** (ATP) from adenylyl cyclase. This increase in cAMP causes the release of kinase which in turn leads to a breakdown of the triglycerides in BAT, which releases fatty acids to be combusted by the **mitochondria**. The fatty acids are readily available on the outer membrane of the mitochondria. Premature infants have inefficient heat production by non-shivering thermogenesis and have an inability to exhibit peripheral vasoconstriction either due to immaturity or poor vasomotor tone.

Non-shivering thermogenesis is also dependent on a source of energy from glucose and fatty acids; therefore, if the body is unable to generate new glucose, this source of heat production will be affected. **Gluconeogenesis** is the process that converts proteins and lipids into glucose to meet requirements. Corticotrophin released from the anterior pituitary gland stimulates the release of glucocorticoid hormone from the adrenal cortex to free proteins within the cells to be metabolised into glucose. In the preterm or small for GA infant, the stores may be depleted, thus inhibiting gluconeogenesis. Hormonal levels may also be inadequate, such as thyroid-stimulating hormone (TSH) and adrenocorticotropic hormone (ACTH), which influence thyroxine release from the thyroid gland as well as hormones from the adrenal cortex, both impacting on gluconeogenesis.

Although neonates possess a greater number of sweat glands than adults, their capacity to regulate temperature through sweating is restricted. This is because the hypothalamus controls the sweat glands through the nervous system, which in neonates is not yet sufficiently myelinated. In preterm neonates, the sweat glands are not fully developed; both the secretory coils of the glandular segment and the physiological response to external temperature stimuli are diminished (Boyar et al., 2025). Additionally, underdeveloped musculature prevents preterm and low birthweight (LBW) neonates from repositioning themselves to conserve body heat.

RISK FACTORS FOR IMPAIRED THERMOREGULATION

Preterm and LBW neonates, and those affected by intrauterine growth restriction (IUGR) experience impaired heat conservation due to reduced subcutaneous fat and immature skin function (Ralphe et al., 2020). Heat loss, GA and weight are inversely proportional; therefore, the smaller and earlier gestation neonate will be at the highest risk of thermoregulation disturbances. Birth weight is often categorised into LBW (<2,500g) and VLBW neonates (<1,500g; Ralphe et al., 2020). Subcutaneous fat is deposited from around 26 weeks of gestation and continues until 36–40 weeks of gestation, when it accounts for approximately 15% of body weight.

ACTIVITY

Consider why the following situations are risk factors for impaired thermoregulation in the neonate:

- Prematurity
- Low birthweight
- Intrauterine growth restriction
- Neurological impairment
- Environmental factors

Skin maturity and keratinisation are severely limited in the extremely preterm baby. Initial keratinisation in the stratum corneum begins around 22–24 weeks of gestation; however, complete keratinisation and functional barrier formation of the epidermis may not occur until 34–36 weeks of gestation. The lack of keratinisation leads to increased permeability to water and heat. Transepidermal water loss (TEWL; Figure 13.2) through an underdeveloped stratum corneum results in a

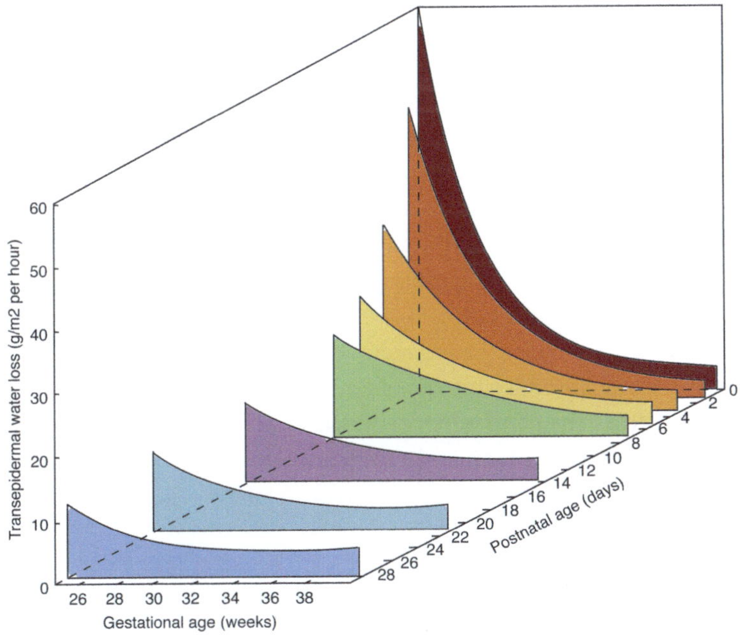

Figure 13.2 The regression of transepidermal water loss at different postnatal ages (adapted from Hammarlund et al., 1983, with permission from Wiley Blackwell Publishers)

decrease in temperature, as water evaporating from the skin also loses energy (heat), known as evaporative cooling. In the preterm neonate, 560 calories of heat are lost for each millilitre of water evaporating from the skin's surface (Boyar et al., 2025). Additionally, the large surface area-to-body mass ratio results in a greater surface area exposed to the environment, allowing for increased heat loss to occur. Combined with the reduction of insulating subcutaneous fat and an immature skin barrier, these variations increase the risk of heat loss.

The preterm cohort of neonates also has an autonomic immaturity, resulting in reduced ability to execute peripheral vasoconstriction and non-shivering thermogenesis (Ralphe et al., 2020). BAT typically develops after 28 weeks of gestation and reaches its peak near term. The preterm neonate also has immature sympathetic nervous system function, and the sympathetic pathways responsible for initiating non-shivering thermogenesis via the release of noradrenaline may not be fully developed (Kyokan et al., 2023). The limited energy stores of preterm or LBW neonates impact the metabolic process of non-shivering thermogenesis. Finally, peripheral vasoconstriction may be limited by the impaired autonomic responses and reduced vascular response in preterm neonates. Neonates who have received a central nervous system injury, such as intraventricular haemorrhage, periventricular leukomalacia, or hypoxic-ischaemic encephalopathy, may have compromised thermoregulatory control. This may result in hypothermia or hyperthermia without an environmental cause.

Environmental factors significantly impact the thermoregulation of the neonate. The intrauterine environment is thermally controlled, and neonates are vulnerable to hypothermia directly following birth. Environmental factors include the four mechanisms of heat loss: convection, conduction, radiation, and evaporation, which are significantly impacted by the ambient room temperature. Failure to dry and provide warmth following birth, as well as bathing too early or in cool environments, can result in iatrogenic causes of hypothermia in the neonatal cohort (Fawke et al., 2025). Neonates who are born unplanned outside of a standard midwifery setting have an increased risk of hypothermia and subsequently worse outcomes. Neonatal thermal care aims to achieve a **thermoneutral zone**, otherwise called **neutral thermal environment** (NTE), resulting in minimal energy expenditure and optimal growth and development (Ralphe et al., 2020).

CONSEQUENCES OF THERMAL INSTABILITY

Hypothermia

The **energy triangle**, coined by Aylott (2006), linked hypothermia to the complications of hypoglycaemia and hypoxia. Non-shivering thermogenesis, whereby BAT is metabolised, utilises and ultimately depletes glucose stores,

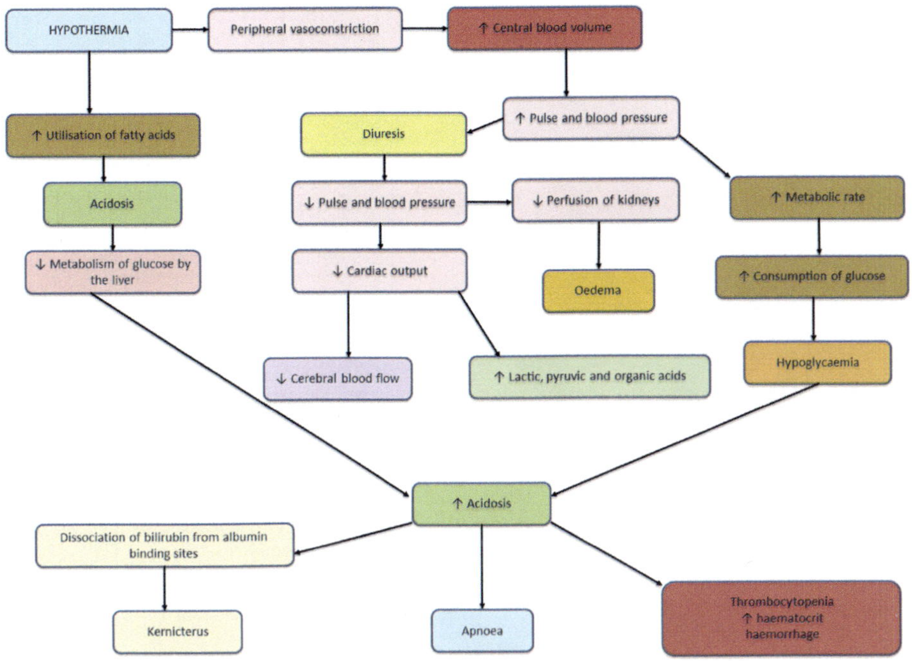

Figure 13.3 The effects of cold stress (adapted from Brueggemeyer, 1993)

resulting in potential hypoglycaemia. Cold stress also increases oxygen demand, leading to anaerobic respiration and a buildup of lactic acid, which results in an increased oxygen requirement, often first observed as tachypnoea (Figure 13.3). Hypothermia can impair various bodily systems, including the immune system, thereby increasing the risk of infection. Additionally, surfactant production can be hindered by cold stress, resulting in impaired gaseous exchange. This increased oxygen consumption, lactic acid and respiratory compromise may result in signs of respiratory distress and metabolic acidosis (Figure 13.4).

Hyperthermia

Hyperthermia can be harmful for preterm and LBW neonates due to their underdeveloped compensatory mechanisms. Overheating has been linked to sudden infant death syndrome in the wider neonatal population and, therefore, should be avoided with all cohorts of neonates (Jhun et al., 2017). Hyperthermic neonates can exhibit irritability and lethargy, tachycardia and tachypnoea. Tachycardia can exacerbate the already increased metabolic rate and oxygen consumption due to increased function of the myocardial muscle. Hypoglycaemia can also be caused by hyperthermia, due to the increased metabolic rate associated with elevated

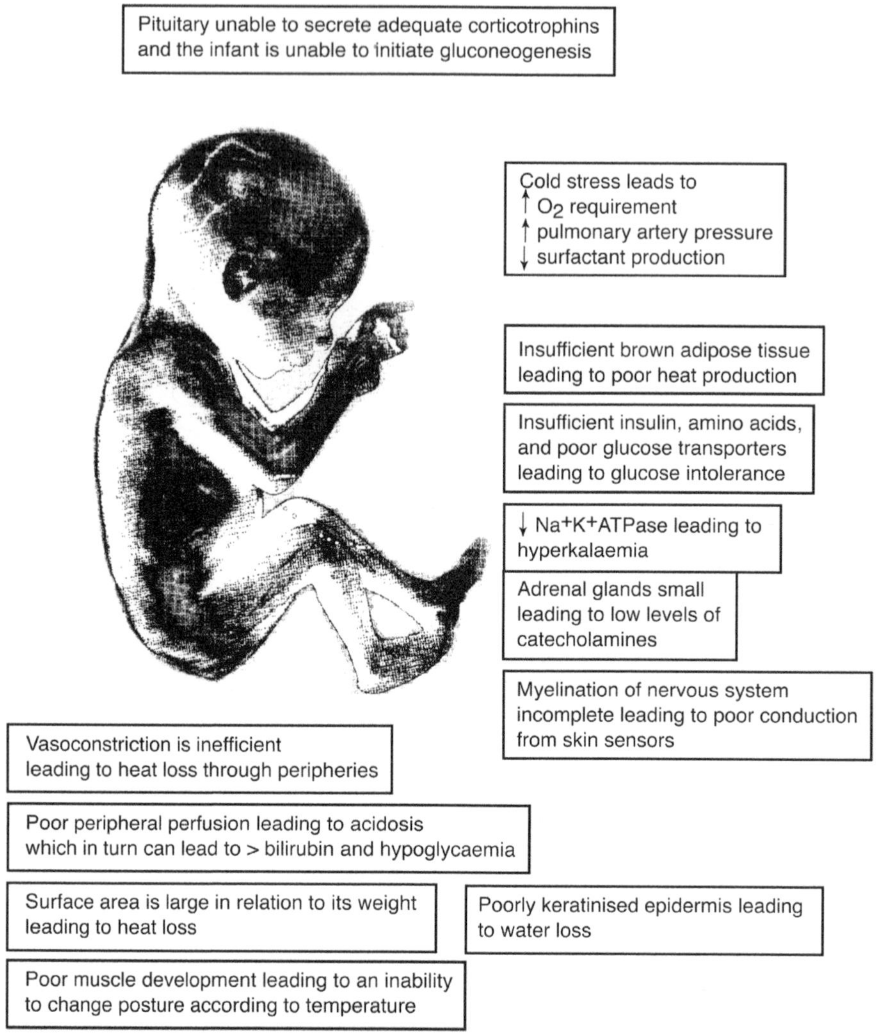

Figure 13.4 Thermal problems facing vulnerable infants

temperatures. Additionally, hyperthermia increases insensible water losses through the skin and respiration, increasing the risk of dehydration and electrolyte imbalance (Chiu et al., 2024). Hyperthermia in preterm and VLBW neonates is associated with an increased incidence of cranial ultrasound abnormalities; further research is required to determine if this is a causative relationship or related to the aetiology of neonatal infection (Brophy et al., 2022).

Neonatal hyperthermia may often have an iatrogenic origin, primarily if heat loss barriers and multiple heat sources are used in conjunction (McCall et al., 2018). There have been cases of skin injury due to the application of heat products, including exothermic gel mattresses such as Transwarmers® and hot water-filled gloves. Injuries from prolonged contact have been reported to cause burns, and therefore, frequent skin assessment is required when in direct contact with any thermal device (Toennesen et al., 2023).

Long-term complications

Neonatal admission temperatures are considered an indicator of the quality-of-service delivery in neonatal care, as a clear inverse relationship exists between preterm and LBW temperatures and morbidity and mortality (Demtse et al., 2020). Temperature instability in VLBW neonates, including hypothermia and hyperthermia, has been associated with increased risk of chronic lung disease. However, further research is needed to determine if the respiratory morbidity and temperature instability have a causal relationship or are coexisting signs of physiological instability (Ralphe et al., 2020). Although observational studies have identified increased mortality of preterm neonates with hypothermia, there is insufficient evidence of mortality reduction following implementation of thermal care strategies across all comparison groups (McCall et al., 2018). There may be an argument that the relationship between neonatal mortality and hypothermia is associative rather than a causal one. However, the literature does demonstrate a link between thermal instability and increased risk of neurological impairment, growth impairment, increased susceptibility to infection, and chronic respiratory issues (Demtse et al., 2020).

THERMOREGULATION MANAGEMENT STRATEGIES AT BIRTH

Assessment of neonatal temperature

Regardless of the clinical context, effective management of hypothermia requires the neonatal nurse to possess a thorough understanding of the physiological systems responsible for initiating and maintaining thermal stability. Additionally, practitioners must be equipped to support the neonate during the critical transitional period immediately following birth. The neonatal nurse plays a pivotal role in minimising heat loss at birth and in creating an environment that supports the neonate's thermal needs and overall wellbeing. Neonatal temperature assessment is necessary to measure, monitor and guide interventions for neonatal thermoregulation. Limitations of various temperature assessment methods can include the risk of cross-infection, site variations, and user error, which can result in the under detection of hypothermia or hyperthermia. The most common method of assessment is via an intermittent digital or chemical-dot axillary thermometer. This is a reliable and non-invasive measurement method, considered an accurate indicator of core body temperature. Digital or chemical-dot axillary thermometers have been proven to be the safest and most precise option, compared to mercury and non-contact infrared temporal scanners (Prashanth et al., 2023). The accuracy of the infrared thermometer scanner can be affected by user errors, including distance, angle of measurement, and neonatal factors such as skin thickness and moisture content. Additionally, mercury thermometers also pose a risk of exposure to toxic substances and should be avoided whenever possible.

Transcutaneous monitoring is often utilised for continuous temperature assessment during the neonatal period, particularly in high-risk neonatal populations, and throughout clinical interventions. Although this method provides continuous up-to-date information, it may not be as accurate as an axillary assessment. User error also remains an issue if the probe's positioning on the skin is incorrect or becomes detached from the skin surface. Additionally, continuous temperature monitoring, used in conjunction with servo control of warming devices such as incubators, relies on a secure thermometer probe to respond accurately.

Rectal thermometer measurement is an accurate option for core body temperature and was traditionally, a valuable route of measurement. However, more recently, is a recognition of this as an invasive monitoring assessment method carrying a risk of infection and rectal injury; therefore, it is generally avoided. Specific contraindications for this method include neonates with anorectal malformations, necrotising enterocolitis, rectal bleeding and recent rectal surgery. However, rectal temperature measurement may be utilised in neonates undergoing therapeutic hypothermia as a management strategy for hypoxic-ischaemic encephalopathy, where accurate core body temperature is essential at low body temperatures. Table 13.2 outlines the key points in relation to assessing thermal instability.

TABLE 13.2 ASSESSING FOR THERMAL INSTABILITY

Hypothermia	*Signs/symptoms*
Visual/touch	Cool, mottled, pallor
Neurological	Lethargy, weak cry, poor feeding, hypotonia
Cardiovascular	Bradycardia and hypotension
Respiratory	Respiratory distress
Metabolic	Hypoglycaemia and metabolic acidosis
Hyperthermia	*Signs/symptoms*
Visual/touch	Warm, flushed, sunken fontanelle, dry mucous membranes, poor skin turgor
Neurological	Irritability, jitteriness, high-pitched cry
Cardiovascular	Tachycardia
Respiratory	Tachypnoea

> **PRACTICE POINT**
>
> It is essential to note that thermal instability can often be an early indicator of infection in the neonate. Abnormal temperature recordings should prompt further investigation into underlying causes, including environmental factors, equipment malfunctions, and potential pathologies such as infection or neurological issues.

Preparing for birth

Preparation for birth is a key step in the thermal protection of the neonate. For neonates <28 weeks' gestation, the delivery room or theatre ambient temperature should be > 25°C. The ambient temperature for neonates over >28 weeks of gestation should be 23–25°C. The delivery setting should be draught-free, and heating devices should be prepared with pre-warmed towels and a hat available (Fawke et al., 2025). Families should be included in pre-delivery discussions to ensure they have a clear understanding of the importance of maintaining the birth environment at a specific temperature. The benefits of skin-to-skin contact following birth should be explained in advance to help prepare them for this essential aspect of neonatal care. These discussions should address the practical arrangements, expected timeframes, and the associated benefits for both the neonate and the family.

Optimal cord management

Optimal cord management or deferred cord clamping (DCC) allows for additional blood transfer from the placenta to the neonate, increasing iron stores and reducing the risk of iron deficiency. According to guidance from BAPM, DCC also supports cardiovascular stability by reducing the sudden drop in blood pressure that can occur when the cord is clamped immediately after birth. BAPM (2020) and the National Institute for Health and Care Excellence (2023) recommend waiting at least 1 minute before clamping the cord, except where there are concerns about the integrity of the cord or the neonate's heart rate. Thermoregulation must be considered when carrying out DCC to ensure that the neonate is not compromised, by utilising warmed towels, radiant heaters or other external heat sources (Fawke et al., 2025). For more discussion on OCM, see Chapter 2.

Immediate interventions at birth >32 weeks of gestation

Immediately following birth, drying the neonate with a warmed towel will prevent evaporative heat loss and stimulate the neonate, supporting a smooth circulatory transition. Prompt removal of the wet towel is essential for thermoregulatory care, or heat will be lost through skin contact with the damp material (Fawke et al., 2025). The neonate should be covered in a warm towel and a head covering in situ. OCM practices should be observed whenever possible, and warming strategies should be maintained. If there is no requirement for resuscitative measures, then the neonate should be placed skin-to-skin on the mother's chest and covered with a warm towel. If the mother is compromised and unavailable, another family member can provide skin-to-skin care. This should be a routine part of immediate post-delivery management for all neonates, unless contraindicated due to stabilisation or resuscitation requirements (WHO, 2017). If the neonate does require resuscitation or stabilisation, then they should be placed on a pre-warmed surface with radiant heat, such as a Resuscitaire® or LifeStart™ trolley.

Following birth, normothermia should be maintained and monitored to ensure prompt action is taken if needed (Fawke et al., 2025). The neonate's temperature should be measured within the first hour of birth and reassessed regularly to enable intervention if required. Early initiation of feeding to prevent hypoglycaemia will support normothermia. Bathing of the neonate should be delayed until at least twenty-four hours after birth. If this is not possible due to religious or cultural reasons, then delayed bathing for up to six hours post birth should be recommended (WHO, 2017; Nyandiko et al., 2021).

Immediate interventions at birth <32 weeks of gestation

The neonate born below 32 weeks of gestation should immediately following birth be covered with a polyethylene wrapping, excluding the face, in conjunction with the use of a radiant warmer (Fawke et al., 2025). If using polyethene wrapping, then drying the neonate is not recommended. However, the head should be dried and a hat placed in situ, due to the increased surface area and risk of heat loss. The aim of care for the neonate is to have minimal energy expenditure in maintaining their temperature within the identified range of 36.5°C and 37.5°C. A Cochrane review with a meta-analysis of over 1,000 preterm infants on the use of polyethylene wrapping concluded that plastic wrapping significantly reduced the rate of hypothermia in neonates <32 weeks of gestation (McCall et al., 2018). Polyethylene wrapping, however, has been associated with hyperthermia; therefore, regular assessment and monitoring are required.

External heat sources in the delivery setting, such as the radiant warmer, often have the option of servo control. There is currently insufficient evidence to support or refute the use of servo control on radiant heaters versus manual mode (International Liaison Committee on Resuscitation Neonatal Life Support Task Force (ILCOR), 2025); however, adhering temperature probes to the skin in neonates following birth may be challenging. OCM may require the use of a radiant warmer or an alternative measure of thermal protection in preterm or compromised neonates. The use of portable thermal equipment, such as a LifeStart™ may provide a safe surface to commence stabilisation alongside a heat source for thermal protection. Exothermic gel mattresses emit latent heat of crystallisation when activated and reach temperatures of 38–42°C in approximately 90 seconds. The thermal mattress must be activated prior to use to prevent any unnecessary heat losses that may occur as a consequence of placing an infant on a non-activated mattress (McCarthy et al., 2013).

Utilising heated humidified gas sources for respiratory support decrease evaporative losses from the epithelium and preventing convective losses during the inspiration of cold air (Trevisanuto & Sedin, 2018).

Skin-to-skin contact may still be advised, but caution is needed for preterm and growth-restricted neonates, to ensure adequate monitoring and prevention of hypothermia. However, it remains a viable thermoregulatory option in preterm neonates where limited alternative options are available, and is globally advocated, particularly in low-resource settings (WHO, 2022; ILCOR, 2025).

IN THE NEONATAL UNIT

A key objective during the first hour following admission to a neonatal unit (NNU) is to establish and maintain normothermia. This is accomplished through preparation and a combination of external heat sources and effective heat loss prevention strategies. Upon admission, neonates are placed in pre-warmed incubators, and admission digital temperatures are recorded. The WHO (1997) recommends the use of incubators or radiant heaters for unstable neonates weighing less than 2,000g. Preterm neonates may rely on this heat source until they reach a target weight; however, the compromised term neonate will also be nursed in an incubator for thermoregulatory control, assessment, and to allow for interventions.

A review of neonatal warming devices used in low-resource settings where skin-to-skin contact is not feasible concluded that there is no significant difference in effectiveness among neonatal warming devices, including incubators, radiant heaters, and conductive thermal mattresses. However, radiant heaters were found to have association with increased insensible water losses (Kyokan et al., 2023). Humidified air in the incubator reduces evaporative heat loss from the permeable skin surface of the preterm neonate, reducing hypothermia and insensible water loss, which can contribute to hypovolemia, hypernatremia and other electrolyte disturbances. A preterm neonate will require nursing in an incubator with humidity. The exact amount and duration are widely disputed; however, high levels of humidity (>70%) have been associated with increased bacterial infections, likely due to the enhanced growth of microorganisms (Chen et al., 2025). Although there remains a lack of consensus, a 2021 systematic review suggested that a humidity level of 60% to 70% is appropriate until the skin is keratinised, at approximately ten to fourteen days, depending on skin maturation and condition, to support normothermia and reduce TEWL (Glass & Valdez, 2021). Chapter 5 has further detail on incubator humidity according to gestation and age.

Clustering of care and interventions can be a viable method for reducing heat loss in neonatal care. Neonatal admissions experience up to 70 stressful interventions per day in a NNU, many of which necessitate opening the incubator porthole doors (Weber & Harrison, 2019; Campbell-Yeo et al., 2024). A study on body temperature and respiratory care in preterm neonates, examined care events as a secondary outcome. The risk for hypothermia was found to be increased 2.6 times during a care event compared to when the portholes of the incubator were closed (Ralphe et al., 2020), suggesting that careful consideration of how often the incubator portholes are opened and for how long is needed to maintain a thermally neutral environment.

Heated and conductive mattresses support thermoregulation by providing a consistent conductive heat source for the neonate. This method may be an alternative to an incubator or radiant heater or utilised in a step-down approach to the neonate achieving independent normothermia. Care is required to ensure safe use, including avoiding direct skin contact with the heated mattress source, wearing suitable layers of clothing where necessary, and closely monitoring to prevent overheating or heat-related injuries. Practitioner competence in operating warming equipment is a critical priority, as errors in use can significantly compromise the effectiveness of the intervention and potentially place the neonate at risk of harm.

Humidified gases in respiratory support

Preterm and compromised neonates are often dependent on respiratory support following birth due to pulmonary immaturity or underlying pathology. Respiratory therapies can disrupt the anatomical processes of the upper respiratory tract, which act by humidifying and heating inhaled gas. Where respiratory support bypasses these physiological processes and clinicians fail to humidify gases, pulmonary epithelial damage and thermal instability can ensue (Ralphe et al., 2020). Consequently, the exploration of the impact of respiratory support on thermal stability has been a growing area of research. ILCOR (2025) recommends using heated, humidified gases in the delivery room environment for resuscitation and stabilisation, as well as on the NNU when the risk of hypothermia is present and resources permit. The incidence of moderate hypothermia has been reduced by 36% with the implementation of heated and humidified respiratory gases as standard care in the delivery room management of neonates (Madar et al., 2021).

Skin-to-skin

Neonates without complications should receive skin-to-skin care within the first hour after birth, as recommended by the WHO. This practice supports thermoregulation and promotes the initiation of breastfeeding, bonding, and attachment. ILCOR's systematic review of thermoregulatory care for infants born at <34 weeks' gestation included a comparison of skin-to-skin versus no skin-to-skin contact. The review found insufficient evidence to make a definitive recommendation for or against immediate post-birth skin-to-skin care in this population, although the authors note that it may be beneficial when other warming strategies are unavailable (WHO, 2023). The WHO has long advocated the use of skin-to-skin care for clinically stable neonates weighing more than 1,200 g in the immediate post-birth period (1997). More recent updates from ILCOR (2025) and the Resuscitation Council UK continue to support the intervention (Fawke et al., 2025).

Post-resuscitation care

Following neonatal resuscitation, the compromised neonate will be at risk of hypothermia, hypoglycaemia, and hypoxia; therefore, the aim is to maintain the neonatal temperature between 36.5°C and 37.5°C (Fawke et al., 2025). All resuscitation should be undertaken in a warm environment, and the utilisation of external heat sources may be required when interventions necessitate access to the neonate. Only once stabilised should consideration be given to conducting therapeutic hypothermia for eligible neonates (Madar et al., 2021). Neonates who have undergone resuscitative measures are already at risk of neurological impairment; there may also be an increased risk of hypothermia and hypoglycaemia due to increased metabolic rates and oxygen and glucose utilisation (Demtse et al., 2020; Luo et al., 2024). Therefore, thermal protective interventions, as well as monitoring of blood sugar and oxygen levels, are required alongside preventive measures for hypoglycaemia through enteral or intravenous routes (Luo et al., 2024).

INTERNAL TRANSFER AND THERMAL CARE OUTSIDE OF NEONATAL CARE SETTINGS

Neonatal thermoregulation research has traditionally focused on birth and admission care, as this period is associated with a high risk of thermoregulation challenges.

However, the international guidance on supporting thermoregulation during internal transfer is lacking. In a primary research study on neonatal hypothermia in magnetic resonance imaging and surgical interventions, 90% of neonates were found to be normothermic when leaving the NNU, compared with only 52% displaying temperatures in the normal range on their return, signifying a deficit in thermal care for this neonatal cohort outside the sphere of the NNU. The study also found hypothermia persisted after infants returned to the neonatal setting, despite access to standard thermal care practices (Don Paul et al., 2018). A further study by Zhao et al. (2023) of over 500 neonates found an intraoperative rate of hypothermia of >83%. The increasing body of evidence suggesting a deficit in practice warrants further research and quality improvement work to bridge this gap. Interventions to address hypothermia outside standard neonatal settings are now being explored, with active prewarming and warming of intravenous fluids being examples of interventions being investigated (Zhao et al., 2023). Further research and education are needed to support thermoregulation outside our standard neonatal settings.

External transport

Thermal protection strategies implemented at birth and within neonatal care settings are rendered ineffective if thermoregulation is not sustained during interhospital transfer. The transportation of compromised neonates poses challenges for thermal protective care in external environments and during transport. The requirement to prevent heat loss while also allowing access for interventions can conflict with each other. Recent research has examined the use of access port covers and their effectiveness in supporting thermoregulation during neonatal transport, particularly in situations where access ports must remain open to facilitate urgent interventions such as ventilatory support (Fukuyama & Arimitsu, 2023). In low-resource settings and where clinically appropriate, skin-to-skin contact could be utilised during interhospital transfer, particularly for more stable neonates, as it supports thermoregulation and promotes physiological stability.

OUT-OF-HOSPITAL BIRTHS

Neonates born unexpectedly, outside of a delivery environment, are at increased risk of hypothermia and associated morbidities (Madar et al., 2021). The use of food-grade plastic bags may be considered in preterm or low birthweight neonates, in conjunction with skin-to-skin contact, if an incubator is unavailable. As in neonatal care settings, neonates born out of hospital and greater than 30 weeks of gestation, once dried, may be nursed in skin-to-skin contact to support normothermia during transfer to a healthcare facility.

RESOURCE-LIMITED SETTINGS

In settings with limited resources, maintaining neonatal thermoregulation presents several challenges, which may include a lack of access to thermal equipment. Alternatives such as food-grade plastic wrapping and water-filled mattresses have been shown to improve rates of hypothermia with minimal financial implications (McCall et al., 2018). Human resource limitations are also common, with a shortage of appropriately trained healthcare professionals and limited awareness of thermal protection guidelines and educational strategies to support both clinical care and family education on preventive practices. A multicentre study on risk factors for neonatal hypothermia in low-resource NNUs determined that, alongside the known risk factors of GA, birthweight, and resuscitation, the presence at delivery of a trained birth attendant also impacted neonatal hypothermia risk.

Additionally, cultural practices that conflict with evidence-based care, such as early bathing and inadequate or excessive covering and wrapping, may further compromise thermal stability (Sanni et al., 2024). Cultural aspects of adherence to adequate clothing, such as placing of a hat and delayed breastfeeding, impacted hypothermia rates in neonates. To maintain normal body temperature in neonates within low-resource environments, a foundational understanding of thermal care is essential, as is an awareness of the cultural practices in the local population. The use of low-cost yet effective interventions, such as skin-to-skin contact and wrapping the neonate, plays a crucial role in improving outcomes.

To successfully implement these strategies, it is essential to build therapeutic relationships with families and engage the wider community, promoting education and encouraging adherence to thermoregulatory care practices. Two-thirds of families were not equipped with education or training on neonatal thermal care, and this was a statistically significant factor associated with admission hypothermia (Nyandiko et al., 2021). In circumstances where external warming equipment is unavailable, continuous skin-to-skin care, commonly referred to as kangaroo care, should be provided for neonates weighing less than 2,000 grams (Nyandiko et al., 2021; WHO, 2023; Sanni et al., 2024). However, prolonged kangaroo care may be logistically challenging if mothers have to return to caring and work responsibilities shortly after birth.

Overcrowding and issues with shared equipment, such as thermal mattresses and thermometers, can also increase the risk of cross-infection (Konlan et al., 2024). It is worth considering that traditions and cultural practices of over-bundling may also risk the health of the neonate, as overheating has been associated with sudden infant death (Ahn et al., 2021). There may be some instances where cultural adaptation may offset some environmental risks of hypothermia, such as co-sleeping in colder climates. There may, however, also be a reluctance to adopt new practices, which is why engagement and respectful community-based education are essential for implementing new evidence-based practices.

NURSING ROLES AND RESPONSIBILITIES

Family education and family integrated care

The desire to keep their baby safe and warm is a biological imperative for families. Therefore, they should be offered the opportunity to learn how they can support their baby's thermoregulation. This includes both methods for reducing heat loss and maintaining normothermia. Improved involvement equips the family to recognise signs of temperature instability, such as mottled skin or cool peripheries and intervene or escalate appropriately. There is evidence of enhanced autonomic regulation in neonates whose families have participated in family integrated care, due to the calming and regulating impact of close caregiver contact (Porges et al., 2019). Skin-to-skin or kangaroo care should not be restricted to a maternal activity; fathers, partners and the wider family can also contribute to this practice. Empowered and educated families are better equipped to monitor their babies' thermoregulation, enabling early intervention when needed.

Quality improvement with multidisciplinary working

Quality improvement programmes are systematic and continuous approaches to enhancing the quality of healthcare services. The process involves multidisciplinary teams identifying issues in the local area, measuring data to establish a baseline, and implementing targeted interventions. It is recognised that for these complex thermal care challenges, a collaborative multidisciplinary approach is required involving obstetric, maternity, neonatal, and paediatric teams (McCall et al., 2018). A thermal care quality improvement programme highlighted the use of standardised checklists and continuous feedback to the multidisciplinary team as key factors in reducing neonatal admission hypothermia, emphasising the importance of involving the broader team in quality improvement work (Madar et al., 2021).

THINK POINT

Reflect on how effectively you anticipate heat loss rather than simply responding to it. Are there moments in your practice, such as transfers, procedures, or early postnatal care, where thermal protection could be strengthened? Consider how small, proactive adjustments could significantly improve neonatal outcomes.

Chapter takeaways

- Preterm and LBW infants are highly vulnerable to heat loss. Their immature skin, reduced subcutaneous fat, and limited brown fat stores make it difficult to conserve heat. These physiological limitations mean they become hypothermic far more quickly than term infants, increasing their risk of complications.
- Heat loss occurs through evaporation, conduction, convection, and radiation. These mechanisms act immediately after birth, especially when the neonate is wet, exposed, or placed on cold surfaces. Effective thermal care requires anticipating each mechanism and putting preventative strategies in place from the moment of delivery.
- Hypothermia and hyperthermia both carry serious risks. Hypothermia increases oxygen and glucose consumption, leading to hypoxia, hypoglycaemia, metabolic acidosis, and respiratory distress. Hyperthermia can cause dehydration, tachycardia, and neurological instability, and is often iatrogenic when multiple heat sources are used.
- Immediate thermal interventions at birth are critical. Drying, wrapping, skin-to-skin contact, and maintaining a warm delivery environment significantly reduce heat loss in term infants. For babies <32 weeks, polyethylene wraps and radiant warmers are essential because they prevent evaporative heat loss and support stabilisation.
- Incubator care, humidity, and minimising handling help maintain normothermia. Humidity reduces transepidermal water loss in preterm infants, while pre-warmed incubators and closed incubator doors help maintain a stable thermal environment. Clustering care reduces unnecessary exposure and prevents repeated drops in temperature.
- Transfers, procedures, and imaging are high-risk periods for temperature instability. Babies often become hypothermic during movement between departments or when incubators are opened for prolonged procedures. Proactive planning, such as pre-warming equipment and maintaining heat sources, is essential to prevent avoidable temperature drops.
- Family involvement and multidisciplinary teamwork strengthen thermal care. Educating families about skin-to-skin care and temperature monitoring empowers them to support thermal stability. Collaboration between maternity, neonatal, and obstetric teams ensures consistent, high-quality thermal protection across the entire care pathway.

CASE STUDY

CASE STUDIES

Case study 1: Thermal care for a term neonate

Baby Grace is a term female born at 39 weeks' gestation via spontaneous vaginal delivery to a 28-year-old mother. The labour was uncomplicated, and membranes ruptured spontaneously one hour before birth. The neonate was vigorous at birth, with Apgar scores of 8 and 9 at 1 and 5 minutes, respectively. The delivery room temperature was 22°C. The neonate was dried but left uncovered for several minutes while awaiting routine weighing and assessment. Delayed skin-to-skin contact was initiated about 20 minutes after birth. No hat or warm wrap was applied initially.

The initial assessment at 30 minutes of life, during routine neonatal observations in the postnatal ward, is as follows:

- Axillary temperature: 35.6°C
- Heart rate: 160 bpm
- Respiratory rate: 52 breaths/min
- Grace appears slightly pale but alert, with good tone and spontaneous movement
- Blood glucose: 2.5 mmol/L

Q1. What are the likely contributing factors to this neonate's hypothermia, and how could this have been prevented immediately after birth?

Q2. What are the early signs of hypothermia in a term neonate, and what investigations might need to be implemented?

Q3. In line with cold stress, what interventions are needed for Grace?

Q4. Why is skin-to-skin care considered a frontline intervention for mild hypothermia in term infants?

Case study 2: Thermal care for a premature neonate

Baby Amar was delivered at 29 weeks of gestation by emergency caesarean section due to maternal pre-eclampsia. Birthweight was 1.20 kg. Apgar scores were 7 at 1 minute and 9 at 5 minutes. Upon admission to the neonatal intensive care unit, the neonate's axillary temperature was 35.5°C. The baby appeared lethargic, with mottled skin and a weak cry. The delivery room temperature was 21°C, and there was a delay in placing Amar in a polythene wrap or under a radiant warmer immediately after birth.

CASE STUDY

Q1. What are the ways this infant will lose heat?
Q2. Why is Amar at risk of hypothermia?
Q3. What complications can arise from neonatal hypothermia, particularly in preterm neonates such as Amar?
Q4. Identify and explain at least three evidence-based strategies that should have been implemented immediately after birth to prevent hypothermia in a preterm neonate.

Case study 3: Transition towards going home

Premature twins born growth restricted at 25 weeks are now 10 weeks old (35 weeks corrected) and have come off all respiratory support except for low flow oxygen. Time has arrived to prepare them towards discharge home, but they are still being nursed in incubators. Their respective weights are 1.56kg and 1.52kg.

Q1. How would you assess the twins' readiness to be nursed in a cot or hot cot?
Q2. What factors now require consideration for both the infants' thermal care and that of the family needs, moving towards going home?

For suggested answer guides to the questions posed in these case studies, please refer to the web-based companion site specific to this chapter. See www.routledge.com/cw/petty

References

Ahn, Y. M., Yang, K. M., Ha, H. I., & Cho, J. A. (2021). Cultural variation in factors associated with sudden infant death during sleep. *BMC Pediatrics*, *21*, 443. https://doi.org/10.1186/s12887-021-02894-8

Aylott, M. (2006). The neonatal energy triangle. Part 1: Metabolic adaptation. *Paediatric Nursing*, *18*(6), 38–42. https://doi.org/10.7748/paed.18.6.38.s30

Boyar, V., Visscher, M., Lund, C., Narendran, V., the Tiny Baby Collaborative Steering Committee, Rysavy, M., Kribs, A., Bell, E., Kusuda, S., Younge, N., Adren, J., Batterbee, A., Vier, K., & Backes, C. (2025). Seeing beyond the obvious: Pragmatic skin care guidance for infants 22–24 weeks gestational age. *Journal of Perinatology*. https://doi.org/10.1038/s41372-025-02375-1

British Association of Perinatal Medicine (BAPM). (2019). *Normothermia toolkit*. https://www.bapm.org/pages/105-normothermia-toolkit

British Association of Perinatal Medicine (BAPM). (2020). *Optimal cord management toolkit*. https://www.bapm.org/pages/197-optimal-cord-management-toolkit

Brophy, H., Tan, G. M., & Yoxall, C. W. (2022). Very low birth weight outcomes and admission temperature: Does hyperthermia matter? *Children*, *9*(11), 1706. https://doi.org/10.3390/children9111706

Brueggemeyer, R. (1993). *Effects of cold stress in the newborn*. In American Academy of Pediatrics and American Heart Association (Eds.), *Neonatal Resuscitation Textbook*. American Academy of Pediatrics.

Campbell-Yeo, M., MacNeil, M., & McCord, H. (2024). Pain in neonates: Perceptions and current practices. *Critical Care Nursing Clinics of North America*, *36*(2), 193–210. https://doi.org/10.1016/j.cnc.2023.11.004

Chen, Z., Lin, R., Wang, H., Shi, B., & Chen, Q. (2025). The effect of incubator humidity on morbidity and mortality in preterm infants: A systematic review. *BMC Pediatrics*, *25*, 262 https://doi.org/10.1186/s12887-025-05538-3

Chiu, M., Mir, I., Adhikari, E., Heyne, R., Ornelas, N., Tolentino-Plata, K., Thomas, A., Burchfield, P., Simcik, V., Ramon, E., Brown, L S., Nelson, D. B., Wyckoff, M. H., & Kakkilaya, V. (2024). Risk factors for admission hyperthermia and associated outcomes in infants born preterm. *The Journal of Pediatrics*, *265*. https://doi.org/10.1016/j.jpeds.2023.113842

Dang, R., Patel, A. I., Weng, Y., Schroeder, A. R., Lee, H. C., Aby, J., & Frymoyer, A. (2023). Incidence of neonatal hypothermia in the newborn nursery and associated factors. *JAMA Network Open*, *6*(8), e2331011.

Demtse, A. G., Pfister, R. E., Nigussie, A. K., McClure, E. M., Ferede, Y. G., Tazu Bonger, Z., Mekasha, A., Demisse, A. G., Gidi, N. W., Metaferia, G., Worku, B., Goldenberg, R. L., & Muhe, L. M. (2020). Hypothermia in preterm newborns: Impact on survival. *Global Pediatric Health*, 7. https://doi.org/10.1177/2333794X20957655

Don Paul, J. M., Perkins, E. J., Pereira-Fantini, P. M., Suka, A., Farrell, O., Gunn, J. K., Rajapaksa, A. E., & Tingay, D. G. (2018). Surgery and magnetic resonance imaging increase the risk of hypothermia in infants. *Journal of Paediatrics and Child Health*, *54*(4), 426–431.

Dunne, E. A., O'Donnell, C. P. F., Nakstad, B., McCarthy, L. K., & European Society for Paediatric Research (ESPR) Neonatal Resuscitation Section Writing Group. (2024). Thermoregulation for very preterm infants in the delivery room: A narrative review. *Pediatric Research*, *95*(6), 1448–1454. https://https://doi.org/10.1038/s41390-023-02902-w

Fawke, J., Alexander-Elborough, E., Benson Clarke, A., Bradfield, M., Cusack, J., Hamilton-Bower, I., Madar, J., Monnelly, V., Reeves, N., Tinnion, R., Wood, T., & Wyllie, J. (2025). *Newborn life support* (6th ed.). Resuscitation Council (UK).

Ferede, Y. A., Chekol, W. C., & Tassew Zeleke, A. M. (2025). Neonatal hypothermia and its determinants among neonates admitted to the neonatal intensive care unit in Ethiopia: A systematic review and meta-analysis, *Journal of Neonatal Nursing*, *31*(1). https://doi.org/10.1016/j.jnn.2024.07.019

Frazer, M., Ciarlo, A., Herr, J., & Briere, C. E. (2018). Quality improvement initiative to prevent admission hypothermia in very-low-birth-weight newborns. *Journal of Obstetric, Gynecologic & Neonatal Nursing*, *47*(4), 520–528.

Fukuyama, T., & Arimitsu, T. (2023). Use of access port covers in transport incubators to improve thermoregulation during neonatal transport. *Scientific Reports*, *13*(1). https://https://doi.org/10.1038/s41598-023-30142-9

Glass, L., & Valdez, A. (2021). Preterm infant incubator humidity levels: A systematic review. *Advances in Neonatal Care: Official Journal of the National Association of Neonatal Nurses*, *21*(4), 297–307. https://doi.org/10.1097/ANC.0000000000000791

Hammarlund, K., Nilsson, G. E., Oberg, P. A., & Sedin, G. (1983). Transepidermal water loss in newborn infants. I. Relation to ambient temperature and humidity. *Acta Paediatrica Scandinavica*, *72*(5), 721–728.

International Liaison Committee on Resuscitation. (2025). *Maintaining normal temperature immediately after birth in late preterm and term infants (NLS 5100/NRP 599)*. Evidence Update

Worksheet. https://costr.ilcor.org/assets/images/photos/2025-NLS-5100Maintaining-normal-temperature-Term-or-Late-PT2024-EvUp-TF-and-SAC-approved.pdf

Jhun, I., Mata, D. A., Nordio, F., Lee, M., Schwartz, J., & Zanobetti, A. (2017). Ambient temperature and sudden infant death syndrome in the United States. *Epidemiology*, *28*(5), 728–734.

Konlan, K. D., Nukpezah, R. N., & Doat, A. R. (2024). Nurses' experiences in neonatal sepsis prevention and management: A qualitative cross-sectional study at selected hospitals in a metropolitan area. *BMC Health Services Research*, *24*, 1298. https://doi.org/10.1186/s12913-024-11811-5

Kyokan, M., Bochaton, N., Jirapaet, V., & Pfister, R. (2023). Early detection of cold stress to prevent hypothermia: A narrative review. *SAGE Open Medicine*. https://https://doi.org/10.1177/20503121231172866

Lubkowska, A., Szymański, S., & Chudecka, M. (2020). Neonatal thermal response to childbirth: Vaginal delivery vs. caesarean section. *PLoS ONE*, *15*(12), e0243453. https://doi.org/10.1371/journal.pone.0243453

Luo, K., Tang, J., Zhang, M., & He, Y. (2024). Systematic review of guidelines on neonatal hypoglycemia. *Clinical Endocrinology (Oxford)*, *100*, 36–49. https://doi.org/10.1111/cen.14995

Madar, J., Roehr, C. C., Ainsworth, S., Ersdal, H., Morley, C., Rüdiger, M., Skåre, C., Szczapa, T., Te Pas, A., Trevisanuto, D., Urlesberger, B., Wilkinson, D., & Wyllie, J. P. (2021). European resuscitation council guidelines 2021: Newborn resuscitation and support of transition of infants at birth. *Resuscitation*, *161*, 291–326. https://doi.org/10.1016/j.resuscitation.2021.02.014

McCall, E. M., Alderdice, F., Halliday, H. L., Vohra, S., & Johnston, L. (2018). Interventions to prevent hypothermia at birth in preterm and/or low birth weight infants. *Cochrane Database of Systematic Reviews*, *2*(2), CD004210. https://doi.org/10.1002/14651858.CD004210.pub5

McCarthy, L. K., Molloy, E. J., Twomey, A. R., Murphy, J. F., & O'Donnell, C. P. (2013). A randomized trial of exothermic mattresses for preterm newborns in polyethylene bags. *Pediatrics*, *132*(1), e135–141. https://doi.org/10.1542/peds.2013-0279

McGregor, J. (2025). *Thermoregulation*. https://oercollective.caul.edu.au/neonatal-care-essentials/chapter/thermoregulation/

National Institute for Health and Care Excellence. (2023). *Intrapartum care [N] evidence reviews for the position of the baby during cord clamping*. NICE Guideline NG235. NG235 Intrapartum Care: Evidence Review N.

National Neonatal Audit Programme (NNAP). (2025*). National neonatal audit programme (NNAP) summary report on 2024 data*. https://www.rcpch.ac.uk/resources/NNAP-summary-report-2024-data

Nyandiko, W. M., Kiptoon, P., & Lubuya, F. A. (2021). Neonatal hypothermia and adherence to World Health Organisation thermal care guidelines among newborns at Moi Teaching and Referral Hospital, Kenya. *PLoS ONE*, *16*(3), e0248838. https://doi.org/10.1371/journal.pone.0248838

Osilla, E. V., Marsidi, J. L., Shumway, K. R., & Sharma, S. (2025). Physiology, temperature regulation [Updated 2023 Jul 30]. In *StatPearls* [Internet]. StatPearls Publishing. https://www.ncbi.nlm.nih.gov/books/NBK507838/

Porges, S. W., Davila, M. I., Lewis, G. F., Kolacz, J., Okonmah-Obazee, S., Hane, A. A., Kwon, K. Y., Ludwig, R. J., Myers, M. M., & Welch, M. G. (2019). Autonomic regulation of preterm infants is enhanced by Family Nurture Intervention. *Developmental Psychobiology*, *61*(6), 942–952.

Prashanth, M. R., Pavithra Shree, B. E., & Namratha, K. B. (2023). Temperature assessment in newborn: A better method. *International Journal of Contemporary Paediatrics*, *10*(12), 1801–1805. https://https://doi.org/10.18203/2349-3291.ijcp20233600

Ralphe, J. L., Silva, S. G., Dail, R. B., & Brandon, D. H. (2020). The association between very premature infant body temperatures over time and respiratory care. *Biological Research for Nursing*, *23*(3), 331–340. https://https://doi.org/10.1177/1099800420969865

Sanni, U. A., Usman, F., Ogunkunle, T. O., Adamu, A. S., Lamidi, A. I., Lawal, T. O., Bello, S. O., Na'uzo, A. M., Ibrahim, T. L., Naphtal, N., Shehu, S., Jibrin, A., Farouk, Z. L., Bashir, M. F., Adedeji, I. A., Abdulsalam, M., Abdullahi, Y., & Imam, A. (2024). Hypothermia in preterm infants admitted to low-resource neonatal units in northern Nigeria: An observational study of occurrence and risk factors. *BMC Pediatrics*, *24*, 471. https://doi.org/10.1186/s12887-024-04960-3

Solvang, T. A. W., Herstad, V. B., Størdal, K., Tveiten, L., Lang, A., Eriksen, B. H., Rønnestad, A., & Stensvold, H. J. (2025). Admission temperature in very preterm infants 2012–2021: A nationwide quality registry study, Norway. *BMJ Paediatrics Open*, *9*, e003263. https://doi.org/10.1136/bmjpo-2024-003263

Toennesen, U. L., Kierkegaard, H., Kofoed, P.-E., Madsen, J. S., Fenger-Gron, J., Noergaard, B., & Soerensen, P. D. (2023). Warming prior to heel stick. Blood sample quality and infant comfort: A randomised controlled trial. *Advances in Neonatal Care*, *23*(6), E129–E138. https://doi.org/10.1097/ANC.0000000000001110

Trevisanuto, D., & Sedin, G. (2018). Physical environment for newborns: The thermal environment. In G. Buonocore, R. Bracci & M. Weindling (Eds.), *Neonatology*. Springer.

van de Kamp, E., & Daanen, H. (2025). Narrative review on infants' thermoregulatory response to heat. *International Journal of Environmental Research and Public Health*, *22*(8), 1265.

Weber, A., & Harrison, T. M. (2019). Reducing toxic stress in the neonatal intensive care unit to improve infant outcomes. *Nursing Outlook*, *67*(2), 169–189. https://https://doi.org/10.1016/j.outlook.2018.11.002

World Health Organization. (1997). *Thermal protection of the newborn: A practical guide*. http://apps.who.int/iris/bitstream/10665/63986/1

World Health Organization. (2017). *WHO recommendations on Newborn Health guidelines approved by the who guidelines review committee*. WHO Recommendations on Newborn Health: Guidelines Approved by the WHO Guidelines Review Committee.

World Health Organization. (2022). *WHO recommendations for care of the preterm or low-birth-weight infant*. https://www.who.int/publications/i/item/9789240058262

World Health Organization. (2023). *Kangaroo mother care: A transformative innovation in health care*. World Health Organization.

Yip, W. Y., Quek, B. H., Fong, M. C. W., Thilagamangai, Ong, S. S. G., Lim, B. L., Lo, B. C., & Agarwal, P. (2017). A quality improvement project to reduce hypothermia in preterm infants on admission to the neonatal intensive care unit. *International Journal for Quality in Health Care*, *29*(7), 922–928.

Zhao, J., Le, Z., Chu, L., Gao, Y., Zhang, M., Fan, J., Ma, D., Hu, Y., & Lai, D. (2023). Risk factors and outcomes of intraoperative hypothermia in neonatal and infant patients undergoing general anesthesia and surgery. *Frontiers in Paediatrics*, *11*, 1113627. https://doi.org/10.3389/fped.2023.1113627

14 MANAGEMENT OF NEONATAL RESPIRATORY DISORDERS

Dr Sabin Roy and Lisa Kaiser

CONTENTS

DOI: 10.4324/9781003591405-18

GUIDANCE ON HOW TO ENHANCE PERSONAL LEARNING FROM THIS CHAPTER

Key points covered in this chapter

- Common neonatal respiratory conditions.
- An overview of respiratory/ventilation strategies.
- Nursing care and assessment of infants requiring respiratory support.

Reflection

Reading through the chapter, you are encouraged to engage with the key points and related literature in an enquiring way. Ask these questions:

- Which common respiratory conditions have you seen in practice and how should these be managed?
- How will the content in this chapter inform or change your practice in caring for infants requiring respiratory support?
- How can parents be involved in the respiratory care of their baby?

Implications for nursing care

- Finally: how will this chapter enable you to consider best, evidence-based practice in the respiratory care of the high-risk infant in neonatal care? Consider the implications of what you learn for your nursing care relating to this area.

INTRODUCTION AND BACKGROUND

Despite advances in the treatment of respiratory disease in the newborn, respiratory compromise remains a very common cause for admission to the neonatal unit (NNU; Sweet et al., 2023). In this chapter, the most common respiratory disorders in the newborn will be presented, incorporating the pathophysiology of the conditions and the strategies that can be utilised in their management. Even less invasive methods of managing respiratory disease in the neonate are complex and not without risk and complications. As respiratory support now available is more varied, an overview of non-invasive interventions, mechanical ventilation, and related nursing care are also included.

THE PHYSIOLOGICAL BASIS OF NEONATAL RESPIRATORY CARE

Gas exchange is essential for life. Although fetal lungs are not fully mature at birth, they must reach sufficient developmental stages to support independent respiration.

Fetal Lung Development

Lung development progresses through five overlapping stages:

- Embryonic (3–6 weeks): Formation of the laryngotracheal groove, tracheo-oesophageal separation, and primitive bronchi.
- Pseudoglandular (5–18 weeks): Branching of narrow tubules, formation of terminal bronchioles, and development of connective tissue, muscle, and vasculature.
- Canalicular (16–25 weeks): Expansion of respiratory bronchioles, rich vascularisation, and emergence of type I and type II **pneumocyte** precursors.

By ~24 weeks, limited gas exchange becomes possible. Type I cells form most of the gas-exchange surface; type II cells synthesise surfactant.

- Saccular (22–32 weeks into term): Expansion and thinning of terminal air sacs, improving capillary proximity and enabling greater gas exchange.
- Alveolar (32 weeks to early adulthood): Formation and multiplication of true alveoli, continuing through early childhood (Kallapur & Jobe, 2024).

FETAL LUNG FLUID AND TRANSITION

Before birth, the lungs are filled with ~40 mL/kg of actively secreted fluid. This fluid maintains lung expansion and is intermittently swallowed or added to amniotic fluid. Near term, rising **catecholamines** reduce secretion and promote resorption; mechanisms less effective in preterm infants. During labour and in the first breaths after delivery, fluid rapidly moves into interstitial tissue and pulmonary circulation; remaining fluid clears over hours. Clearance depends on epithelial sodium channels, enhanced by antenatal glucocorticoids. Impaired fluid removal contributes to early respiratory difficulties (Kallapur & Jobe, 2024).

SURFACTANT

Surfactant, produced by type II cells, is a complex mix of phospholipids, lipids, and proteins that reduces alveolar surface tension and prevents atelectasis, reducing the work of breathing (Kallapur & Jobe, 2024). Its production is regulated by hormonal pathways as follows: Glucocorticoids accelerate maturation, supporting the rationale for antenatal corticosteroids in preterm labour (Sweet et al., 2023). Catecholamines increase surfactant release, explaining why small-for-gestational age (SGA) infants often breathe well. Insulin suppresses surfactant synthesis, increasing risk of respiratory distress syndrome (RDS) in infants of diabetic mothers (Lagoski et al., 2024). Hypothermia and acidosis depress surfactant production, reinforcing the need for normothermia and early correction of acidaemia (Hogeveen et al., 2025; Dhugga et al., 2025).

Respiratory changes at birth

The first breaths are triggered primarily by:

- Umbilical cord clamping, causing an asphyxial stimulus
- Rapid cooling at delivery
- Tactile stimulation (Hogeveen et al., 2025)

A term infant (~3 kg) clears ~100 mL of airway fluid as strong negative intrathoracic pressures draw air into the lungs. Crying further enhances pressure gradients, promoting fluid movement into pulmonary vessels and helping establish **functional residual capacity** (FRC).

Infants born by rapid labour or caesarean section before labour lack these preparatory hormonal and mechanical changes, increasing the likelihood of conditions such as transient tachypnoea of the newborn (TTN) and RDS (Kallapur & Jobe, 2024; Hogeveen et al., 2025).

RESPIRATORY CONDITIONS IN THE NEONATE

Respiratory distress syndrome

RDS is primarily a pulmonary disorder linked to neonatal lung immaturity. Its presentation has evolved with new treatments and early prophylaxis (Sweet et al., 2023). The condition results from insufficient surfactant, with incidence and severity inversely related to gestational age (GA), reflecting the natural rise in surfactant production as term approaches. RDS typically presents within the first six hours of life, with tachypnoea (>60 breaths/minute), nasal flaring, and subcostal or sternal recession due to a compliant ribcage. Infants predominantly use diaphragmatic breathing. An expiratory grunt is often present, caused by exhalation against a partially closed glottis to maintain alveolar pressure and reduce atelectasis (Lagoski et al., 2024). Classic signs are less commonly observed now because high-risk infants receive early management with exogenous surfactant, continuous positive airway pressure (CPAP), or mechanical ventilation. Surfactant-deficient lungs often need higher pressures to maintain gas exchange, which can promote inflammation, protein leak, and formation of hyaline membranes that further impair gaseous exchange.

Diagnosis is based on clinical findings supported by imaging. Chest X-rays typically show a '**ground-glass**' or 'reticulogranular' pattern with air bronchograms. Severe cases may show near-total atelectasis or complete opacification. Reduced lung volume may be seen in non-intubated infants. Lung ultrasound is increasingly used, and point-of-care gastric aspirate testing offers promising prediction of disease severity (Sweet et al., 2023). Blood gases usually show acidosis; respiratory (from hypercapnia), metabolic (from tissue hypoxia), or mixed. Congenital pneumonia can appear similar. During acute illness, protein loss and reduced renal perfusion can lead to oedema. As surfactant synthesis begins at around 36–48 hours, infants usually improve, often marked by spontaneous diuresis.

The primary aim of RDS management is to ensure effective gaseous exchange and prevent complications until type II pneumocytes regenerate and produce surfactant. Strategies focus on minimising **chronic lung disease** (CLD)/bronchopulmonary dysplasia (BPD). Mild RDS with good respiratory effort may be managed with supplemental oxygen. Despite increasing use of non-invasive support, around half of infants <28 weeks still require intubation (Sweet et al.,

2023). Surfactant has traditionally been delivered via an endotracheal tube (ETT) over a few seconds as prophylaxis. It spreads across the alveoli, reducing surface tension (Kallapur & Jobe, 2024). Concerns about intubation risks led to the INSURE technique (intubate–surfactant–extubate). More recently, less invasive surfactant administration (LISA), also called minimally invasive surfactant treatment (MIST), uses a thin catheter, with or without Magill's forceps (Herting et al., 2020). Thin-catheter delivery has shown improved outcomes over INSURE (Abdel-Latif et al., 2021). Nebulised surfactant is under investigation, with limited evidence of benefit in higher-gestation infants, though existing studies are underpowered (Nancarrow, 2025).

European guidelines recommend surfactant for infants ≤30 weeks' gestation, preferably via LISA, when the fraction of inspired oxygen (FiO_2) exceeds 0.30 (Sweet et al., 2023), replacing previous rescue-based approaches. The National Institute for Care and Healthcare Excellence (NICE, 2019) now advises using minimally invasive administration whenever possible. Early in the illness, infants may require IV fluids or parenteral nutrition, as enteral feeding can worsen respiratory compromise. Small-volume feeds, ideally breastmilk, can begin once ventilatory needs stabilise. The clinical course may be influenced by other complications of prematurity, such as intraventricular haemorrhage (IVH), infection, or necrotising enterocolitis (NEC).

Bronchopulmonary dysplasia

BPD, also known as CLD, is the most common long-term morbidity associated with prematurity, linked with increased mortality and later neurodevelopmental and pulmonary problems (Katz et al., 2025). With improved survival of extremely preterm infants, its incidence has risen despite advances in management. Global prevalence varies due to differing definitions and populations, though pooled data suggest broadly comparable overall rates. Regional variation exists; Europe and South America report lower rates, though data from South America remain limited. National cohort studies provide the most reliable estimates, highlighting how local practices influence incidence (Moreira et al., 2024).

The definition of BPD remains debated. Prior to the late 1980s, it described premature infants with RDS who required prolonged ventilation and high oxygen, leading to CLD with characteristic radiological changes. The National Institutes of Health definition shifted to oxygen dependency at 36 weeks postmenstrual age (Jobe & Bancalari, 2001). With gentler ventilation now common, classic BPD is less frequently seen. The Jensen et al. (2019) classification (see Box 14.1) is widely used because it is based on mode of support and better predicts long-term outcomes (Katz et al., 2025).

BPD is understood as a complex, multifactorial disease influenced by both antenatal and postnatal factors. It is associated with positive pressure ventilation and is inversely related to GA and birthweight. Inflammation is central to the lung injury that precedes BPD. Additional risk factors include male sex, maternal smoking, chorioamnionitis, significant hypothermia on admission, infection, and formula feeding (NICE, 2019; Schmidt & Bancalari, 2024). *Ureaplasma* spp. colonisation may contribute, but a recent multicentre RCT showed that routine antibiotics do not prevent BPD (Lowe et al., 2024).

BOX 14.1 BPD DEFINITION ACCORDING TO JENSEN ET AL., 2019 – TIME POINT OF ASSESSMENT 36 WEEKS PMA

No BPD: on room air/no respiratory support
Grade 1: Nasal cannula ≤2 L/min
Grade 2: Nasal cannula >2 L/min or nasal CPAP or nasal intermittent positive pressure ventilation (nIPPV)
Grade 3: Invasive ventilation

Management of BPD begins with prevention, including antenatal efforts to prolong pregnancy. Delivery room care is crucial: avoiding intubation and invasive ventilation where possible, administering early surfactant followed by non-invasive support, or using gentle, preferably volume-targeted ventilation if intubation is required (Schmidt & Bancalari, 2024). A short tapering course of low-dose dexamethasone may facilitate extubation for infants still ventilated after 1–2 weeks. Early prophylactic hydrocortisone can reduce BPD in selected infants; although risks such as spontaneous intestinal perforation and hyperglycaemia are concerns (Baud et al., 2016, PREMILOC), no adverse neurodevelopmental impact has been reported (Baud et al., 2017). Future care may be informed by genomics, proteomics, transcriptomics, metabolomics, and microbiomics, helping to identify susceptibility and personalise management (Kim et al., 2024).

Nursing responsibilities focus on minimising oxygen exposure and carefully titrating respiratory support. Optimal early nutrition supports lung growth and reduces BPD risk and severity (Schmidt & Bancalari, 2024). Parents should receive clear information and emotional support, particularly regarding long-term implications such as potential growth impairment, neurodevelopmental delay, and, in severe cases, mortality. Infants with BPD may be discharged on home oxygen; implementation should follow local/national guidelines, supported by strong community and outreach services (NICE, 2019; Schmidt & Bancalari, 2024).

Transient tachypnoea of the newborn

TTN is a lung disorder characterised by pulmonary oedema due to delayed reabsorption and clearance of fetal lung fluid. It is one of the most common causes of perinatal dyspnoea. TTN is a common cause of respiratory distress in the immediate newborn period, and infants usually present with tachypnoea and increased work of breathing lasting for 24 to 72 hours. Chest X-rays reveal excess fluid in the interstitial space, and occasionally **pleural effusions** (Bruschettini et al., 2022). Lung ultrasound has been suggested as a more sophisticated diagnostic tool, allowing for better prognostication of disease duration (Jiang et al., 2025). Management is supportive, likely including supplemental oxygen, and frequently CPAP is necessary to assist in maintaining alveolar patency and driving fluid into the infant's circulation. Blood gases may reveal a mild respiratory acidosis and hypoxaemia. The course of TTN is self-limiting and does not usually require mechanical ventilation (Bruschettini et al., 2022).

Pulmonary interstitial emphysema

Pulmonary interstitial emphysema (PIE) is a recognised complication of RDS, usually resulting from terminal bronchiole rupture after exposure to high-pressure ventilation. Air escapes into the interstitial spaces rather than remaining in the alveoli. This decreases lung compliance, raises residual volume, and enlarges dead space. These changes impair pulmonary blood flow, leading to hypoxaemia and hypercapnia. PIE may be localised or widespread; more commonly the latter. Clinical features include respiratory acidosis, significant hypoxaemia, and progressive deterioration. Chest X-ray shows hyperinflation with characteristic cystic lucencies, and advanced cases may form large bullae. Transillumination may show increased brightness similar to pneumothorax. Localised PIE can resolve spontaneously; widespread disease often takes weeks to improve (Gardner et al., 2020). Management focuses on reducing barotrauma and includes lowering positive inspiratory pressure (PIP), optimising positive end-expiratory pressure (PEEP), selective intubation of the healthy lung, positioning the affected lung downwards, and use of high frequency oscillatory ventilation (HFOV). Emerging evidence suggests that neurally adjusted ventilatory assist (NAVA) may help improve established PIE (Chen et al., 2024).

Pneumothorax

Spontaneous pneumothorax occurs occasionally but is more frequent in preterm infants and those requiring mechanical ventilation, especially when high inspiratory pressures are used. Clinical signs include:

- Pallor
- Worsening oxygenation
- Bradycardia and hypotension
- Asymmetric chest movement and breath sounds, rapidly evolving in **tension pneumothorax**.

Transillumination is useful, particularly in preterm infants. Diagnosis can be confirmed by chest X-ray, but treatment should not be delayed in unstable infants. Lung ultrasound, where available, allows rapid bedside diagnosis. Management includes needle decompression and/or thoracostomy drain insertion connected to an underwater seal. The drain remains in place until the air leak resolves, the lung re-expands, and the infant is clinically stable.

Pulmonary haemorrhage

Small amounts of blood in tracheal aspirates may follow traumatic intubation, but massive pulmonary haemorrhage is an acute, often catastrophic event caused by leakage of blood from the pulmonary microvasculature into the alveoli and airways. It presents with sudden respiratory collapse and bloody fluid from the oropharynx or ETT. It is more common in extremely preterm or growth-restricted infants, those receiving ventilation and surfactant, and infants with a patent ductus arteriosus (DA). Management includes surfactant, HFOV, and increasing mean airway pressure (MAP), alongside ventilation adjustments, fluid and nutritional support, blood products, vitamin K, vasopressors, inotropes, and endotracheal adrenaline. Correction of coagulopathy (see Chapter 17) is essential. Despite treatment, mortality may reach 50%, depending on the severity of respiratory and systemic compromise (Barnes et al., 2022).

Pneumonia

Neonatal pneumonia may be an isolated focal infection but is usually part of a more widespread illness. As pneumonia can be difficult to distinguish from RDS, all infants with respiratory symptoms at birth should be carefully evaluated and, if deemed necessary, treated with appropriate antibiotics. Pneumonia in the neonatal period falls into two general categories: congenital pneumonia, originating *in utero* or via the birth canal, and acquired/late onset (or **nosocomial**) pneumonia; see Table 14.1 for details of causative organisms based on timing of onset.

Congenital pneumonia usually occurs because of ascending infection and chorioamnionitis following premature or prolonged rupture of membranes. It can be difficult to distinguish from TTN on presentation, but the clinical course is different, with affected infants displaying higher morbidity and requiring treatment for longer. Congenital pneumonia has a mortality rate of around 10%. Group B

TABLE 14.1 PATHOGENS IN NEONATAL PNEUMONIA

Congenital pneumonia	*Acquired pneumonia*
Bacteria	Bacteria
■ *Streptococcus agalactiae* (Group B streptococcus)	■ *Escherichia coli*
■ *Escherichia coli*	■ *Klebsiella*
■ *Treponema pallidum* (Syphilis)	■ *Serratia marcescens*
■ *Ureaplasma urealyticum*	■ *Pseudomonas aeruginosa*
■ *Chlamydia trachomatis*	■ *Staphylococcus aureus*
■ *Listeria monocytogenes*	■ *Streptococcus pneumoniae*
■ *Haemophilus influenzae*	■ *Staphylococcus epidermidis*
Fungi	Fungi
■ *Candida albicans*	■ *Candida albicans*
Viruses	Viruses
■ *Herpes simplex*	■ *Respiratory syncytial virus*
■ *Varicella zoster*	■ *Enterovirus*
■ *Cytomegalovirus*	■ *Parainfluenza virus*
	■ *Adenovirus*

streptococcus (GBS) is the most common pathogen accounting for many cases. Apart from respiratory signs, the infant may also display general lethargy and poor tone, temperature instability and hypoglycaemia (Gardner et al., 2020).

Acquired pneumonia occurs after 48 hours of life and is usually acquired nosocomially. It is most common in preterm infants who require some form of ventilatory support, with ventilator-associated pneumonia (VAP) carrying an incidence of 1.4–7 per 1000 ventilator days in high-income countries, and 16–89 per 1000 ventilator days in low- and middle-income countries. It has a significant impact with regard to overall morbidity and prolongation of hospital stay (Rangelova et al., 2024), and mortality is estimated at 50%.

Onset of illness may be gradual or rapid, depending on the organism. There is usually a significant increase in endotracheal secretions, alongside increased work of breathing, worsening gas exchange, tachypnoea, or apnoea, as well as systemic deterioration, which may include tachy- or bradycardia, and temperature instability (Gardner et al., 2020).

The treatment for all forms of neonatal pneumonia is predominantly supportive and involves the administration of antimicrobial agents depending on the causative organism identified or suspected. Ventilatory support required during the acute illness will be determined by the degree of respiratory compromise and may vary from supplemental oxygen to full mechanical ventilation. In congenital pneumonia, ventilated preterm or late preterm infants may be considered for surfactant administration, as pneumonia may lead to surfactant inactivation (Gardner et al., 2020).

> **THINK POINT**
>
> Can you remember the case of an infant in your care who was diagnosed with congenital pneumonia? How did they present compared to babies with TTN or RDS you may have looked after? How did the course of their illness, and treatment, differ?

Meconium aspiration syndrome

Meconium-stained amniotic fluid (MSAF) occurs in around 8% of births, with significant variation (0.07–10%) in how many infants develop meconium aspiration syndrome (MAS; Gardner et al., 2025). Although incidence may be decreasing due to evolving obstetric practice, MAS still carries a risk of death and short- and long-term morbidity (Tillery & Connor, 2023). MAS predominantly affects term and post-term infants, with risk increasing beyond term. Fetal passage of meconium is usually a sign of chronic or acute compromise caused by hypoxic stress, which may trigger gasping and inhalation of meconium into the lungs (Gardner et al., 2020). Postnatal **aspiration** can occur, but most cases result from perinatal fetal compromise (Tillery & Connor, 2023). MSAF in preterm infants is no longer considered a marker of *Listeria monocytogenes*; instead, it is usually associated with uterine infection and higher neonatal morbidity (Abu Shqara et al., 2025). Once in the respiratory tract, meconium causes several pulmonary problems:

- Obstruction; complete obstruction can cause alveolar collapse, whereas partial obstruction leads to air trapping, over-distension, air leak, and pneumothorax.
- Surfactant inactivation due to damage to type II pneumocytes, reducing lung compliance.
- Chemical pneumonitis and parenchymal injury from the inflammatory response, which also increases **pulmonary vascular resistance** (PVR).
- Inflammation linked to phospholipase A2.

These mechanisms contribute to V/Q mismatch, making oxygenation and ventilation difficult, and MAS is strongly associated with persistent pulmonary hypertension of the newborn (PPHN). Most infants develop respiratory distress; tachypnoea, nasal flaring, sternal recession, cyanosis, and grunting within 12 hours. The chest may appear hyperinflated. Signs may be delayed, so infants born through MSAF require close respiratory assessment.

Around 30–50% of infants with MAS develop respiratory failure and can be challenging to manage. Conventional care focuses on supporting ventilation and oxygenation while maintaining normal pH. CPAP or mechanical ventilation may be necessary, but over-distended areas combined with lung injury increase the risk of air leak. Infants often 'fight' the ventilator, requiring sedation or muscle relaxants to optimise ventilation. Because acidosis raises pulmonary vascular resistance (PVR), maintaining normal pCO_2 helps stabilise pH, although high PIP may be needed. HFOV and surfactant therapy may reduce MAS severity and decrease the need for **extracorporeal membrane oxygenation** (ECMO; Gardner et al., 2020). Early evidence suggests that LISA may reduce the necessity for mechanical ventilation (Prasath et al., 2025).

Frequent suctioning and physiotherapy may be required if imaging shows collapse or consolidation, though infants with MAS may be poorly tolerant of handling. Severe hypoxic-ischaemic insult may affect other organ systems. Inotropes may be required, and echocardiography can guide choice by assessing cardiac output, myocardial function, and severity of PPHN. It also confirms normal cardiac structure and helps determine whether inhaled nitric oxide (iNO) or vasodilators may be beneficial. Hypotension and poor perfusion may cause metabolic acidosis, which can be corrected with bicarbonate (Gardner et al., 2020). If conventional management is insufficient, specialist advice should be sought and transfer to a centre offering iNO or ECMO may be required.

Persistent pulmonary hypertension of the newborn

PPHN is the failure of the normal cardiopulmonary transition after birth and is characterised by raised PVR with right-to-left shunting through the foramen ovale and DA, causing severe hypoxaemia (Coletti et al., 2024). Incidence ranges from 0.4–7 per 1000 live births, with a mortality of 7–11%, and survivors are at risk of adverse neurodevelopmental outcomes.

PPHN often arises secondary to other disease processes and may result from:

- Idiopathic PPHN, with profound hypoxia and minimal lung disease.
- Severe intrapartum asphyxia, where hypoxia and acidosis cause pulmonary vasoconstriction and prevent postnatal circulatory transition; hypotension from myocardial injury can worsen right-to-left shunting.
- MAS, due to obstruction and inflammation.
- Infection, most commonly GBS.
- Pulmonary hypoplasia, such as in congenital diaphragmatic hernia.
- Excessive pulmonary muscularisation.
- Congenital heart disease producing right-to-left shunts (Mandell et al., 2020).

Clinically, infants present with respiratory distress and cyanosis, typically within 24 hours and almost always by 72 hours of age. They are critically ill and may remain hypoxic and acidotic despite ventilation and 100% oxygen (Gardner et al., 2020). Pre- and post-ductal oxygen saturations assist diagnosis: with ductal right-to-left shunting, pre-ductal (right hand) saturations exceed post-ductal (feet). A difference >10% indicates shunting (Mandell et al., 2020). Invasive sampling will show corresponding PaO_2 differences (Gardner et al., 2020).

Severity is often assessed using the **oxygenation index** (OI):

$$OI = (MAP \times FiO_2 \times 100)/PaO_2$$

Values of 30–40 reflect severe disease; OI >40, or persistently >20 after 24 hours of maximal therapy, indicates the need to consider ECMO. As OI requires arterial sampling, recent studies have explored correlation with the non-invasive oxygen saturation index, with moderate concordance (Slaughter et al., 2025).

Investigations include full blood count; anaemia or polycythaemia can worsen PPHN; white cell counts help identify infection; platelet levels are often low in MAS or asphyxia. Chemistry screens monitor for hypoglycaemia and hypocalcaemia. Chest X-rays assess underlying lung disease; idiopathic PPHN shows clear lung fields with reduced vascular markings and normal or slightly enlarged cardiac size (Gardner et al., 2020). Echocardiography is essential to rule out congenital heart disease, confirm PPHN, assess shunting, evaluate ventricular function, and aid prognosis (Breinig et al., 2021).

Management requires meticulous monitoring, oxygenation, blood pressure (BP) and perfusion support. Mechanical ventilation, and sometimes HFOV, may be needed. Surfactant reduces surface tension and work of breathing. Minimal handling, sedation, analgesia and sometimes muscle relaxation help maintain ventilator synchrony. Systemic BP is supported using inotropes such as adrenaline and dobutamine (see Chapter 15). Historically, high systemic BP was targeted to reverse shunting, but this approach is now considered outdated due to the risk of worsening cardiac strain. Pulmonary vasodilation aims to lower PVR. Agents include milrinone (also inotropic), prostacyclin, sildenafil, and bosentan, though systemic effects may cause hypotension. iNO remains the most specific pulmonary vasodilator for neonatal PPHN. Evidence for combined therapy with iNO and systemic vasodilators remains inconclusive due to challenges in completing sufficiently powered trials (Coletti et al., 2024).

TRENDS IN NEONATAL RESPIRATORY CARE

It is now widely accepted that positive pressure ventilation in the neonatal period can result in lung injury which increases the risk of respiratory morbidity including air leak and CLD. This has resulted in an increase in the use of non-invasive methods of respiratory support. Several mechanisms for **ventilator-induced lung injury** have been proposed:

- Volutrauma, where the alveoli are over-distended by the delivery of too much gas.
- Barotrauma, where high airway pressures cause alveolar rupture.
- Biotrauma, resulting from the injurious effects of inflammation, infection, and oxidative stress.
- Atelectotrauma, where there is alveolar collapse at the end of expiration, requiring re-recruitment with every breath, with necessary shear forces causing micro-tears.
- Rheotrauma, caused by high inspiratory or expiratory flow rates creating shear stress in airways and alveoli (Donn et al., 2024).

Current practice in ventilating preterm newborns is to provide those who need it with the gentlest invasive ventilation possible for the shortest time possible. A strategy for protecting the lungs can be achieved through permissive hypercapnia, where the target $PaCO_2$ is higher than the previously accepted norm (usually defined together with a target pH). These strategies may decrease volutrauma and the duration of positive pressure ventilation. The small group of term infants who require mechanical ventilation have different pathophysiology and require different targets. Example targets for both groups are shown in Table 14.2.

ACID-BASE BALANCE, GAS TRANSPORT AND MONITORING

Healthy infants maintain blood pH within a narrow range through coordinated cardiorespiratory, neurological and renal mechanisms. Unwell infants are vulnerable

TABLE 14.2 ACCEPTABLE BLOOD GAS RESULTS FOR INFANTS REQUIRING RESPIRATORY SUPPORT

Parameter	*Normal*	*Ventilated preterm infants**	*Term targets*
pH	7.35–7.45	>7.25	7.3–7.4
$PaCO_2$	4.6–6 kPa	4.5–8.5 kPa (up to 10kPa from day 4)	4.5–6 kPa
PaO_2	7.9–11 kPa	6.5–9.5 kPa	>8 kPa
SaO_2	100%	90–94%	>95%

(adapted from NICE, 2019; Barry et al., 2020; Nock & Olicker, 2024)
*Targets with permissive hypercapnia

to disturbances caused by disease or treatment, so nurses caring for ventilated infants must understand acid–base balance to recognise abnormalities and intervene appropriately. Blood pH must be tightly regulated because enzyme and protein function is highly pH-sensitive. Disturbances arise from:

- CO_2 retention → low pH (respiratory acidosis)
- Low CO_2 → raised pH (respiratory alkalosis)
- Poor perfusion → anaerobic metabolism (metabolic acidosis)
- Loss of hydrogen ions (e.g. gastric losses) leads to metabolic alkalosis (Barry et al., 2020)

The underlying cause of a pH disturbance must guide management. Respiratory acidosis requires increased ventilation, whereas metabolic acidosis with normal CO_2 suggests a systemic cause such as hypotension, possibly requiring cautious bicarbonate administration. Sodium bicarbonate is hyperosmolar and may increase IVH risk if given rapidly; it may also raise CO_2 levels (Dhugga et al., 2025). Over-correction risks metabolic alkalosis. **Hypocapnia** must be avoided because it increases cerebral vascular resistance and reduces cerebral perfusion (Donn et al., 2024).

CO_2 is transported dissolved in plasma (5%), bound to haemoglobin (10%), and as part of the bicarbonate buffer system (85%; Travers & Ambalavanan, 2022). CO_2 retention results in respiratory acidosis; hypocapnia produces **alkalosis** and reduces cerebral blood flow.

Four methods assess CO_2:

- Arterial sampling: gold standard but invasive
- Capillary sampling: reasonable estimate but affected by perfusion
- Transcutaneous monitoring: useful for trends; requires calibration and site rotation
- Capnography: limited accuracy in neonates but useful to confirm ETT placement

Oxygen diffuses across the alveoli into blood, mostly binding to haemoglobin. Adequate oxygenation is essential for aerobic metabolism and adenosine triphosphate (ATP) production; poor perfusion triggers anaerobic metabolism and lactate-driven metabolic acidosis. Hyperoxia is harmful, carrying risks to eyes, lungs, and brain (Vento, 2022).

Monitoring oxygenation:

- Arterial sampling- direct PaO_2 measurement
- Pulse oximetry- continuous, widely used, but affected by motion, light, and perfusion; requires regular probe repositioning (Travers & Ambalavanan, 2022)

- Near-infrared spectroscopy (NIRS)- a non-invasive, continuous monitoring technique using light (700–1000nm) to measure regional tissue oxygen saturation in haemoglobin, reflecting tissue-specific oxygenation. This is increasingly used but without proven outcome benefit

RESPIRATORY SUPPORT STRATEGIES IN NEONATAL CARE

It is vital to follow the latest national guidance for the respiratory care of premature infants (NICE, 2019; Sweet et al., 2023) which will be referred to, where applicable in the following discussion of respiratory support strategies. However, it must be remembered that not all infants requiring ventilatory support are premature, and so all modes of ventilation will be discussed.

Oxygen therapy

Oxygen therapy is a common aspect of care in the NNU. Oxygen can be administered by several methods depending on the infant's clinical condition and specific requirements. For those requiring low concentrations, ambient oxygen can be administered via the incubator for short periods, or for longer-term administration via low flow nasal cannula (< 1 L/minute).

For infants with increased work of breathing, oxygen may be delivered via the chosen mode of ventilation. Oxygen administered to neonates for prolonged episodes needs to be warmed and humidified, particularly at flow rates exceeding 2L/minute (NICE, 2019). Oxygen therapy contributes greatly to neonatal care but is not without its risks (Vento, 2022). It is necessary to treat oxygen as the drug that it is, identify correctly the baby that needs oxygen, assess the baby's condition to administer the correct dose, use the most appropriate method of administration, and administer oxygen for the correct duration in order that the baby receives the greatest therapeutic benefit with the least risk. Oxygen administration requires careful consideration in preterm infants, as the correct therapeutic range has proven difficult to establish. A meta-analysis of data from five international trials comparing infants born at less than 28 weeks' gestation targeted to receive SpO2 85–89% with similar infants targeted to receive SpO_2 90–95% included data from 4965 infants worldwide. The lower SpO_2 target range was associated with a higher risk of death and NEC, but a lower risk of retinopathy of prematurity treatment (Askie et al., 2018). The most recent guidelines recommend that in preterm infants receiving oxygen the target SpO_2 level should be 91–95% (Sweet et al., 2023).

Non-invasive respiratory support

Infants who are at high risk of developing RDS and those who display an increase in their work of breathing associated with hypercapnia and an increase in oxygen requirements will benefit from non-invasive respiratory support in the form of CPAP, nasal intermittent positive pressure ventilation (NIPPV), or high-flow nasal cannula (HFNC). Non-invasive support can be considered if the infant has a reasonable spontaneous respiratory effort with mild hypercapnia. CPAP is comparable with intubation and mechanical ventilation as a treatment for RDS, even in very preterm infants, and even confers some benefits over invasive ventilation (Lagoski et al., 2024).

The relative merits of HFNC and CPAP have been debated for many years, but recent evidence suggests that CPAP may be more effective in preventing CLD. Findings for NIPPV remain inconclusive at present (Schmidt & Bancalari, 2024). Those infants who 'fail' non-invasive support, either because they present with a decreased respiratory drive or apnoeas with a raised $PaCO_2$ and reduced PaO_2 will need to be intubated and ventilated, and in these cases volume-targeted ventilation should be used. In line with the recent aim to provide protective lung strategies to prevent BPD, non-invasive ventilation strategies must be considered wherever possible (NICE, 2019; Sweet et al., 2023; Schmidt & Bancalari, 2024).

An overview of the options available will now be discussed.

CONTINUOUS POSITIVE AIRWAY PRESSURE

CPAP is a method of delivering a predetermined continuous pressure and supplementary oxygen to the airways of a spontaneously breathing infant (Figure 14.1). CPAP helps reduce upper airway occlusion and decreases upper airway resistance by mechanically splinting the airways open. This improves ventilation by providing FRC (preventing alveolar collapse) and increasing the surface area available for gas exchange. It also stabilises the chest wall and reduces the work of breathing (Donn et al., 2024). It is the modality of choice for primary respiratory support as well as post extubation. The starting pressure for CPAP is usually in the range of 6–8cmH_2O. Bi-level CPAP (BiPAP) is sometimes used, with small differences in pressure generated at the inspiratory and expiratory phases of respiration. This has not been shown to confer greater benefit than traditional CPAP (Sweet et al., 2023). CPAP can be administered in a variety of ways. While it is possible to deliver CPAP through an ETT, and indeed historically an ETT was fashioned into a single nasal prong, the most common mode is the application of a nasal interface, such as binasal prongs or a mask (Donn et al., 2024) As newborn infants are inherent nasal breathers, nasal CPAP (nCPAP) is easily facilitated and usually well tolerated. Underwater bubble CPAP (BCPAP) is a continuous-flow

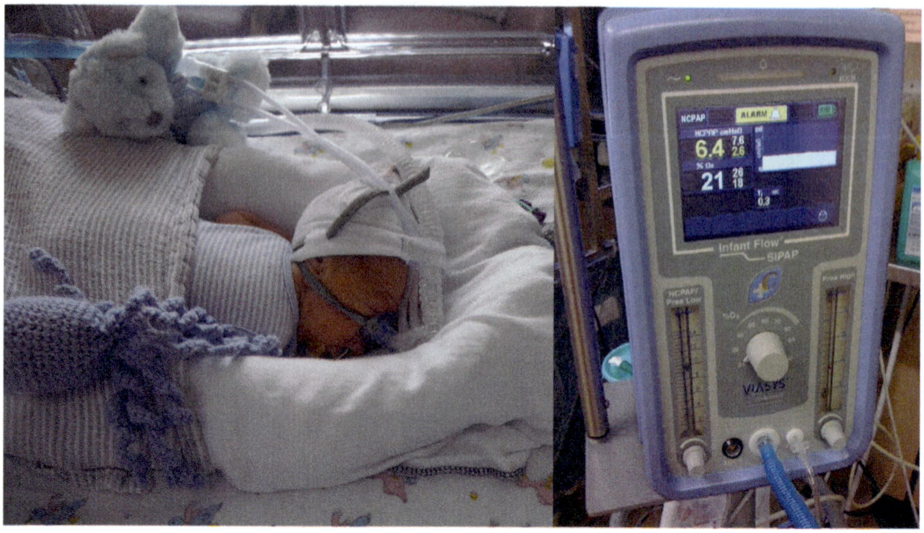

Figure 14.1 Preterm infant receiving continuous positive airway pressure and CPAP driver

respiratory support system first used in the early 1970s. Heated, humidified gas is delivered to the infant through a nasal interface, while the expiratory tubing is submerged in water so that the depth of immersion determines the pressure. The bubbling may also create chest vibrations that aid gas exchange. BCPAP remains an effective, low-cost method for supporting premature infants' breathing.

Problems associated with the delivery of nCPAP include:

- Nasal trauma, ranging from mild redness and indentation to erosion of the nasal septum. Correct sizing of the interface, regular pressure relief, and alternation of CPAP prongs and masks are measures preventing this and the potential resultant facial disfigurement.
- Loss of pressure due to poorly fitting prongs or an open mouth. Chinstraps can be used with caution, as they prevent the infant from clearing the mouth in the event of vomiting or regurgitation, and therefore increase the risk of aspiration. Pacifiers can be utilised, with parental permission.
- Gastric distension increases when a baby is on CPAP and can be overcome by having an orogastric tube in situ and either leaving on free drainage or aspirating the tube on a regular basis to decompress the stomach.
- Reduced cardiac output due to excessive intrathoracic pressure, impacting venous return.
- Air leak or pneumothorax can be a particular issue in the larger infant with RDS. Any infant suddenly deteriorating or having a significant increase

in their oxygen requirements while on CPAP should be immediately investigated for pneumothorax (Donn et al., 2024).

Weaning practices from CPAP will vary, but in many NNUs pressures are gradually weaned until the baby is either switched to HFNC or may attempt breathing without support or in nasal cannula oxygen only. Historically, time periods off CPAP were trialled and subsequently extended as tolerated. This has been demonstrated to be less effective at keeping babies off CPAP and is now uncommon practice in the UK (Donn et al., 2024). Evaluation of histograms can guide weaning management (Gentle et al., 2020).

NON-INVASIVE NASAL VENTILATION

Non-invasive ventilation methods, including NIPPV, synchronised NIPPV (SNIPPV) and/or synchronised CPAP (or SiPAP), and NAVA, augment nasal CPAP by allowing adjustment of PEEP, PIP, respiratory rate, and inspiratory time, though terminology across systems is often inconsistent. SiPAP, for example, is also referred to as biphasic, bilevel CPAP, or BiPAP. NIPPV is thought to work through the same mechanisms as CPAP, helping maintain FRC, prevent alveolar collapse, improve tidal volume and gas exchange, and reduce work of breathing. Clinically, NIPPV has been studied as primary support for premature infants with RDS, for preventing post-extubation failure and for treating apnoea, though comparisons are complicated by device variability. Meta-analyses suggest NIPPV reduces extubation failure compared with CPAP but does not consistently decrease apnoea events; synchronised NIPPV appears more effective than non-synchronised modes in reducing the need for mechanical ventilation and improving extubation success, though SNIPPV technology is currently limited to Europe (Donn et al., 2024). Ventilator-generated, synchronised NIPPV may reduce the risk of BPD when used as either primary or post-extubation support in preterm infants but is not associated with a decrease in mortality (Rüegger et al., 2021).

Newer approaches such as non-invasive (NIV-)NAVA aim to improve synchrony by using diaphragmatic electrical activity to trigger and proportionally assist breaths, with backup settings available for apnoea. This strategy, apart from offering more comfort and better patient-ventilator interaction than conventional triggers, has been shown to reduce significant bradycardia and desaturation events in infants with apnoea of prematurity, though NIV-NAVA cannot be used in infants without respiratory drive or in those unable to accommodate the catheter (Donn et al., 2024). A small study showed reduced duration of invasive ventilation and length of stay but not rates of BPD or home oxygen therapy (Shetty et al., 2021).

HIGH FLOW NASAL CANNULA

This non-invasive method of respiratory support (see Figure 14.2) allows for the administration of flows >1 L/min oxygen or a blend of air and oxygen as an alternative to other non-invasive ventilatory interfaces. It is unclear whether HFNC works because some CPAP is generated through the high flow of gas in relatively small infant nares, but the level of pressure can be variable and unpredictable and is not measurable. Its goal is to optimise spontaneous breathing through the reduction of dead space and the creation of positive distending airway pressure. The interface is often preferred by parents and nursing staff, and it is an effective post-extubation modality (Donn et al., 2024). A recent systematic review argues for HFNC as a primary modality of respiratory support in preterm babies despite a higher risk of treatment failure, considering no difference in intubation rates and a lower rate of nasal trauma using HFNC compared with CPAP (Bruet et al., 2021).

Modes of invasive ventilation

Decision-making regarding the most appropriate respiratory mode and parameters must be individualised and undertaken collaboratively with parents, with neonatal nurses playing a central role. Advances in invasive ventilation technology now allow real-time monitoring of inspiratory and expiratory flow, displayed as

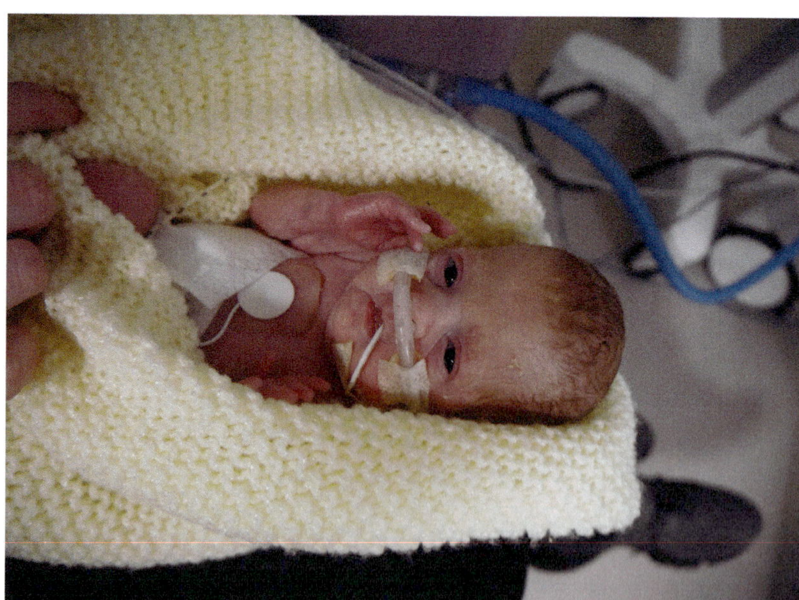

Figure 14.2 Preterm infant on high flow nasal cannula support

loops and waves (see Figures 14.3–14.4 and Box 14.2). These visualisations illustrate infant–ventilator interaction and support optimisation of ventilatory support. Modern ventilation modes permit infant-regulated, breath-by-breath adjustments in peak pressures, tidal volumes, inspiratory times, and rate. This is clinically important because mean airway pressure influences PaO_2, while tidal volume governs $PaCO_2$ (Keszler, 2022). Fluctuating or elevated $PaCO_2$ levels

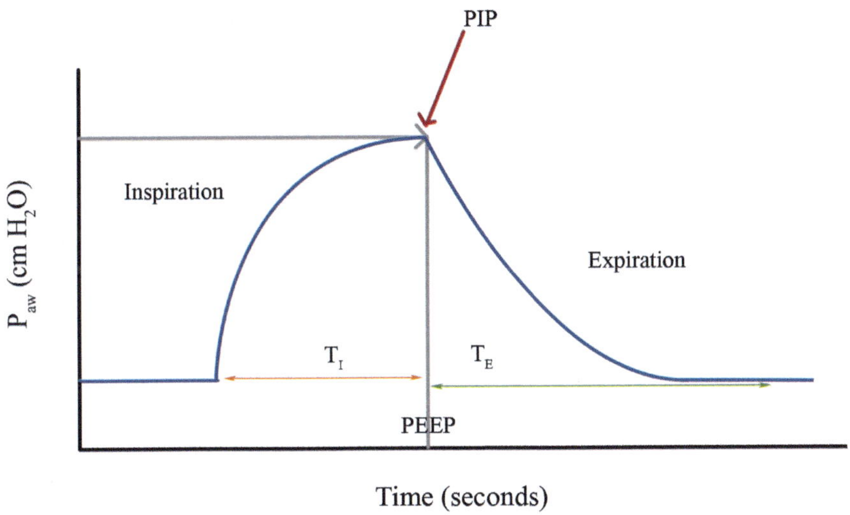

Figure 14.3 Pressure/time scalar

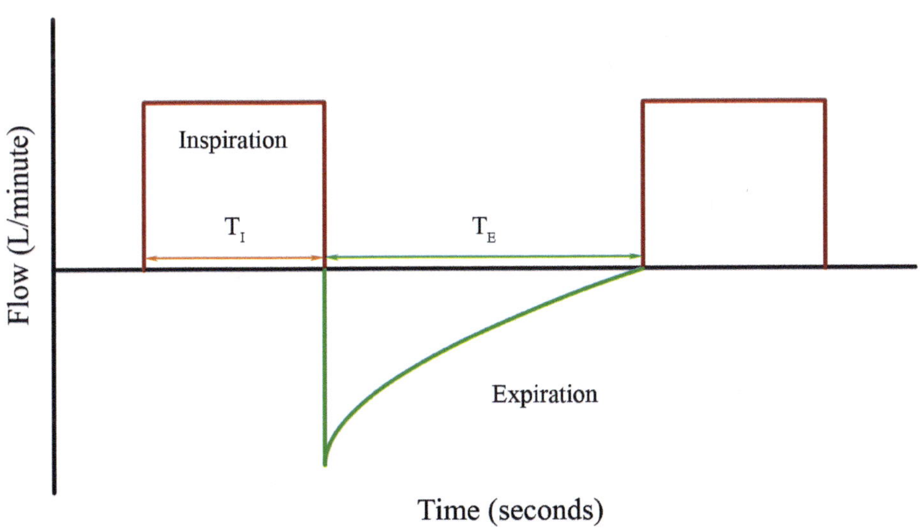

Figure 14.4 Flow/time scalar

are strongly associated with severe intracranial haemorrhage, BPD, and adverse neurodevelopment, independent of PaO_2 (Donn et al., 2024). Contemporary ventilators enable tighter control of both gases while supporting infant comfort (Figures 14.6 and 14.7). Because terminology varies between manufacturers, practitioners must understand their specific equipment. Synchronised time-cycled pressure-limited modes without targeted tidal volumes are no longer recommended (NICE, 2019; Keszler, 2022).

PRACTICE POINT

With advances in neonatal care, intubations are nowhere near as common as they used to be, which can pose challenges for neonatal teams in terms of skills maintenance.

Does your place of work have any strategies in place to overcome this issue, i.e. simulation/skills drills, clear guidelines and/or local safety standards for invasive procedures (LocSSIPs)? Can you think of any others?

BOX 14.2 TERMINOLOGY RELATING TO RESPIRATORY FUNCTION MONITORING THROUGH A VENTILATOR CYCLE (READ IN CONJUNCTION WITH FIGURES 14.3 AND 14.4)

- During inspiration, circuit pressure rises to PIP, driving gas through the ETT into the infant – this is inspiratory flow. Gas entering the lungs or leaking around the ETT is measured as the inspiratory tidal volume (VTi).
- During expiration, pressure falls to PEEP, the baseline pressure maintained in the lungs. Gas returning from the infant to the ventilator constitutes expiratory flow, and the ventilator calculates the expiratory tidal volume (VTe).
- The difference between VTi and VTe indicates leak. Because less gas escapes during expiration, VTe is generally the more accurate reflection of true tidal volume (VT).
- At end-expiration, the lungs retain gas known as the FRC.
- Minute volume (MV) is the total tidal volume delivered in one minute (VT × rate).

- Lung and chest wall compliance influence the pressure needed to achieve the set VT; the stiffer the lung, the higher the required pressures (see Figure 14.5).
- Airway characteristics (ETT and bronchi) affect gas flow: increasing length or decreasing diameter raises resistance, slowing flow and altering VT.

CONTINUOUS MANDATORY VENTILATION

Also known as intermittent mandatory ventilation (IMV) or intermittent positive-pressure ventilation (IPPV), continuous mandatory ventilation (CMV) is the longest-established invasive ventilation mode. It is typically time-cycled, pressure-limited, and continuous-flow, with clinician-set inspiratory time (Ti), rate, PIP, and PEEP. Settings do not respond to infant effort, so this mode is most suitable for infants who are sedated or muscle-relaxed to avoid asynchrony. CMV can be

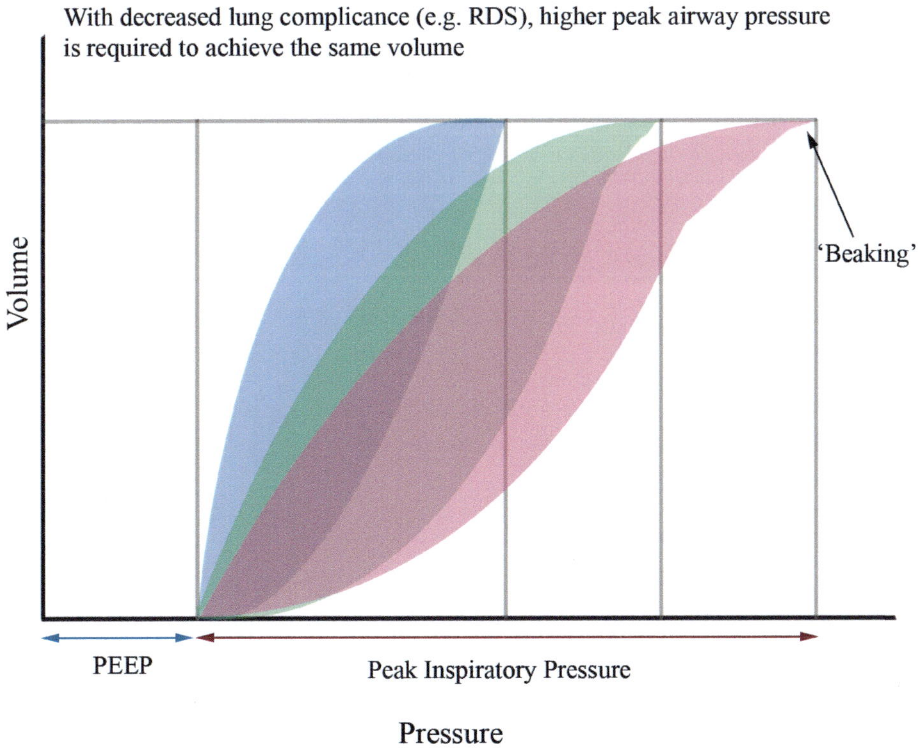

Figure 14.5 Pressure/volume loop

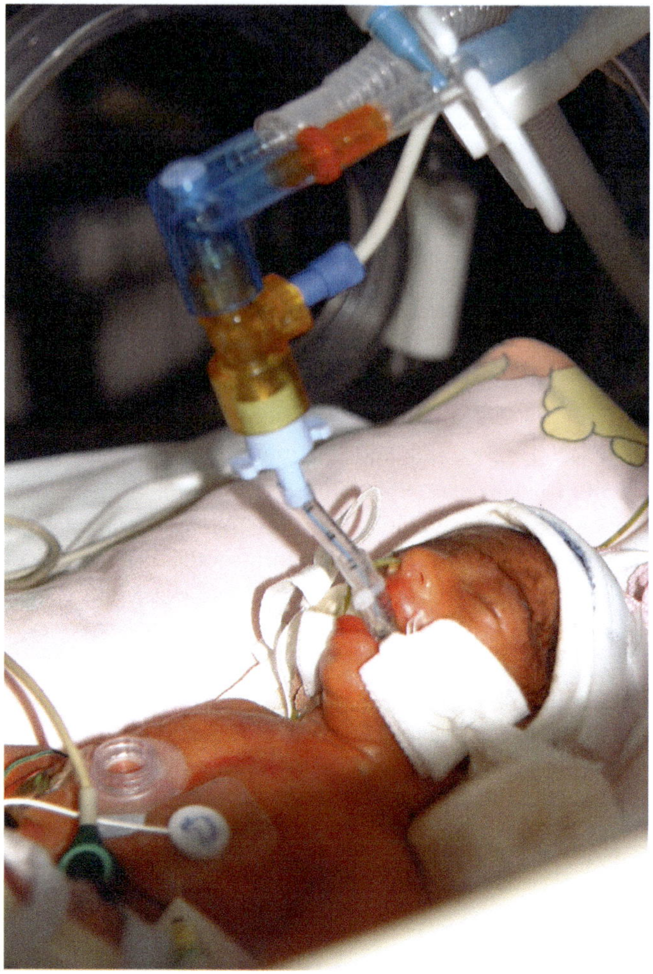

Figure 14.6 Ventilated neonate

uncomfortable during weaning and has largely been replaced by synchronised ventilation modes (Keszler, 2022).

VOLUME-TARGETED VENTILATION

Volume-targeted ventilation (VTV) improves survival without lung injury (Donn et al., 2024) and is recommended for preterm infants (NICE, 2019). This mode provides time-cycled, pressure-limited breaths but adjusts pressure to achieve a clinician-set tidal volume, aiming for stable ventilation and reduced pCO_2 variability.

Advantages include reduced volutrauma, a contributing factor in BPD; prevention of excessive pressures when compliance improves (e.g. after surfactant); automatic PIP weaning; and more consistent tidal volumes. Tidal volume targets

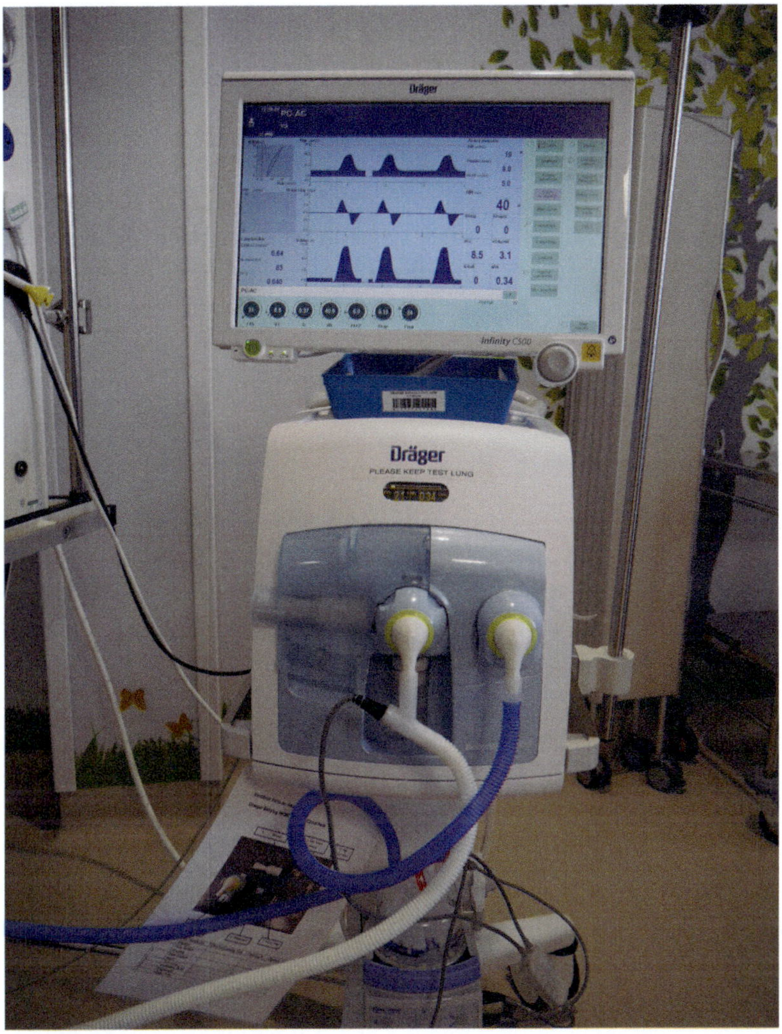

Figure 14.7 Ventilator

are typically 4–6mL/kg in preterm infants and 5–8mL/kg in term infants. Leak around the uncuffed ETT can affect accuracy, but modern ventilators use leak compensation (Donn et al., 2024).

ASSIST-CONTROL VENTILATION

Also termed patient-triggered ventilation (PTV) or synchronised intermittent positive pressure ventilation (SIPPV), this mode uses the infant's inspiratory flow to trigger each breath. Clinicians set PIP or tidal volume, PEEP, Ti, a back-up rate, and trigger sensitivity. Sensitivity must be adjusted to avoid missed triggers or auto-triggering from water or secretions. Every triggered breath receives full support; if the infant becomes apnoeic, the back-up rate ensures ventilation continues (Keszler, 2022).

SYNCHRONISED INTERMITTENT MANDATORY VENTILATION

This modality delivers a set number of mandatory synchronised breaths per minute. Additional spontaneous breaths receive only PEEP, resulting in variable tidal volumes. Synchronised intermittent mandatory ventilation (SIMV) provides less support than assist-control ventilation and is commonly used during weaning (Keszler, 2022).

PRESSURE SUPPORT VENTILATION

This provides a clinician-set pressure boost to every spontaneous breath, reducing work of breathing and improving comfort. The infant determines breath onset and inspiratory duration; the ventilator ends inspiration once flow falls to 5–10% of peak. Pressure support ventilation (PSV) depends on adequate respiratory drive and may be combined with SIMV or VTV (Keszler, 2022).

ACTIVITY

Research how the compliance curve displayed on the ventilator is affected by different respiratory disease states. This online resource may assist you: https://pressbooks.lib.vt.edu/pulmonaryphysiology/chapter/lung-volumes-and-compliance/.

Next time you look after a ventilated baby, evaluate their compliance curve and think about the information about their lungs you can take from this. How does it change over time, and what caused the changes?

HIGH-FREQUENCY OSCILLATORY VENTILATION

HFOV delivers very small tidal volumes at supraphysiologic rates (e.g. 10Hz = 600 breaths/minute) and improves gas exchange in severe respiratory failure (Figure 14.8). Active expiration reduces gas-trapping, and advantages include lower-pressure ventilation, reduced volutrauma and barotrauma, and more uniform lung inflation (Donn et al., 2024). HFOV is recommended when VTV is ineffective (NICE, 2019), may modestly reduce BPD in preterm infants, and in term infants with MAS can reduce the need for ECMO, with or without iNO. Disadvantages

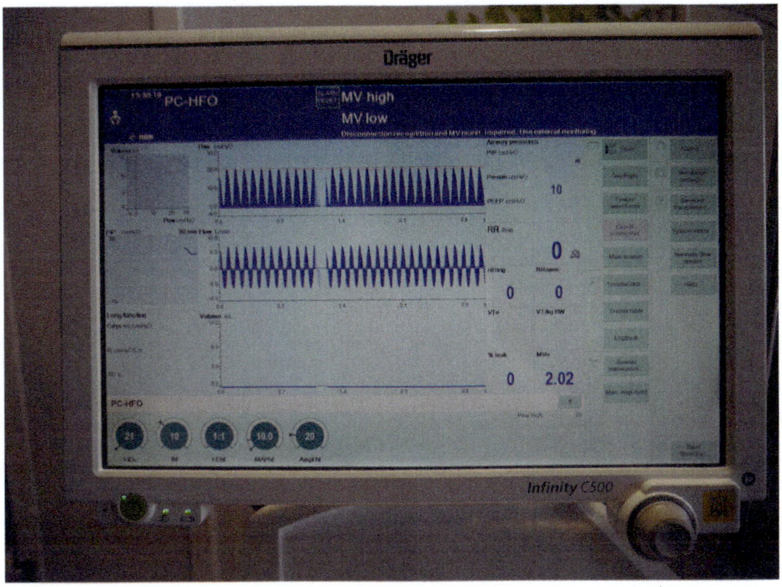

Figure 14.8 High-frequency oscillatory ventilation

include rapid reductions in $PaCO_2$, risking altered cerebral blood flow, and decreased venous return causing lower cardiac output (van Kaam, 2022). A blood gas should be checked within 30 minutes of starting HFOV, and chest X-ray is used to identify over- or under-expansion (see Table 14.3; Gardner et al., 2020).

HFOV uses low-volume strategies for non-homogeneous disease such as air leaks, pulmonary hypoplasia, and PPHN, and high-volume strategies for homogeneous disease such as severe RDS. When used as rescue therapy, MAP is set 1–2 cm H_2O above conventional settings (Gardner et al., 2020). CO_2 clearance depends on amplitude (ΔP), frequency, and inspiratory time, with ΔP increased until adequate 'chest wiggle' is seen (Yasmeen & Ansary, 2024).

BOX 14.3 THE 'OPEN LUNG STRATEGY'

Also known as an *optimal lung volume strategy*, is a lung-protective approach that aims to recruit and maintain alveolar expansion using adequate MAP and optimal PEEP, while avoiding overdistension. The goal is to keep as many alveoli open as possible throughout the respiratory cycle to improve oxygenation and reduce ventilation-induced lung injury (VILI). This strategy emphasises alveolar recruitment, stabilisation, and minimal tidal volumes to maintain FRC and protect fragile neonatal lungs (van Kaam, 2022).

TABLE 14.3 BLOOD GAS PARAMETERS ON HFOV AND POSSIBLE CAUSES (ADAPTED FROM YASMEEN & ANSARY, 2024)

pO_2	Low	■ Review ETT position/patency ■ 'Rain-out' in the ventilator circuit ■ Pneumothorax ■ Increase FiO_2 ■ Underinflation – increase MAP by 1–2cm H_2O ■ Overinflation – check BP, reduce MAP, consider chest x-ray
	High	■ Decrease FiO_2
pCO_2	Low	■ Review ETT position/patency ■ Increase amplitude (ΔP) and look for improved 'chest wiggle' ■ Overinflation will lead to hypercapnia over time ■ Consider reducing frequency
	High	■ Decrease amplitude (ΔP) ■ Increase frequency if this has been previously decreased

Nursing care includes maintaining a neutral neck position, ensuring regular suctioning, supporting parents, managing hypotension in low-volume states, applying the DOPE algorithm (Box 14.4) if deterioration occurs, and assisting with blood gas-guided troubleshooting (Yasmeen & Ansary, 2024).

BOX 14.4 DOPE ALGORITHM – TROUBLESHOOTING SEQUENCE FOR VENTILATED INFANTS (ADAPTED FROM BRITISH ASSOCIATION OF PERINATAL MEDICINE, 2024)

D – Displaced ETT

O – Obstructed airway (check for particulate matter or secretions)

P – Pneumothorax

E – Equipment failure

Inhaled nitric oxide

iNO is delivered as a gas mixed into the breathing circuit of a ventilator via a delivery system (Figure 14.9) and through the ETT, diffusing to pulmonary vascular smooth muscle where it causes vasodilation and improves V/Q matching. It is rapidly inactivated by haemoglobin, limiting systemic effects. iNO improves short-term

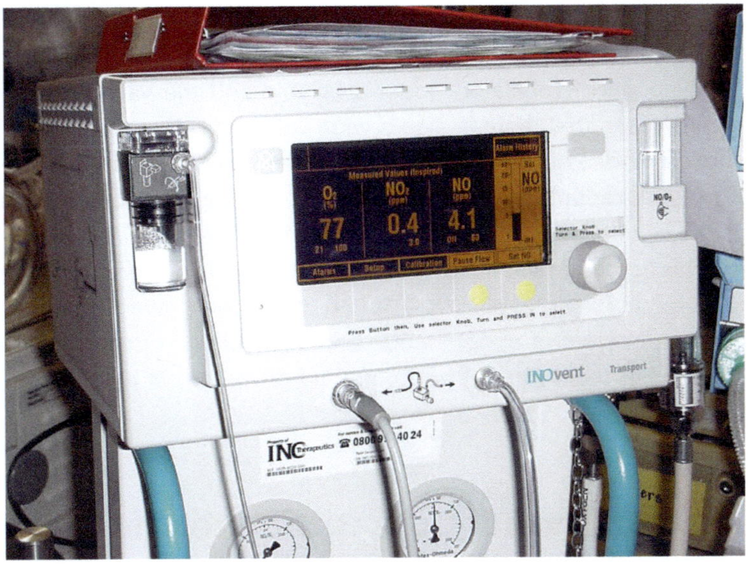

Figure 14.9 Nitric oxide delivery system

oxygenation and reduces ECMO need in term and near-term infants, especially those with PPHN (Gardner et al., 2020). Its use in preterm infants remains controversial and should be limited to specific pathology (NICE, 2019). The recommended starting dose is 20 parts per million (ppm) in infants ≥34 weeks; higher doses rarely improve oxygenation. Responders can be weaned rapidly once stable. Risks of this therapy include methaemoglobinaemia (monitoring of MetHb on blood gases is required) and impaired platelet aggregation (Gardner et al., 2020).

Extracorporeal membrane oxygenation

ECMO provides cardiopulmonary support for severe but reversible respiratory failure. Criteria include:

- BW >2.0 kg, GA >34 weeks
- No major coagulopathy or significant intracranial haemorrhage
- <12 days of ventilation
- No lethal anomalies
- OI >40 or >25 for >4 hours (Gardner et al., 2020), or >20 despite 24 hours maximal therapy (Slaughter et al., 2025).

ECMO is unsuitable for preterm infants due to anticoagulation risks. It improves mortality and morbidity, though long-term neurodevelopment remains influenced largely by underlying disease severity (Gardner et al., 2020).

WEANING FROM INVASIVE VENTILATION

The large selection of ventilator modes available and the variation in their use between units mean that there is also a wide variation between individual NNUs in weaning methods. As blood gases, lung mechanics and respiratory efforts improve, gradual reductions in the level of ventilation support are made (i.e. lowering PIP or tidal volume and rate, introducing SIMV and/or PSV, reducing sedation). This is commonly followed by extubation to a non-invasive respiratory support mode (Donn et al., 2024). There have been several attempts to use measurable parameters of spontaneous breathing trials to determine readiness for extubation, but these do not appear superior to clinical judgement (Shalish et al., 2020).

FAMILY INTEGRATED CARE IN THE CONTEXT OF NEONATAL RESPIRATORY DISORDERS

The family must be a prime consideration for any infant cared for on the NNU, and respiratory care is no exception. Parents with a baby who requires respiratory support must be made aware of the rationale for interventions performed and be fully informed and included in the care of their baby (NICE, 2019). Beyond this, there is evidence that some of the quantifiable benefits of family integrated care, such as enhanced weight gain and breastfeeding rates, as well as reports of reduced parental stress, apply also to infants receiving non-invasive respiratory support (O'Brien et al., 2018). When parents are furthermore actively involved in their baby's respiratory care activities, skill acquisition of these has been observed to be significantly quicker than anticipated (Moreno-Sanz et al., 2021).

NURSING CARE OF THE INFANT RECEIVING RESPIRATORY SUPPORT

Caring for a ventilated infant is complex, as most are initially unstable and vulnerable to rapid deterioration. Nurses must remain vigilant to subtle clinical changes, as early recognition can prevent significant collapse. Infants receiving respiratory support require continuous monitoring of heart rate, BP, and oxygen saturation. Additional tools, such as transcutaneous monitoring and end-tidal CO_2, can aid management, though end-tidal monitoring can be challenging due to the weight of the equipment attached to the ETT, increasing the risk of accidental extubation. The neonatal nurse is often the infant's most reliable monitor; therefore, no ventilated baby should ever be left unattended.

Respiratory assessment is a critical nursing skill, requiring knowledge of clinical signs, vital-sign interpretation, and blood gas analysis (see Chapter 4). ETT size and position must be documented clearly. Evidence regarding the safest fixation method is limited; a 2014 Cochrane review was unable to make recommendations (Lai et al., 2014). However, suboptimal fixation is the most common cause of unplanned extubation, and quality-improvement projects report up to 80% reductions with consistent standardisation (Nair & Smith, 2020; Igo et al., 2021).

Maintaining ETT patency is essential. The tube should be the largest appropriate size: smaller tubes increase airway resistance and leak risk, whereas larger tubes carry a greater risk of laryngeal or tracheal trauma. Correct placement is just below the larynx and above the **carina** (approximately T2–3), though this distance is small in very low birthweight infants, increasing displacement risk. Mucociliary clearance is suppressed with an ETT in situ, so suctioning is required, but only according to clinical need, not routinely.

Indications for suctioning include visible secretions, reduced or coarse breath sounds, desaturation, deteriorating blood gases, altered pulmonary graphics, increased work of breathing, bradycardia, or rising PIP to achieve target volumes. Potential complications include hypoxia, bradycardia, raised intracranial pressure, atelectasis, trauma, infection, and accidental extubation. To avoid mucosal injury, catheter insertion depth must be measured accurately to prevent deep suctioning beyond the ETT tip. Routine use of saline to loosen secretions is not recommended; it does not improve pulmonary function, may worsen oxygen saturation, and increases the risk of bacterial colonisation. Instead, optimal humidification is essential to maintain secretion mobility and prevent mucosal drying. Inspired gases should be delivered at 37°C and close to 100% relative humidity (Gardner et al., 2020). Suctioning may be performed using either open or closed techniques. Evidence comparing the two remains mixed, but closed suction reduces the severity and duration of hypoxaemia and may reduce fluctuations in cerebral blood flow. Elevating the head by 15–30° may help reduce aspiration of oropharyngeal secretions and the risk of ventilator-associated pneumonia (Rangelova et al., 2024).

Nurses should document the amount and nature of secretions, as this may influence clinical decisions. Comfort measures, including swaddling, maternal breastmilk, sucrose, and non-nutritive sucking, reduce pain and support cardiorespiratory stability during suctioning. Adequate rest following procedures is vital (Gardner et al., 2020).

Chapter takeaways

- Neonatal respiratory disease remains a major cause of NNU admission, making an understanding of fetal lung development, birth transition, and early physiology essential. Lung maturity determines viability and vulnerability: infants born before the late saccular stage have limited gas-exchange capacity and a high risk of respiratory failure.

- RDS results from surfactant deficiency, causing alveolar collapse and reduced FRC. Management focuses on supporting gas exchange while minimising injury, with early minimally invasive surfactant delivery (LISA/MIST) preferred, and antenatal corticosteroids vital for prevention.
- Non-invasive ventilation, particularly CPAP, is first-line, while extremely preterm infants may require mechanical ventilation using gentle, volume-targeted strategies.
- BPD is a multifactorial lung disease influenced by inflammation, antenatal factors, ventilatory injury, and disrupted lung growth. Prevention centres on minimising invasive ventilation, optimising oxygen, and supporting nutrition.
- Acute conditions such as TTN, PIE, pneumothorax, pulmonary haemorrhage, and pneumonia require rapid recognition, targeted management, and vigilant nursing to prevent deterioration and minimise lung injury.

CASE STUDY

CASE STUDIES

For the three case studies below, consider the following questions:

Q.1. Considering the current literature and guidelines on neonatal respiratory management, what are the strategies required for these three cases below?

Q.2. What are your reasons for your answer to Q.1, for each case?

Q.3. What factors will benefit these infants' outcomes and why?

Q.4. What are the risks associated with respiratory management in these cases and how can these be minimised?

Case study 1: Ventilatory management of the premature infant

Nubia is 27+3 weeks' gestation and weighs 810g. She was delivered by caesarean section for maternal pregnancy-induced hypertension. Her mother is a primigravida and received a full course of antenatal steroids prior to delivery. At birth, Nubia had a heart rate over 100 and required a period of ventilation breaths for weak respiratory effort, after which she was switched to delivery room CPAP.

Following admission to NNU, her blood gas showed a pH 7.16, $PaCO_2$ 8.6kPa, PaO_2 2.4kPa. Bicarbonate 14mmol/L, base excess = −7, and she is in 32% supplemental oxygen on a CPAP of 6cm H_2O with occasional apnoeas responding to stimulation.

CASE STUDY

Case study 2: Weaning from ventilation

Gabriella was born at 30 weeks' gestation, birthweight 900g, and required respiratory intervention at birth due to marked work of breathing. She was diagnosed with an early onset infection and has required invasive ventilation as she did not have adequate respiratory drive. She has failed one previous attempt at extubation at 4 days old. She is now 7 days old and her blood gas shows a pH 7.49, $PaCO_2$ 3.4 kpa PaO_2 10.5kPa, Bicarbonate 20mmol/L, base excess +3.

Case study 3: Weaning from CPAP

Sanjeet, born at 24 weeks' gestation, has x-ray changes consistent with evolving chronic lung disease and has been on bi-level CPAP for 5 weeks after an unstable period of ventilation. He has an oxygen requirement of 55%. He is now 9 weeks old and the decision is made to wean and discontinue the CPAP as soon as his condition allows. His blood gas shows pH 7.33, $PaCO_2$ = 9kpa, PaO_2 8.6kPa, Bicarbonate 30 mmol/L and Base excess = +4.

For suggested answer guides to the questions posed in these case studies, please refer to the web-based companion site specific to this chapter. See www.routledge.com/cw/petty

References

Abdel-Latif, M. E., Davis, P. G., Wheeler, K. I., De Paoli, A. G., & Dargaville, P. A. (2021). Surfactant therapy via thin catheter in preterm infants with or at risk of respiratory distress syndrome. *Cochrane Database of Systematic Reviews*, *2021*(5). https://doi.org/10.1002/14651858.CD011672.pub2

Abu Shqara, R. A., Hoffman, N., Lowenstein, L., & Frank Wolf, M. (2025). Preterm meconium-stained amniotic fluid: A red flag for infection and adverse perinatal outcomes. *International Journal of Gynecology and Obstetrics*, *172*(1), 420–427.

Askie, L. M., Darlow, B. A., Finer, N., Schmidt, B., Stenson, B., Tarnow-Mordi, W., . . . & Das, A. (2018). Association between oxygen saturation targeting and death or disability in extremely preterm infants in the neonatal oxygenation prospective meta-analysis collaboration. *Jama*, *319*(21), 2190–2201.

Barnes, M. E., Feeney, E., Duncan, A., Jassim, S., MacNamara, H., O'Hara, J., Refila, B., Allen, J., McCollum, D., Meehan, J., Mullaly, R., O'Cathain, N., Roche, E., & Molloy, E. J. (2022). Pulmonary haemorrhage in neonates: Systematic review of management. *Acta Paediatrica*, *111*(2), 236–244. https://doi.org/10.1111/apa.16127

Barry, J. S., Deacon, J., Hernandez, C., & Jones, M. D. (2020). Acid-base homeostasis and oxygenation. In S. L. Gardner, B. S. Carter, M. E. Hines & J. A. Hernandez (Eds.), *Merenstein & Gardner's handbook of neonatal intensive care: An interprofessional approach* (9th ed., pp. 186–200). Elsevier.

Baud, O., Maury, L., Lebail, F., Ramful, D., El Moussawi, F., Nicaise, C., Zupan-Simunek, V., Coursol, A., Beuchée, A., Bolot, P., Andrini, P., Mohamed, D., & Alberti, C. (2016). Effect of early low-dose hydrocortisone on survival without bronchopulmonary dysplasia in extremely preterm infants (PREMILOC): A double-blind, placebo-controlled, multicentre, randomised trial. *The Lancet, 387*(10030), 1827–1836.

Baud, O., Trousson, C., Biran, V., Leroy, E., Mohamed, D., Alberti, C., & for the PREMILOC Trial Group. (2017). Association between early low-dose hydrocortisone therapy in extremely preterm neonates and neurodevelopmental outcomes at 2 years of age. *JAMA, 317*(13), 1329. https://doi.org/10.1001/jama.2017.2692

Breinig, S., Dicky, O., Ehlinger, V., Dulac, Y., Marcoux, M.-O., & Arnaud, C. (2021). Echocardiographic parameters predictive of poor outcome in persistent pulmonary hypertension of the newborn (PPHN): Preliminary results. *Pediatric Cardiology, 42*(8), 1848–1853. https://doi.org/10.1007/s00246-021-02677-z

British Association of Perinatal Medicine. (2024). *BAPM neonatal airway safety standard.* British Association of Perinatal Medicine. Retrieved January 9, 2026, from https://www.bapm.org/resources/BAPM-Neonatal-Airway-Safety-Standard

Bruet, S., Butin, M., & Dutheil, F. (2021). Systematic review of high-flow nasal cannula versus continuous positive airway pressure for primary support in preterm infants. *Archives of Disease in Childhood – Fetal and Neonatal Edition, 107*, 56–59.

Bruschettini, M., Hassan, K.-O., Romantsik, O., Banzi, R., Calevo, M. G., & Moresco, L. (2022). Interventions for the management of transient tachypnoea of the newborn – An overview of systematic reviews. *Cochrane Database of Systematic Reviews.* https://doi.org/10.1002/14651858.CD013563.pub2

Chen, C.-M., Chung, M.-Y., Kang, H.-Y., Ou-Yang, M.-C., Wang, T.-M., & Hsu, C.-T. (2024). Case Report: Neurally adjusted ventilatory assist as an effective rescue treatment for pulmonary interstitial emphysema in extremely low birth weight infants. *Frontiers in Pediatrics, 12*, 1332332. https://doi.org/10.3389/fped.2024.1332332

Coletti, K., Wild, K. T., Foglia, E. E., Otter, S. C., & Kirpalani, H. (2024). Randomized controlled trials of pulmonary vasodilator therapy adjunctive to inhaled nitric oxide for persistent pulmonary hypertension of the newborn. *Clinics in Perinatology, 51*(1), 253–269. https://doi.org/10.1016/j.clp.2023.11.009

Dhugga, G., Sankaran, D., & Lakshminrusimha, S. (2025). ABCs of base therapy in neonatology: Role of acetate, bicarbonate, citrate and lactate. *Journal of Perinatology, 45*(3), 298–304. https://doi.org/10.1038/s41372-024-02169-x

Donn, S. M., Stepanovich, G. E., & Attar, M. A. (2024). Assisted ventilation and its complications. In R. J. Martin, A. A. Fanaroff & M. C. Walsh (Eds.), *Fanaroff and Martin's neonatal-perinatal medicine: Diseases of the fetus and infant* (12th ed., pp. 1240–1270). Elsevier.

Gardner, S. L., Enzman-Hines, M., & Nyp, M. (2020). Respiratory diseases. In S. L. Gardner, B. S. Carter, M. E. Hines & J. A. Hernandez (Eds.), *Merenstein & Gardner's handbook of neonatal intensive care: An interprofessional approach* (9th ed., pp. 729–835). Elsevier.

Gentle, S. J., Ambalavanan, N., & Carlo, W. A. (2020). Oxygen saturation histograms predict nasal continuous positive airway pressure-weaning success in preterm infants. *Pediatric Research, 88*(4), 637–641. https://doi.org/10.1038/s41390-020-0772-2

Herting, E., Härtel, C., & Göpel, W. (2020). Less invasive surfactant administration: Best practices and unanswered questions. *Current Opinion in Pediatrics, 32*(2), 228–234.

Hogeveen, M., Monnelly, V., Binkhorst, M., Cusack, J., Fawke, J., Kardum, D., Roehr, C. C., Rüdiger, M., Schwindt, E., Solevåg, A. L., Szczapa, T., te Pas, A., Trevisanuto, D., Wagner,

M., Wilkinson, D., & Madar, J. (2025). European Resuscitation Council guidelines 2025 Newborn resuscitation and support of transition of infants at birth. *Resuscitation*, *215*, 110766.

Igo, D. A., Kingsley, K. M., Malaspina, E. M., & Picarillo, A. P. (2021). Decreasing unplanned extubations in the neonatal ICU. *Respiratory Care*, *66*(7), 1059–1062.

Jensen, E. A., Dysart, K., Gantz, M. G., McDonald, S., Bamat, N. A., Keszler, M., Kirpalani, H., Laughon, M. M., Poindexter, B. B., Duncan, A. F., Yoder, B. A., Eichenwald, E. C., & DeMauro, S. B. (2019). The diagnosis of bronchopulmonary dysplasia in very preterm infants. An evidence-based approach. *American Journal of Respiratory and Critical Care Medicine*, *200*(6), 751–759. https://doi.org/10.1164/rccm.201812-2348OC

Jiang, P., Wei, J., & Han, M. (2025). Lung ultrasound to evaluate the outcome and prognosis of transient tachypnea of the newborn. *Frontiers in Pediatrics*, *12*, 1536992. https://doi.org/10.3389/fped.2024.1536992

Jobe, A. H., & Bancalari, E. (2001). Bronchopulmonary dysplasia. *American Journal of Respiratory and Critical Care Medicine*, *163*(7), 1723–1729.

Kallapur, S. G., & Jobe, A. H. (2024). Lung development and maturation. In R. J. Martin, A. A. Fanaroff & M. C. Walsh (Eds.), *Fanaroff and Martin's neonatal-perinatal medicine: Diseases of the fetus and infant* (12th ed., pp. 1190–1209). Elsevier.

Katz, T. A., de Ridder, R., Bancalari, E., Higgins, R. D., Isayama, T., Jensen, E. A., Offringa, M., Pillow, J. J., Shah, P. S., Soll, R. F., Stoecklin, B., Daams, J. G., van Kaam, A. H., Onland, W., & Mugie, S. M. (2025). Prognostic accuracy of BPD definitions for long-term outcomes in preterm infants: A systematic review. *Pediatrics*, *156*(5), e2025070741. https://doi.org/10.1542/peds.2025-070741

Keszler, M. (2022). Overview of assisted ventilation. In M. Keszler & G. K. Suresh (Eds.), *Goldsmith's assisted ventilation of the neonate* (7th ed., pp. 221–231). Elsevier.

Kim, J., Villarreal, M., Arya, S., Hernandez, A., & Moreira, A. (2024). Bridging the gap: Exploring bronchopulmonary dysplasia through the lens of biomedical informatics. *Journal of Clinical Medicine*, *13*(4), 1077. https://doi.org/10.3390/jcm13041077

Lagoski, M., Hamvas, A., & Wambach, J. A. (2024). Respiratory distress syndrome in the neonate. In R. J. Martin, A. A. Fanaroff & M. C. Walsh (Eds.), *Fanaroff and Martin's neonatal-perinatal medicine: Diseases of the fetus and infant* (12th ed., pp. 1226–1239). Elsevier.

Lai, M., Inglis, G. D. T., Hose, K., Jardine, L. A., & Davies, M. (2014). Methods for securing endotracheal tubes in newborn infants. *Cochrane Database of Systematic Reviews*, *7*, Article CD007805. https://doi.org/10.1002/14651858.CD007805.pub2

Lowe, J., Gillespie, D., Aboklaish, A., Lau, T. M. M., Consoli, C., Babu, M., Goddard, M., Hood, K., Klein, N., Thomas-Jones, E., Turner, M., Hubbard, M., Marchesi, J., Berrington, J., & Kotecha, S. (2024). Azithromycin therapy for prevention of chronic lung disease of prematurity (AZTEC): A multicentre, double-blind, randomised, placebo-controlled trial. *The Lancet Respiratory Medicine*, *12*(8), 608–618. https://doi.org/10.1016/S2213-2600(24)00079-1

Mandell, E., Kinsella, J. P., & Abman, S. H. (2020). Persistent pulmonary hypertension of the newborn. *Pediatric Pulmonology*, *56*(3), 661–669. https://doi.org/10.1002/ppul.25073

Moreira, A., Noronha, M., Joy, J., Bierwirth, N., Tarriela, A., Naqvi, A., Zoretic, S., Jones, M., Marotta, A., Valadie, T., Brick, J., Winter, C., Porter, M., Decker, I., Bruschettini, M., & Ahuja, S. K. (2024). Rates of bronchopulmonary dysplasia in very low birth weight neonates: A systematic review and meta-analysis. *Respiratory Research*, *25*, 219. https://doi.org/10.1186/s12931-024-02850-x

Moreno-Sanz, B., Montes, M. T., Antón, M., Serrada, M. T., Cabrera, M., & Pellicer, A. (2021). Scaling up the family integrated care model in a level IIIc neonatal intensive care unit: A systematic approach to the methods and effort taken for implementation. *Frontiers in Pediatrics*, *9*, 682097. https://doi.org/10.3389/fped.2021.682097

Nair, V., & Smith, H. (2020). Phased quality improvement interventions in reducing unplanned extubation in the neonatal icu. *Respiratory Care, 65*(10), 1511–1518. https://doi.org/10.4187/respcare.07643

Nancarrow, L. (2025). Neonatal respiratory outcomes following nebulised surfactant administration: A literature review. *Journal of Neonatal Nursing, 31*(2), 101618. https://doi.org/10.1016/j.jnn.2025.101618

National Institute for Health and Care Excellence. (2019). *Specialist neonatal respiratory care for babies born preterm. NG124*. NICE.

Nock, M. L., & Olicker, A. L. (2024). Tables of normal values. In R. J. Martin, A. A. Fanaroff & M. C. Walsh (Eds.), *Fanaroff and Martin's neonatal-perinatal medicine: Diseases of the fetus and infant* (12th ed., pp. 2118–2166). Elsevier.

O'Brien, K., Robson, K., Bracht, M., Cruz, M., Lui, K., Alvaro, R., Da Silva, O., Monterrosa, L., Narvey, M., Ng, E., Soraisham, A., Ye, X. Y., Mirea, L., Tarnow-Mordi, W., Lee, S. K., O'Brien, K., Lee, S., Bracht, M., Caouette, G., . . . Hales, D. (2018). Effectiveness of Family Integrated Care in neonatal intensive care units on infant and parent outcomes: A multicentre, multinational, cluster-randomised controlled trial. *The Lancet Child & Adolescent Health, 2*(4), 245–254. https://doi.org/10.1016/S2352-4642(18)30039-7

Prasath, A., Chotzoglou, E., Ahmad, A., Diaz, E., Burchfield, P., Brown, L. S., Nelson, D. B., Stumpf, K., & Kakkilaya, V. (2025). Less invasive surfactant administration for meconium aspiration syndrome. *BMJ Paediatrics Open, 9*, e003317. https://doi.org/10.1136/bmjpo-2025-003317

Rangelova, V., Kevorkyan, A., Raycheva, R., & Krasteva, M. (2024). Ventilator-associated pneumonia in the neonatal intensive care unit – Incidence and strategies for prevention. *Diagnostics, 14*(3), 240. https://doi.org/10.3390/diagnostics14030240

Rüegger, C. M., Owen, L. S., & Davis, P. G. (2021). Nasal intermittent positive pressure ventilation for neonatal respiratory distress syndrome. *Clinics in Perinatology, 48*(4), 725–744. https://doi.org/10.1016/j.clp.2021.07.004

Schmidt, A. F., & Bancalari, E. H. (2024). Bronchopulmonary dysplasia in the neonate. In R. J. Martin, A. A. Fanaroff & M. C. Walsh (Eds.), *Fanaroff and Martin's neonatal-perinatal medicine: Diseases of the fetus and infant* (12th ed., pp. 1330–1345). Elsevier.

Shalish, W., Kanbar, L., Kovacs, L., Chawla, S., Keszler, M., Rao, S., Latremouille, S., Precup, D., Brown, K., Kearney, R. E., & Sant'Anna, G. M. (2020). Assessment of extubation readiness using spontaneous breathing trials in extremely preterm neonates. *JAMA Pediatrics, 174*(2), 178. https://doi.org/10.1001/jamapediatrics.2019.4868

Shetty, S., Evans, K., Cornuaud, P., Kulkarni, A., Duffy, D., & Greenough, A. (2021). Neurally adjusted ventilatory assist in very prematurely born infants with evolving/established bronchopulmonary dysplasia. *American Journal of Perinatology Reports, 11*(4), e127–e131. https://doi.org/10.1055/s-0041-1739458

Slaughter, J., Sites, J., Ballard, H., Bauer, J., Schadler, A., & Severyn, N. (2025). Comparison of the oxygenation index and the oxygen saturation index as clinical indicators for neonatal ECMO. *Frontiers in Pediatrics, 13*, 1586985. https://doi.org/10.3389/fped.2025.1586985

Sweet, D. G., Carnielli, V. P., Greisen, G., Hallman, M., Klebermass-Schrehof, K., Ozek, E., Te Pas, A., Plavka, R., Roehr, C. C., Saugstad, O. D., Simeoni, U., Speer, C., Vento, M., Visser, G. H. A., & Halliday, H. L. (2023). European consensus guidelines on the management of respiratory distress syndrome: 2022 update. *Neonatology, 120*(1), 3–23.

Tillery, M., & Connor, D. (2023). Delivery room care of newborns with meconium-stained amniotic fluid. *Journal of Neonatal Nursing, 29*(3), 423–428. https://doi.org/10.1016/j.jnn.2022.08.001

Travers, C., & Ambalavanan, N. (2022). Blood gases: Technical aspects and interpretation. In M. Keszler & G. K. Suresh (Eds.), *Goldsmith's assisted ventilation of the neonate* (7th ed., pp. 94–110). Elsevier.

Van Kaam, A. H. (2022). Principles of lung-protective ventilation. In M. Keszler & G. K. Suresh (Eds.), *Goldsmith's assisted ventilation of the neonate* (7th ed., pp. 241–248). Elsevier.

Vento, M. (2022). Oxygen therapy. In M. Keszler & G. K. Suresh (Eds.), *Goldsmith's assisted ventilation of the neonate* (7th ed., pp. 185–195). Elsevier.

Yasmeen, T., & Ansary, A. (2024). *High frequency oscillatory ventilation (HFOV): A guide to the use of HFOV in the neonate (888)*. Greater Glasgow and Clyde Paediatrics Guideline. Retrieved January 9, 2026, from https://www.clinicalguidelines.scot.nhs.uk/ggc-paediatric-guidelines/ggc-paediatric-guidelines/neonatology/high-frequency-oscillatory-ventilation-hfov-a-guide-to-the-use-of-hfov-in-the-neonate-888/#S26

15 MANAGEMENT OF NEONATAL CARDIOVASCULAR DISORDERS

Nicky McCarthy and Jonathan O'Keeffe

CONTENTS

DOI: 10.4324/9781003591405-19

GUIDANCE ON HOW TO ENHANCE PERSONAL LEARNING FROM THIS CHAPTER

Key points covered in this chapter

- An overview of embryological development of the cardiovascular system, fetal circulation, and physiology of the heart.
- Types of congenital heart disease and their diagnosis and management.
- Cardiovascular disorders such as blood pressure disturbances and dysrhythmias and their management.

Reflection

Reading through the chapter, you are encouraged to engage with the key points and related literature in an enquiring way. Ask these questions:

- How does what you have learnt about embryology and cardiac function help you understand the problems of the cardiovascular system newborns can present with?
- How can you carry out a comprehensive assessment of the cardiovascular system, which may help with the diagnosis of any problems?
- What do you need to know about the management strategies of the various conditions to provide good nursing care to affected babies?

Implications for nursing care

- Finally: how will this chapter enable you to approach the assessment, management, and nursing care of neonates with cardiac problems? Consider the implications of what you learn for your daily practice relating to this area.

INTRODUCTION AND BACKGROUND

Cardiovascular disorders are among the most common challenges encountered during the neonatal period. A thorough understanding of cardiac anatomy and physiology is essential, as the cardiovascular system undergoes rapid changes during this time; changes that do not occur at any other stage of life. Understanding the implications of this transition is crucial. While structural heart disease occurs in 7–12 per 1000 live births (British Heart Foundation, 2025), the number of newborns affected by acquired heart disease such as endocarditis, metabolic disorders which may involve the heart muscle, and neonatal arrhythmias have no reliable data, and therefore the true incidence of all neonatal heart disease is as yet unquantifiable. This chapter will review embryology, anatomy and physiology, while also exploring common cardiovascular disorders, congenital heart disease (CHD), and current management strategies.

EMBRYOLOGY OF THE HEART

The heart is the first functioning organ, beating rhythmically as early as day 21 (Schoenwolf et al., 2021). The heart functions as an efficient organ providing oxygen and nutrients and disposing of carbon dioxide and waste to and from the mother's blood (Torchia & Persaud, 2024). Most of the development, remodelling, and separation occurs while the heart is pumping blood (Schoenwolf et al., 2021). The development of the heart begins with the formation of two endocardial tubes which fuse, forming a thin endothelial tube which is separated from a thick myocardium by a gelatinous matrix of connective tissue, the cardiac jelly (Torchia & Persaud, 2024).

Between weeks 4 and 8, the primitive heart tube undergoes a process of looping, remodelling, realignment, and separation that transforms the single lumen into four regions which will further develop into the more recognised chambers of the adult heart. As the heart tube lengthens, it develops a series of expansions and shallow sulci that will subdivide into heart chambers at the earliest stages of their development (Schoenwolf et al., 2021). Starting at the **caudal** end, which is towards the tail of the embryo, these sections of the primitive heart are the sinus venosus, the primitive atrium, the primitive ventricle, the bulbus cordis, and the truncus arteriosus (see Figure 15.1).

The bulbus cordis and the ventricles grow more rapidly than the other regions, which are restricted by the pericardium. This causes the tube to loop and fold, resulting in an S- shaping. Essentially, the heart folding involves the bulbus cordis and truncus arteriosus traveling forwards and downwards, and the primitive atrium and primitive ventricles being pushed upwards and backwards. The end result of this cardiac modulation is to bring the four chambers of the future heart into the correct position (Figure 15.2). The remainder of the heart development consists of remodelling these chambers, developing the septa and valves between them and forming the epicardium, coronary vasculature, and cardiac innervation and conducting system.

Partitioning of the heart into four chambers is accomplished through the formation of walls (septa) in the primitive atrium, ventricles and outflow tract (Schoenwolf et al., 2021). By the 5th week, endothelial cushions appear and

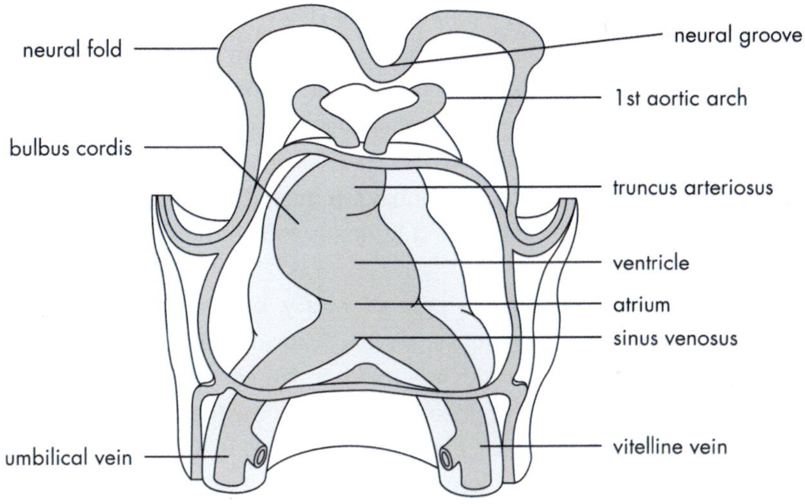

Figure 15.1 Differentiation of the regions in the primitive heart tube

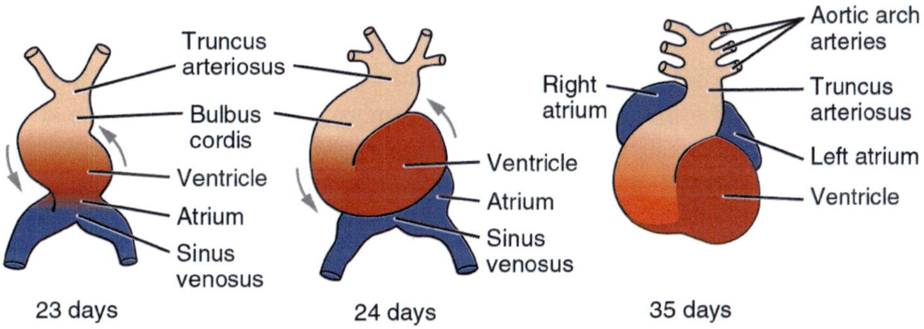

Figure 15.2 Bending of the primitive heart and orientation of the atria and ventricles in their final adult position (Source: Creative Commons)

function as primitive valves that assist the forward propulsion of blood (Carlson, 2023). The primitive atrium is divided into the right and left atria by the formation of two septa: the septum primum and septum secundum. The septum primum develops downwards from the roof of the common atrium towards the endocardial cushions. Before a complete closure of the connection between the right and left atrium, an opening develops in the mid-section in this newly formed wall; this is called the foramen secundum (Torchia & Persaud, 2024). As the septum secundum, a more muscular structure, then begins a similar descent from the roof alongside the septum primum, a communication between both atria remains open; this is called the foramen primum. Once both septa have formed, they leave an oval-shaped orifice, the patent foramen ovale (PFO), through which for the rest of fetal development, blood shunts from the right atrium across to the left atrium. Blood cannot travel back in the opposite direction, as the foramen secundum acts as a block when pushed against the muscular septum secundum (Schoenwolf et al., 2021; Torchia & Persaud, 2024).

While the interatrial septa are forming, a muscular interventricular septum begins to grow between the ballooning right and left ventricle towards the atrioventricular cushions.

The intraventricular foramen is present initially, but this is obliterated by the growth of the muscular interventricular septum (Carlson, 2023). The protrusion of the muscular interventricular septum is formed as the expanding walls of the right and left ventricles become more closely opposed to each other. The formation of the outflow tracts begins with the single lumen, the bulbus cordis. By the time the interventricular septum begins to form, this single tube has elongated and divided. Although initially there is a single channel within this tube, due to the direction of flow through it, the tract divides into separate aortic and pulmonary channels. As they are shaped by the spiral flow of blood during the partitioning, they develop into a helical arrangement, the ridges finally meeting and separating the lumen into two channels (Figure 15.3). The sinus venosus becomes integrated with the right atrium and forms the **inferior** vena cava (IVC) and **superior** vena cava (SVC) by the end of the fifth week (Schoenwolf et al., 2021). Aortic and pulmonary artery valves and the atrioventricular valves, namely the mitral and tricuspid valves, form from subendothelial tissue, and their function is to prevent blood from washing back (Carlson, 2023).

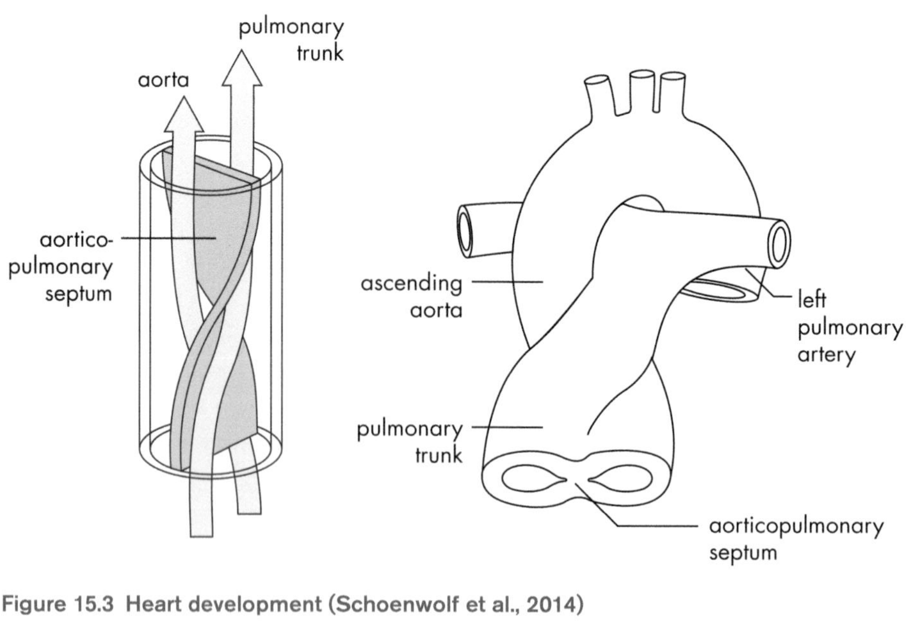

Figure 15.3 Heart development (Schoenwolf et al., 2014)

The heart has to function as soon as it forms. Rhythmic waves of electric depolarisation that trigger the myocardium to contract spontaneously arise from the cardiac muscle itself and spread from cell to cell. This results in the primitive heart tube cardiomyocytes contracting asynchronously. A cluster of cells that migrate from the sinus venosus into the right atrium take over the pacemaker activity and develop into the sinoatrial node. Soon after the development of the sinoatrial node, cells within the atrioventricular junction begin to form a secondary pacemaker: the atrioventricular node. This node regulates the conduction of impulses from the atrium to the ventricles. Simultaneously, from the atrioventricular node, the bundle of His is then formed, and this is followed by the development of the Purkinje fibres. This produces a conductive system for the heart (Schoenwolf et al., 2021).

PHYSIOLOGY

The understanding of cardiovascular physiology will assist our ability to assess, interpret, and plan management for the neonate displaying signs and symptoms of a congenital or an acquired cardiovascular disorder.

Fetal circulation

The fetal circulation is quite different from the neonatal circulation; it comprises two umbilical arteries bringing deoxygenated blood to the placenta, and a single umbilical vein carrying oxygenated blood back to the heart. Oxygenated blood travels from the placenta through the umbilical vein, where it meets the first of three fetal shunts. the ductus venosus which diverts the blood away from the liver. The blood then moves to the right atrium, where most of it flows through the second fetal shunt, the FO, straight into the left atrium. This fetal shunt effectively bypasses the pulmonary circulation. The blood then flows into the left ventricle, where it is pumped into the aorta and around the body. Not all of the blood that enters the right atrium is shunted through the FO; instead, it enters the right ventricle and leaves the heart via the pulmonary artery, where it meets the third and final fetal shunt, the ductus arteriosus (DA). This shunt directs most of the blood away from the lungs and into the aorta (Figure 15.4). Only 7% of the combined ventricular output of blood actually passes into the lungs. The mechanism allowing blood to be shunted away from the lungs is facilitated by the high pulmonary pressure as a result of the fluid-filled fetal lung. Therefore, the blood is taking the path of least resistance in every case. Consequently, unlike in the adult heart, the right ventricle is the dominant chamber in utero and is ejecting 66% of the combined ventricular output.

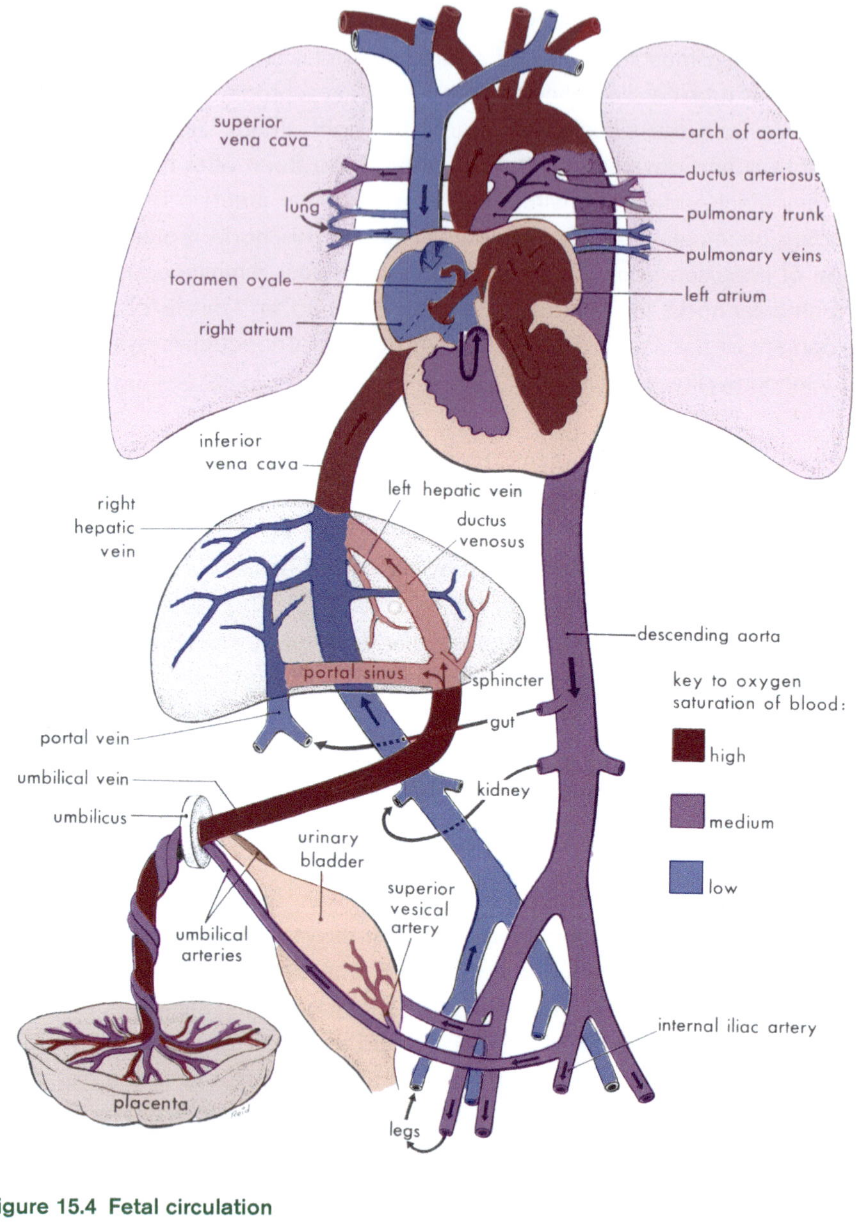

Figure 15.4 Fetal circulation

Cardiovascular adaptations are required to survive extrauterine life. When an infant breathes for the first time at birth, the fluid in the lungs is expelled by the generation of significant negative pressures (60–90cmH_20). This fluid is absorbed through the pulmonary lymphatics and capillaries over the first 6–12 hours of life. Lung aeration triggers the cardiovascular transition at birth by decreasing pulmonary vascular resistance, which allows for increased pulmonary blood flow. There is a decrease in the pressure on the right side of the heart due to the reduction in pulmonary pressure. As a consequence of this pressure change, blood no longer crosses from the right to the left atrium through the FO, which results in its closure. Hereafter it is referred to as the fossa ovalis. There is decreased blood flow in the IVC resulting in the closure of the ductus venosus, which becomes the ligamentum teres. The umbilical vessels take longer to become obliterated and may still be cannulated up to 10 days after birth (Strainic, 2024). The increase in concentration of oxygen in the blood leads to a decrease in circulating prostaglandins and causes closure of the DA. Blood is now prevented from bypassing the pulmonary circulation, and the newly operational lungs must oxygenate the infant's blood.

> **THINK POINT**
>
> How does your knowledge of the transition from fetal to neonatal circulation influence the way you interpret changes in colour, pulses, or oxygen saturation during the first 24 hours?

Cardiac cycle

A single cardiac cycle includes all of the events associated with one heartbeat. One full cardiac cycle consists of **systole** and **diastole** of the atria, plus systole and diastole of the ventricles. During atrial systole, the atria are contracting, and at the same time the ventricles are relaxed. During atrial diastole the atria are relaxed while at the same time ventricular systole is occurring, which means the ventricles are contracting. Blood fills both atria simultaneously: the IVC and SVC fill the right atrium, and the pulmonary veins fill the left atrium. The sinoatrial node is stimulated and sends an impulse to contract across the atria; this causes the blood to be ejected into the ventricles through the atrioventricular valves. The atrioventricular node is then stimulated by this contraction, and it in turn emits an impulse of contraction down the Purkinje fibres, stimulating the contraction of the ventricles and the expulsion of the blood into the pulmonary artery and aorta. The heart relaxes, and this is the completion of one cardiac cycle (Tortora & Derrickson, 2020).

Cardiac output

Cardiac output (CO) is the amount of blood ejected from both ventricles and is dependent upon **stroke volume** (SV) and heart rate (HR)

$$CO = SV \times HR$$

SV is the total amount of blood leaving the ventricles in one heartbeat and is dependent upon the stretch undergone by individual heart myofibres.

$$SV = \text{preload} + \text{afterload} + \text{contractility}$$

Preload represents the passive stretching of the resting heart prior to ventricular filling. The myocardium contracts efficiently at certain preload volumes. If filling increases, the cardiac muscle fibres are stretched, leading to an increase in the force of the ventricular muscle contraction. This is known as the Frank-Starling law. Overfilling or underfilling can cause the contractions to be less effective (Koeppen et al., 2024).

Afterload is pressure against which the heart has to work to eject the blood from both ventricles. The afterload effect on the left ventricle is determined by the aortic pressure, and the afterload effect on the right ventricle must exceed the pressure in the pulmonary trunk. Essentially, afterload is the resistance the heart must pump against and is dependent on peripheral vascular resistance and the viscosity of the blood (Sinha et al., 2018).

Contractility is the metabolic state of the heart muscle itself and is independent of pre- and afterload. CO can be increased by increasing myocardial contractility (inotropy) or increasing the HR (chronotropy). These changes are mediated through adrenergic receptors, either α, β, or dopaminergic receptors. β_1 stimulation increases myocardial contractility and heart rate; β_2 stimulation increases pulmonary and systemic vasodilation; and stimulation causes arteriolar constriction. Dopaminergic stimulation causes vasodilation in vascular beds such as the kidney, brain and gut (Sinha et al., 2018). The increased contractility produced by β-adrenoceptor stimulation can be mimicked by drugs such as dopamine and dobutamine, which are described as positive **inotropes**. A complete list of drugs used in the management of cardiovascular disorders appears in Table 15.1.

TABLE 15.1 ADRENERGIC RECEPTORS AND THEIR AGONISTS AND ANTAGONISTS

	α_1	α_2	β_1	β_2	β_3
Adrenaline	+	+	+	+	+
Noradrenaline	+	+	+		
Isoprenaline			+	+	+
Dopamine	+	+	+		
Dobutamine			+		
Salbutamol				+	
Propranolol			-	(-)	
Labetalol	-		-	-	

Heart rate

Cardiac excitation originates in the sinoatrial node, spreads through the atrial muscle to the atrioventricular node and after a short delay progresses down the bundle of His to bring about depolarisation of the ventricular muscle (Noble, 2009). The individual parts of the heart each have an intrinsic rhythm of their own, but the rate of the heart is dominated by the part with the faster rhythm, the sinoatrial node. The sympathetic and parasympathetic nerves modify HR (Koeppen et al., 2024). The accelerans nerve provides sympathetic input to the heart by releasing noradrenaline onto the cells of the sinoatrial node, which in turn increases HR, while the vagus nerve provides parasympathetic input on the sinoatrial node by releasing acetylcholine, reducing HR (Tortora & Derrickson, 2020). This effect can be mimicked by agonists such as adrenaline and isoprenaline and can be blocked by propranolol (see Table 15.1). Other sensory receptors that provide input into the cardiovascular centre include **chemoreceptors** which monitor chemical changes in the blood, and **baroreceptor**s which monitor stretching of major arteries and veins (Tortora & Derrickson, 2020). Receptors in the arch of the aorta and carotid arteries detect changes in blood pressure and provide this information to the cardiovascular centre. There are also chemicals that regulate HR: hypoxia, acidosis, and alkalosis all depress cardiac activity. Cations (positively charged ions) modulate HR. Sodium and potassium are crucial for the production of action potentials in all nerve and muscle fibres; it is important to know that ionic imbalances can quickly compromise the pumping effectiveness of the heart (Tortora & Derrickson, 2020).

PRACTICE POINT

Reflect on aspects of neonatal care such as medications, pain, as well as environmental factors that may impact neonatal HR.

How can you contribute to maintaining this in an optimal range?

Blood pressure

Blood pressure (BP) is the product of flow and resistance according to the formula

$$\text{Blood pressure} = \text{blood flow} \times \text{peripheral resistance}$$

The resistance in peripheral circulation is controlled by the pressure in the arterioles. They constitute the greatest resistance to flow of any segment of the circulation. This means that the peripheral circulatory control is dependent on arteriolar smooth muscle contraction (Koeppen et al., 2024). They are stimulated to contract or dilate by various endothelial factors, local metabolites, blood-borne hormones, and neuronal stimulus.

- *Endothelial factor* Nitric oxide (NO) has a vasodilator action and is produced continuously in the blood vessel walls. The main stimulus is the friction of the blood flowing within the vessels, as well as some blood-borne agonists such as acetylcholine, bradykinin and thrombin. Chemical mediators such as cytokines also stimulate NO. Cytokines are released during an inflammatory response, as for example in septic shock; if substantial amounts are released, cytokines cause excessive vasodilation, which can in turn cause the blood pressure to drop. This is seen commonly in babies with sepsis.
- *Local metabolites* During periods of increased metabolic activity, accumulation of hydrogen, carbon dioxide, and lactic acid will have a local effect and relax the smooth muscle around it, leading to increased blood flow in that area, which will flush out these accumulated metabolites.
- *Blood-borne hormones* The renin-angiotensin system is a potent systemic pressor. The renin system is functional in the fetus, and activity increases at birth helping to maintain BP. Figure 15.5 details the function of the renin-angiotensin system.
- *Neural control* The baroreceptor reflex is guided by the major receptors of high pressure located in the carotid sinus and the aortic arch. Baroreceptors are modified nerve endings sensitive to stretch; when arterial pressure rises, the vessel becomes inflated, and the nerve endings are stretched. In the glossopharyngeal nerve for example, the increase in stretch passes along via the cranial nerve into the medulla of the brain. The medulla and hypothalamus process this information and organise an autonomic response (Koeppen et al., 2024).

CONGENITAL HEART DISEASE

Congenital heart defects are the most common type of birth defect, affecting about 1% of live births. This represents 123 live births (LB) per 10,000 globally, 81 LB per 10,000 in Europe and within the United Kingdom (UK) the latest figures suggest 66 LB per 10,000 (British Heart Foundation, 2025).

These figures include inherited and non-inherited CHD. Such structural problems of the heart, present at birth, can significantly impact blood flow and overall health. Defects vary widely, from minor defects needing little or no intervention to severe, life-threatening malformations requiring urgent surgical and intensive medical care in the first weeks of life (Chan & Singh, 2022).

Renin-angiotensin system

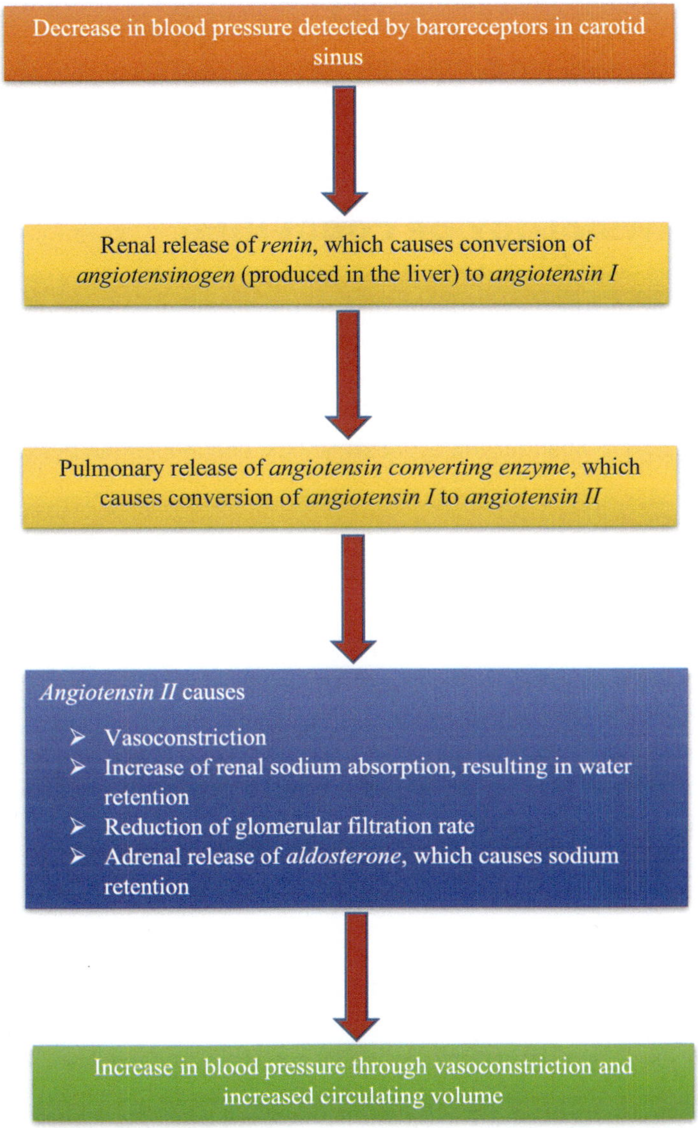

Figure 15.5 The renin-angiotensin system (adapted from Gordan et al., 2015)

Classification and types

CHD encompasses a wide range of abnormalities, but the most common types include;

1. Septal Defects: Including atrial septal defect (ASD) and ventricular septal defect (VSD) – incomplete formation of the heart's walls separating chambers.

2. Obstructive Defects: For example, coarctation of the aorta (CoA) and aortic valve **stenosis**, which restrict blood flow.
3. Cyanotic Defects: For example, Tetralogy of Fallot (ToF) and transposition of the great arteries (TGA), which can lead to low oxygen saturation and cyanosis.
4. Single Ventricle Pathways: Examples include hypoplastic left heart syndrome (HLHS).

PATHOPHYSIOLOGY OF CONGENITAL HEART DISEASE

The impact of CHD depends on the defect's size and location, and how it affects blood flow through the heart and to the rest of the body. Defects may cause too much (over-circulation) or too little (under circulation) blood flow to the lungs and/or body, leading to heart failure, cyanosis, shock, and multiorgan dysfunction.

Clinical presentation

Neonates may present with;

- Respiratory distress and feeding difficulties
- Cyanosis (blue-tinted skin, lips, or nail beds)
- Poor growth and failure to thrive
- Heart murmurs
- Signs of heart failure or shock, especially as the ductus arteriosus closes in **duct-dependent** lesions (Alkhushi, 2023)

DYSMORPHIC FEATURES

The presence of **dysmorphic** features in a newborn can be a source of considerable anxiety for both parents and healthcare professionals. These features may be subtle or striking, and their recognition should prompt a thorough and sensitive clinical evaluation. When dysmorphic traits are noted, particularly those known to be associated with CHD, a full cardiac examination is essential, including auscultation, pulse assessment, and consideration of echocardiography (Jones et al., 2022).

If CHD is confirmed, the infant should be carefully assessed for additional anomalies across other organ systems. Identifying a constellation of defects may suggest an underlying genetic or chromosomal syndrome (see Table 15.2 for common associations between CHD and genetic syndromes). Early recognition of syndromic patterns enables timely referral for genetic evaluation, multidisciplinary care planning, and appropriate family counselling.

Recent studies have shown that dysmorphology scoring systems can help stratify the likelihood of a genetic diagnosis in infants with CHD. For example, Helm et al. (2024) demonstrated that each incremental increase in dysmorphology

TABLE 15.2 COMMON GENETIC SYNDROMES AND THEIR ASSOCIATION WITH CONGENITAL HEART DISEASE

Disorder	*Most common CHD*	*Percentage affected*
Trisomy 21	Atrioventricular septal defect (AVSD)	45% of babies with trisomy 21 have an AVSD, but 80% of babies with AVSD will have trisomy 21
Turner syndrome (XO)	Coarctation of the aorta, aortic stenosis, HLHS	50% have CHD, of which 15% will have coarctation of the aorta
22q11 deletion syndrome	Tetralogy of Fallot, interrupted aortic arch, VSD	74% have CHD, of which 20% have Tetralogy of Fallot Up to 90% of patients with interrupted aortic arch will have 22q11 deletion
Williams syndrome (7q11.23 deletion)	Supravalvular aortic stenosis, branch pulmonary artery stenosis	80% have CHD, of which 75% have aortic stenosis
Noonan's syndrome	Pulmonary stenosis, hypertrophic cardiomyopathy	60% have pulmonary stenosis

(adapted from Mitchell, 2024)

score was associated with a 17–20% increased risk of identifying a genetic disorder, even among infants with isolated CHD. Similarly, Dykes et al. (2016) found that 79% of neonates with chromosomal abnormalities and CHD exhibited dysmorphic features, highlighting their diagnostic value.

This integrated approach supports holistic care, improves diagnostic accuracy, and ensures that both cardiac and extracardiac needs are addressed from the outset (Pierpont et al., 2018)

CYANOSIS

Cyanosis, which is a bluish or purple discolouration of the skin, lips, or mucous membranes typically becomes visible when arterial oxygen saturation falls below approximately 85%. In neonates, this threshold may vary depending on haemoglobin concentration and skin pigmentation. Cyanosis is classified into two types:

- *Peripheral cyanosis* (acrocyanosis): Common in healthy newborns, especially in the first 24–48 hours, due to immature peripheral circulation.
- *Central cyanosis* Involves the tongue and mucous membranes and is a clinical red flag for hypoxaemia, often caused by structural congenital heart disease, persistent pulmonary hypertension of the newborn (PPHN), or severe respiratory pathology (Singh et al., 2022b).

It is essential to differentiate true cyanosis from other conditions that mimic its appearance;

- *Facial petechiae* from birth trauma may resemble cyanosis but lack mucosal involvement.
- *Polycythaemia* can deepen skin colour, giving a dusky or ruddy appearance that may be mistaken for cyanosis.
- *Anaemia* may present with pallor rather than cyanosis, but in cases of desaturation, the skin may appear grey rather than blue.
- *Methaemoglobinaemia*, a rare but serious cause of neonatal hypoxaemia, can produce a slate-grey or blackish hue. It should be considered when oxygen saturation remains low despite normal arterial oxygen tension and imaging.

Accurate assessment requires integration of clinical signs, pulse oximetry, and blood gas analysis. When central cyanosis is suspected, urgent evaluation for cardiac, pulmonary, or haematological causes is warranted.

MURMURS

A heart murmur is an additional sound heard between the normal heart sounds, typically described as a 'whooshing' or 'swishing' noise caused by turbulent blood flow. In newborns, murmurs may be classified as either:

- *Innocent (physiological)* Resulting from normal blood flow through structurally normal cardiac chambers and valves.
- *Pathological* Indicative of underlying structural abnormalities such as CHD.

Murmurs are detected during routine neonatal examination in approximately 2.6–4.0% of newborns. Of these, up to 50% may be due to CHD, particularly if the murmur is persistent, loud, or associated with other clinical signs such as cyanosis, poor feeding, or respiratory distress (Gonzalez et al., 2021).

During auscultation, four key areas of the chest are examined, corresponding to the anatomical positions of the aortic, pulmonary, tricuspid, and mitral valves. The characteristics of the murmur are evaluated systematically, including:

- *Timing* (systolic, diastolic, continuous)
- *Intensity* (graded I–VI)
- *Pitch* (high or low frequency)
- *Quality* (harsh, blowing, musical)
- *Radiation* and *associated sounds* (e.g. clicks)

Certain features, such as a harsh systolic murmur, diastolic murmur, or continuous machinery-like murmur, are more suggestive of pathological causes and warrant further investigation.

Importantly, serious cardiac lesions (e.g. TGA, total anomalous pulmonary venous return (TAPVR)) may present with minimal or no murmur. Therefore, absence of a murmur does not exclude CHD. A careful clinical assessment, including pulse oximetry and echocardiography when indicated, is essential in all cases (Pierpont et al., 2018).

PULSES

In the neonatal period, peripheral pulse assessment is a vital component of cardiovascular examination. Pulses should be equal in strength across all four limbs; right and left, upper and lower. Discrepancies may indicate underlying pathology and should prompt further evaluation.

- *Weak or absent pulses* may suggest systemic hypoperfusion, as seen in shock, left-sided obstructive lesions (e.g. CoA), or severe cardiac dysfunction.
- *Upper limb pulses stronger than lower limb pulses* are a hallmark of CoA or interrupted aortic arch (IAA). Simultaneous palpation of brachial and femoral pulses is essential to detect this gradient.
- *Bounding pulses* are typically associated with wide pulse pressure, often seen in conditions with left-to-right shunting such as patent DA (PDA), arteriovenous malformations, or aortic regurgitation. These may be more easily appreciated in the palmar and pedal arteries than in the femoral region (Grosse-Wortmann & Al-Otay, 2023).

Pulse quality should be interpreted alongside other signs such as capillary refill, blood pressure, oxygen saturation, and clinical appearance. In duct-dependent lesions, changes in pulse character may be subtle until the DA begins to close, underscoring the importance of early and repeated assessments (Bocks et al., 2020).

FAILURE TO THRIVE

Infants with CHD often have increased metabolic demands due to chronic hypoxaemia, elevated cardiac workload, and inefficient circulation. As a result, one of the presenting signs, particularly in longer-stay neonatal unit (NNU) patients or those discharged home, may be failure to thrive (FTT; McGinn et al., 2023). FTT is typically not apparent in the immediate neonatal period but may become evident when the infant fails to regain birthweight within the expected timeframe or shows poor postnatal growth velocity. In duct-dependent lesions or cyanotic CHD, feeding may be compromised by breathlessness, fatigue, and poor coordination of sucking and swallowing (Chan et al., 2025).

SWEATING (DIAPHORESIS)

Neural and hormonal mechanisms are activated to maintain the increased CO, and this results in tachycardia and sweating. **Diaphoresis** occurs mainly on the forehead and scalp when the baby is feeding (Singh et al., 2022c).

HEPATOMEGALY

Infants with congenital heart defects that cause increased pulmonary blood flow, such as VSD, atrioventricular septal defect (AVSD), or PDA, typically present with signs of heart failure within the first 2–6 weeks of life. This timing coincides with the physiological fall in pulmonary vascular resistance, which leads to a surge in pulmonary blood flow and volume overload of the left heart. The excess volume returning to the systemic circulation results in hepatomegaly, as the liver becomes engorged to accommodate increased venous pressure and fluid retention (Giesinger & McNamara, 2020).

Diagnosis of congenital heart disease

- Pulse oximetry screening (POS): Universal screening in neonates helps detect critical CHDs before symptoms worsen.
- Echocardiography: The gold standard for diagnosis.
- Other investigations: Chest X-ray (CXR), electrocardiogram (ECG), and cardiac catheterisation as needed.

Apart from an understanding of the features of the different CHDs, there are some important considerations relating to history taking, assessment, and examination of infants with a suspected CHD. Not all infants are born in tertiary cardiac centres with accessibility to cardiology input; therefore it is important to understand what information is required to assist with forming a differential diagnosis of a CHD and where to find it.

RELEVANT HISTORY

A detailed pregnancy history and family history of CHD or infant deaths provide helpful background information, and furthermore there are specific risk factors to consider (see Table 15.3).

ANTENATAL SCANS

Fetal ultrasound scans are a routine and essential component of antenatal care in the UK. Pregnant women are offered two standard scans:

- *The dating scan* (performed between 8–14 weeks gestation) confirms gestational age and includes nuchal translucency measurement as part of the

TABLE 15.3 RISK FACTORS FOR CONGENITAL HEART DEFECTS

Maternal health and lifestyle factors	*Ethnic and socioeconomic disparities*	*Environmental factors*	*Inherited/ non-inherited*
■ Diabetes ■ Obesity ■ Smoking ■ Alcohol consumption ■ Substance misuse	■ Ethnic variations ■ Exposure to air pollution ■ Poor housing quality	■ Air pollution and toxins ■ Workplace chemical exposure	■ Family history ■ Genetic syndrome ■ Prematurity

(Adapted from Lui et al., 2024; Yu et al., 2024; Nair, 2025)

combined screening for **trisomies** 13, 18, and 21 (Patau's, Edwards', and Down's syndrome, respectively).

- *The anomaly scan* (performed between 18–21 weeks' gestation) systematically assesses fetal anatomy, including a screening view of the heart.

Cardiac screening during the anomaly scan typically includes a four-chamber view, which visualises the atria and ventricles. However, this view alone detects fewer than 50% of structural heart defects, even in experienced hands. Lesions such as CoA, TGA, and TAPVR are particularly challenging to identify prenatally due to subtle or evolving anatomical features.

Detection rates improve significantly when outflow tract views (including the left and right ventricular outflows) are added to the standard four-chamber view. These extended views allow better visualisation of **conotruncal** anomalies and great vessel relationships.

On average, 92% of CCHDs can be detected when a structured approach to mid-trimester fetal anatomy ultrasound is used (100% detection rate of right/pulmonary duct-dependent lesions, 85% left/systemic duct-dependent lesions, and 93% detection in mixed pulmonary/systemic lesions).

When cardiac abnormalities are suspected, either due to scan findings or associated extracardiac anomalies, referral is made for a fetal echocardiogram, typically performed by a specialist in fetal cardiology. This detailed assessment enables early diagnosis, parental counselling, and planning for delivery in a centre equipped for neonatal cardiology care, thus improving mortality and morbidity (Cody et al., 2024).

NEWBORN INFANT PHYSICAL EXAMINATION

In the UK, all babies undergo the newborn infant physical examination (NIPE) within the first 72 hours of life, often prior to discharge from hospital (see

Chapter 4 for details). This structured assessment includes evaluation of the cardiovascular system, with particular attention to:

- Auscultation for heart murmurs
- Palpation of femoral pulses

While these components are essential, they have limitations in detecting CHD. Studies show that clinical examination alone identifies only around 50% of CHD cases, as:

- *Murmurs may be absent* in serious defects such as TGA or TAPVR.
- *Many murmurs are innocent,* reflecting normal flow dynamics rather than structural pathology.
- *Femoral pulses may remain palpable* in duct-dependent lesions (e.g. CoA) until the DA closes, often after discharge, delaying recognition of systemic outflow obstruction.

PULSE OXIMETRY SCREENING

To address the abovementioned limitations, pulse oximetry screening (POS) has been incorporated into newborn cardiovascular assessment. It enhances detection of critical CHD (CCHD) by identifying hypoxaemia that may not be clinically apparent. When combined with NIPE, POS improves sensitivity and supports timely referral for echocardiography and specialist care. Although there is currently no mandatory national policy in the UK for routine POS in newborns, its implementation has significantly improved early detection of CCHDs. These defects may lead to sudden circulatory collapse within the first week of life, particularly when the DA closes and compensatory shunting ceases (Grosse-Wortmann & Al-Otay, 2023).

POS involves measuring oxygen saturation at two sites: the right hand (pre-ductal) and either foot (post-ductal). A normal result is defined as saturations ≥95% in both limbs, with a difference of <3% between them. A discrepancy or low SpO_2 may indicate impaired oxygen due to underlying cardiac pathology (Jullien, 2021). In the UK, POS is often performed between 4–6 hours after birth. While this early timing facilitates prompt identification before discharge, it is associated with a higher false positive rate compared to countries that screen after 24 hours. This is due to the transitional physiology of the newborn; elevated pulmonary vascular resistance and incomplete postnatal circulatory adaptation can transiently lower oxygen saturations, mimicking pathology. POS is particularly effective in identifying cyanotic heart defects such as TGA, pulmonary atresia, or ToF. In these cases, low saturations are present from birth, but clinical signs may be subtle due to duct-dependent pulmonary blood flow. Conversely, POS is less sensitive for left-sided obstructive lesions (e.g. CoA, HLHS), where systemic perfusion remains adequate while the DA is patent, and saturations may appear normal (Singh et al., 2022a).

Despite limitations, when POS is combined with antenatal anomaly scans and thorough postnatal examination, it significantly enhances early detection of CCHD. This integrated approach reduces the risk of undiagnosed duct-dependent lesions and potential collapse after discharge, improving outcomes through timely intervention (UK National Screening Committee, 2019).

RESPIRATORY ASSESSMENT

Distinguishing between cardiac and respiratory causes of distress in neonates can be clinically challenging, as both may present with overlapping signs. Infants with CHD, particularly those with duct-dependent or cyanotic lesions, may exhibit classic respiratory features such as tachypnoea, subcostal and intercostal recession, and nasal flaring. These signs reflect increased work of breathing but are not specific to pulmonary pathology.

Importantly, infants with reduced pulmonary blood flow (e.g. pulmonary atresia or ToF) may demonstrate a distinctive breathing pattern: slow respiratory rate with deep, laboured breaths. This contrasts with the rapid, shallow breathing typically seen in primary pulmonary disease (McGinn et al., 2023).

Grunting is more commonly associated with respiratory conditions such as transient tachypnoea of the newborn, respiratory distress syndrome, or meconium aspiration. Its presence in a baby with suspected CHD may indicate acute decompensation, such as hypoxaemia or acidosis, and should prompt urgent evaluation for both cardiac and pulmonary causes. A structured approach combining clinical signs, pulse oximetry, chest imaging, and echocardiography is essential to differentiate between these pathologies and guide appropriate management (Bocks et al., 2020).

HYPEROXIA TEST

Once a widely used bedside tool, the hyperoxia test is now less commonly employed but may still support the diagnosis of cyanotic CHD in resource-limited settings or during initial assessment. The infant is administered 100% oxygen for 10 minutes, and arterial blood gases are measured. A $PaO_2 < 15$ kPa (113mmHg) suggests a right-to-left shunt or impaired pulmonary oxygenation, consistent with cyanotic CHD (Bocks et al., 2020)

CHEST X-RAY, ELECTROCARDIOGRAM, AND ECHOCARDIOGRAPHY

Chest X-rays remain a low-cost, widely available tool that can provide valuable anatomical insights, including:

- Visceral situs (e.g. **situs inversus** or **heterotaxy**)
- Cardiac position, size, and silhouette

- Pulmonary vascular markings
- Thoracic skeletal abnormalities

A 12-lead ECG offers information on:

- Cardiac rhythm
- Atrial and ventricular axis
- Chamber enlargement
- Signs of hypertrophy or ischaemia

However, both investigations may appear normal in life-threatening duct-dependent lesions, such as HLHS or critical CoA, and are therefore not reliable for ruling out CCHD (Giesinger & McNamara, 2020).

Echocardiography remains the gold standard for diagnosing congenital heart defects. It is non-invasive and provides real-time visualisation of:

- Cardiac anatomy (chambers, valves, septa, great vessels)
- Function (contractility, shunting, flow patterns)
- Ductal and foramen ovale patency

Most NNUs in the UK have access to echocardiography and trained staff capable of performing urgent scans. Early echocardiographic assessment is critical for timely diagnosis and management of duct-dependent and cyanotic lesions (Gardiner, 2023).

Management principles

IMMEDIATE AND PRE-OPERATIVE CARE

- *Maintain ductal patency* In duct-dependent lesions (e.g. HLHS, TGA, pulmonary atresia; see Figure 15.6), intravenous prostaglandin E1 (PGE1) is administered to keep the DA open and ensure systemic or pulmonary blood flow until definitive intervention (see Box 15.1).
- *Oxygen therapy* Oxygen is not always beneficial; in some defects, too much oxygen may worsen pulmonary over-circulation and lower systemic perfusion. Some CHDs may necessitate acceptance of lower-than-normal saturation levels, which will be explored further below.
- *Monitor and support* Vigilant monitoring of vital signs, oxygen saturation, perfusion, and fluid/electrolyte balance. Address respiratory failure with ventilatory support if needed.
- *Nutrition* via feeding tubes/intravenously as oral feeding may not be possible pre-operatively.
- *Family support* Early, clear communication with families about diagnosis, prognosis, and treatments is essential.

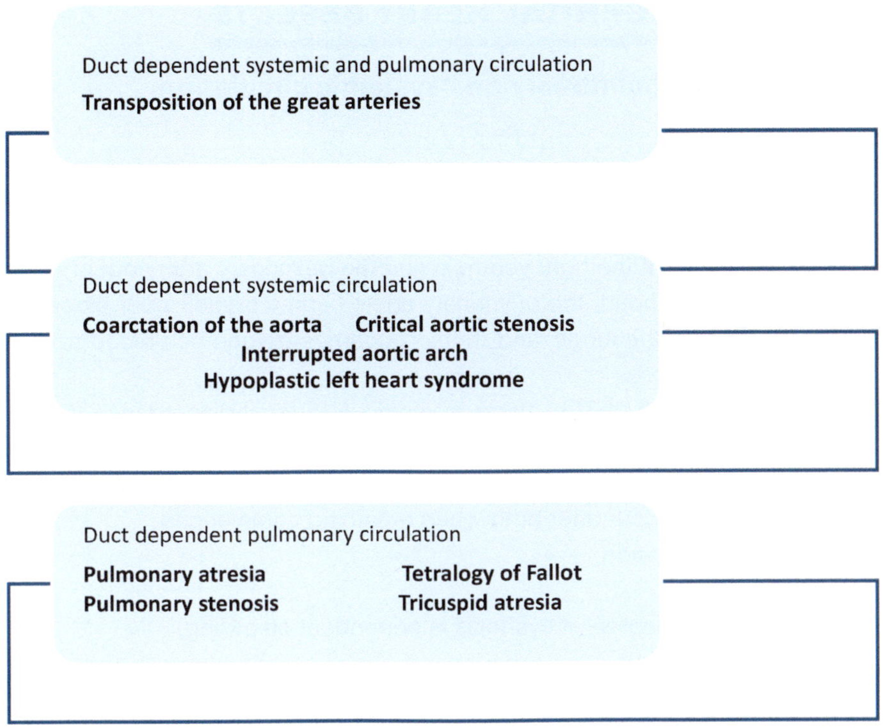

Figure 15.6 Duct-dependent critical congenital heart defects

Whilst some defects can be apparent immediately at delivery or within the first few hours after birth, there are some lesions that can present at a later time; in some instances after the baby has had a NIPE, or even after discharge, with the baby subsequently presenting at a children's emergency department. This occurs when some of the fetal circulation structures do not close immediately, which enables the body to compensate for the defect (Bakker et al., 2019). This is why it is vital for newborns to have their NIPE before discharge so that heart murmurs or any signs of cardiovascular compromise, as well as failed POS, may be detected (Neonatal Network South East, 2023).

In some situations, babies with CHD are delivered outside tertiary units, where appropriate intervention is not immediately available, resulting in higher mortality rates (Cody et al., 2024). In these scenarios expedient communication with the tertiary cardiology team, and uplift once it is safe to transfer the neonate, are paramount (Alkhushi, 2023). Improved outcomes for babies who not so long ago died in infancy mean that there is now a population of adult CHD survivors who outnumber the children born with CHD. Many of these adults have lifelong health problems (American Heart Association, 2025).

SPECIFIC CONGENITAL HEART DEFECTS

Duct-dependent pulmonary and systemic circulation

TRANSPOSITION OF THE GREAT ARTERIES

TGA (see Figure 15.7) is a CCHD which occurs as a result of failure in the spiralling phase in week 5 of embryological development. If the truncus does not spiral, the aorta comes out of the right ventricle and the pulmonary artery out of the left ventricle. In a normal heart, the pulmonary artery carries oxygen-poor blood from the right ventricle to the lungs, and the aorta carries oxygen rich blood from the left ventricle to the body.

As a direct result of TGA there is ventriculo-arterial discordance (reversal of the great vessels), causing separate parallel circulations (see Figure 15.8). *In utero* this causes no problems as the fetus does not need to use their lungs, so that symptoms only occur after birth when breathing commences.

Clinical presentation

- Cyanosis (the degree of cyanosis is dependent on mixing)
- Tachypnoea
- Poor feeding/lethargy

Albeit rare, some of these babies do not present immediately after birth if this lesion was not detected antenatally. Survival and presentation of TGA is dependent on mixing. If a baby is known to have TGA antenatally, an important consideration prior to attending the delivery is whether antenatal scans suggest whether the septum is complete or incomplete.

Management at birth

As survival is dependent on mixing, a PGE1 infusion needs to be readily available. Close liaison with the cardiology team is important, as a balloon atrial septostomy will need to be performed soon after birth. Longer term, these infants will require a 'switch procedure,' which involves relocating the great vessels to their correct anatomical sites and realigning the coronary arteries (Dorobantu et al., 2023).

PULMONARY ATRESIA AND CRITICAL PULMONARY STENOSIS

Pulmonary atresia (PA; see Figure 15.9) and critical pulmonary stenosis (CPS) are defects resulting from the narrowing or blocking of blood flow from the heart to the lungs. This defect affects the pulmonary valve which allows deoxygenated blood to reach the lungs to be oxygenated.

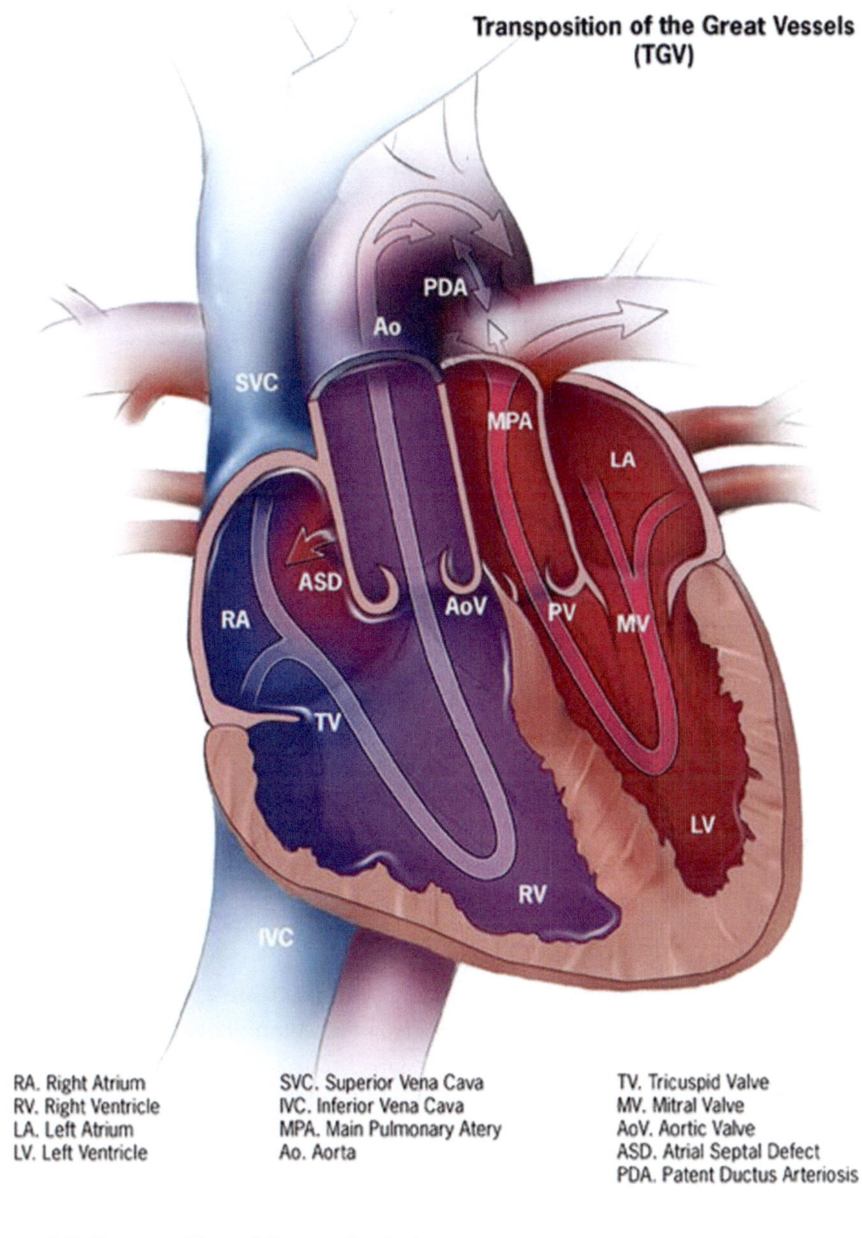

Figure 15.7 Transposition of the great arteries

Pulmonary atresia: During the initial 8 weeks of embryological development due to a disruption of unknown cause, the valve fails to form properly, which results in blood being unable to flow from the right ventricle into the pulmonary artery. Blood must then find an alternate route by means of congenital shunts, primarily the PDA, or via an ASD or VSD.

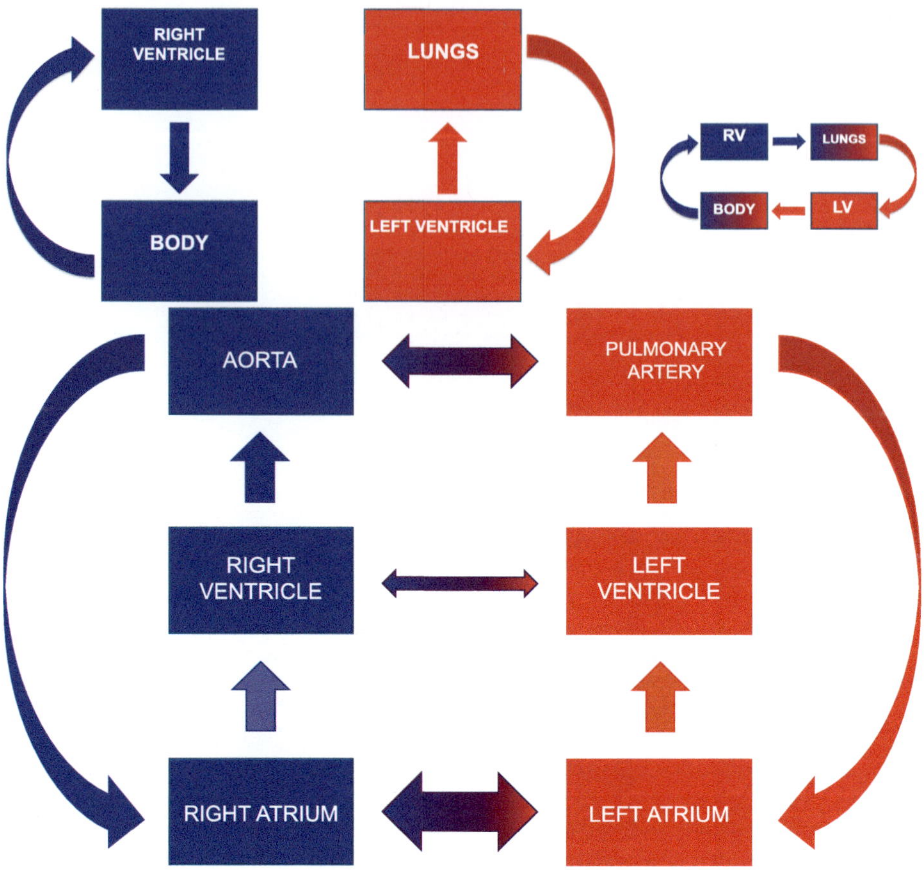

Figure 15.8 Levels of mixing in transposition of the great arteries

Critical pulmonary stenosis: The pulmonary valve is present but either abnormally thickened or fused allowing very limited blood flow. This creates a high pressure load on the right ventricle which can lead to enlargement (hypertrophy) and reduced cardiac function over time.

Clinical presentation

Both conditions often present in the neonatal period; signs may include:

- Cyanosis
- Tachypnea
- Fatigue when feeding
- Poor perfusion and acidosis in severe cases

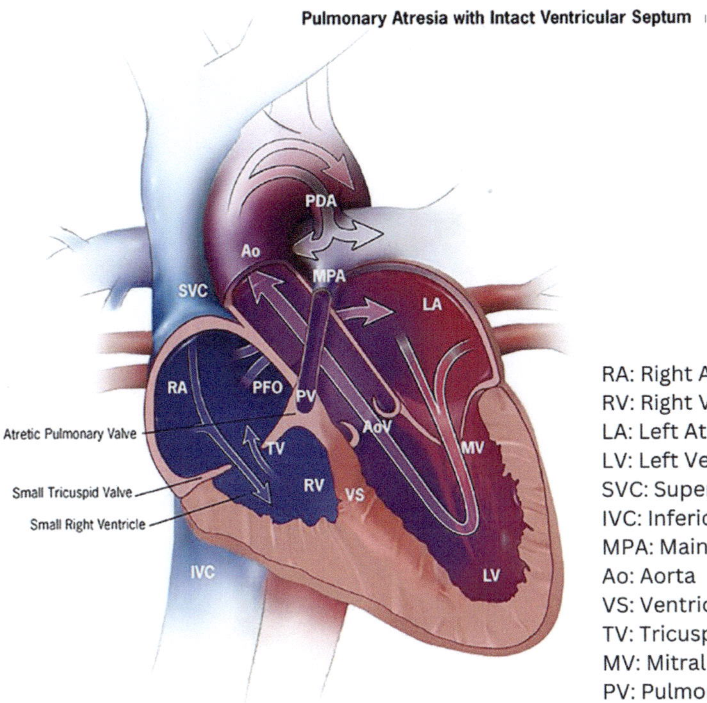

RA: Right Atrium
RV: Right Ventricle
LA: Left Atrium
LV: Left Ventricle
SVC: Superior Vena Cava
IVC: Inferior Vena Cava
MPA: Main Pulmonary Artery
Ao: Aorta
VS: Ventricular Septum
TV: Tricuspid Valve
MV: Mitral Valve
PV: Pulmonary Valve
AoV: Aortic Valve
PDA: Patent Ductus Arteriosis
PFO: Patent Foramen Ovale

Figure 15.9 Pulmonary artresia with intact ventricular septum

Immediate management

It is necessary to inform the local cardiologist team of pending delivery to prompt a quick review.

For both defects, the following are needed:

- Having reliable access to a PGE1 infusion (prepare before delivery)
- Quick vascular access
- Standard neonatal life support at birth

PA requires a shunt in early infancy, while CPS is treated with a balloon valvuloplasty to expand the valve (Haddad et al., 2019)

TETRALOGY OF FALLOT

ToF (Figure 15.10) is one of the more common congenital heart defects. 'Tetra' is Greek for four, so that the term tetralogy refers to four abnormalities that result in disrupted blood flow and oxygenation (see Table 15.4).

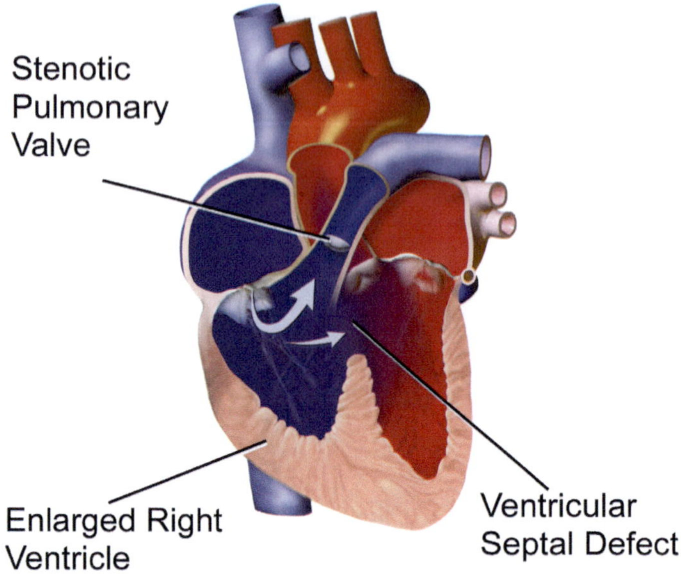

Figure 15.10 Tetralogy of Fallot

TABLE 15.4 FOUR KEY FEATURES OF TETRALOGY OF FALLOT

Ventricular septal defect	Opening in the lower chambers of the heart, which causes mixing of oxygenated and de-oxygenated blood.
Pulmonary stenosis	Narrowing of the pulmonary valve, which restricts the blood flow from the right ventricle to the lungs.
Right ventricular hypertrophy	Thickening of the right ventricle muscle wall due to the ventricle working against increased pressure.
Overriding aorta	The aorta is located above the VSD; this results in the aorta receiving blood from both ventricles.

(Adapted from Anderson et al., 2010)

Clinical presentation

- Cyanosis
- Heart murmur
- Clubbing of fingers and toes (mainly in older children)
- **Tet spells** – sudden episodes of deep cyanosis, irritability, and/or fainting due to desaturations

Management

- Management of Tet spells
- Lower target SpO_2 to avoid pulmonary over-circulation
- Surgery

TRICUSPID ATRESIA

Albeit rare, this is a serious CHD, where the tricuspid valve fails to form properly. This valve separates the right atrium from the right ventricle, so that blood flow between the two, and subsequently normal circulation, can be impeded.

Pathophysiology

- The tricuspid valve is absent which results in the right ventricle being underdeveloped.
- When blood returns to the right atrium it needs to find its way to the left ventricle, typically via the ASD, and then toward the lungs via a VSD or PDA.

Clinical presentation

- Typically early, in the first few days of life
- Severe cyanosis (this can vary depending on the levels of mixing)
- Dyspnoea
- Fatigue when feeding
- FTT
- Heart murmur

Management

- Readily available PGE1 infusion to maintain patency of shunts.
- Long term surgery, beginning with a temporary Blalock-Taussig shunt, followed by a bidirectional Glenn procedure and a Fontan procedure (Lai et al., 2015).

Duct-dependent systemic lesions

COARCTATION OF THE AORTA

CoA (Figure 15.11) is a CCHD where there is narrowing (coarctation) of the aorta, the major blood vessel which carries oxygen rich blood around the body. This results in increased blood pressure in the upper half of the body compared to the lower part of the body.

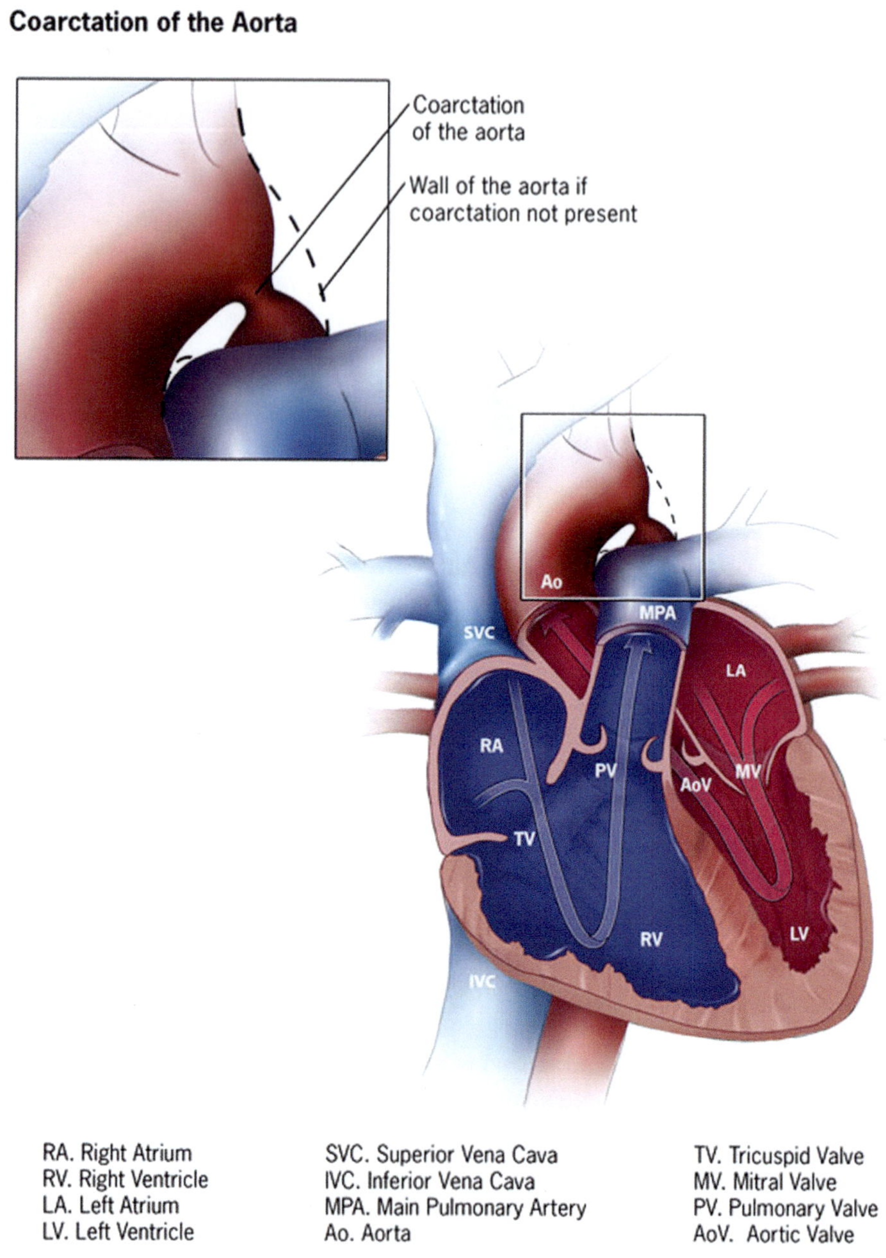

Figure 15.11 Coarctation of the aorta (Source: Creative Commons)

Pathophysiology

- There is a tight constriction to the aorta, typically close to the ductus arteriosus (DA) where it joins the arch. This becomes problematic postnatally, when the DA begins to close secondary to commencement of breathing (ductal tissue is sensitive to oxygen).

- The left ventricle then needs to work harder to try to push blood beyond the defect, which can lead to hypertension and result in heart failure.

Clinical presentation

- Murmur
- Absent femoral pulses
- Breathlessness on feeding
- Heart failure/shock if DA closes
- Pre- and post-ductal oxygen saturation difference
- Lower limb blood pressure lower than those of the upper limbs

Management

If there is suspicion antenatally

- May require PGE1 infusion from birth
- If there is uncertainty from antenatal scans, a 'watch and wait' approach may be adopted, with admission to NNU and monitoring without PGE1 infusion
- Balloon angioplasty and stenting are the definitive treatment

If not known antenatally

- Some clinical features may be present after birth or during the NIPE, but if the DA has not closed prior to discharge, signs may not become apparent until later, so that the infant presents to the emergency department (Gossett, 2024).

INTERRUPTED AORTIC ARCH

IAA is a rare, life-threatening CHD that results in incomplete connection of the aorta, i.e. there is a gap between the ascending and descending portions. This interruption inhibits the flow of oxygen-rich blood from reaching the lower body, which is a medical emergency post-delivery.

Pathophysiology

- The gap between the upper and lower portion of the aorta inhibits blood flow to the lower half of the body
- Malposition of the subclavian artery
- Circulation needs to be maintained by shunting of blood via PDA or VSD if present
- Can be associated with 22q11 (DiGeorge syndrome)

Clinical presentation

- Severe cyanosis
- Weak/absent femoral pulses
- Poor perfusion/cold extremities
- Metabolic acidosis
- Shock
- Heart failure

Management

- PGE1 infusion
- Correct acidosis
- Manage shock
- Surgery within the neonatal period

HYPOPLASTIC LEFT HEART SYNDROME

HLHS (see Figure 15.12) is a severe and complex CHD because of underdevelopment of left-sided cardiac structures. This involves the left ventricle, mitral valve, aortic valve, and ascending aorta, all essential for supplying the body with oxygenated blood. These are either too small or absent, so that normal circulation cannot occur. This is life threatening from birth if not managed appropriately.

Pathophysiology

- Left ventricle too small to function
- Mitral and aortic valves may be stenosed or closed
- Ascending aorta is extremely small; this limits blood flow
- Issues arise after birth when DA and PFO close

Clinical presentation

- Profound cyanosis
- Weak pulses, especially in lower limbs
- Cold, mottled skin and poor perfusion
- Lethargy on feeding
- Shock/heart failure

Management

- PGE1 infusion

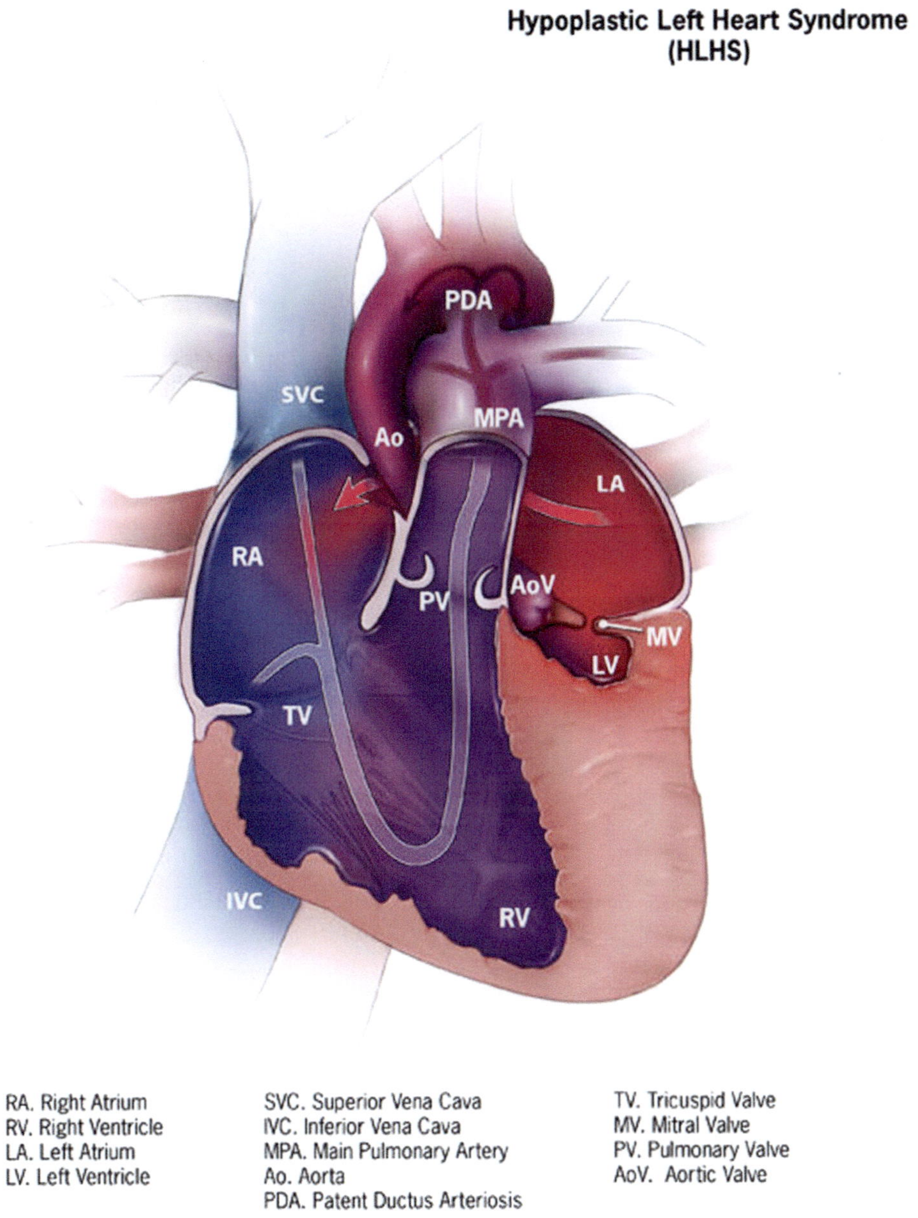

Figure 15.12 Hypoplastic left heart syndrome

- Ventilation
- Metabolic support
- Inotropes
- Ultimately multiple surgeries are required: Norwood procedure, Glenn procedure, and a Fontan procedure (Cheung, 2023)

ACTIVITY

Find out the side effects of prostaglandin and devise a care plan for a baby on a PGE1 infusion taking them into consideration

Non-duct dependent lesions

TOTAL ANOMALOUS PULMONARY VENOUS RETURN

TAPVR (Figure 15.13) is a rare CHD in which the veins that usually carry oxygen-rich blood from the lungs are not connected to the left atrium; they instead drain into the right side of the heart, mixing oxygenated with deoxygenated blood. This is a critical lesion with different types (Table 15.5).

TABLE 15.5 TYPES OF TOTAL ANOMALOUS PULMONARY VENOUS RETURN

Type	*Pathophysiology*	*Info*
Supracardiac	Pulmonary veins drain above the heart into the superior vena cava	Most common
Cardiac	Veins drain directly into the right atrium or coronary sinus	Moderately severe
Infradiaphragmatic	Veins drain below the heart into the abdominal veins	Often obstructed and life threatening
Mixed	Combination of all the above	Complex and life threatening

Clinical presentation

- Tachypnoea
- Cyanosis (particularly around lips and fingertips)
- Poor feeding
- Lethargy
- Heart murmur

This condition can typically present similar to PPHN. Prostaglandin infusions can offer some temporary support in unobstructed or mixed lesions, but if obstructed, pulmonary congestion will worsen (Tsoi et al., 2023).

Total Anomalous Pulmonary Venous Return

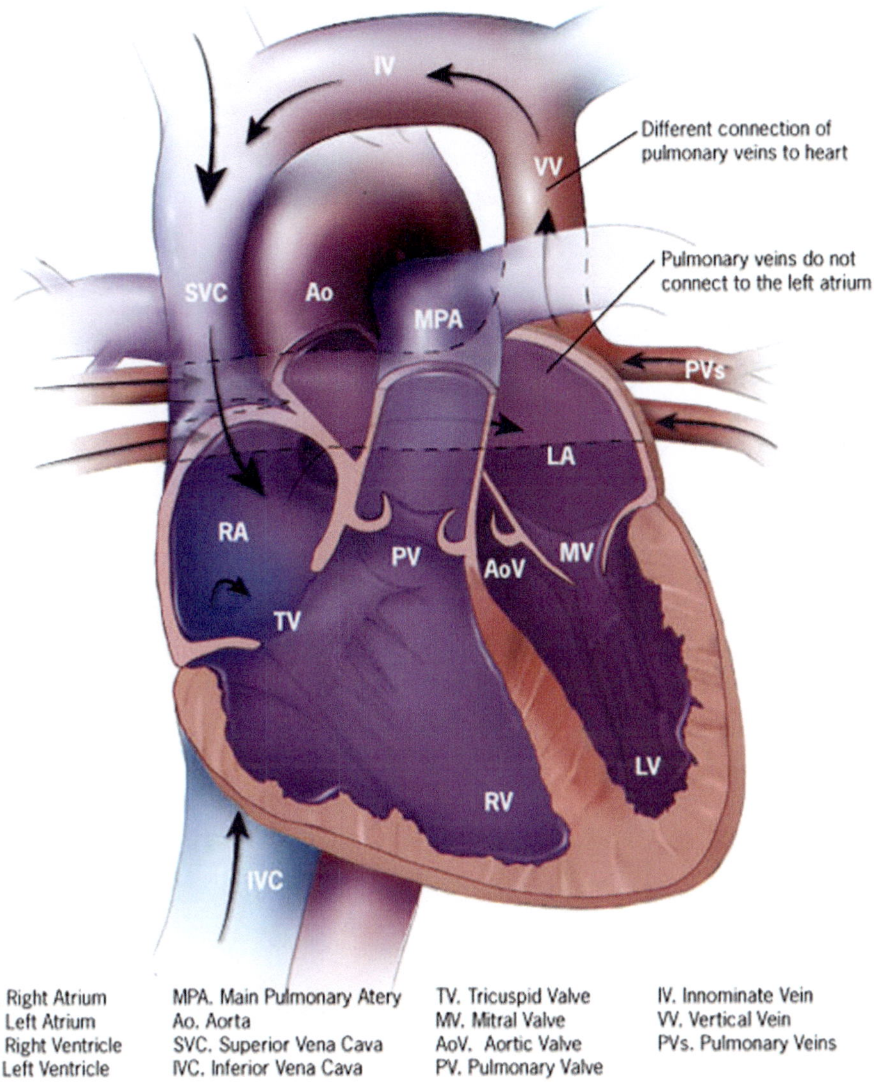

Figure 15.13 Total anomalous pulmonary venous return

VENTRICULAR SEPTAL DEFECT

VSD (Figure 15.14) is the incomplete formation of the cardiac wall that separates the right and left ventricles. This can result in mixing of oxygenated blood from the left ventricle with oxygen-poor blood in the right ventricle. Some smaller lesions may be insignificant and close spontaneously, whereas larger defects can lead to pulmonary over-circulation, respiratory problems, and heart failure and will require surgery. The principal presentation of this lesion is a heart murmur.

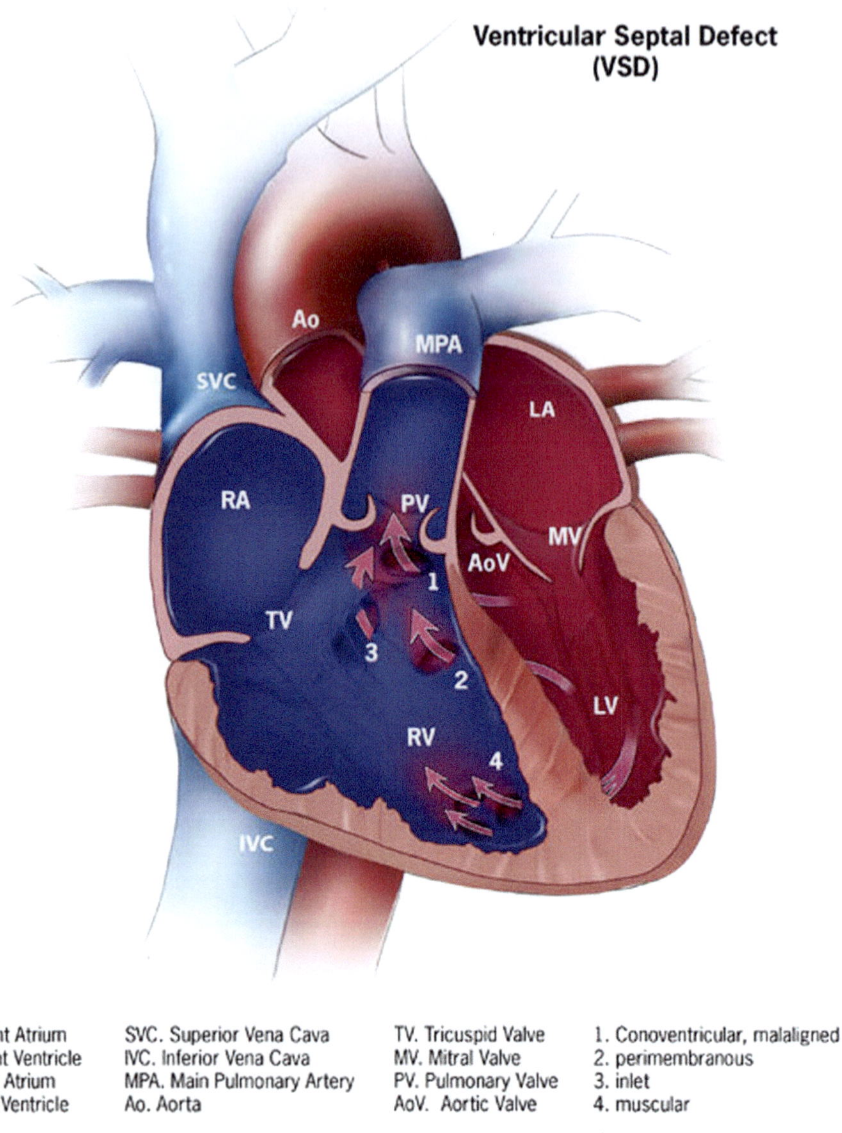

Figure 15.14 Ventricular septal defect

ATRIAL SEPTAL DEFECT

ASD (Figure 15.15) a lesion which allows for communication between the atria and increases blood flow in the pulmonary circuit, and symptoms may be subtle. It may present as a systolic murmur, smaller lesions even potentially asymptomatic, while larger defects can lead to volume overload.

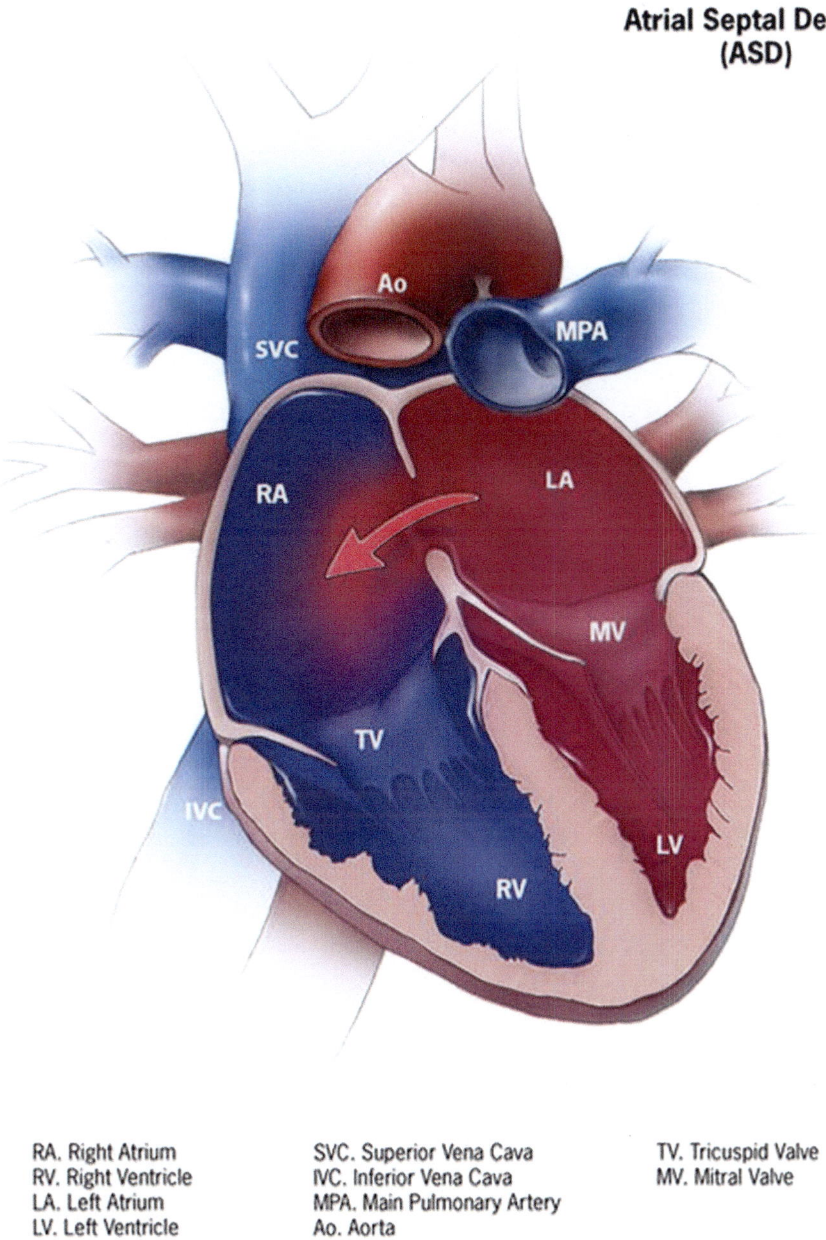

Figure 15.15 Atrial septal defect (Source: Creative Commons)

ATRIOVENTRICULAR SEPTAL DEFECT

AVSD (Figure 15.16) is a congenital cardiac anomaly characterised by incomplete formation of both the atrial and ventricular septa.

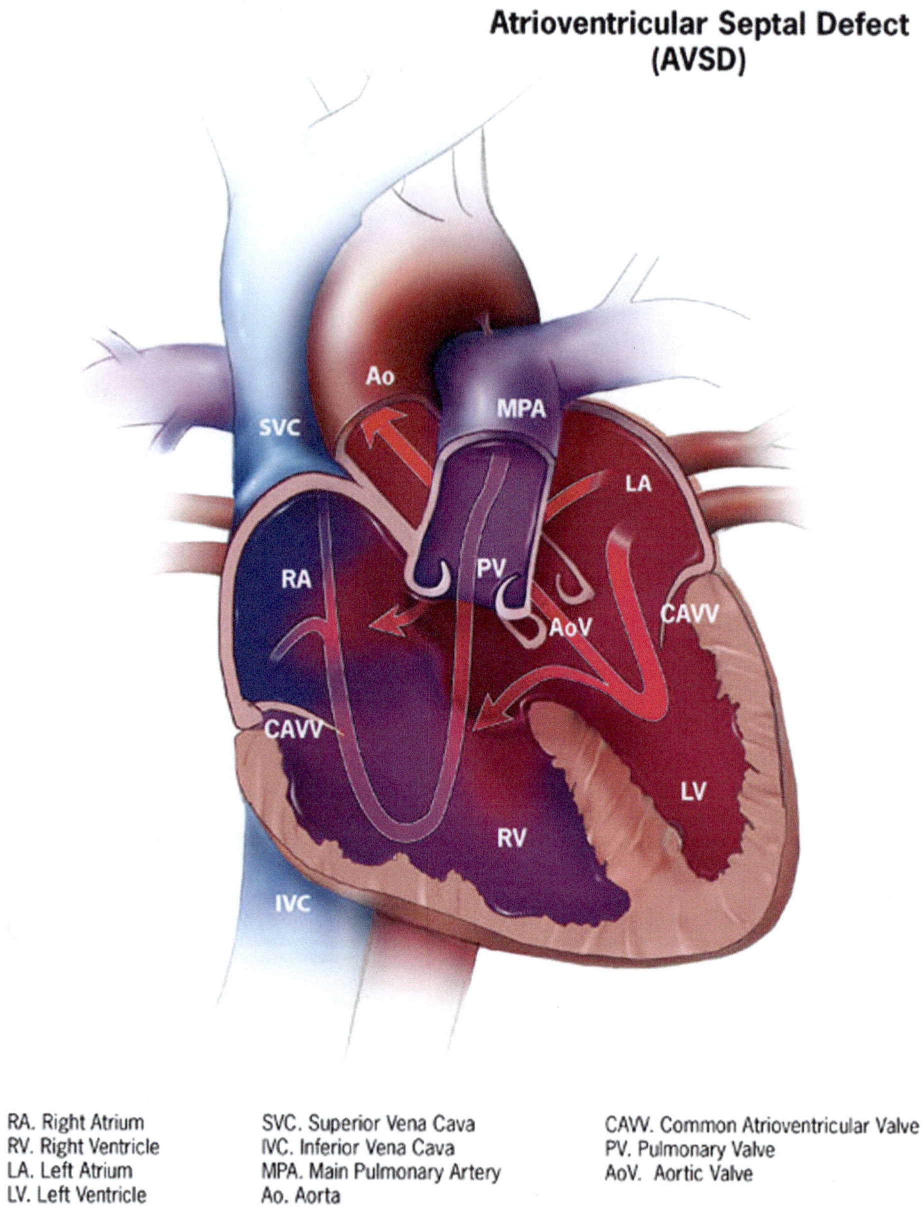

Figure 15.16 Atrioventricular septal defect (Source: Creative Commons)

BOX 15.1 PROSTAGLANDIN INFUSION

1. Starting dose typically 5 nanograms/kg/min
2. If no improvement, this can be escalated to 10–15 nanograms/kg/min in increments of 5 nanograms/kg/min

3. Maximum dose is 100 nanograms/kg/min, but this should be only in discussion with cardiology

   Important to note: one of the principal side effects of PGE1 is apnoea and mostly documented to occur > 12.5nanograms/kg/min but can occur at any dosing.

   - *Access considerations* Ideally, the infusion should have a dedicated line, and if peripheral rather than central access is being used, a second cannula should be sited in the event of extravasation or loss of cannula, so the infusion can be quickly transferred across.

Administration notes Some recommendations suggest an infusion rate of no less than 1mL/hr; if the infusion is running at a rate less than this, consider making up the difference with a supplementary infusion of compatible fluid. This increases the likelihood of occlusion detection and prevention of backflow, optimising PGE1 delivery.

OTHER CARDIOVASCULAR DISORDERS AND THEIR MANAGEMENT

Hypotension

Hypotension is a critical concern in neonatal care, requiring careful monitoring and clinical judgment. Traditionally, blood pressure (BP) management in preterm infants was guided by the concept that the mean arterial blood pressure (MAP) should match the infant's gestational age in weeks (e.g. a 25-week infant should have a MAP of 25mmHg or above). However, this approach was not evidence-based, and in many cases, aggressive intervention to meet these arbitrary thresholds may have done more harm than good (Murphy et al., 2023).

Nurses play a vital role in assessing and managing neonatal blood pressure, using both invasive (arterial lines) and non-invasive (oscillometric/cuff) methods to monitor BP. However, BP alone is not a definitive indicator of adequate circulation. Relying solely on numerical values has led to overtreatment, including excessive administration of volume and inotropes, which may have contributed to fluid overload, intraventricular haemorrhage, and other complications (Abdul Aziz et al., 2020).

A more individualised approach to neonatal perfusion is now encouraged, integrating BP measurements with cotside assessments (Dore et al., 2024). Key indicators such as; capillary refill time (CRT), peripheral perfusion (skin:shin gap), lactate, and urine output have been used provide a more accurate picture of circulatory health (see Box 15.2), but these parameters can be subjective (Murphy et al., 2023). This change in practice acknowledges that a 'low' BP number alone does not always signify compromised circulation, and conversely, a 'normal' BP does not guarantee adequate organ perfusion.

BOX 15.2 CLINICAL SIGNS OF POOR ORGAN PERFUSION

- Skin and superficial tissue perfusion: in low CO states, blood supply to the skin is diverted to vital organs. Skin perfusion can be assessed by timing capillary refill and measuring central-peripheral temperature gap. Both of these can be affected by the thermal environment.
- Metabolic acidosis: tissue hypoxia leads to anaerobic metabolism and lactate production.
- Reduced urine output: a urine output < 1 ml/kg/hour is indicative of inadequate kidney perfusion (Murphy et al., 2023).
- Reduced conscious level: with severe hypotension comes a loss of autoregulation of blood flow in the brain so that babies may become encephalopathic (Sinha et al., 2018).

In addition, BP can be assessed by:

Functional echocardiography: Performed at the bedside, functional echocardiography evaluates CO, ductal shunting, and myocardial function, offering a more direct assessment of hemodynamic stability. While again inter-operator variability has been described as a potential issue, in the context of structured training programmes and clearly defined procedures for execution and treatment escalation echocardiography leads to significantly more targeted and individualised management of hypotension than BP thresholds.

Near-infrared spectroscopy (NIRS): A non-invasive method that measures regional tissue oxygenation (e.g. cerebral and splanchnic perfusion), helping to identify cases where BP is 'normal,' but tissue perfusion is inadequate.

Although not standard investigations for guiding treatment, these tools may provide valuable data to be considered in the clinical context of the baby (Murphy et al., 2023). By combining traditional monitoring, new technology with hands-on clinical assessment, neonatal nurses play a crucial role in recognising true circulatory compromise and ensuring interventions are guided by the infant's overall physiological status rather than an arbitrary BP mean target.

Management of hypotension must be targeted to the underlying cause. If the aetiology is a diminished preload as seen in hypovolemia and septic shock, then the first action would be to fill the vascular compartment with volume. If afterload has been compromised, for example by depleted vascular resistance in septic shock/necrotising enterocolitis (NEC), then adrenaline (epinephrine) may cause a sufficient increase in peripheral vascular resistance. If the myocardium is in a poor metabolic state and contractility is diminished, as seen in hypoxic injury, then dobutamine is an inotrope which improves cardiac function. Finally, if HR is not adequate to sustain a good CO, noradrenaline (norepinephrine) may be indicated to induce tachycardia as well as increase contractility and vascular resistance.

VOLUME REPLACEMENT

Cautious volume administration of a normal saline bolus is reasonable and has been shown to transiently improve left ventricular output. Sick premature infants may become hypovolaemic due to insensible water loss; however, overall hypovolemia is a less common cause in the preterm infant. Volume replacement will be beneficial mostly to preterm infants with a background of blood loss, or vasoactive shock, as is seen in sepsis or necrotising enterocolitis. Importantly, overzealous administration of fluids to premature infants may be harmful (Mullaly & El-Khuffash, 2024).

INOTROPES AND VASOPRESSORS

Adrenaline Low to moderate-dose adrenaline is now more frequently used instead of dopamine to treat hypotension, including in very low birthweight (VLBW) infants. At these doses, its β-adrenergic effects predominate, increasing CO and BP despite some vasodilation. In contrast, higher doses trigger stronger α-adrenergic activity, raising vascular resistance, reducing CO, and risking impaired organ perfusion. Short-term side effects include tachycardia, raised lactate, reduced bicarbonate, and hyperglycemia. Importantly, cautious dose escalation in hypotensive VLBW infants has not been linked to adverse outcomes such as death or neurodevelopmental problems (Goldsmith & Keels, 2022).

Dobutamine has mainly β_2 effects, raising BP by increasing myocardial contractility, but with some reduction in systemic vascular resistance. Compared with dopamine it is thought to lead to improved end-organ perfusion due to increased ventricular output (Goldsmith & Keels, 2022).

Noradrenaline has not been extensively studied in the neonatal population but there is evidence of its good effect in septic shock. It has both α- and ß-receptor effects, equating to increased contractility and tachycardia. The main effect is vasoconstriction, thus increasing systemic vascular resistance. The use of noradrenaline has been associated with compromised peripheral perfusion, so that the baby needs to be carefully monitored for signs of this (Garegrat et al., 2024).

Dopamine produces a mixture of cardiovascular effects, the main being vasodilation in the renal circulation as well as increased CO. In low doses, it has a primary dopaminergic effect and vasodilates renal, coronary and possibly cerebral circulation. In higher doses, it stimulates β_1 receptors, which enhances myocardial contractility and increases HR. At the highest dose (10–20mcg/kg/minute), the effects are almost exclusively α_1-adrenergic. For many years the first choice to treat hypotension, dopamine is now less favoured as it is recognised to negatively impact end organ perfusion and myocardial function at higher doses. It is also contraindicated in infants with suspected or confirmed pulmonary hypertension, as it can worsen pulmonary vasoconstriction (Goldsmith & Keels, 2022).

CORTICOSTEROIDS

Preterm infants often have limited cortisol production due to an immature hypothalamic–pituitary axis, resulting in a reduced stress response. Hydrocortisone can be considered in cases of refractory hypotension or when major blood loss or asphyxia may compromise adrenal perfusion but should be used with caution due to a link with NEC and intestinal perforation (Mullaly & El-Khuffash, 2024).

NURSING CONSIDERATIONS

A proportion of significantly hypotensive newborns will require invasive ventilation, which increases their risk of pneumothorax or pneumopericardium, both of which impair venous return. It is imperative that if nursing a baby who is not responding to inotropes, other possible causes of hypotension be considered (see Box 15.3).

BOX 15.3 POTENTIAL CAUSES OF HYPOTENSION

- Prescription or administration error (check all infusions and doses)
- Pneumothorax
- Pericardial tamponade
- Extreme hypovolemia

- High mean airway pressure (especially on high frequency oscillatory ventilation)
- Hidden blood loss (intra-ventricular haemorrhage (IVH) or scalp, bowel, twin-to-twin transfusion, or feto-maternal haemorrhage)
- PPHN (check pre- and post-ductal oxygen saturation)
- Congenital heart defect
- Drug side effects

Adapted from Mullaly and El-Khuffash (2024)

Hypertension

Neonatal hypertension is being recognised with increasing frequency, a trend largely driven by advances in neonatal intensive care, improved survival of extremely premature infants, and a more sophisticated understanding of neonatal cardiovascular physiology. BP regulation in this population is multifactorial, with gestational age, birthweight, and postmenstrual age exerting significant influence, yet normative reference ranges (see Table 15.6) remain poorly defined, complicating diagnostic thresholds. Careful evaluation often reveals an underlying aetiology, with umbilical catheter-associated thrombosis, renal parenchymal disease, and chronic lung disease representing the most common causes. Diagnosis typically involves perinatal history, targeted imaging such as renal ultrasound and Doppler studies, and laboratory assessment of renal function and electrolytes. Therapeutic decision-making is challenging, as evidence supporting antihypertensive pharmacotherapy in neonates is sparse, necessitating reliance on clinical expertise and

TABLE 15.6 BLOOD PRESSURE VALUES IN INFANTS

Postconceptional age		*95th percentile*	*99th percentile*
40 weeks	Systolic BP	95 mmHg	100 mmHg
	Diastolic BP	65 mmHg	70 mmHg
	MAP	75 mmHg	80 mmHg
30 weeks	Systolic BP	80 mmHg	85 mmHg
	Diastolic BP	55 mmHg	54 mmHg
	MAP	65 mmHg	63 mmHg
26 weeks	Systolic BP	72 mmHg	77 mmHg
	Diastolic BP	50 mmHg	56 mmHg
	MAP	57 mmHg	63 mmHg

(adapted from Dionne et al., 2012)

extrapolation from older paediatric cohorts; agents including calcium channel blockers, beta-blockers, and angiotensin-converting enzyme (ACE) inhibitors may be considered, though dosing and safety data are limited. Despite these complexities, the long-term outlook is generally favourable, with hypertension resolving in the majority of affected infants as they mature (Starr & Flynn, 2019).

Patent ductus arteriosus

Patency of the DA (Figure 15.17) is maintained *in utero* through prostaglandins and low levels of oxygen; thus, following birth increased oxygenation and lower concentrations of prostaglandins lead to constriction of the DA, usually within 72 hours in well term infants. In preterm infants, however, ductal closure is often delayed due to immaturity-related physiological differences. Postnatal changes to the pressure gradients within the neonatal cardiovascular system subsequently lead to shunting of blood from the systemic to the pulmonary circulation across the DA. This results in reduced renal, gastrointestinal and cerebral perfusion, associated with increased risks of NEC, intestinal perforation and IVH. Simultaneously, there is circulatory overload of the lung leading potentially to a prolonged need for mechanical ventilation, pulmonary haemorrhage, exacerbation

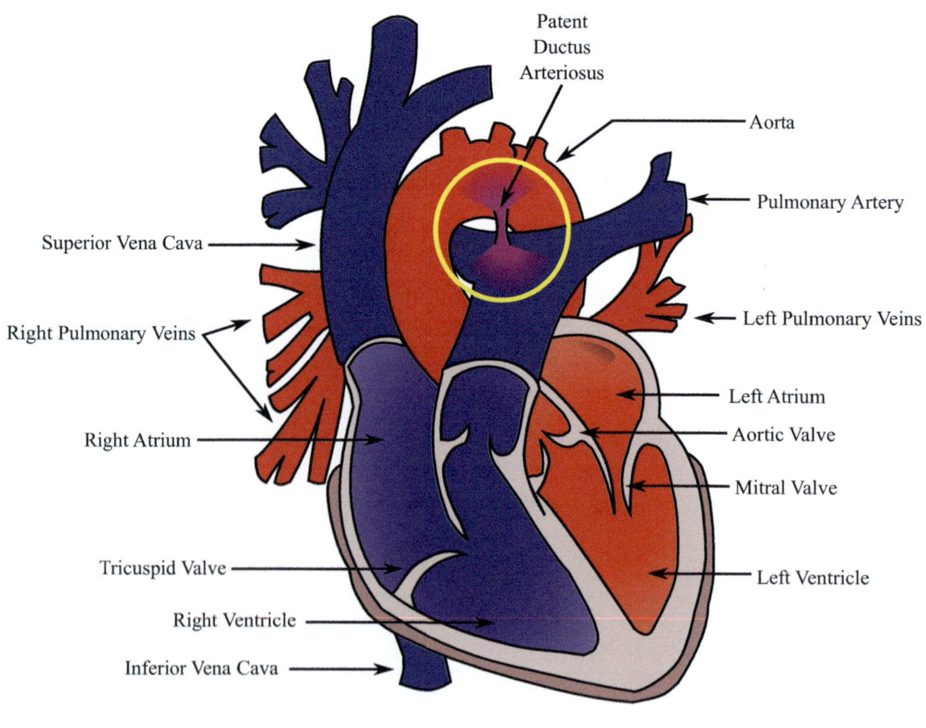

Figure 15.17 Patent ductus arteriosus

of respiratory distress syndrome, and possibly chronic lung disease (Ohlsson et al., 2020; Benitz & Bhombal, 2024).

Symptoms of a PDA include a heart murmur, apnoeas, bounding pulses, an active precordium, significant systolic/diastolic BP difference, and fluctuating oxygen saturations (Benitz & Bhombal, 2024). Asymptomatic infants should be monitored for any evidence of heart failure, failure to thrive, increasing oxygen requirements, or other complications (Swanson & Erickson, 2020).

Controversy remains as to whether active treatment of a PDA is preferable to no intervention (Ohlsson et al., 2020), with emerging evidence suggesting improved outcomes with early treatment of a haemodynamically significant PDA (Gillam-Krakauer and Reese, 2024). PDA management consists of pharmacological or surgical treatment, with the latter generally implemented when drug therapy has been unsuccessful (Benitz & Bhombal, 2024).

There are currently three options for pharmacological management: indomethacin, ibuprofen or paracetamol. Indomethacin and ibuprofen function via inhibition of prostaglandin synthesis. Paracetamol has a similar but weaker effect on the same enzymes as the above, so its effect on the DA may be secondary to yet unidentified mechanisms (Jasani et al., 2022).

As reduced prostaglandin synthesis results in vasoconstriction not only of the DA, the risks associated with pharmacological treatment are similar to those posed by the PDA itself, i.e. NEC/bowel perforation, poor renal function and increased risk of IVH. A side effect observed with indomethacin and ibuprofen is thrombocytopenia, so this therapy should not be commenced in infants with low platelet levels (Ohlsson et al., 2020).

In view of potentially hazardous side effects, prophylactic pharmacological management of the PDA has not become standard practice, as an improvement of long-term outcomes has not been demonstrated (Mitra et al., 2023).

Multiple trials have shown ibuprofen to be as effective as indomethacin in achieving ductal closure, but with less severe adverse effects (Ohlsson et al., 2020). The efficacy of paracetamol needs yet to be addressed in further research trials, but there is evidence that it causes ductal constriction with fewer renal and gastrointestinal side effects than ibuprofen or indomethacin, even in infants where these drugs have not been effective. Further research, particularly taking into consideration long-term neurodevelopmental outcomes, is required in light of suggestions of an association of prolonged paracetamol use and autism spectrum disorders (Jasani et al., 2022).

Surgical intervention, historically ligation involving thoracotomy, is not without risk: potential side effects include chylothorax, left vocal cord paresis, and prolonged period of intensive care. More recently, transcatheter ductal closure has been successfully implemented in infants as small as 700 grams, with fewer adverse effects. Long-term outcome data are still pending (Benitz & Bhombal, 2024).

From a nursing perspective, careful observation of the infant throughout the duration of treatment, including monitoring for abdominal concerns, any signs of bleeding and measurements of urine output, is vital. Surgical intervention is reserved for infants with hemodynamically significant PDAs, for example ventilator-dependent babies; those who are not eligible for medical treatment; where this is not effective; or where the DA reopens following initial pharmacological closure.

Persistent pulmonary hypertension of the newborn

This subject is covered in detail in Chapter 14.

Dysrhythmias

Disorders of HR and rhythm may occur in the antenatal or postnatal period. It is important for neonatal nurses to be able to detect an abnormal HR or rhythm, to enable swift remedial or supportive action, if required, the majority of neonatal dysrhythmias do not require intervention. The three commonest dysrhythmias encountered in the neonatal period are described below.

SUPRAVENTRICULAR TACHYCARDIA

Supraventricular tachycardia (SVT) is considered a HR greater than 220 beats per minute and can be a result of either a congenital cause, such as an aberrant electrical pathway re-entering the atrioventricular node causing it to depolarise in asynchrony with the cardiac cycle, or an iatrogenic cause, for example, a misplaced umbilical catheter in the right atrium stimulating the sinoatrial node. Recurrent SVTs can also affect the fetus during pregnancy, often lead to the development of hydrops, and can result in death (Swanson & Erickson, 2020). To avoid heart failure in the neonate, remedial action (see Box 15.4) is required.

BOX 15.4 MANAGEMENT OF SVT

1. Vagal stimulation
2. Adenosine (150–300microgram/kg) by rapid intravenous/intraosseous injection.
3. Direct current cardioversion (0.5–1J/kg; adapted from Swanson & Erickson, 2020).

CONGENITAL ATRIOVENTRICULAR BLOCK

Congenital heart block can be due to a cardiac abnormality, such as TGA (see above), or damage to the conducting system from maternal antibodies secondary to connective tissue disorders such as systemic lupus erythematosus. Third degree heart block, known as complete heart block, presents as profound bradycardia. Mostly these infants recover without further intervention; some, however, will require a pacemaker (Swanson & Erickson, 2020).

VENTRICULAR TACHYCARDIA

Ventricular tachycardia (VT) is rare in the neonate and often presents with cardiac arrest rather than notable tachycardia. It usually occurs with pathologies such as hypoxaemia, electrolyte disturbances, or shock and is not always easy to differentiate from SVT, even with the aid of an ECG. Pulseless VT, where the infant presents arrested, requires full resuscitation and direct current cardioversion. In infants who appear otherwise well, pharmacological management with lidocaine can be attempted; maintenance therapy is with lidocaine, amiodarone, or propranolol (Swanson & Erickson, 2020).

Chapter takeaways

- A solid grasp of cardiac embryology and fetal circulation helps neonatal nurses understand how structural defects arise and how newborns may present. This knowledge underpins accurate assessment during the critical transition from fetal to neonatal circulation.
- Symptoms such as central cyanosis, tachypnoea, feeding fatigue, diaphoresis, weak or absent femoral pulses, and hepatomegaly should raise suspicion for CHD. Many duct-dependent lesions deteriorate rapidly as the ductus arteriosus closes, making early recognition essential.
- Pulse oximetry screening, antenatal anomaly scans, and echocardiography form the backbone of early CHD detection. Supporting investigations such as CXR, ECG, and blood gases help differentiate cardiac from respiratory causes of instability.
- Lesions such as TGA, HLHS, pulmonary atresia, and severe CoA rely on a patent ductus arteriosus for survival. Prostaglandin E1 infusion, careful ventilation, and avoidance of excessive oxygen are key stabilisation strategies before transfer to a cardiac centre.
- Conditions such as hypotension, hypertension, PDA, and arrhythmias require nuanced interpretation of perfusion, blood pressure trends, and functional echocardiography. Management often involves balancing preload, afterload, and contractility while avoiding iatrogenic harm.

- Neonatal nurses are pivotal in detecting subtle deterioration through continuous monitoring, pulse assessment, auscultation, and evaluation of feeding tolerance. Their observations guide escalation, intervention, and multidisciplinary decision-making.
- Infants with CHD often expend significant energy on breathing and circulation, leading to poor feeding endurance and failure to thrive. Early nutritional planning, including nasogastric feeds, high-calorie formulas, or feeding support, can significantly improve outcomes.

CASE STUDY

CASE STUDIES

Case study 1: The term baby with failed pulse oximetry screening

Neil is a 6-hour-old term baby who has failed pulse oximetry screening, with both upper and lower saturation reading 78%. He is tachypnoeic but has no other signs of respiratory distress.

Q.1. What are the cyanotic defects presenting with failed pulse oximetry?
Q.2. What defect can present with higher post-ductal saturations compared to pre-ductal?

Neil is started on a prostaglandin infusion.

Q.3. What is the aim of the prostaglandin infusion in this case?
Q.4. What are the side effects of prostaglandin?
Q.5. What particular nursing care does this baby need?

Case study 2: The term baby with absent femoral pulses

Ryan is a 5-day-old term baby who is completing a course of antibiotics for pneumonia on the postnatal ward. On his discharge examination, the femoral pulses cannot be felt. The baby is otherwise well and feeding normally.

Q.1. What congenital heart defect is most commonly associated with absent femoral pulses?
Q.2. Is the pulmonary or systemic circulation affected?
Q.3. What could you do to provide more information regarding the possible diagnosis before the echocardiogram is performed?

A prostaglandin infusion is commenced.

Q.4. What is the aim of the prostaglandin infusion in this case?
Q.5. What would you expect to happen once prostaglandin is commenced?

Case study 3: Hypotension in a preterm infant

Kiyomi is a 25-week gestation infant who is now 8 hours old. She has been stable since admission, minimally ventilated, has commenced parenteral nutrition, and has umbilical lines in situ. You notice that for the past 10 minutes her MABP has been reading 22–24mmHg.

Q.1. What are your first steps to verify if this is a true reflection of Kiyomi's BP? What else would your clinical assessment include?
Q.2. What would the initial pharmacological management of her hypotension be?

Kiyomi has been started on a dobutamine infusion. There is suboptimal response to this at 15mcg/kg/minute, so a dopamine infusion is also started at initially 5mcg/kg/minute.

Q.3. Other than the desired increase in BP, what other changes in Kiyomi's parameters might you observe?
Q.4. In the case of a poor response, what other causes of hypotension would you need to consider? Which investigations could aid in the diagnosis of these?

Case study 4: The baby with a VSD

Shelley is a 2-week-old term baby admitted for poor feeding and has been found to have a heart murmur due to a ventricular septal defect (VSD). Over the past few days she has become increasingly tachypnoeic and in need of nasal cannula oxygen.

Q.1. What is happening and why?
Q.2. What other signs would you expect to see?
Q.3. What medical treatment would you expect this baby to have?
Q.4. What are the principles of nursing care for this baby?

For suggested answer guides to the questions posed in these case studies, please refer to the web-based companion site specific to this chapter. See www.routledge.com/cw/petty

References

Abdul Aziz, A. N., Thomas, S., Murthy, P., Rabi, Y., Soraisham, A., Stritzke, A., Kamaluddeen, M., Al-Awad, E., & Mohammad, K. (2020). Early inotrope use is associated with higher risk of death and/or severe brain injury in extremely premature infants. *The Journal of Maternal-Fetal & Neonatal Medicine*, *33*(16), 2751–2758.

Alkhushi, N. (2023). The management of newborns with critical congenital heart diseases prior to transport to a cardiac center. *The Cardiothoracic Surgeon*, *31*(1). Retrieved September 26, 2025, from https://cts.springeropen.com/articles/10.1186/s43057-022-00090-7

American Heart Association. (2025). *As people born with congenital heart defects now live longer, challenges evolve over time*. Retrieved September 26, 2025, from https://www.heart.org/en/news/2025/01/10/as-people-born-with-congenital-heart-defects-now-live-longer-challenges-evolve-over-time

Anderson, R. H., Baker, E. J., Penny, D. J., Redington, A. N., & Rigby, M. L. (2010). *Paediatric cardiology* (3rd ed.). Churchill Livingstone Elsevier.

Bakker, M. K., Bergman, J. E. H., Krikov, S., Amar, E., Cocchi, G., Cragan, J., De Walle, H. E. K., Gatt, M., Groisman, B., Liu, S., Nembhard, W. N., Pierini, A., Rissmann, A., Chidambarathanu, S., Sipek Jr., A., Szabova, E., Tagliabue, G., Tucker, D., Mastroiacovo, P., & Botto, L. D. (2019). Prenatal diagnosis and prevalence of critical congenital heart defects: An international retrospective cohort study. *BMJ Open*, *9*(7), e028139. Retrieved September 26, 2025, from https://doi.org/10.1136/bmjopen-2018-028139

Benitz, W. E., & Bhombal, S. (2024). Patent ductus arteriosus. In R. J. Martin, A. A. Fanaroff & M. C. Walsh (Eds.), *Fanaroff and Martin's neonatal-perinatal medicine: Diseases of the fetus and infant* (12th ed., pp. 1401–1410). Elsevier.

Bocks, M. L., Boe, B. A., & Galantowicz, M. E. (2020). Neonatal management of congenital heart disease. In R. J. Martin, A. A. Fanaroff & M. C. Walsh (Eds.), *Fanaroff and Martin's neonatal-perinatal medicine* (11th ed., pp. 1393–1414). Elsevier.

British Heart Foundation. (2025). *UK cardiovascular disease statistics factsheet*. Retrieved September 26, 2025, from https://www.bhf.org.uk/what-we-do/our-research/heart-statistics

Carlson, B. M. (2023). *Human embryology and developmental biology* (7th ed.). Elsevier.

Chan, B., & Singh, Y. (2022). Beyond prostaglandin E1: Management of infants with critical congenital heart defects. *NeoReviews*, *23*(5), e257–e267.

Chan, B., Woodbury, A., Hazelwood, L., & Singh, Y. (2025). Feeding approach to optimizing nutrition in infants with congenital heart disease. *Journal of Cardiovascular Development and Disease*, *12*(2), 38. https://doi.org/10.3390/jcdd12020038

Cheung, C. (2023). *Stage III Norwood procedure or fenestrated Fontan*. Congenital Heart Defects UK. Retrieved November 19, 2025, from http://www.congenital-heart-defects.co.uk/types-of-chd-and-operations/stage-iii-norwood-procedure-or-fenestrated-fontan

Cody, F., Franklin, O., Mc Cay, N., Molphy, Z., Dicker, P., & Breathnach, F. M. (2024). Critical congenital heart disease: Contemporary prenatal screening performance and outcomes in a multi-centre perinatology service. *BMC Pregnancy and Childbirth*, *24*(1), 163. Retrieved September 26, 2025, from https://doi.org/10.1186/s12884-024-06350-0

Dionne, J. M., Abitbol, C. L., & Flynn, J. T. (2012). Hypertension in infancy: Diagnosis, management and outcome. *Pediatric Nephrology*, *27*(1), 17–32. https://doi.org/10.1007/s00467-010-1755-z

Dore, R., Barnes, K., Bremner, S., Iwami, H. I., Apele-Freimane, D., Batton, B., Dempsey, E., Ergenekon, E., Klein, A., Pesco-Koplowitz, L., Dionne, J. M., & Rabe, H. (2024). Neonatal blood pressure by birth weight, gestational age, and postnatal age: A systematic review. *Maternal Health, Neonatology and Perinatology*, *10*(1), 9.

Dorobantu, D.-M., Espuny Pujol, F., Kostolny, M., Brown, K. L., Franklin, R. C., Crowe, S., Pagel, C., & Stoica, S. C. (2023). Arterial switch for transposition of the great arteries: Treatment timing, late outcomes, and risk factors. *JACC: Advances*, *2*(5), 100–104.

Dykes, J. C., Al-Mousily, M. F., Abuchaibe, E.-C., Silva, J. N., Zadinsky, J., Duarte, D., & Welch, E. (2016). The incidence of chromosome abnormalities in neonates with structural heart disease. *Heart*, *102*(8), 634–637.

Gardiner, H. M. (2023). Postnatal imaging of congenital heart disease: Evolving standards and technologies. *Archives of Disease in Childhood – Fetal and Neonatal Edition*, *108*(2), F121–F128.

Garegrat, R., Patnaik, S., Suryawanshi, S., Chetan, C., Banait, N., Singh, P., Kallimath, A., Soni, N. B., Singh, Y., & Suryawanshi, P. (2024). A pilot randomized controlled trial comparing noradrenaline and adrenaline as a first-line vasopressor for fluid-refractory septic shock in neonates. *Frontiers in Pediatrics*, *12*, 1443990. https://doi.org/10.3389/fped.2024.1443990

Giesinger, R. E., & McNamara, P. J. (2020). Hemodynamic consequences of PDA in preterm infants. *Neonatology*, *117*(3), 233–245.

Gillam-Krakauer, M., & Reese, J. (2024). We still don't know when to close a patent ductus arteriosus in infants born very premature. *The Journal of Pediatrics*, *265*, 113817. https://doi.org/10.1016/j.jpeds.2023.113817

Goldsmith, J. P., & Keels, E. (2022). Recognition and management of cardiovascular insufficiency in the very low birth weight newborn. *Pediatrics*, *149*(3), e2021056051. https://doi.org/10.1542/peds.2021-056051

Gonzalez, V. J., Kyle, W. B., & Allen, H. D. (2021). Cardiac examination and evaluation of murmurs. *Pediatrics In Review*, *42*(7), 375–382. https://doi.org/10.1542/pir.2020-000604

Gordan, R., Gwathmey, J. K., & Xie, L. H. (2015). Autonomic and endocrine control of cardiovascular function. *World Journal of Cardiology*, *7*(4), 204.

Gossett, J. (2024). *BMJ best practice. Aortic coarctation*. Retrieved September 23, 2025, from https://bestpractice.bmj.com/topics/en-gb/698

Grosse-Wortmann, L., & Al-Otay, A. (2023). Diagnostic approach to cyanosis in neonates: Revisiting the hyperoxia test. *Pediatric Cardiology*, *44*(1), 101–109.

Haddad, R. N., Hanna, N., Charbel, R., Daou, L., Chehab, G., & Saliba, Z. (2019). Ductal stenting to improve pulmonary blood flow in pulmonary atresia with intact ventricular septum and critical pulmonary stenosis after balloon valvuloplasty. *Cardiology in the Young*, *29*(4), 492–498.

Helm, B. M., Helvaty, L. R., Conboy, E., Geddes, G. C., Graham, B. H., Lah, M., Wetherill, L., Landis, B. J., & Ware, S. M. (2024). Performance of dysmorphology-based screening for genetic disorders in pediatric congenital heart disease supports wider genetic testing. *Molecular Genetics & Genomic Medicine*, *12*(11), e70040.

Jasani, B., Mitra, S., & Shah, P. S. (2022). Paracetamol (acetaminophen) for patent ductus arteriosus in preterm or low birth weight infants. *Cochrane Database of Systematic Reviews*, *12*, Art. No.: CD010061. Retrieved December 1, 2025, from https://doi.org/10.1002/14651858.CD010061.pub5

Jones, K. L., Jones, M. C., & Campo, M. del. (2022). *Smith's recognizable patterns of human malformation* (8th ed.). Elsevier.

Jullien, S. (2021). Newborn pulse oximetry screening for critical congenital heart defects. *BMC Pediatrics*, *21*(Suppl 1), Article 305.

Koeppen, B. M., Stanton, B. A., Hall, J. A., & Swiatecka-Urban, A. (Eds.). (2024). *Berne & Levy physiology* (8th ed.). Elsevier.

Lai, L., Starnes, V. A., & Alejos, J. C. (2015). Surgical management of congenital heart disease: Staged palliation for single ventricle physiology. In M. Gersony (Ed.), *Pediatric cardiology for practitioners* (6th ed., pp. 245–260). Elsevier Saunders.

Liu, Y., Yue, L., & Chang, L. (2024). Maternal gestational diabetes mellitus and congenital heart disease in offspring: A meta-analysis. *Hormone and Metabolic Research*, *56*(8), 574–584.

McGinn, C., Casey, F. A., Watson, C., & Morrison, L. (2023). Paediatric heart failure – understanding the pathophysiology and the current role of cardiac biomarkers in clinical practice. *Cardiology in the Young*, *33*(4), 503–513. https://doi.org/10.1017/S1047951123000331

Mitchell, A. L. (2024). Congenital anomalies. In R. J. Martin, A. A. Fanaroff & M. C. Walsh (Eds.), *Fanaroff and Martin's neonatal-perinatal medicine: Diseases of the fetus and infant* (12th ed., pp. 504–528). Elsevier.

Mitra, S., De Boode, W. P., Weisz, D. E., & Shah, P. S. (2023). Interventions for patent ductus arteriosus (PDA) in preterm infants: An overview of Cochrane Systematic Reviews. *Cochrane Database of Systematic Reviews, 2023*(4). https://doi.org/10.1002/14651858.CD013588.pub2

Mullaly, R., & El-Khuffash, A. F. (2024). Haemodynamic assessment and management of hypotension in the preterm. *Archives of Disease in Childhood – Fetal and Neonatal Edition, 109*(2), 120–127. https://doi.org/10.1136/archdischild-2022-324935

Murphy, E., Healy, D. B., Chioma, R., & Dempsey, E. M. (2023). Evaluation of the hypotensive preterm infant: Evidence-based practice at the bedside? *Children (Basel), 10*(3), 519.

Nair, M. (2025). *Ethnic disparities in congenital heart disease among infants in the UK and the underlying maternal risk factors.* Nuffield Department of Population Health, University of Oxford. Retrieved September 26, 2025, from https://www.ndph.ox.ac.uk/study-with-us/dphil-population-health/choose-a-dphil-project-2025/ethnic-disparities-in-congenital-heart-disease-among-infants-in-the-uk-and-the-underlying-maternal-risk-factors

Neonatal Network South East. (2023). *Pulse oximetry screening – Routine SpO_2 screening.* Thames Valley & Wessex Neonatal Operational Delivery Network. Retrieved September 26, 2025, from https://neonatalnetworkssoutheast.nhs.uk/professionals/guidelines/tvw-guidelines/pulse-oximetry-screening/

Noble, A. (2009). The cardiovascular system. In M. Hall, A. Noble, & S. Smith (Eds.), *A foundation for neonatal care.* Radcliffe.

Ohlsson, A., Walia, R., & Shah, S. S. (2020). Ibuprofen for the treatment of patent ductus arteriosus in preterm or low birth weight (or both) infants. *Cochrane Database of Systematic Reviews, 2*(2), CD003481. https://doi.org/10.1002/14651858.CD003481.pub8

Pierpont, M. E., Brueckner, M., Chung, W. K., Garg, V., Lacro, R. V., McGuire, A. L., Mital, S., Priest, J. R., Pu, W. T., Roberts, A., Ware, S. M., Gelb, B. D., Russell, M. W., & On behalf of the American Heart Association Council on Cardiovascular Disease in the Young; Council on Cardiovascular and Stroke Nursing; and Council on Genomic and Precision Medicine. (2018). Genetic basis for congenital heart disease: Revisited: A scientific statement from the American heart association. *Circulation, 138*(21). https://doi.org/10.1161/CIR.0000000000000606

Schoenwolf, G. C., Bleyl, S. B., Brauer, P. R., & Francis-West, P. H. (2014). *Larsen's human embryology* (5th ed.). Elsevier.

Schoenwolf, G. C., Bleyl, S. B., Brauer, P. R., & Francis-West, P. H. (2021). *Larsen's human embryology* (6th ed.). Elsevier Health Sciences.

Singh, Y., Roehr, C. C., & Tissot, C. (2022a). Point-of-care echocardiography in neonatal intensive care: Clinical utility and diagnostic yield. *Archives of Disease in Childhood – Fetal and Neonatal Edition, 107*(5), F545–F550.

Singh, Y., Roehr, C. C., & Tissot, C. (2022b). Clinical signs and bedside tools for evaluating neonatal cyanosis. *Archives of Disease in Childhood – Fetal and Neonatal Edition, 107*(5), F539–F544.

Singh, Y., Roehr, C. C., & Tissot, C. (2022c). Recognising cardiac causes of respiratory distress in neonates. *Archives of Disease in Childhood – Fetal and Neonatal Edition, 107*(4), F420.

Sinha, S., Miall, L., & Jardine, L. (2018). *Essential neonatal medicine* (6th ed.). Wiley.

Starr, M. C., & Flynn, J. T. (2019). Neonatal hypertension: Cases, causes, and clinical approach. *Pediatric Nephrology, 34*(5), 787–799.

Strainic, J. (2024). Prenatal diagnosis of congenital heart disease. In R. J. Martin, A. A. Fanaroff & M. C. Walsh (Eds.), *Fanaroff and Martin's neonatal-perinatal medicine: Diseases of the fetus and infant* (12th ed., pp. 1387–1400). Elsevier.

Swanson, T., & Erickson, L. (2020). Cardiovascular diseases and surgical interventions. In S. L. Gardner, B. S. Carter, M. E. Hines & J. A. Hernandez (Eds.), *Merenstein & Gardner's handbook of neonatal intensive care: An interprofessional approach* (9th ed., pp. 836–885). Elsevier.

Torchia, M. G., & Persaud, T. V. N. (2024). *The developing human: Clinically oriented embryology* (12th ed.). Elsevier.

Tortora, G. J., & Derrickson, B. (2020). *Principles of anatomy and physiology* (16th ed.). Wiley.

Tsoi, S. M., Nawaytou, H., Almeneisi, H., Steurer, M., Zhao, Y., Fineman, J. R., & Keller, R. L. (2023). Prostaglandin-E1 infusion in persistent pulmonary hypertension of the newborn. *Pediatric Pulmonology*, *59*(2), 379–388.

UK National Screening Committee. (2019). *Consultation on the use of pulse oximetry as an additional test in the newborn and infant physical examination*. Public Health England. Retrieved November 19, 2025, from https://www.gov.uk/government/consultations/pulse-oximetry-in-newborn-physical-screening

Yu, W., Xu, R., Ye, T., Abramson, M. J., Morawska, L., Jalaludin, B., Johnston, F. H., Henderson, S. B., Knibbs, L. D., Morgan, G. G., Lavigne, E., Heyworth, J., Hales, S., Marks, G. B., Woodward, A., Bell, M. L., Samet, J. M., Song, J., Li, S., & Guo, Y. (2024). Estimates of global mortality burden associated with short-term exposure to fine particulate matter (PM2·5). *The Lancet Planetary Health*, *8*(3), e146–e155. https://doi.org/10.1016/S2542-5196(24)00003-2

16 NEONATAL BRAIN INJURY

Rebecca Drescher

CONTENTS

DOI: 10.4324/9781003591405-20

GUIDANCE ON HOW TO ENHANCE PERSONAL LEARNING FROM THIS CHAPTER

Key points covered in this chapter

- An overview of neonatal conditions affecting the brain and neurological system.
- Physiological basis and vulnerability of the neonatal brain.
- Nursing care and assessment of infants with neurological compromise.

Reflection

Reading through the chapter, you are encouraged to engage with the key points and related literature in an enquiring way. Ask these questions:

- How have neurological problems affected the condition of babies you have encountered in your clinical practice?
- How can you minimise potential insults to the neurological system and brain?
- How might neurological compromise influence infants' outcomes?

Implications for nursing care

- Finally: how will this chapter enable you to consider and understand the nature of vulnerability of the neonatal brain and nervous system? Consider the implications of what you learn for your nursing care relating to this area, both in the short term and in relation to long-term outcomes.

INTRODUCTION AND BACKGROUND

Normal function of the central nervous system (CNS) is critical to the working of all other organs and systems in the body and therefore any injury to the brain will have implications for both physical and cognitive outcomes. Despite great advances in the understanding of the mechanisms of injury to the developing brain and the many attempts at prevention, perinatal cerebral injury remains a major cause of neonatal morbidity and mortality. Of preterm survivors, 5–10% have minor motor disability and up to half have significant cognitive, behavioural or social impairment. Preterm infants are particularly at risk of intraventricular haemorrhage (IVH), periventricular haemorrhagic infarction (PVHI) and periventricular leukomalacia (PVL). With magnetic resonance imaging (MRI) becoming more widely available, white matter injury (WMI) is now recognised as a key contributor to adverse neurological outcomes in preterm infants (de Bruijn et al., 2023). There is active debate over whether neurodevelopmental outcomes in preterm infants stem primarily from impaired brain maturation or from discrete brain injuries, for example white matter lesions. With recent MRI and diffusion-tensor studies suggesting both mechanisms play critical roles, it is increasingly recognised that the relationship between delayed developmental trajectories and focal injuries contributes to the varied outcomes observed in this population (Parikh et al., 2021). In addition, in the term infant, encephalopathy occurs in approximately 1.7 per 1,000 live births in high-income countries, but up to 20 per 1,000 live births in low- and middle-income countries (LMIC). Neonatal encephalopathy (NE) is defined as a condition of disturbed neurological function in the newborn period that may be identified through altered tone or consciousness, abnormal reflexes, cardiorespiratory compromise or seizures (Chakkarapani et al., 2025). A variety of causes can result in encephalopathy; hypoxic-ischaemic perinatal events are the most common, but other causes such as cerebral haemorrhage, infection and metabolic disturbances should be considered, particularly if a history for hypoxic-ischaemic encephalopathy (HIE) is not clear or does not fit the clinical picture.

This chapter provides an overview of both the preterm and term infant in relation to a range of neurological conditions with reference to how they can be prevented to minimise any impact on future outcomes.

VULNERABILITY OF THE NEONATAL BRAIN

To better understand neonatal brain injury, it is important to recognise that the immature brain is very different to the adult brain. Brain development begins early, at approximately 4–8 weeks gestation, and continues through childhood, via proliferation, migration, differentiation and maturation of neurons, ending in **myelination** dependent on **oligodendrocyte** function. During the third trimester and early neonatal period, pre-myelinating oligodendrocytes are prevalent but highly vulnerable to hypoxia-ischaemia, inflammation, excitotoxicity and oxidative stress, which impair their maturation and disrupt myelination. Environmental and systemic insults such as drugs, poor nutrition, infection and elevated cortisol from stress can cause further compromise to oligodendrocyte development by altering neuroactive steroid-mediated protection (Shaw et al., 2021).

In premature infants (<32 weeks), the fragile germinal matrix is a richly vascularised ventricular region (Figure 16.1) which is prone to haemorrhage due to lack of autoregulation and fluctuating blood pressure (BP). Germinal matrix haemorrhage (GMH), often extending into intraventricular spaces, induces oxidative stress and impacts cerebrospinal fluid dynamics, contributing to WMI (Cizmeci & De Vries, 2024). Neurons in the preterm brain may exhibit relative resilience to hypoxic–ischaemic damage compared with term neurons; WMI remains the predominant concern in this vulnerable population (Shaw et al., 2021).

For infants of any gestation who spend their first few weeks or even months on a neonatal unit (NNU), there is the added issue of being in a non-nurturing environment during a critical period of brain development, which may have implications for later life. Synaptic connections in the cortical plate increase at a rate of 4% per week until around 26–28 weeks' gestation, when there is acceleration in synaptogenesis, so that by 34 weeks' gestation it is estimated that there are 40,000 new synapses being formed every second (Sarnat, 2023). Exposure to an increased number of stressful events secondary to neonatal care is associated with decreased brain size in the frontal and parietal regions and corresponding poorer neurodevelopmental scores (van Dokkum et al., 2021).

The importance of this crucial period of brain development, which lasts from conception to the age of 2 years, and how this impacts the future of the child, is well recognised. Nursing and medical management must aim to support vulnerable infants and their families during this time; for example, developmental care strategies as seen in Chapter 7. All infants spending time on a NNU are at risk of developing neurological sequelae due to the harsh environment and possible delayed attachment to a specific primary caregiver.

Strong epidemiological data link maternal infection with neonatal brain injury. Chorioamnionitis is associated with premature delivery and low gestational age (GA).

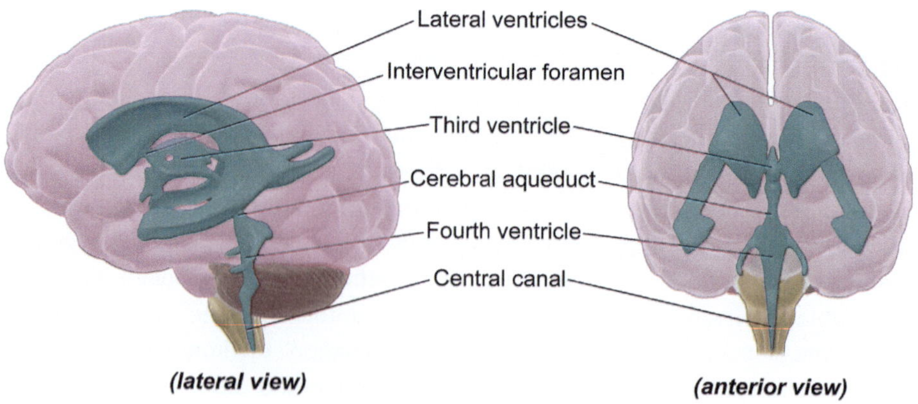

Figure 16.1 Ventricular system of the brain (Source: Creative Commons)

Cytokines play a part in this process. These are produced by, or act on, the immune system mediating responses associated with infection, inflammation and tissue injury. Recent work links increased amniotic fluid or blood concentrations of cytokines with perinatal brain injury. It is thought that maternally or fetally derived circulating inflammatory mediators may cross the immature blood–brain barrier, either directly injuring neurons or increasing their vulnerability to subsequent hypoxic-ischaemic insults. Alternatively, intrauterine infection could initiate injury by producing septic shock *in utero* with its resultant decreased cerebral perfusion. The neurological outcome linked most commonly with chorioamnionitis is cerebral palsy (Gall et al., 2021).

INTRAVENTRICULAR HAEMORRHAGE AND PERIVENTRICULAR HAEMORRHAGIC INFARCTION

Intraventricular haemorrhage (IVH) is the most common type of intracranial haemorrhage seen in the neonatal period and is almost exclusively confined to infants <32 weeks or <1500g. It is the leading cause of neurological and cognitive impairment in preterm infants with an incidence that increases with increasing prematurity. In the preterm infant, haemorrhage arises from the subependymal germinal matrix, while in the rarer cases of near-term IVH/PVHI it stems from the **choroid plexus**. IVH/PVHI was previously classified into grades I–IV, this grading system has more recently been revisited (see Box 16.1; Cizmeci & de Vries, 2024).

BOX 16.1 CATEGORIES OF INTRAVENTRICULAR HAEMORRHAGE

Grade I: The bleed is confined to the periventricular germinal matrix, a highly vascularised area which supports the development of the brain. It contains neurons and glial cells which migrate out during embryological development.

Grade II: The bleed has extended from the germinal matrix into the ventricles, but there is no evidence of ventricular dilatation (VD).

Grade III: Either due to a large volume of blood, or subsequent outflow obstruction of the ventricular system, this haemorrhage leads to significant distension of the ventricles.

Periventricular haemorrhagic infarction (previously grade IV): The bleed was thought to extend into the parenchyma, but it has more recently been recognised that parenchymal haemorrhage occurs due to periventricular haemorrhagic infarction secondary to the extent of the initial bleed.

The outcome for grades I and II was previously reported as good; more recent studies have shown an increased incidence in cerebral palsy and neurosensory impairment. The outcome for grade III is dependent on white matter involvement and the flow of cerebrospinal fluid (CSF); if this is blocked by blood clots at the aqueduct of Sylvius or foramen of Monro causing further VD, outcome is much worse, as these infants usually go on to develop post-haemorrhagic **hydrocephalus**. PVHI carries a higher incidence of poor neurodevelopmental outcome (Cizmeci & De Vries, 2024).

The term hydrocephalus refers to a progressive dilatation of the cerebral ventricular system due to a production of CSF that exceeds the absorption rate. In the infant suffering an IVH, a particulate blood clot may occlude or obliterate the microscopic arachnoid villi rendering them non-functional, resulting in insufficient absorption of CSF. In many infants, VD occurs slowly. Increased intracranial pressure does not usually occur due to the neonate's soft malleable skull, open sutures and fontanelles that, for a period of time, allow head size to increase without an appreciable rise in pressure. In approximately half of all infants, VD spontaneously arrests within about 30 days. However, for the remainder, dilatation continues with accompanying signs of rising intracranial pressure such as bulging fontanelles, setting sun eye sign, dilated scalp veins and widely spaced sutures. Progressive VD may be managed with a ventriculo-peritoneal shunt or temporary ventricular drainage via needle aspiration if the infant is too small or unwell for surgery.

It is important to note that grade IV is not simply blood in the ventricles bursting out into the parenchyma but a consequence of a secondary ischaemic injury. Although IVH occurs in about 20–25% of very low birthweight infants, PVHI affects approximately 10% of those weighing <750 g (roughly 3–4% of all VLBW infants) and carries a poor prognosis, making it a clinically significant diagnosis (Depala et al., 2023).

Aetiology

The pathophysiology of IVH/PVHI involves a combination of intravascular, vascular and extravascular factors. The germinal matrix is a transient structure which involutes by 36 weeks' gestation. Here, neuroectodermal cells (precursors for neurons) and glial cells develop before migrating to the cerebral cortex. Due to the high activity in this region during fetal life, the area is highly vascularised, with a significant proportion of cerebral blood flowing through. In the preterm brain normal cerebral autoregulation may not be developed enough to maintain a steady blood flow with changes in systemic BP resulting in possible under- or over-perfusion of this delicate area. Increased venous pressure can also directly affect the capillaries of the germinal matrix, impeding venous return and leading to reduced cerebral blood flow. The combination of these events, compounded by episodes of hypoxia and fragility of the immature and extremely thin-walled, irregularly shaped vessels of the germinal matrix lead to rupture of the area with various degrees of haemorrhage. Antenatal events that increase the risk of IVH include antepartum haemorrhage, fetal compromise/hypoxia, prolonged labour and malpresentation. Following birth, hypoxic events such as respiratory problems, apnoea and hypotension are associated with an increased risk.

Episodes of high systemic BP, linked to increased cerebral blood flow, can be caused by noxious stimuli, spontaneous over-activity or handling, crying, tracheal suctioning, excessive light and noise, over-infusion of inotropes, hypercapnia, pneumothorax and rapid volume expansion. Systemic hypotension significantly decreases cerebral blood flow and can be caused by cardiac dysfunction, sepsis and hypovolaemia (Depala et al., 2023). As gestation increases, the capillary walls thicken, and from 32 weeks onwards, cell proliferation and migration reduce as does the risk of IVH.

Diagnosis

IVH is usually detected within the first week of life, with diagnosis at the bedside. In the newborn infant, the anterior fontanelle provides an ideal window through which cranial ultrasound scanning (CUSS) may be performed. CUSS is especially helpful in identifying brain injury in newborn infants and allows grading of the injury according to the location and severity of the haemorrhage. For more than 90% of newborn infants with IVH, bleeding occurs within the first 72 hours after birth, with 50% of haemorrhages occurring in the first 24 hours. For approximately 10–20% of infants, there is a progressive increase in the size of the haemorrhage over a 24–48-hour period. Late haemorrhages may be seen after a few days or weeks in a small number of infants; however, these are seen primarily in those preterm infants with a more complicated history, such as severe, prolonged respiratory problems.

The clinical manifestations of IVH are non-specific. Three classic syndromes are described: catastrophic, saltatory or silent. The catastrophic syndrome occurs most infrequently but is one of sudden dramatic deterioration with a decrease in BP and haematocrit, a full fontanelle and seizure activity. Catastrophic deterioration usually involves major haemorrhages that evolve rapidly over several minutes or hours. Some infants exhibit a more protracted or saltatory course where symptoms fluctuate over a period of time. Findings include changes in alertness and tone, abnormal eye position and movement, an abnormally tight popliteal angle, with respiratory distress progressing to apnoea. These signs evolve over many hours and may cease, only to begin again. They may also be so subtle they are missed. Infants with a clinically silent syndrome, the most common of the three, fail to show any neurological signs but may have an unexplained fall in haematocrit or failure of haematocrit to rise following red blood cell transfusion. Diagnosis of silent haemorrhages is usually by CUSS (Cizmeci & De Vries, 2024).

PERIVENTRICULAR LEUKOMALACIA AND WHITE MATTER INJURY

PVL occurs following necrosis of the white matter behind and to the sides of the **lateral** ventricles. The area is susceptible to ischaemic damage from reduced blood flow, as this border zone is furthest away from arterial supply. PVL can be classified as cystic or non-cystic. In cystic PVL, early CUSS shows a bright area (periventricular brightness, also called 'flare') that later develops into macroscopic cysts which can be detected on ultrasound. In non-cystic PVL the damage is diffuse, and the microscopic cysts cannot be seen and evolve into glial scars (de Bruijn et al., 2023). In later MRI scans this non-cystic PVL may manifest itself with reduced growth of the cerebellum and is thought to be a possible cause of poor neurodevelopment in preterm infants, especially when earlier CUSS showed little or no abnormality (Volpe, 2021).

Previously, cystic PVL was a common occurrence on NNUs, but with improving perinatal care, most preterm WMI is non-cystic and diffuse. Impaired glial cell function, along with the heightened vulnerability of oligodendrocyte precursors to inflammation and ischaemia, is believed to contribute to hypomyelination, which is a common feature of WMI seen on MRI. This highlights the growing recognition that contemporary neonatal brain injury often reflects disrupted maturation processes rather than discrete focal lesions (Shaw et al., 2021).

PREVENTION OF PRETERM BRAIN INJURY

- *Preventing preterm birth* This is the single most important method of preventing brain injury of any type.
- *Perinatal optimisation* The British Association of Perinatal Medicine (BAPM), in collaboration with the Royal College of Obstetricians and Gynaecologists (RCOG) and other professional bodies, has developed a seven-element perinatal optimisation pathway aimed at reliably implementing evidence-based interventions during the antenatal, intrapartum and early neonatal periods to improve outcomes for preterm infants (NB not all these measures are aimed at neuroprotection; see Chapter 2 for more details).
    - Place of birth – delivery in units adjacent to Neonatal Intensive Care Units (NICUs) should be aimed for in all babies expected to be born before 27 weeks' GA.

   - Antenatal corticosteroids – Antenatal administration of corticosteroids is associated with a 45% reduction of IVH incidence, as this aids maturation of the fetal lungs, decreasing the occurrence of respiratory distress syndrome (RDS) with its concomitant acid-base balance disturbances (McGoldrick et al., 2020). Additionally, antenatal corticosteroids may also decrease IVH by promoting cardiovascular stability postnatally and may contribute to maturation of the germinal matrix itself.
   - Magnesium sulphate for neuroprotection – This has been shown in many studies to be protective of the fetal brain and is now recommended practice (BAPM and the National Neonatal Audit Programme (NNAP), 2020). This occurs in a few ways: magnesium sulphate reduces excitotoxicity from glutamate release in the immature brain during hypoxic–ischaemic episodes through blocking some receptors. This prevents calcium influx into neurons, reducing oxidative stress and cellular injury. Magnesium sulphate also contributes to a reduction in fluctuations in cerebral perfusion and furthermore has anti-inflammatory properties that can mitigate damage to developing brain structures (Crowther et al., 2017).
   - Intrapartum antibiotic prophylaxis.
   - Optimised umbilical cord clamping – Deferred cord clamping (DCC) for up to 2 minutes has been shown to be associated with a lower incidence of IVH, as DCC improves cardiovascular stability by boosting blood volume and cardiac output, which helps stabilise BP, thus reducing cerebral blood flow fluctuations. Increased red blood cell mass leads to better oxygen delivery, lowering the risk of hypoxic-ischaemic injury that can contribute to IVH (Fogarty at et al., 2018).
   - Maintaining normothermia.
   - Initiating early maternal breastmilk feeding (BAPM & NNAP, 2020).
- *Caffeine* This is one of the most widely used drugs in NNUs, its primary objective being the prevention of apnoea of prematurity. However, in the trial designed to investigate its use, it was found that infants in the caffeine arm had a lower incidence of cerebral palsy and cognitive delay at 18–21 months and improved motor function at 5 years of age (Schmidt et al., 2017).
- *Homeostasis* Maintaining normotension, optimised fluid balance and blood gases within the normal range are all neuroprotective measures. Sodium bicarbonate should be used cautiously as a buffer due to its effect of causing an abrupt rise in arterial carbon dioxide following administration that leads to vasodilation of the cerebral arteries and a subsequent increase in cerebral perfusion.
- *Comfort measures and family integrated care (FiCare)* Traditionally seen as nursing responsibilities, good positioning, careful handling, pain management and working with families to ensure FiCare models are all contributing

factors towards better neurological outcomes. These practices represent a crucial element of neuroprotective care and must therefore be endorsed by the entire multidisciplinary team to reduce morbidity and enhance long-term neurodevelopmental outcomes (Alsadaan et al., 2023).

> **THINK POINT**
>
> Review the elements of neuroprotective nursing care in Table 16.4 and consider whether these form part of your unit's culture and everyday practice already. If not, what steps could you take to facilitate a change in practice?

MANAGEMENT OF PRETERM BRAIN INJURY

Acute management of the infant once IVH has occurred is supportive in nature, with control of ventilation, fluids, metabolic and nutritional states, temperature and, if a catastrophic bleed has occurred, management of seizures. The outcome for an infant suffering an IVH is largely determined by the severity and extent of the haemorrhage and the presence of associated problems, such as RDS, perinatal hypoxic-ischaemic injury and sepsis, which all increase morbidity and mortality. Parents should be kept fully updated and be aware that their child may have some developmental delay; assurance should be given that close follow-up will identify any specific needs promptly and early intervention will be given if required. Community support and follow-up should be coordinated, and the importance of attending follow-up appointments must be stressed.

BRAIN INJURY IN THE TERM INFANT

As previously mentioned, the most common cause of NE in the term infant is HIE. Hypoxic perinatal brain injury is caused by a decrease in the amount of oxygen supplied to an infant's brain close to the time of birth or early neonatal period. It can result in stillbirth or neonatal death, and infants who survive may develop HIE, which can lead to severe lifelong disability or death. Hypoxic perinatal brain injury may be associated with multi-organ failure affecting the heart, lungs, liver and kidneys in some infants (Chakkarapani et al., 2025). The potential causes of hypoxia can be seen in Table 16.1.

TABLE 16.1 CAUSES OF HYPOXIC BRAIN INJURY

Failure of gas exchange across the placenta	Prolonged or excessive uterine contractions placental abruption Ruptured uterus
Interruption of umbilical blood flow	Cord compression (including tight nuchal cord, shoulder dystocia, cord prolapse, true knots)
Inadequate placental perfusion	Maternal hypo-/hypertension
Impaired maternal oxygenation	Asthma Pulmonary embolism Pneumonia
Compromised fetus	Intrauterine growth restriction Anaemia
Failure of cardiorespiratory adaptation at birth	

A diagnosis of HIE can be difficult to make, so that health professionals need to adopt a structured approach in their examination and consider the following.

- History of a sentinel event such as abruption or uterine rupture
- Evidence of fetal/intrapartum compromise or acidosis
- Low Apgar scores and/or delayed onset of respiration requiring resuscitation (considering that Apgar scores are subjective)
- Signs of encephalopathy
- Evolution of the condition: Babies are in poor condition initially and then get better. This will require regular assessment and documentation by an experienced practitioner using a standardised neurological examination template which should include the nationally used Sarnat scoring tool (see Box 16.2)
- Signs of multi-organ involvement usually occurs in association with moderate to severe encephalopathy
- Measurement of lactate levels: An initial cord or admission lactate of ≥12 mmol/L or persisting high lactate levels on subsequent measurements correlate with the severity of HIE and may provide a useful adjunctive marker
- Exclusion of other likely causes of encephalopathy (BAPM, 2020). Other causes of NE include neonatal stroke, sepsis, metabolic, neuromuscular or cardiac disorders. When a sentinel event to cause HIE is not apparent, further diagnostic tests should be undertaken.

HYPOXIC-ISCHAEMIC ENCEPHALOPATHY

Pathophysiology

The hypoxic-ischaemic event results in primary injury that significantly depletes adenosine triphosphate (ATP) stores and increases lactate production. The low ATP causes disruption of cell function, particularly to the sodium-potassium pump and the mechanism to maintain low intracellular calcium. The failure of the sodium-potassium pump results in depolarisation of neurons and the release of the neuro-transmitter glutamate that further increases intracellular calcium and sodium. The detrimental effects of this process include cerebral oedema and microvascular damage leading to necrosis and **apoptosis**. Around 6 hours following this initial period of damage there is a latent period where many of the damaged neurons partially recover and there is a transient improvement in cerebral metabolism. This is followed by a secondary phase of injury, characterised by excitotoxicity, mito-chondrial impairment, intracellular calcium regulation, oxidative stress and inflam-mation, which all contribute to the process of further and possible catastrophic cell death (Wu et al., 2024). A tertiary phase, lasting weeks to months, may show chronic inflammation and subsequently compromised maturation (Chakkarapani et al., 2025).

Treatment

Following results of three large trials (TOBY, CoolCap, NICHD) there is now robust evidence that moderate hypothermia following a perinatal hypoxic-ischaemic event results in improved neurodevelopmental outcome for survivors. Furthermore, the TOBY study group has shown that this improvement continues into middle childhood. These interventions, however, have not demonstrated the same effects in LMIC (Chakkarapani et al., 2025). Criteria for **therapeutic hypothermia** (TH) have been identified in the 2020 BAPM framework. Three areas of assessment determine if TH is to be commenced. These can be seen in Box 16.2.

BOX 16.2 CRITERIA FOR THERAPEUTIC HYPOTHERMIA

Criteria A

Infants ≥36* completed weeks' gestation admitted to the NNU with at least one of the following:

- Apgar score of <5 at 10 minutes after birth
- Continued need for resuscitation†, at 10 minutes after birth
- Acidosis defined as any occurrence of:
- pH <7.00
- Base deficit ≥16mmol/L in any cord or baby gas sample within 60 minutes of birth

Criteria B

Infants that meet criteria A will be assessed for whether they meet the neurological abnormality entry criteria (B) by trained personnel only.

Moderate to severe encephalopathy, consisting of altered state of consciousness (lethargy, stupor or coma) AND at least one of the following:

- Hypotonia
- Abnormal reflexes including oculomotor or pupillary abnormalities
- Absent or weak suck
- Clinical seizures

Criteria C

Infants that meet criteria A and B will be assessed by **amplitude integrated electroencephalogram** (aEEG; read by trained personnel)

At least 30 minutes duration of aEEG recording that shows abnormal background aEEG activity or seizures. There must be one of the following.

- Normal background with some seizure activity
- Moderately abnormal activity
- Suppressed activity
- Continuous seizure activity (BAPM, 2020)

* *Infants with GA between 35 and 36 weeks should be managed using the same initial steps but should be discussed with a tertiary centre before any TH is commenced.*

† *Continued resuscitation = continued need for resuscitation including mask or endotracheal ventilation excluding infants who are receiving positive end-expiratory pressure alone.*

TH is now standardised treatment for HIE in infants >36 weeks' gestation and should be followed in all NNUs (BAPM, 2020). Recent evidence indicates that TH does not, however, significantly reduce the risk of death or moderate neurodevelopmental disability in infants born between 33+0 and 35+6 weeks, and there is insufficient safety data for those below 35+0 weeks. Consequently,

TH is not recommended for infants born at or below 34+6 weeks gestation. For infants born between 35+0 and 35+6 weeks, if they meet eligibility criteria, the decision to proceed with TH should involve a clear discussion with the local tertiary centre (if in a local NNU or special care baby unit) and further discussions with the family. It should be explained that, while current evidence suggests TH is likely safe in this group, it has not been shown to improve survival or reduce moderate disability (Faix et al., 2025).

Active cooling to a core temperature of 33–34°C for a period of 72 hours with a servo-control mattress should be commenced as soon as diagnosis is confirmed, so transport to a tertiary centre is time-critical. The aim of treatment is to prevent the secondary phase of damage and therefore cooling started within six hours of birth is crucial. Current evidence indicates that TH is most effective when initiated within three hours of the hypoxic-ischaemic insult, with limited benefit beyond six hours (Chakkarapani et al., 2025). Infants who exceed the six-hour threshold but otherwise meet all eligibility criteria may still be considered for TH, if target temperature can be reached by 12 hours of age. In practical terms, this requires the cooling decision to be made by no later than nine hours after birth.

There are several hypothesised mechanisms by which hypothermia is thought to be neuroprotective. It may safeguard neurons by reducing cerebral metabolic rate, attenuating the release of excitatory amino acids, ameliorating the ischaemia-impaired uptake of glutamate and lowering production of toxic nitric oxide and free radicals. Hypothermia may also modify cells programmed for apoptosis, leading to their survival.

Hypothermia appears to be well tolerated. Adverse effects such as sinus bradycardia, increased BP and increased oxygen requirement are generally transient and reversible with re-warming. Due to the potential effect of hypoxia on other body organs, the infant being treated for HIE should be closely monitored; poor renal, hepatic and intestinal function, deranged clotting and cardiac and respiratory deficiencies are all commonly seen. Pain management and sedation must be considered. Once at a tertiary centre, EEG monitoring should be continued.

Maintaining physiological stability in a critically ill, hypothermic infant is challenging, requiring labour-intensive and skilful care (Ranjan & Gulati, 2023). A large retrospective cohort study using data from UK NNUs found that babies who received enteral feeds (mostly maternal breastmilk) during TH had lower rates of NEC, shorter hospital stays and higher rates of breastfeeding at discharge, compared with matched babies who did not receive enteral feeding (Gale et al., 2021). Perceptions of patient discomfort during cooling, with anecdotal experiences of restlessness and shivering, have arisen in those caring for these infants. Clinicians have acknowledged this as a major barrier for nursing staff and provision for providing comfort with sedation is standard in protocols. Support of the family, especially following the often-traumatic events of a hypoxic-ischaemic insult, is paramount (BAPM, 2020).

> **PRACTICE POINT**
>
> The CoolCuddle study found that allowing parents to hold their babies for up to two hours during therapeutic hypothermia was associated with minor changes in body temperature, CFM trace, and pCO_2 levels. However, it also resulted in lower rates of postnatal depression and improved breastfeeding outcomes (Odd et al., 2021).

The most effective intervention against hypoxic-ischaemic brain injury remains prevention with vigilant intrapartum monitoring to help detect fetuses at risk. The hallmarks of intrapartum hypoxia-ischaemia are the occurrence of fetal heart rate abnormalities and the passage of meconium *in utero*. Robust intrapartum assessment allows appropriate obstetric management and effective resuscitation following delivery (Chakkarapani et al., 2025).

Cerebral function monitoring

Cerebral function monitoring (CFM) using aEEG is almost universally used in the NNU today. aEEG uses a limited number of channels to record raw EEG signals which are filtered and displayed on an amplitude and time-compressed scale (see Figure 16.2). This can be monitored continuously at the bedside without interruption of daily care, and extensive formal training is not required.

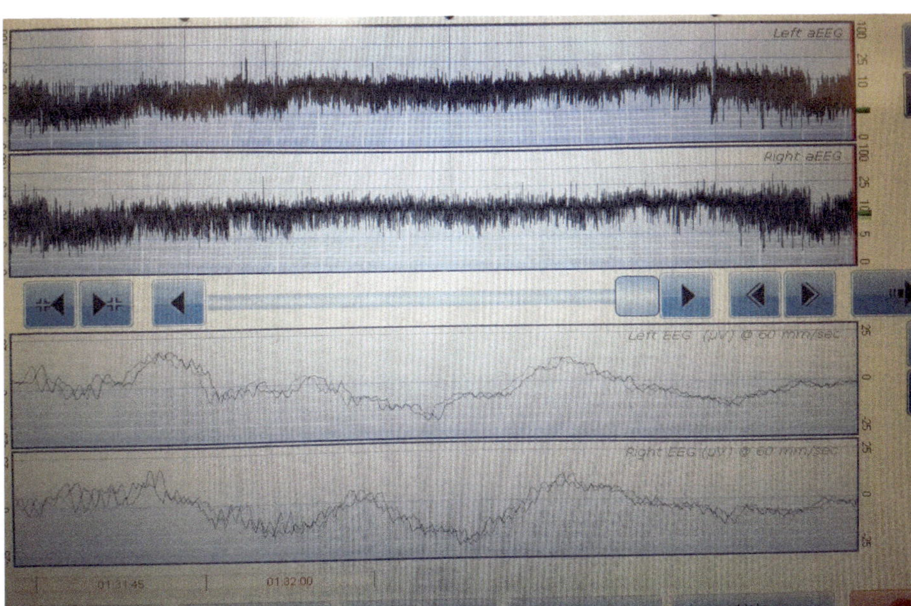

Figure 16.2 Normal aEEG trace with sleep–wake cycling (Source: Wikimedia Commons)

Primarily, the aEEG is used to detect seizure activity, to gauge response to anticonvulsant therapy and as part of routine clinical monitoring, especially for those infants pharmacologically paralysed.

Studies have shown that the aEEG is very accurate in outcome prediction of term infants with HIE between 3 and 48 hours postnatal age, especially when the early aEEG is combined with clinical evaluation. Continuous activity with a lower amplitude of around 5 microvolts (μV) and maximum up to 50μV is considered normal; sleep-wake cycling should be seen. An abnormal background pattern persisting beyond the first 12–24 hours after birth is known to carry a poor prognosis (Glass et al., 2023).

Outcome

The severity of HIE grading can be assessed using the adapted Sarnat and Sarnat criteria in Box 16.3.

BOX 16.3 HIE GRADING

Category	*Stage I (Mild)*	*Stage II (Moderate)*	*Stage III (Severe)*
Level of consciousness	Hyperalert	Lethargic/obtunded	Stuporous or comatose
Spontaneous activity	Normal	Decreased	None
Posture	Normal	Distal flexion	Decerebrate (extension)
Muscle tone	Normal/ increased	Hypotonia	Flaccid
Primitive reflexes	Strong (e.g. suck, Moro)	Weak	Absent
Pupillary reaction	Dilated and reactive	Constricted and reactive	Non-reactive or unequal
Heart rate	Normal	Bradycardia possible	Variable or severely depressed
Seizures	None	Common (frequent clinical seizures)	Uncommon or subtle (may be subclinical)
EEG findings	Normal	Abnormal (slow wave, discontinuous)	Severely abnormal or isoelectric
Duration	<24 hours	Days (often >5–7 days)	Prolonged or fatal

Utilising this grading system, for those term infants with mild neonatal encephalopathy in the first few days of life, there is a high likelihood of being completely normal at follow-up. For those with moderate encephalopathy there is a 20–35% risk of neurological sequelae, although those with normal neurological examination and effective feeding within two weeks of birth are likely to have normal outcomes. Infants with severe encephalopathy have a 75% risk of dying with coma persisting or progressing to brain death by 72 hours of life. If the infant survives for longer than 72 hours without losing all cerebral function, a variable amount of improvement may be seen; however, there is an almost universal risk of poor neurological outcome in survivors (Wu et al., 2024). Permanent sequelae may be mild, such as learning difficulties or attention deficit disorder, or may be severe and disabling, including cerebral palsy, epilepsy, visual impairment and severe cognitive and developmental disorders.

Clinical evaluation including aEEG, neurological examination and MRI are useful means of long-term prognostication. However, they should not be relied on in isolation; all the details of a baby's individual case, including antenatal and perinatal history, clinical course and neurological status at discharge must be taken into consideration to allow for as accurate a prognosis as possible (BAPM, 2020).

ACTIVITY

Consider watching resources 2 and 3 on https://learn.nes.nhs.scot/62008, which has some excellent suggestions of how to communicate difficult messages to parents around the diagnosis and prognosis of HIE.

OTHER MECHANISMS OF BRAIN INJURY

Subdural haemorrhage

Subdural and subarachnoid haemorrhages in neonates are frequently underdiagnosed by routine CUSS due to their subtle or posterior position, and up to one third of asymptomatic term infants show birth-related subdural haemorrhages on MRI that are often missed on standard scans. Traditionally linked to birth trauma such as instrument-assisted vaginal deliveries, prolonged labour or breech presentation, improvements in obstetric care have significantly reduced the incidence of major clinically significant haemorrhages. Signs, when present, may include lethargy, apnoea, seizures and a tense or bulging fontanelle, and diagnosis typically requires MRI or CT imaging, as CUSS lacks sensitivity for small extra-axial bleeds. Management is generally supportive, focused on stabilisation, seizure control and serial imaging, with neurosurgical intervention reserved for large haematomas causing mass effect. Close developmental follow-up is essential to monitor potential sequelae such as post-haemorrhagic hydrocephalus or neurodevelopmental delay (Cizmeci & De Vries, 2024).

Neonatal stroke

Neonatal stroke is a rare occurrence presenting in the first 48 hours of life in the majority of infants. It can be defined as a focal disruption of cerebral blood flow secondary to arterial ischaemia or sinovenous thrombosis (Cizmeci & De Vries, 2024), which can occur secondary to the fact that the neonate is relatively thrombophilic. Conditions such as polycythaemia, dehydration, congenital vascular or cardiac anomalies, meningitis and transplacental passage of an **embolus** have been described as causative of neonatal stroke. Symptoms can be subtle and non-specific or sudden and dramatic, ranging from lethargy and poor feeding to seizures. If suspected, an EEG and CUSS should be carried out as soon as possible followed by MRI when practical. Management is primarily symptom control and ensuring stability of all body systems as required (Chakkarapani et al., 2025).

Metabolic disorders

When a newborn infant presents with a sudden illness which may include signs from almost every system, inborn errors of metabolism should be considered. Although rare, outcome is very much linked to speed of diagnosis and initiation of treatment. When neurological symptoms are present with no explanation from antenatal or perinatal history, then metabolic screening should be carried out and advice sought from a specialist paediatrician. Relevant symptoms include hypotonia, encephalopathy, seizures and sudden respiratory collapse (Chakkarapani et al., 2025).

Neonatal seizures

Seizures are the most common neurological sign during the neonatal period resulting from abnormal electrical impulses generated by the brain. Excessive synchronous electrical discharge or depolarisation in the brain produces stereotypic, repetitive behaviours which may be the first, and at times only, sign of CNS dysfunction. Although the precise mechanism that causes neonatal seizures is unknown, they are thought to result from one or more of these mechanisms: disturbances in the sodium-potassium pump, altered neuronal permeability to sodium or imbalance in excitatory (glutamate) and inhibitory (GABA) neurotransmitters. Seizures are important, as they indicate a potentially serious underlying disease process and may have a detrimental effect on the developing brain. They also interfere with supportive care and result in an increase in glucose metabolism and altered cerebral blood flow. Repetitive seizures may eventually alter brain lipid, protein and energy metabolism or result in damage from hypoxia or oedema; however, although neonates have a lower seizure threshold than children or adults, it is thought that the developing neurons are more resistant to the toxic effects of seizure activity.

Seizures occur more often in the newborn infant than at any other period of life, with the incidence in term infants being 1 to 3.5 per 1000 live births, and it is more common than this in the preterm population. The clinical manifestations of neonatal seizures differ from those of older children with five major varieties described: **subtle, generalised tonic, multifocal clonic, focal clonic** and **myoclonic** (see Table 16.2). Seizures generally indicate an underlying, potentially treatable, aetiology. Therefore,

TABLE 16.2 NEONATAL SEIZURES

Type of seizure	*Manifestation*	*Comments*
Subtle seizures	Horizontal deviation of the eyes or repetitive blinking/fluttering of eyelids. Drooling, sucking and/or tongue thrusting, lip smacking, yawning. Swimming or rowing movements of limbs or cycling movements of legs.	Most common seizure in newborns especially preterm infants. Difficult to distinguish from normal movements; therefore, may be missed.
Tonic seizures	Tonic extension or flexion (less common) of all extremities or may be limited to one. May be accompanied by eye deviations, apnoea, occasional clonic movements.	Generalised tonic seizures may be mistaken for decerebrate (extension of arms and legs) or decorticate posturing (extension of legs, flexion of arms) where there are no EEG changes. Seizure most frequently seen in preterm infant especially following IVH and asphyxia.
Clonic seizures	Rhythmic jerky movements. Multifocal – migration in non-ordered fashion. Focal – usually focal injury.	More frequent in term infants. More frequent in term infants. Often associated with: ■ CNS injury ■ Severe acidosis ■ Asphyxia.
Myoclonic seizures	Sudden single or multiple jerks with flexion of upper (more common) or lower extremities.	Uncommon in term infants. Rarely seen in preterm infants. Often associated with: ■ inborn errors of metabolism, ■ other metabolic problems.
Benign myoclonic seizures	Brief, intermittent jerk (no EEG changes).	Seen during sleep only.

determining and treating the cause of the seizures are priorities in preventing further seizures and neurological injury. Timing of the onset of seizures (Figure16.3) may provide insight into possible aetiology (Kayyal & Inder, 2024).

The timing of seizure onset in infants with HIE is highly variable and most often occurs within the first 24 hours after birth, typically between 4 and 20 hours of age. Although previous literature suggested that earlier seizures might indicate a pre-labour insult and later seizures a peripartum event, contemporary studies demonstrate considerable overlap in seizure timing and poor correlation with the precise onset of injury. Many infants experience subclinical seizures, and therapeutic hypothermia can further modify the natural timing of seizure presentation. For these reasons, the age at first seizure is no longer considered a reliable indicator of the timing of the hypoxic–ischaemic insult (Pisani et al., 2024).

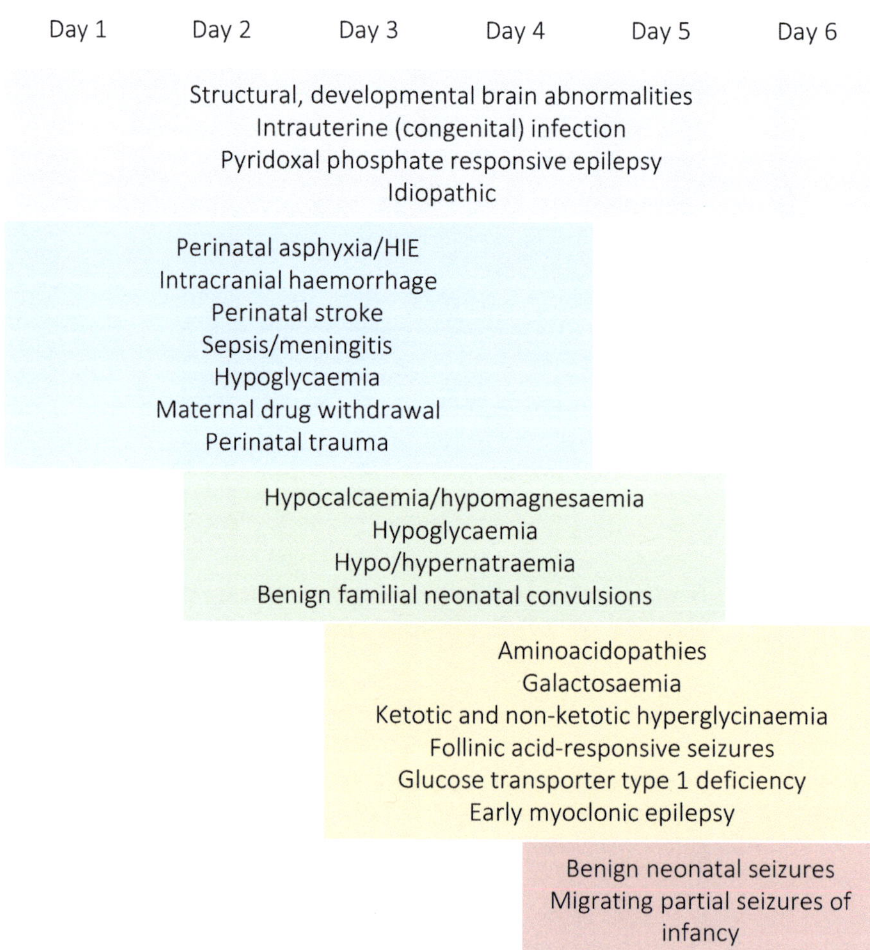

Figure 16.3 Timing of onset of seizures (adapted from Kumar et al., 2024)

The issue of when to treat with anticonvulsant drugs and for how long, however, remains controversial. Generally, UK guidelines suggest treatment if a seizure is longer than 3 minutes' duration or occurs at a frequency of more than three per hour (Kumar et al., 2024), while internationally treatment of any electrical seizures is recommended. The first-line anticonvulsant remains phenobarbital, despite the known long-term effects on brain growth. Other drugs often used include phenytoin and benzodiazepines such as midazolam (Kayyal & Inder, 2024). A systematic review conducted in 2023 suggested agents, such as levetiracetam showed results to be non-inferior to phenobarbitone for managing neonatal seizures. Considering a better safety profile and marginally better neurodevelopment in the short term, levetiracetam may be considered an initial choice for managing neonatal seizures in future seizure management (Kumar et al., 2025). As anticonvulsants can be respiratory, myocardial and CNS depressants, the baby's respiratory effort and heart rate must be assessed to maintain adequate ventilation and perfusion. Anticonvulsants also compete with bilirubin for albumin binding sites, so the infant must be monitored for signs of jaundice.

Neonatal seizures must be differentiated from non-seizure behaviours of the newborn, which can at times be problematic. Normal behaviour such as stretching, yawning, jitteriness, startling and clonus may raise suspicions of seizure activity. Traditionally, diagnosis in the NNU has been based upon clinical observation; however, in recent years, continuous CFM has become increasingly acknowledged as a method for evaluation of brain activity in neonates and may now be a part of clinical surveillance of sick newborn infants. Overall, accurate and prompt diagnosis is pivotal in providing optimal outcomes for infants with neonatal seizures. As clinical signs may be subtle or lacking altogether, effective management should involve continuous aEEG or EEG monitoring (see Table 16.3)

TABLE 16.3 CLASSIFICATION OF AEEG TRACES IN FULL-TERM INFANTS

Continuous normal voltage pattern	Continuous activity with lower margin of amplitude around 5 to 10μV and maximum amplitude around 10 to 25μV (up to 50). Sleep–wake cycling should be present.
Discontinuous normal voltage pattern	Discontinuous background, with variable minimal amplitude, but < 5μV and maximum amplitude greater than 10μV.
Burst suppression	Discontinuous background with minimum amplitude without variability at 0 to 2μV.
Continuous low voltage	Continuous background pattern of extremely low voltage (less than or around 5μV).
Inactive flat trace	Mainly inactive (isoelectric tracing) background less than 5μV.

depending on local availability and identification of the underlying potential cause (Kayyal & Inder, 2024).

NURSING CARE OF INFANTS WITH NEUROLOGICAL COMPROMISE

Nursing and medical care in relation to the neonatal brain and nervous system should focus on preventative, protective and supportive strategies. In more detail, minimising brain injury in premature infants should start in the perinatal period with the prevention of preterm birth, birth trauma and hypoxic events. After birth, nurses have a key role in the prevention of brain injury in premature infants during the neonatal period and the worsening of injuries that have occurred already. Nursing management includes interventions to reduce activities that can lead to hypoxic events, rapid changes to cerebral BP, flow and pressures. Recognition and management of pain and stress are furthermore of vital importance, as well as developmentally supportive care, including handling and positioning techniques (European Standards of Care for Newborn Health, 2018). These interventions can promote physiological stability during and after caregiving and reduce environmental stress and so protect the infant. Table 16.4 outlines examples in relation to these areas. Parents must also be consistently involved in any individualised developmental care programmes that aim to reduce any external stressors on their vulnerable baby and promote the best future outcomes.

Chapter takeaways

- CNS injury affects all organ systems and has significant developmental consequences.
- Preterm infants have a high risk of IVH, PVHI, PVL and WMI. IVH arises from fragile vasculature, poor autoregulation and fluctuating pressures and both antenatal and postnatal hypoxic events increase risk. Acute management of IVH is supportive. Severity, associated conditions and complications influence outcome. Parent communication and coordinated follow-up are essential.
- Extended NNU stays expose infants to a non-ideal environment during rapid synaptic growth and the stressful experience in NNU can reduce brain growth and impair neurodevelopment, which is also impacted by hypoxia, inflammation and poor nutrition. The first 2 years form a critical neurodevelopmental window and developmental care, alongside family partnership is key to mitigating environmental risks.
- HIE evolves in phases: primary insult → latent recovery → secondary injury → tertiary phase. Mechanisms include excitotoxicity, oxidative stress and

TABLE 16.4 NEUROPROTECTIVE NURSING CARE

Type of care	*Strategies*	*Rationale*
Preventative care	■ Assessment of oxygenation and perfusion. ■ Optimise ventilation and oxygenation levels, avoiding fluctuations in pressure and oxygen.	To avoid sudden changes to oxygenation, BP and volume.
	■ Avoid routine endotracheal tube suctioning. ■ Careful fluid bolus administration. ■ Close monitoring – EEG.	To prevent potentially catastrophic sequelae of this and improve the clinical outcome.
	■ Assist with preparation of the infant for regular scanning and/or timely brain imaging.	To identify any problem as early as possible and any worsening of injuries that have occurred already. Brain imaging is an important step in the diagnosis and management of sick infants: e.g. post-haemorrhagic VD, encephalopathy, seizures and suspected structural brain abnormalities (Cizmeci & De Vries, 2024; Chakkarapani et al., 2025).
Protective care	■ Neurological assessment including tone, consciousness, activity level, behaviour changes as well as vital signs: BP, oxygenation, blood gases. Correction of imbalances. ■ Avoid unnecessary handling, stress/pain and stimulation. ■ Careful handling. ■ Avoid transportation if possible.	As above, to identify any changes early and ensure appropriate care is given. To protect the immature, vulnerable brain. The seven neuroprotective core measures are ■ healing environment ■ partnering with families ■ positioning and handling ■ safeguarding sleep ■ minimising stress and pain ■ protecting skin ■ optimising nutrition.
Supportive care	■ Optimise the environment. ■ Give developmentally supportive care in partnership with parents. ■ Ensure comfortable and supportive positioning. ■ Reduce and manage stress and pain (e.g. containment and pain relief) during procedures.	To provide a nurturing supportive environment without undue stress that optimises the developmental capabilities of the developing infant. Noise, light, invasive treatment and caring activities are among disturbing factors in the NNU (Altimier & Phillips, 2016). See also Chapters 7 and 8.

mitochondrial dysfunction. HIE treatment is TH and is evidence-based for ≥36 weeks with limited benefit for late preterm infants. It requires strict eligibility criteria and early initiation.

- Neonatal stroke is rare but serious and diagnosis uses EEG, CUSS, MRI; treatment is supportive.
- Seizures are common and often subtle. It is important to treat the underlying cause and control seizures. Phenobarbital is the first-line anticonvulsant, with levetiracetam posing a promising alternative. aEEG is crucial for accurate diagnosis. Careful and ongoing neurological nursing assessment is key.

CASE STUDY

CASE STUDIES

Case study 1: The infant with IVH

Vihaan is a 26-week gestation infant born by a quick vaginal delivery, weighing 675g. During pregnancy, there had been some intermittent vaginal bleeding at 12–16 weeks' gestation and then again at 25weeks. However, before Diya, his mother, could be transferred to a tertiary perinatal centre, she began to feel unwell with uterine tenderness and fever, and on admission to her local hospital, Vihaan was delivered without receiving antenatal steroids and had a loading dose of magnesium sulphate. Diya also experienced a significant antepartum haemorrhage. Vihaan required resuscitation at birth including intubation and positive-pressure ventilation and after being given a dose of surfactant, he was transferred to the neonatal intensive care unit (NICU). On admission to NICU, he was commenced on volume-targeted ventilation and in the first 24 hours of life, his BP was problematic, requiring two doses of volume expansion followed by inotropic support. Due to his weight, gestation and current condition, Vihaan was transferred to a level 3 neonatal intensive care unit, 10 miles from the local hospital. His parents Diya and Kavi are married and have one other child.

Q.1. What antenatal factors placed Vihaan at risk of brain injury?
Q.2. What antenatal optimisation measures could have been considered before delivery?
Q.3. What postnatal factors in the first few hours of life placed Vihaan at further risk of brain injury?

On day 3 of life, Vihaan became more hypotensive, and a murmur presented on auscultation. A patent ductus arteriosus was confirmed on cardiac echo.

On day 7, a head ultrasound scan identified evidence of intraventricular haemorrhage (IVH) with blood present in both right and left ventricles (grades 3 and 2, respectively).

Q.4. Describe the mechanisms for injury that were present in this situation.
Q.5. What potential caregiving practices need addressing in the prevention and management of IVH?

Follow-up head ultrasound scan at 14 days of age revealed further bleeding on the left side and ventricles were slightly dilated. However, he was extubated to continuous positive airway pressure (CPAP) on day 15 and further regular ultrasounds were planned as the parents had been told there was a risk of post-haemorrhagic hydrocephalus. Successive scans did show progressive dilation of the ventricles. He also remained on low flow oxygen for chronic lung disease.

Q.6. How should the team prepare Diya and Kavi for Vihaan's discharge and how can they all work together to optimise his outcome?
Q.7. What is Vihaan's likely long-term outcome?

Case study 2: The infant with HIE

Sireesha is a 40+5-week gestation female infant born by emergency category 1 caesarean section, due persistent fetal bradycardia presenting during prolonged second stage of labour. She was born in a local special care baby unit. Sireesha was born pale, floppy, with no respiratory effort and a heart rate of less than 60. She required inflation breaths followed by bag and mask ventilation, chest compressions, intubation and adrenaline. A fluid bolus of 10mL/kg of normal saline was given for poor perfusion. Her first spontaneous respiration was noted at 10 minutes of age. Apgar scores were 1, 1, 5 and 7 at 1, 5, 10 and 15 minutes, respectively. On admission to NICU her breathing pattern was stabilising, but she remained significantly floppy. On the first arterial gas obtained, her pH was 6.9 with a base deficit of 16mEq/L.

Q.1. Why is therapeutic cooling likely to be beneficial to Sireesha and what are the initial actions that must be taken at this point?
Q.2. Describe the reasons for this in line with the criteria for this treatment and why it is important for her to be transferred to a tertiary centre?
Q.3. What should be explained to the parents?

CASE STUDY

The aEEG initially showed a discontinuous pattern without sleep–wake cycling; at 2h of age she was noted to have repetitive jerky movements of her upper extremities with eye flickering lasting 45 seconds. She was given a loading dose of phenobarbital for recurrent episodes of jerking movements correlating to seizure activity on aEEG.

Q.4. Describe the significance of seizures including their nature and timing.

Q.5. Identify and explain caregiving practices required while Sireesha is being cooled.

Over the next 12 hours Sireesha's seizures stopped. She was re-warmed after 72 hours of cooling and was extubated to room air. Over the course of the next 10 days Sireesha established breastfeeding well.

Q.6. What is Sireesha's long-term outcome likely to be and what do the parents need to be told?

Case study 3: The infant with uncertain neurological outcome

Austin is one of triplets born at 25 weeks' gestation and is now 12 weeks old. Following a long period of respiratory support and stabilisation, he is now progressing in the special care area of the neonatal unit along with the other triplets, Hunter and Aidan, who are due to go home in the next few days. Austin, however, has been much slower to get to this point and suffered periods of being much more unstable both from a ventilation and BP perspective. He also has two periods of infection requiring antibiotics which set his progress back. Austin's mother Danielle also showed signs of infection during her pregnancy. The last few head ultrasound scans show that there are bilateral white echogenic areas, cystic appearances around the ventricular areas of the brain. He is presenting with some abnormal neurological signs.

Q.1. What is the significance of the information presented here in relation to a possible diagnosis relating to the brain?

Q.2. What factors leading up to this point have predisposed Austin to neurological compromise?

Q.3. In relation to the 'abnormal' neurology mentioned above, what might this be in relation to your nursing assessment of this infant?

Q.4. What is the potential long-term outcome for Austin?

Q.5. What should the parents be told about this situation and how will they be facilitated/supported to improve future outcome?

For suggested answer guides to the questions posed in these case studies, please refer to the web-based companion site specific to this chapter. See www.routledge.com/cw/petty

CASE STUDY

References

Alsadaan, N., Ramadan, O. M. E., Alqahtani, M., Shaban, M., Elsharkawy, N. B., Abdelaziz, E. M., & Ali, S. I. (2023). Impacts of integrating family-centered care and developmental care principles on neonatal neurodevelopmental outcomes among high-risk neonates. *Children*, *10*(11), 1751. https://doi.org/10.3390/children10111751

Altimier, L., & Phillips, R. M. (2016). The Neonatal Integrative Developmental Care Model: Advanced clinical applications of the seven core measures for neuroprotective family-centered developmental care. *Newborn and Infant Nursing Reviews*, *16*(4), 230–244.

British Association of Perinatal Medicine. (2020). *Therapeutic hypothermia for neonatal encephalopathy: A BAPM framework for practice*. Retrieved July 25, 2025, from https://www.bapm.org/resources/237-therapeutic-hypothermia-for-neonatal-encephalopathy

British Association of Perinatal Medicine (BAPM) & National Neonatal Audit Programme (NNAP). (2020). *Antenatal optimisation for preterm infants less than 34 weeks: A quality improvement toolkit*. BAPM & NNAP.

Chakkarapani, E., de Vries, L., Ferriero, D. M., & Gunn, A. J. (2025). Neonatal encephalopathy and hypoxic-ischaemic encephalopathy: The state of the art. *Pediatric Research*. Retrieved July 25, 2025, from https://doi.org/10.1038/s41390-025-03986-2

Cizmeci, M. N., & De Vries, L. S. (2024). Intracranial hemorrhage and stroke in the neonate. In R. J. Martin, A. A. Fanaroff & M. C. Walsh (Eds.), *Fanaroff and Martin's neonatal-perinatal medicine: Diseases of the fetus and infant* (12th ed., pp. 1033–1058). Elsevier.

Crowther, C. A., Middleton, P. A., Voysey, M., Askie, L., Duley, L., Pryde, P. G., Maret, S., & Doyle, L. W. for the AMICABLE Group (2017). Assessing the neuroprotective benefits of antenatal magnesium sulphate: An individual participant data meta-analysis. *PLoS Medicine*, *14*(10), e1002398.

de Bruijn, C. A. M., Di Michele, S., Tataranno, M. L., Ramenghi, L. A., Rossi, A., Malova, M., Benders, M., van den Hoogen, A., & Dudink, J. (2023). Neurodevelopmental consequences of preterm punctate white matter lesions: A systematic review. *Pediatric Research*, *93*(5), 1480–1490.

Depala, K. S., Chintala, S., Joshi, S., Paidipelly, N., Patel, B., Rastogi, A., Madas, N., & Mydam, J. (2023). Clinical variables associated with grade III and IV intraventricular hemorrhage (IVH) in preterm infants weighing less than 750 grams. *Cureus*, *15*(6), e40471.

European Foundation for the Care of Newborn Infants. (2018). *European standards of care for newborn health: Care procedures*. EFCNI. Retrieved October 20, 2025, from https://

newborn-health-standards.org/wp-content/uploads/2022/08/2022_09_01_TEG_Care-procedures_all.pdf

Faix, R. G., Laptook, A. R., Shankaran, S., Eggleston, B., Chowdhury, D., Heyne, R. J., Das, A., Pedroza, C., Tyson, J. E., Wusthoff, C., Bonifacio, S. L., Sánchez, P. J., Yoder, B. A., Laughon, M. M., Vasil, D. M., Van Meurs, K. P., Crawford, M. M., Higgins, R. D., Poindexter, B. B., . . . Shankaran, S. (2025). Whole-body hypothermia for neonatal encephalopathy in preterm infants 33 to 35 weeks' gestation: A randomized clinical trial. *JAMA Pediatrics, 179*(4), 396. https://doi.org/10.1001/jamapediatrics.2024.6613

Fogarty, M., Osborn, D. A., Askie, L., Seidler, A. L., Hunter, K., Lui, K., Simes, J., & Tarnow-Mordi, W. (2018). Delayed versus early umbilical cord clamping in preterm infants: A systematic review and meta-analysis. *American Journal of Obstetrics and Gynecology, 218*(1), 1–18.

Gale, C., Longford, N. T., Jeyakumaran, D., Ougham, K., Battersby, C., Ojha, S., & Dorling, J. (2021). Feeding during neonatal therapeutic hypothermia, assessed using routinely collected National Neonatal Research Database data: A retrospective, UK population-based cohort study. *The Lancet Child & Adolescent Health, 5*(6), 408–416. https://doi.org/10.1016/S2352-4642(21)00026-2

Gall, A. R., Amoah, S. K., Kitase, Y., & Jantzie, L. L. (2021). Placental mediated mechanisms of perinatal brain injury: Evolving inflammation and exosomes. *Experimental Neurology, 347*, 113914. https://doi.org/10.1016/j.expneurol.2021.113914

Glass, H. C., Numis, A. L., Comstock, B. A., Gonzalez, F. F., Mietzsch, U., Bonifacio, S. L., Massey, S., Thomas, C., Natarajan, N., Mayock, D. E., Sokol, G. M., Van Meurs, K. P., Ahmad, K. A., Maitre, N., Heagerty, P. J., Juul, S. E., Wu, Y. W., & Wusthoff, C. J. (2023). Association of EEG background and neurodevelopmental outcome in neonates with hypoxic-ischemic encephalopathy receiving hypothermia. *Neurology, 101*(22), e2223–e2233.

Kayyal, S., & Inder, T. E. (2024). Seizures in the neonate. In R. J. Martin, A. A. Fanaroff & M. C. Walsh (Eds.), *Fanaroff and Martin's neonatal-perinatal medicine: Diseases of the fetus and infant* (12th ed., pp. 1085–1116). Elsevier.

Kumar, D., Hinton, R., Ram, D., Saha, B., & Chandrasekaran, M. (2024). *North West Neonatal Operational Delivery Network seizure guideline*. Retrieved December 9, 2025, from GL-ODN-23-Neonatal-Seizure-Guideline_final.pdf

Kumar, J., Yadav, B., Meena, J., Yadav, J., & Sahu, J. K. (2025). Levetiracetam versus phenobarbitone for management of neonatal seizures: A systematic review and meta-analysis. *Indian Journal of Pediatrics, 92*(1), 29–41.

McGoldrick, E., Stewart, F., Parker, R., & Dalziel, S. R. (2020). Antenatal corticosteroids for accelerating fetal lung maturation for women at risk of preterm birth. *Cochrane Database of Systematic Reviews, 2021*(2). https://doi.org/10.1002/14651858.CD004454.pub4

Odd, D., Okano, S., Ingram, J., Blair, P. S., Billietop, A., Fleming, P. J., Thoresen, M., & Chakkarapani, E. (2021). Physiological responses to cuddling babies with hypoxic–ischaemic encephalopathy during therapeutic hypothermia: An observational study. *BMJ Paediatrics Open, 5*, e001280. https://doi.org/10.1136/bmjpo-2021-001280

Parikh, M. N., Chen, M., Braimah, A., Kline, J., McNally, K., Logan, J. W., Tamm, L., Yeates, K. O., Yuan, W., He, L., & Parikh, N. A. (2021). Diffusion MRI microstructural abnormalities at term-equivalent age are associated with neurodevelopmental outcomes at 3 years of age in very preterm infants. *American Journal of Neuroradiology, 42*(8), 1535–1542. https://doi.org/10.3174/ajnr.A7135

Pisani, F., Facini, C., Pavlidis, E., Spagnoli, C., & Boylan, G. (2024). Treating seizures and improving newborn outcomes for infants with hypoxic–ischemic encephalopathy. *Pediatric Research, 96*(5), 1100–1112.

Ranjan, A. K., & Gulati, A. (2023). Advances in therapies to treat neonatal hypoxic-ischemic encephalopathy. *Journal of Clinical Medicine, 12*(20), 6653.

Sarnat, H. B. (2023). Sequences of synaptogenesis in the human fetal and neonatal brain by synaptophysin immunocytochemistry. *Frontiers in Cellular Neuroscience*, *17*, 1105183. https://doi.org/10.3389/fncel.2023.1105183

Schmidt, B., Roberts, R. S., Anderson, P. J., Asztalos, E. V., Costantini, L., Davis, P. G., Dewey, D., D'Ilario, J., Doyle, L. W., Grunau, R. E., Moddemann, D., Nelson, H., Ohlsson, A., Solimano, A., & Tin, W. (2017). Academic performance, motor function, and behavior 11 years after neonatal caffeine citrate therapy for apnea of prematurity: An 11-year follow-up of the CAP randomized clinical trial. *JAMA Pediatrics*, *171*(6), 564–572.

Shaw, J. C., Crombie, G. K., Palliser, H. K., & Hirst, J. J. (2021). Impaired oligodendrocyte development following preterm birth: Promoting GABAergic action to improve outcomes. *Frontiers in Pediatrics*, *9*, Article 618052.

van Dokkum, N. H., de Kroon, M. L. A., & Reijneveld, S., & Bos, A. F. (2021). Neonatal stress, health, and development in preterms: A systematic review. *Pediatrics*, *148*(4), e2021050414. https://doi.org/10.1542/peds.2021-050414

Volpe, J. J. (2021). Cerebellar underdevelopment in the very preterm infant: Important and underestimated source of cognitive deficits. *Journal of NeonatalPerinatal Medicine*, *14*(4), 451–456.

Wu, L., Zhao, H., & Ma, D. (2024). Regulated cell death in hypoxic-ischaemic encephalopathy: Recent development and mechanistic overview. *Cell Death Discovery*, *10*, Article 277.

17 MANAGEMENT OF NEONATAL HAEMATOLOGICAL DISORDERS

Lynne Wainwright

CONTENTS

DOI: 10.4324/9781003591405-21

GUIDANCE ON HOW TO ENHANCE PERSONAL LEARNING FROM THIS CHAPTER

Key points covered in this chapter

- An overview of the main haematological disorders that present in neonatal care.
- The causes and clinical presentation of these disorders.
- The assessment, management and nursing care associated with caring for neonates with a range of haematological disorders.

Reflection

Reading through the chapter, you are encouraged to engage with the key points and related literature in an enquiring way. Ask these questions:

- Have you observed neonates who have had abnormal blood results? What were these and the underlying causes?
- How did these neonates present?
- How were these neonates managed?

Implications for nursing care

- Finally: how will this chapter enable you to consider how to best care for high-risk neonates with haematological conditions? Consider the implications of what you learn for your nursing care relating to this area.

INTRODUCTION AND BACKGROUND

Caring for babies with haematological disorders presents the neonatal nurse with many challenges. To correctly interpret clinical signs, monitor changes and provide information to support parents, a background knowledge of the haematological system is necessary. This chapter will review a range of common haematological disorders in the newborn: jaundice, polycythaemia, coagulation disorder including vitamin K deficiency bleeding (VKDB, also known as haemorrhagic disease of the newborn), **thrombocytopenia, disseminated intravascular coagulation** (DIC) and finally **anaemia**. The pathophysiology and treatment of each condition will be discussed, to enable the nurse to anticipate problems, assess the effectiveness of treatment and limit complications that may impact on the neonate.

JAUNDICE

Jaundice in a newborn is extremely common, approximately 60% of term and 80% of preterm neonates will develop jaundice during the first week of life. It is usually harmless, but high levels of unconjugated bilirubin can be damaging. Jaundice can also be a sign of serious liver disease. It is vital, therefore, that jaundice is recognised early, to ensure treatment of any underlying condition to be instigated. Jaundice is the yellow discolouration of the skin and sclerae seen when there is a buildup of bilirubin, produced from the breakdown of red blood cells (RBC). If levels of bilirubin in the circulation are high, this is known as hyperbilirubinaemia. Neonates have higher levels of bilirubin than adults due to their higher concentration of RBC, which also have a shorter lifespan. When RBCs break down, unconjugated bilirubin is formed. Unconjugated bilirubin is bound to albumin in the circulation and is then metabolised by the liver to produce conjugated (water-soluble) bilirubin which can subsequently be excreted in the stool (National Institute for Care Excellence (NICE), 2023a). Elevated levels of serum bilirubin (SBR) are common in the newborn and usually harmless. However, jaundice occurring in the first 24 hours of life, lasting for more than 2 weeks or reaching excessive levels is more concerning. This will be discussed in the relevant sections.

Physiology of bilirubin metabolism

In utero, the placenta manages the excretion of unconjugated bilirubin. Following delivery, the neonatal liver assumes responsibility for bilirubin metabolism. The main source of bilirubin is the breakdown of haem-containing proteins; 75% of bilirubin is formed by the breakdown of haemoglobin (Hb), a major constituent of RBC. One gram of Hb produces approximately 600µmol of unconjugated, fat-soluble bilirubin, which cannot be excreted via the gut or kidney but can easily pass through the lipid membranes of cells such as fatty tissue and the brain. Neonates have higher rates of total serum bilirubin than adults due to a higher Hb at birth, their RBC have a short lifespan of 40–70 days compared with 120 days in adults and the neonatal liver has limited conjugating capacity. Newborns produce 6mg/kg/day of bilirubin, double the amount produced by an adult. Bilirubin production is a two-stage process within the reticuloendothelial system. During the first stage, haem is degraded by the enzyme haem oxygenase, which causes the release of iron and the formation of biliverdin and carbon monoxide. Biliverdin is then broken down by biliverdin reductase to form unconjugated bilirubin (Kamath-Rayne et al., 2020).

Unconjugated bilirubin is transported in the circulation bound with albumin. Once bound, bilirubin enters the smooth endoplasmic reticulum in the liver with the help of carrier proteins Y (a ligandin) and Z. A series of reactions then occur, catalysed by the enzyme uridine diphosphate glucuronyl transferase (UGPGT), resulting in the joining of bilirubin with two molecules of glucuronic acid to produce conjugated bilirubin (Figure 17.1). Conjugated bilirubin is a component of bile and enters the gut via the biliary system. During its passage through the intestinal tract, bacterial enzymes convert bilirubin into urobilinogen and stercobilinogen, water-soluble compounds which can be excreted in the stools (Mitra & Rennie, 2017).

ACTIVITY

Consider registering for an account on e-learning for healthcare (https://support.e-lfh.org.uk/home/elfh Support) and completing the session 05_01 *Physiology of Jaundice*.

Physiological jaundice

Neonatal jaundice is classified as either physiological or pathological.

Physiological jaundice can be a result of:

- Increased bilirubin production due to increased RBC volume, decreased RBC life span or increased enterohepatic circulation
- Decreased uptake by the liver because of decreased ligandins or binding of ligandins to other **anions**
- Decreased conjugation in the liver because of decreased uridine diphosphoglucuronyl transferase (UDPGT) activity
- Decreased excretion into bile (Mitra & Rennie, 2017).

Physiological jaundice may be exacerbated by prematurity, administration of albumin-bound medications, bruising, polycythaemia, short life span of fetal red

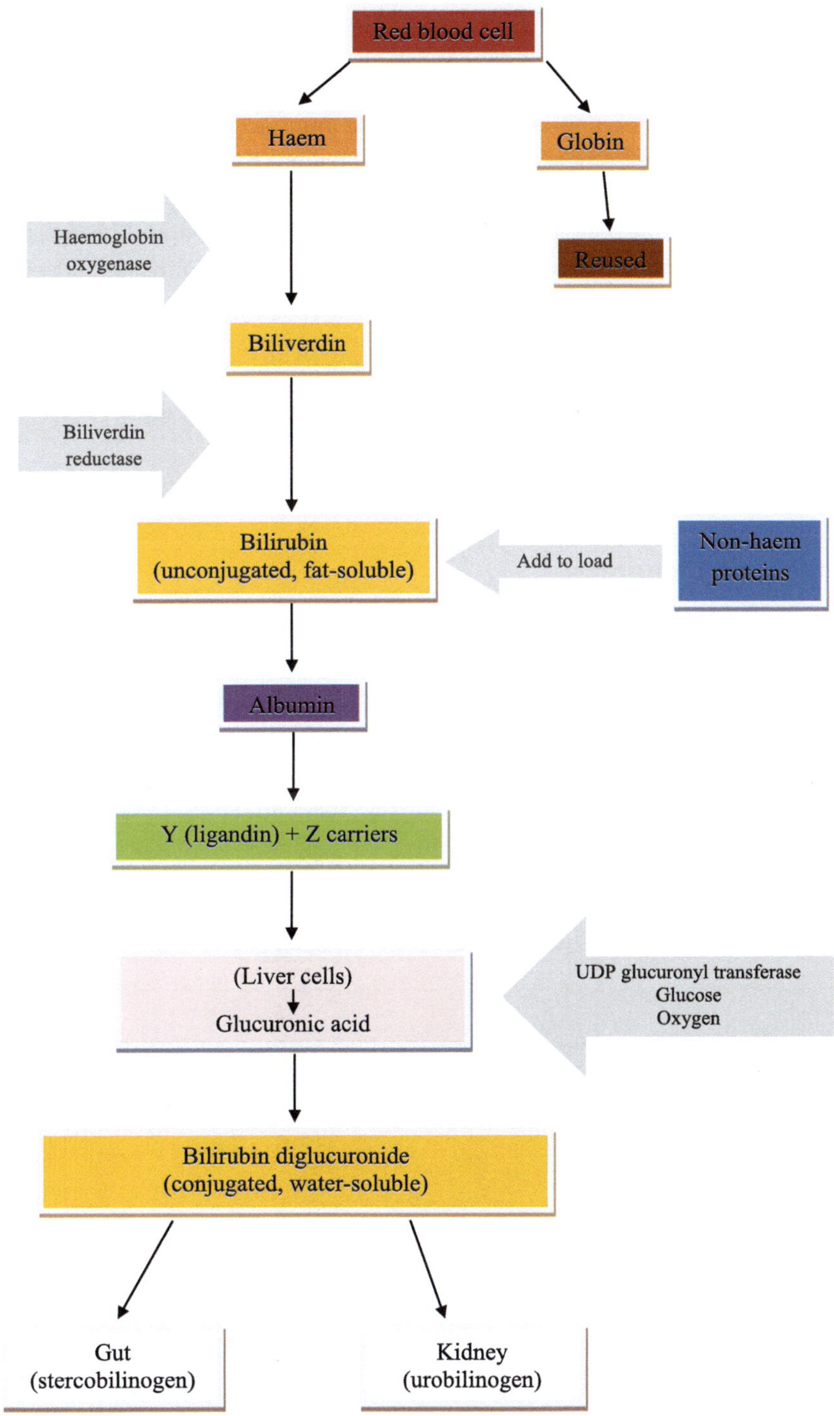

Figure 17.1 Physiology of bilirubin production

blood cells, inadequate oral intake, delayed passage of stool and breastfeeding (Kamath-Rayne et al., 2020).

Sick and premature neonates are more likely to experience neurotoxic effects of hyperbilirubinaemia. It can cause neurological damage including deafness, neurodevelopmental and motor problems. **Kernicterus** occurs when unconjugated bilirubin passes through the blood–brain barrier, resulting in yellow staining of the basal ganglia and causing irreversible damage. The symptoms of this clinical encephalopathy include hypertonia, an abnormally high-pitched cry, poor feeding, seizures and abnormal posture. Risk factors for developing kernicterus are:

- Serum bilirubin >340 μmol/L in a term neonate (>37 weeks)
- A rapid rise in SBR level (>8.5μmol/litre/hour)
- Clinical signs suggestive of bilirubin encephalopathy (Mitra & Rennie, 2017).

Pathological jaundice

Jaundice that occurs within the first 24 hours is likely to be pathological and usually results from the presence of exacerbating factors in addition to the mechanisms leading to physiological jaundice (Kamath-Rayne et al., 2020). Underlying disease processes may cause **haemolysis**, which increases bilirubin levels due to the increased breakdown of RBC; or other conditions may interfere with the normal bilirubin metabolism pathway. This can occur for several reasons (see Table 17.1), the most common being haemolytic disease highlighted below.

TABLE 17.1 CAUSES OF PATHOLOGICAL JAUNDICE

Pathology	*Mechanism*
ABO/rhesus incompatibility (haemolytic disease) Haemoglobinopathies G6PD deficiency	Increased red cell breakdown leading to hyperbilirubinaemia
Trauma	Sequestered blood
Hypothyroidism Galactosaemia	Interfere with metabolism and excretion
Drugs	Need albumin binding sites
Infection	May affect hepatic function +/− increase haemolysis
Biliary atresia Cystic fibrosis Tumours	Impaired ability to excrete conjugated bilirubin

Haemolytic disease of the newborn (HDN) is caused by maternal alloimmunisation against RBC **antigens**. In severe cases, HDN may lead to fetal anaemia with a risk for intrauterine death and to severe forms of neonatal hyperbilirubinaemia with a risk for kernicterus (Kamath-Rayne et al., 2020).

RHESUS INCOMPATIBILITY

Rhesus (Rh) HDN, also known as **erythroblastosis fetalis**, occurs when there is maternal red cell alloimmunisation and is one of the common pathological causes of hyperbilirubinaemia. Maternal **antibodies** are directed against fetal red cells when fetal RBC positive for an antigen (often Rhesus D) pass into the circulation of a mother who is negative for that antigen. Fetal and maternal circulations, although closely positioned in the placenta, are essentially separate from one another, but small tears in the placental capillaries or placental separation during delivery may facilitate the passage of fetal cells into the maternal circulation. Where a mother is Rh-negative and is carrying a Rh-positive fetus, passage of Rh-positive fetal cells into the Rh-negative maternal circulation generates an immune response and the production of anti-Rh antibodies. These maternal antibodies cause destruction of the Rh-positive fetal RBC (see Figure 17.2).

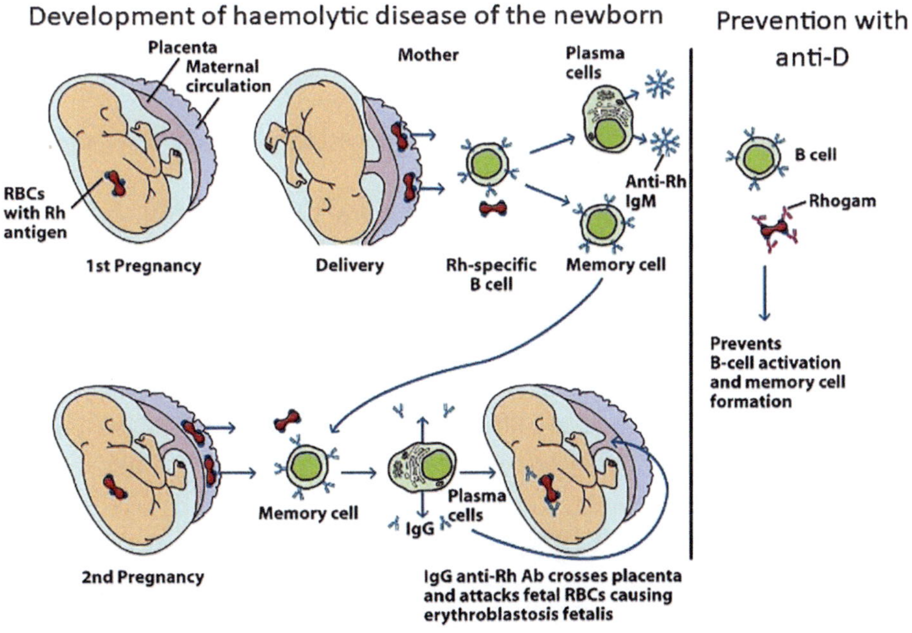

Figure 17.2 Haemolytic disease of the newborn

This maternal sensitisation to fetal Rh antigens occurs when there is fetal-maternal blood transfusion during pregnancy, delivery, miscarriage, termination or **amniocentesis**. During the first pregnancy this does not cause any issues; however, during subsequent pregnancies, the risk of fetal red cell haemolysis is present due to the elevated level of maternal anti-Rh antibodies (Kamath-Rayne et al., 2020). Breakdown of fetal RBC then results in raised bilirubin levels. During pregnancy, this excess bilirubin is excreted via the placenta, but after birth haemolysis continues, and the immature neonatal liver is unable to cope with the conjugation of large amounts of bilirubin, resulting in severe hyperbilirubinaemia appearing in the first 24 hours.

Severe HDN in the fetus due to Rh incompatibility can cause anaemia of the fetus and promotes RBC production from unusual sites such as the liver. The most severe form of HDN causes fetal hypoxia and cardiac failure, which in turn results in hydrops fetalis with generalised oedema and pleural, pericardial and/or peritoneal effusions. Due to the production of therapeutic anti-D **immunoglobulin** that binds to fetal cells and promotes their destruction prior to the initiation of a maternal immune response, this is now a rare occurrence. Routine administration of anti-D was introduced in the 1960s and has dramatically reduced maternal alloimmunisation in subsequent pregnancies. The routine administration of anti-D immunoglobulin to Rh negative mothers during the second trimester (28–34 weeks) and following any high-risk event during pregnancy is now accepted obstetric practice (Kamath-Rayne et al., 2020).

ABO INCOMPATIBILITY

ABO incompatibility occurs in the following situations:

- Maternal blood type is O and neonate's blood type A (most common type) or B (results in most severe haemolysis).
- Maternal blood type is B and neonate's blood type is A or AB.
- Maternal blood type is A and neonate's blood type is B or AB.

Naturally occurring maternal antibodies attach to the antigens on the incompatible fetal RBC, causing haemolysis and the production of bilirubin. The neonate presents with anaemia and jaundice. The direct antiglobulin (Coombs) test (DAT), which detects the presence of antibodies on the surface of RBC, is positive (Kamath-Rayne et al., 2020).

G6PD DEFICIENCY

Glucose-6-phosphate dehydrogenase is an enzyme responsible for maintaining the integrity of the red cell membrane. A deficiency of this enzyme renders the cell liable to haemolyse. This is most common in neonates of Mediterranean, Asian or

African origin. G6PD deficiency presents after 48 hours. In affected individuals, this can occur during ingestion of or exposure to oxidants such as naphthalene (moth balls), sulphonamide medications, fava beans (broad beans) or during periods of infection. Newborns are usually symptom-free until exposed to an oxidant, which triggers haemolysis. This condition has a sex-linked recessive inheritance pattern, which means that heterozygous females are carriers and males are affected. Once diagnosis is established, the family need to be advised on how to avoid the oxidants. G6PD deficiency is usually only clinically significant in infancy where there is a risk of developing kernicterus and is not a clinical problem in adults.

The most frequent clinical manifestations of G6PD deficiency are neonatal jaundice and acute haemolytic anaemia, which is usually triggered by an exogenous agent. Neonates with G6PD are much more likely to develop severe hyperbilirubinaemia than those without. Treatment is based on avoiding triggers and managing jaundice to prevent this (Kamath-Rayne et al., 2020).

Measurement of bilirubin levels

Jaundice becomes clinically evident when SBR levels reach 90µmol/L (Mitra & Rennie, 2017). Assessment of jaundice and bilirubin measurement is an important nursing role. The visual progression of jaundice may indicate the level of bilirubin; however, it should not replace actual SBR measurement. NICE guidance advises checking for signs of jaundice, especially in the first 72 hours. The naked neonate should be viewed in bright, ideally natural light. The sclerae, gums and skin should be examined, but visual inspection alone is not enough to estimate the bilirubin level. Effectiveness of visual assessment may be impacted by the skin tone of the neonate. Jaundice may be harder to detect visually in babies of darker skin tone. There is a lack of definitive evidence related to accuracy of transcutaneous bilirubinometers (TcB) in dark skinned babies, but this does not impact the current guidance (NICE, 2023b). Furness et al. (2024) noted that visual inspection for jaundice is subjective and can be inaccurate which is especially true in babies with darker skin tones where assessment of the sclerae and mucous membranes may be more accurate. Whilst the World Health Organization (WHO) postnatal care guidance (2022) advocates universal screening using TcB on discharge, there is insufficient evidence for the use of universal SBR. Neonates of Asian ethnicity are at increased risk of jaundice, making the issue of undetected jaundice all the more pertinent (Furness et al., 2024). Most healthcare professionals (HCPs) are aware of the difficulties identifying jaundice in dark-skinned babies and therefore focus on detecting yellowing of the sclerae and gums and other assessments. However, the need for improved training to effectively assess neonates of ethnic minorities for jaundice, remains. A further important point is that parents often identify jaundice before HCPs but are not always listened to (Fair et al., 2024).

Transcutaneous bilirubinometers (TcB) appear to be an accurate and non-invasive screening method for clinically significant jaundice in the well term neonate. The device measures the presence of yellow pigment in the skin of the forehead or over the sternum (Okwundu et al., 2017). Although these measurements correlate well with SBR in the lower range, and their use as a screening device to detect clinically significant jaundice decreases the need for frequent blood sampling in the well term neonate, accuracy is reduced above 250μmol/L, so that checking an SBR is recommended above this level. Serum measurement of total bilirubin remains the gold standard for diagnosing and treating hyperbilirubinaemia. SBR should be used for neonates in the first 24 hours of life or in neonates below 35 weeks' gestation. In neonates who are over 35 weeks' gestation and over 24 hours old, TcB can be used, or, in the absence of a bilirubinometer, SBR can be measured. SBR should be measured where bilirubin levels are at or above treatment thresholds and for subsequent measurements (NICE, 2023a). Thresholds are depicted as a line on gestation specific graphs on which SBR levels are plotted over time. A link to the phototherapy threshold graphs provided by NICE, now almost universally used in neonatal units (NNUs) in the UK, can be found in the web-based companion.

Treatment

PHOTOTHERAPY

Developed following recognition that sunshine appeared to reduce the jaundice pigment in the skin of a neonate reported by Cremer et al. (1958), phototherapy is universally used as a safe and convenient way of lowering SBR levels. It causes reactions that convert bilirubin into water-soluble isomers which can then be excreted more easily from the body as the products of breakdown do not need conjugation in the liver. It is effective only once bilirubin enters the skin and the SBR is above 80μmol/L (Mitra & Rennie, 2017). Phototherapy works through a process known as photooxidation to convert the bilirubin into a nontoxic soluble form by adding oxygen, which makes it easier for the liver to manage.

Phototherapy lamps/units emitting visible blue light in the wavelength of 460–490 nanometres are the most effective in reducing serum bilirubin (see Figure 17.3). The efficacy of phototherapy is dependent on dose and wavelength of the light used and the surface area of the neonate's skin which is exposed to the light. The dose can be increased by placing the lights at the minimum safe distance from the neonate, by using more than one unit or by combining overhead lamps with a fibreoptic system under the neonate (Bhutani et al., 2024).

Conventional phototherapy units use fluorescent tubes to administer light at the blue end of the spectrum. These lights are placed above the neonate.

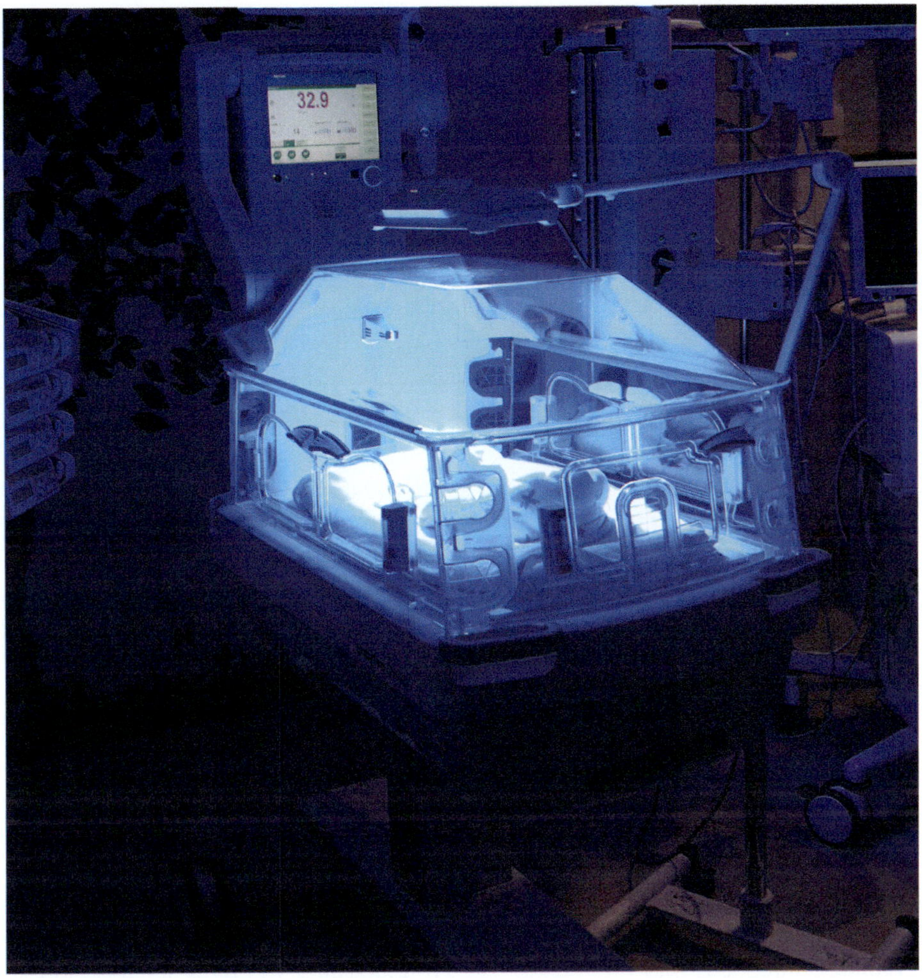

Figure 17.3 Phototherapy

Newer phototherapy units utilise multiple light-emitting diodes (LEDs) which can be used closer to the neonate's skin as they do not generate infrared or ultraviolet radiation (Bhutani et al., 2024). Fibreoptic systems are used via a body pad or wrap and have made phototherapy more versatile. In this case, phototherapy is delivered using a single light source that comprises a light generator, a fibreoptic cable through which the light is carried and a flexible light pad on which the neonate is placed or that is wrapped around the neonate. NICE guidance advises that phototherapy can be delivered with light-emitting diodes, fibreoptic or fluorescent lamps, tubes or bulbs; no specific device is recommended. In lower resource countries, phototherapy is not universally available, so that window-tinting films are used to filter out solar radiation with the potential to cause damage in the treatment of hyperbilirubinaemia (Bhutani et al., 2024).

Gestational age-specific treatment threshold graphs should be used to determine the need for treatment (NICE, 2023a). These graphs show two clear lines indicating the phototherapy and exchange transfusion thresholds for neonates in the first two weeks of life. Term neonates over 24 hours of age who have a bilirubin reading below the treatment line, but within 50μmol/L, should have a SBR measurement repeated within 18 hours if they have risk factors for jaundice (a sibling who required phototherapy or where the mother intends to exclusively breastfeed) or within 24 hours if they have no risk factors (NICE, 2023a).

ACTIVITY

Look up the NICE guidance 'Tools and Resources' on Neonatal Jaundice and download the Treatment Threshold graphs – https://www.nice.org.uk/guidance/cg98/resources Take note of the different graphs according to gestation along with the thresholds for both phototherapy and exchange transfusion treatments.

Nursing management of the jaundiced neonate not only includes assessment, but the administration of phototherapy with its own set of specific care interventions, outlined later.

In neonates who require phototherapy, SBR should be checked 4–6 hours after commencement of treatment and then every 6-12 hours if stable or falling. Phototherapy should be continued until the SBR is at least 50μmol/L below the treatment threshold and rechecked 12–18 hours later to check for rebound. In cases where SBR levels are rising rapidly, are within 50μmol/L below the exchange transfusion threshold after 72 hours or fail to respond to initial phototherapy within 6 hours, intensified phototherapy should be considered. This involves adding a further light source or higher radiance light sources (NICE, 2023a).

Phototherapy is a generally safe treatment, although it may have side effects. These include:

- Diarrhoea has historically been described as a side effect of phototherapy, but this is not reflected in recent evidence.
- Unstable temperature and increased transepidermal water loss should not be an issue when LED units are used, although UK guidance still suggests daily weighing (NICE, 2023a).
- Skin rashes and discolouration (bronze neonate syndrome and tanning): Bronze Neonate Syndrome occurs due to an interaction between cholestatic

jaundice and phototherapy. The brown pigment stains the skin and may linger after discontinuation of treatment for some weeks.

- Potential retinal damage: Early animal studies suggested that retinal damage may occur following exposure to phototherapy lights. Although these studies were conducted over 40 years ago, this risk has never been conclusively disproven in humans, and thus neonates' eyes should be shielded during phototherapy (Bhutani et al., 2024). Eye shields should be removed at regular intervals to check for abrasions or infection. The shields need to be tight enough to prevent slipping and potential airway obstruction, but not so tight as to restrict blood flow or cause tissue damage. Orange-tinted head boxes or shields can be used as an alternative to eye shields in term neonates (NICE, 2023a).
- Concerns regarding an association between phototherapy and later development of childhood epilepsy or cancers have been suggested, mostly affecting extremely preterm neonates. A cycled approach to phototherapy delivery is currently being investigated.
- Parental support during phototherapy is essential, as a diagnosis of jaundice is associated with increased maternal anxiety about their neonate's health during the first weeks (Bhutani et al., 2024). Parents should be encouraged to continue feeding, caring for and visiting their baby and ideally receive written and verbal information. Lactation support should be continued. During single phototherapy, short breaks should be encouraged for feeding and cuddles. If intensified phototherapy is required, it should not be stopped for feeding, but intravenous fluids or enteral feeds of breastmilk should be given dependent on clinical need (NICE, 2023a).

PRACTICE POINT

Although fairly common practice in other countries, such as the USA, home phototherapy is still in its infancy in the UK. Generally, a continuation of phototherapy commenced in hospital for low-risk neonates, it is associated with good effect, low readmission rates and, most importantly, high parental satisfaction (Noureldein et al., 2021).

INTRAVENOUS IMMUNOGLOBULIN

Administration of intravenous immunoglobulin (IVIG) combined with phototherapy has been shown to significantly reduce the need for exchange transfusion, length of phototherapy and overall length of stay in neonates with severe Rhesus or ABO isoimmunisation. Neonates are, however, more likely to need top-up transfusions for late anaemia. It has been suggested that the main role of IVIG is to 'buy time' before commencing exchange transfusion (Mitra & Rennie, 2017). NICE (2023a) guidelines state that 500mg/kg over 4 hours should be given alongside intensified phototherapy when neonates have severe Rhesus or ABO haemolytic disease and the SBR continues to increase by more than 8.5μmol/L per hour. IVIG works by blocking receptors on macrophages, reducing the breakdown of antibody-coated red cells and by increasing the clearance of maternal antibodies (Kamath-Rayne et al., 2020). IVIG is a human-derived blood product and has potential side effects, including transfusion reactions, infection transmission, association with necrotising enterocolitis (NEC) and acute renal failure.

EXCHANGE TRANSFUSION

Exchange transfusion is a specialist procedure with associated risks of morbidity and mortality from vascular injuries, cardiovascular complications, biochemical and haematological disturbances, in addition to a small risk of blood-borne infection. However, exchange transfusions are now infrequently performed in NNUs, mainly due to the use of prophylactic anti-D for Rh negative mothers (Kamath-Rayne et al., 2020).

Aims of exchange transfusion:

- To lower the SBR level and reduce the risk of brain damage and kernicterus
- To correct anaemia and increase the oxygen-carrying capacity of the baby's blood
- To remove damaged and antibody-coated red cells
- To control the blood volume and relieve potential heart failure
- To correct life-threatening electrolyte imbalance.

Double volume exchange transfusion should be used to treat neonates whose SBR indicates its necessity or where there are clinical signs of acute bilirubin encephalopathy. This will remove up to 50% of intravascular bilirubin.

Parents should be fully informed of the rationale for the procedure and its associated risks and consent obtained. An exchange transfusion should normally be undertaken in neonatal intensive care, with the baby under a radiant heater. Intensified phototherapy should be continued (NICE, 2023a). Nursing responsibilities include continuous monitoring and frequent recording of heart rate, respiratory rate, oxygen saturation, blood pressure and temperature during the procedure. A baseline set of observations encompassing colour, tone and blood sugar should be documented before the procedure starts. Enteral feeds should be stopped to reduce the risk of NEC. A specific red cell component for neonatal exchange transfusion is provided by UK Blood Services, usually group O, and should also be compatible with any maternal antibody. Twice the neonate's blood volume should be exchanged (2 × 80mL/kg). Intravenous and arterial access is required via umbilical and/or peripheral lines. Aliquots of less than 5mL/kg are removed over 3–5 minutes with simultaneous continuous infusion of blood to the neonate. After the exchange transfusion, intensified phototherapy should be continued and the SBR measured within 2 hours. Management is then maintained in accordance with the threshold graph (NICE, 2023a).

THINK POINT

Phototherapy can prevent parents from interacting with their baby although having an exchange transfusion is more prohibited as it means that parents are unable to hold their baby for the duration of the procedure. Think how you could promote family integrated care, bonding and closeness when looking after a neonate requiring both phototherapy and, if needed, an exchange transfusion?

Prolonged jaundice

Prolonged jaundice is defined as jaundice that is still evident in a term neonate at 2 weeks of age or in a premature neonate at 3 weeks of age. This is most commonly unconjugated hyperbilirubinaemia, such as that seen in breastfed neonates, with around 9% of breastfed neonates still jaundiced at 28 days of life (Mitra & Rennie, 2017). However, prolonged jaundice may occur due to issues such as dehydration/inadequate intake or congenital hypothyroidism.

Most important to rule out is conjugated hyperbilirubinaemia (a serum conjugated bilirubin greater than 25µmol/L). This is usually associated with underlying pathology (see Table 17.2), which needs to be addressed in order to treat the condition such as infection (Kamath-Rayne et al., 2020).

Suggested initial investigations for prolonged jaundice are as follows:

- Evaluation of urine colour – is it dark and does it stain the nappy?
- Check stool colour – whether yellow or pale and chalky
- Measure total and split bilirubin
- Full blood count, blood group and direct antibody test (Coombs test)
- Liver function test
- Urine culture
- Routine metabolic screening (ensure newborn bloodspot test has been sent)
- Thyroid function test
- G6PD level (NICE, 2023a).

Jaundice associated with breastmilk/breastfeeding

The likelihood of a newborn developing hyperbilirubinaemia has been suggested to increase with the maternal intention to breastfeed exclusively (NICE, 2023a). This type of jaundice usually reaches its peak between 14 and 21 days and is resolved by 3 months. The neonate is generally well and gaining weight. This type of jaundice can occur for two reasons:

- Newborns who are breastfed tend to have a lower fluid intake compared with formula-fed neonates in the first few days and as such have relatively higher levels of SBR. When a newborn has an insufficient intake of breastmilk, their meconium output is decreased, increasing the reabsorption of bilirubin. Newborns have slower intestinal transit times increasing exposure to beta-glucuronidase as well as the unconjugation process via the enterohepatic circulation. A baby who is not feeding well is inclined to be lethargic and less likely to feed, therefore perpetuating the issue. Promotion of good milk supply in the early days will help the neonate to take in sufficient amounts of colostrum, which is important, as it is a natural laxative and is an effective method of ensuring passage of meconium and prevention of a buildup of meconium. Breastfeeding mothers require support and education if they are to be successful.
- The other proposed reason is thought to be due to constituents of breastmilk. Breastmilk is rich in beta-glucuronidase which increases the reuptake of unconjugated bilirubin.

If the neonate is well, and no other pathologies are identified, breastmilk jaundice does not require any intervention, as it is benign and self-limiting (Kamath-Rayne et al., 2020).

Investigations for jaundice are outlined in Table 17.3.

POLYCYTHAEMIA

Neonatal polycythaemia is defined as an excess of RBC. This results in raised haematocrit (>65%), otherwise known as packed cell volume (PCV) which increases blood viscosity, impairing the circulatory flow to and in organs, and can cause neurological, cardiopulmonary and gastrointestinal symptoms. Many neonates may be asymptomatic or present with signs related to the organ affected by decreased perfusion. Polycythaemia can be the result of a physiological condition, such as antenatal or intrapartum hypoxia, or a passive process (from RBC transfusion). Neonates born post-term or small for gestational age, neonates of diabetic mothers, recipient twins in twin-to-twin transfusion syndrome and those where the umbilical cord was milked are all at a higher risk of the condition.

TABLE 17.2 CAUSES OF CONJUGATED HYPERBILIRUBINAEMIA

- Congenital viral infection
- Perinatal hypoxia-ischaemia
- Sepsis
- Severe haemolysis
- Prolonged use of parenteral nutrition
- α-1antitrypsin deficiency
- Cystic fibrosis
- Biliary atresia
- Choledochal cyst
- Spontaneous bile duct perforation
- Cholestasis
- Intrahepatic biliary hypoplasia
- Progressive familial idiopathic cholestasis
- Galactosaemia
- Tyrosinaemia.

TABLE 17.3 INVESTIGATIONS FOR JAUNDICE RELATED TO TIMING OF ONSET

Jaundice in the first 24 hours	Serum bilirubin levels including conjugated fraction (level >20μmol/L may indicate biliary atresia) Full blood count with haematocrit/packed cell volume Blood group and direct antiglobulin test maternal blood group G6PD screening (be aware that this can be false during acute haemolysis) Galactose-l-phosphate uridyl transferase (to detect galactosaemia) Screening for evidence of congenital viral infection (to detect toxoplasmosis, hepatitis, HIV, parvovirus, rubella, cytomegalovirus and herpes)
Jaundice appearing at 2–5 days	Blood cultures Urine metabolic screening looking for metabolic disorders Serum bilirubin, blood group (maternal and neonate), DAT Depending on treatment response, consider investigations as for jaundice in the first 24 hours
'Prolonged' jaundice (persisting for more than 14 days)	Same as for jaundice in first 24 hours, as well as liver function tests and conjugated bilirubin fraction Thyroid function tests

A key nursing responsibility is to observe the affected neonate for potential signs and symptoms and ensure that treatment is started, if applicable, as soon as possible to avoid complications such as diminished blood supply to organs and/or thrombosis. Symptoms include cyanosis, lethargy, poor feeding and tremors, and apnoea may also be present (McKinney et al., 2020). Treatment of polycythaemia is by partial exchange transfusion, which can be undertaken via peripheral or central lines and reduces the PCV without causing hypervolaemia. Partial exchange transfusion is carried out by withdrawing blood from a vein or artery and replacing it with a diluent such as normal saline leading to diluted plasma volume. Normal saline is the diluent of choice, as it does not carry infection risks, which are present if colloids are used.

The calculation used is

$$\text{Partial exchange (mL)} = \frac{\text{Blood volume} \times \text{weight (kg)} \times (\text{observe Hct} - \text{desired Hct})}{\text{observed Hct}}$$

Blood volume is 80–90mL/kg in preterm neonates or 90–100 mL/kg in term neonates. The desired haematocrit is normally 55%. As existing evidence comparing partial exchange transfusion to management with IV fluids alone does not show an improvement in long term outcomes, this should be reserved only for neonates who are symptomatic or whose haematocrit exceeds 70% (McKinney et al., 2020). Further details about nursing care are covered later.

COAGULATION DISORDERS

Neonates are susceptible to bleeding for several reasons, including immaturity of the haemostatic system because of quantitative and qualitative deficiency of coagulation factors; maternal disease and medication use; birth trauma; and conditions such as sepsis and asphyxia. Coagulation disorders include those that involve haemorrhage, such as VKDB, thrombocytopenia and DIC or, conversely, thrombosis. To understand the processes involved in coagulation disorders, it is important to appreciate the underlying physiology.

Coagulation physiology

Coagulation (clotting) and haemostasis (stopping the flow of blood) in the neonatal period are in a unique state of balance, due to the altered levels of procoagulants and anticoagulants common of this age group. Term neonates have immature livers and associated levels of clotting factors in early life. Neonates who are born prematurely or who are sick often present with even lower levels of clotting factors and further deranged clotting processes. The normal process is outlined below.

When blood vessel injury occurs, platelets adhere to the damaged area and release adenosine diphosphate which activates the process of clotting. Platelets are pulled together due to an affinity for the blood protein fibrinogen, and in combination they form a mesh over the injury. In order to prevent the mesh from being pulled away, platelets contribute to the release of thromboxane, which encourages vasoconstriction and decreased blood flow in the damaged area. A process known as the clotting cascade is then initiated, in which a series of proteins and enzymes are activated sequentially through a variety of complex biochemical reactions to produce a blood clot. In addition, vitamin K is essential for the function of several proteins involved in blood coagulation (prothrombin, factors VII, IX and X, protein C, protein S and protein Z; see Table 17.4). The importance of vitamin K in haemostasis arises from the fact that all vitamin K-dependent coagulation factors require carboxylation of glutamic acids to enable binding of calcium and attachment to phospholipid membranes (McKinney et al., 2020).

Vitamin K deficiency bleeding

VKDB can cause bleeding in a neonate in the first few weeks of life. Vitamin K, a fat-soluble vitamin, is necessary for the synthesis of coagulation factors amongst other roles. VKDB is defined as a bleeding disorder in which the coagulopathy is

TABLE 17.4 BLOOD CLOTTING FACTORS

Factor I	Fibrinogen
Factor II*	Prothrombin
Factor III	Thromboplastin
Factor IV	Calcium ions
Factor V	Pro-accelerin
Factor VI	Is no longer recognised in the clotting pathway
Factor VII*	Pro-convertin (Serum prothrombin conversion accelerator)
Factor VIII	Antihaemophilic factor
Factor IX	Plasma thromboplastin component* (Christmas factor)
Factor X*	Thrombokinase (Stuart–Power factor)
Factor XI	Plasma thromboplastin antecedent
Factor XII	Hageman factor
Factor XIII	Fibrin stabilising factor
Other	Platelets

* Vitamin K-dependent

rapidly corrected by vitamin K supplementation. Term neonates, especially those who are exclusively breastfed, are deficient in vitamin K and have minimal reserves in the liver and consequently may develop VKDB (McKinney et al., 2020). Preterm neonates are potentially at greater risk for VKDB because of delayed feeding and subsequent delay in the colonisation of their gastrointestinal system with vitamin K-producing microflora, as well as immature hepatic and haemostatic function (Ardell et al., 2018).

In high income countries, VKDB is very rare with most cases occurring in breastfed neonates whose parents have refused prophylaxis. Globally, however, low and middle-income countries have a higher incidence, suggested to be related to a lower use of vitamin K prophylaxis. Insufficient awareness, unrelated to income status, is also an issue, highlighting the necessity for better education for parents as well as HCPs (Sirachainan et al., 2025).

VKDB is usually classified by aetiology and by the age of onset.

- *Early onset* The least common form of VKDB presents within the first 24 hours and is associated with placental transfer of maternal medications which interfere with vitamin K metabolism. These include anticonvulsants (phenytoin, carbamazepine and barbiturates), antituberculosis drugs (isonizid, rifampicin), some antibiotics (cephalosporins) and vitamin K antagonists (warfarin). The clinical presentation is often severe with cephalic haematoma and intracranial and intra-abdominal haemorrhage. Postnatal administration of vitamin K cannot prevent early neonatal bleeding.
- *Classical onset* This usually presents between 2 and 7 days of life and is associated with delayed or insufficient feeding. The clinical presentation is often mild, with bruises, gastrointestinal blood loss or bleeding from the umbilicus and puncture sites. Blood loss can be significant, and intracranial haemorrhage has been described.
- *Late onset* is associated with exclusive breastfeeding. It occurs between the ages of 2 and 12 weeks. The clinical presentation is severe with a mortality rate of 20% and intracranial haemorrhage occurring in 30–60% of these babies.

Babies who are entirely breastfed have a twentyfold risk of developing VKDB than those who receive formula milk due to the low level of vitamin K in breastmilk and also the low levels of bacteria which help to synthesise vitamin K in the guts of breastfed neonates (McKinney et al., 2020).

If VKDB is suspected, it is important to review certain aspects of the medical history:

- Drugs taken in pregnancy
- Gestation at delivery

- Type and length of delivery
- Feeding history (breastfed or formula-fed)
- Maternal diseases e.g. idiopathic thrombocytopenic purpura, pre-eclampsia and diabetes
- Family history of bleeding disorders
- Previous affected siblings
- Confirmation of vitamin K administration.

Investigations

- Full blood count
- Clotting screen, including prothrombin time (prolonged), coagulation time and partial thromboplastin time, D-dimer
- Chest X-ray or ultrasound may confirm intrathoracic bleed
- CT or MRI scan if intracranial haemorrhage or other major haemorrhage is suspected.

MANAGEMENT OF VITAMIN K DEFICIENCY BLEEDING

Vitamin K is commonly given prophylactically after birth for the prevention of VKDB. Since the 1950s, the use of artificial vitamin K to prevent VKDB has been common practice. Both oral and intramuscular (IM) prophylactic Vitamin K are effective in prevention of classical VKDB. In accordance with current recommendation, healthy newborn neonates who are not at particular risk of bleeding disorders should receive an IM injection of 1mg vitamin K at birth; or 2mg by mouth for 1 dose at birth followed by 2mg at 4–7 days and one month for neonates without bleeding risk who are exclusively breastfed (Paediatric Formulary Committee, 2024). For the preterm neonate, a single dose of 400 micrograms/kg (maximum dose 1mg) is to be given at birth. The intravenous route may be used with very low birthweight neonates if IM injection is not possible. However, it may not provide the prolonged protection of IM administration, and the neonate may require subsequent oral doses. Further research on appropriate dosing and route for preterm neonates is needed (Ardell et al., 2018). Many units require informed parental consent prior to any administration of vitamin K. Those advocating for mandatory IM vitamin K for all newborns suggest that, while parental autonomy would be reduced, newborn care would be enhanced (Sirachainan et al., 2025).

Thrombocytopenia

The normal platelet count of a healthy newborn neonate is 150×10^9/L and above; therefore, a count below this represents thrombocytopenia, which may present with petechiae. The two pathological mechanisms for this condition are decreased production or increased destruction of platelets. Thrombocytopenia that presents early, for example, in the first 72 hours of life, is usually secondary to placental insufficiency, perinatal hypoxia-ischaemia or maternal pre-eclampsia or diabetes leading to reduced platelet production. This can be mild to moderate in severity and should resolve spontaneously. The underlying cause for early thrombocytopenia in a well baby tends to be neonatal alloimmune thrombocytopenia. Presentation after 72 hours of age is more likely secondary to sepsis or more serious conditions such as NEC. This is usually more severe and prolonged (McKinney et al., 2020). Platelet transfusion is the treatment and administered either to prevent or to treat haemorrhage, with recent evidence in the preterm population (PlaNET-2 trial) supporting transfusion at lower levels (Estcourt, 2019).

PRACTICE POINTS

When caring for neonates with thrombocytopenia, nurses should closely monitor for subtle bleeding signs, including petechiae, oozing at cannula sites or gastrointestinal loss and escalate concerns early. Minimising invasive procedures, using gentle handling, and ensuring clear communication with the medical team can significantly reduce bleeding risk and support timely intervention.

Disseminated intravascular coagulation

DIC can be defined as a systemic thrombohaemorrhagic disorder. Endothelial tissue damage from a variety of underlying disorders (sepsis, trauma) activates the coagulation cascade, which promotes fibrin production and consumption of clotting factors (Figure 17.4). Neonates, especially preterm neonates, are one of the highest-risk groups to develop DIC secondary to labile blood pressure and cardiac output, intravascular volume contraction after birth, immature mucosal and skin barriers and multiple invasive procedures.

Clinical manifestations include **petechiae**, unexplained anaemia, bleeding from the gastrointestinal tract and puncture sites. In severe cases, intrapulmonary and intraventricular haemorrhages occur. There may be thrombus formation in the small vessels of the liver, brain, lungs and kidneys. Laboratory investigations should be interpreted in context of normal findings for gestation and postnatal age. Findings include consumption of coagulation factors and platelets and combined prolonged APTT and PT +/- low fibrinogen (McKinney et al., 2020).

MANAGEMENT OF DISSEMINATED INTRAVASCULAR COAGULATION

As DIC is a secondary disease, management of the primary disease is the only way to reverse it. It is important to obtain samples for coagulation factors prior

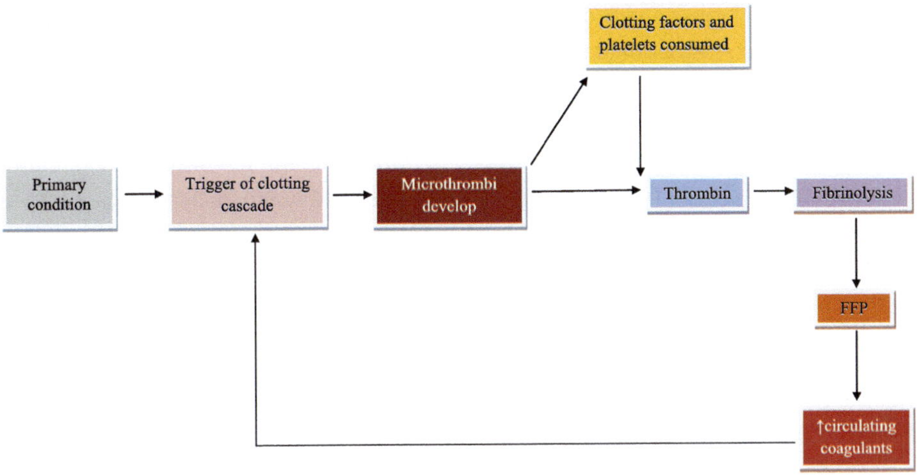

Figure 17.4 Disseminated intravascular coagulation

to transfusing the baby to avoid inaccurate results. Treatment is replacement of clotting factors. FFP can be used to replace all factors, and 10–15ml/kg is the usual dose. Thrombocytopenia is a sensitive sign of DIC. Transfusion of platelets at 10–15ml/kg is indicated in babies who are actively bleeding, otherwise platelet transfusion may worsen the condition. Other factors used may include cryoprecipitate to replace specific clotting factors and especially fibrinogen (McKinney et al., 2020). Nursing care related to DIC is outlined in Table 17.5.

THROMBOSIS

Levels of several coagulation factors are reduced when compared to adults, and this is especially true in preterm babies. Thus, there is an increased incidence of thrombosis in high-risk neonates. Thromboses in neonates are often related to central venous catheters or arterial lines. All intravascular access acts to disrupt blood flow and damage endothelial cells and vessel walls, leading to **thrombus** formation. Treatment is mainly via the use of low molecular weight heparin, with the aim of avoiding end organ damage, but the risk of bleeding must be weighed up individually (McKinney et al., 2020).

ANAEMIA

In the NNU, anaemia is a common challenge. It is a deficiency in the concentration of RBC and Hb in the blood, related to blood loss, reduced red blood cell production and higher levels of erythrocyte breakdown and can result in tissue hypoxia and acidosis. A neonate may be considered anaemic if the Hb or haematocrit value is more than two standard deviations below normal for their gestational age group. All term and preterm neonates experience a degree of physiological anaemia due to the conversion of fetal Hb to adult Hb during the first few weeks of postnatal life. Certain conditions may exacerbate this and lead to acute and chronic anaemia. These include acute or chronic blood loss/sampling and acute or chronic RBC haemolysis (Kollamparambil et al., 2024). Deferred clamping of the umbilical cord (not earlier than 1 minute after birth) has been recommended to improve iron status in the neonate for up to six months after birth (McKinney et al., 2020).

Physiological anaemia

In utero, fetal oxygen saturation is 45%. **Erythropoietin** levels are high, and fetal Hb has a higher affinity for oxygen, meaning that it does not release oxygen easily into the tissues. and therefore, facilitates the transfer of oxygen from mother to neonate in utero compared to adult haemoglobin. During the last weeks of gestation, the transition from production of fetal to adult haemoglobin starts and by 6 months of age most fetal haemoglobin will have been replaced by the adult form. Erythropoiesis decreases after birth as a result of increased tissue oxygenation with the onset of breathing, closure of the ductus arteriosus and a reduced production of erythropoietin (McKinney et al., 2020).

Anaemia of prematurity

Anaemia of prematurity (AOP) is an exaggeration of physiological anaemia and is seen in neonates less than 32 weeks' gestation. The primary cause of AOP is the impaired ability to increase serum erythropoietin appropriately when anaemic, low reticulocyte counts and decreased tissue availability of oxygen. Nutritional deficiencies of iron, vitamin E, vitamin B12 and folic acid may furthermore exaggerate the degree of anaemia (Kollamparambil et al., 2024).

In healthy term babies, the Hb does not often fall below 100g/L at 10–12 weeks and is well tolerated, but in preterm babies the drop in Hb is more rapid, occurring at 4–6 weeks, falling to 80g/L in babies with birth weights of 1–1.5kg and 70g/L in babies born below 1kg. This is associated with clinical signs and the need for RBC transfusions (Chaudhary et al., 2022). Signs associated with AOP include tachycardia, poor weight gain, increased requirement of supplemental oxygen or increased episodes of apnoea and bradycardia. Identification of the cause of anaemia through maternal and perinatal history review, laboratory data analysis and symptoms will guide management and treatment options.

Iatrogenic anaemia due to repeated blood sampling is an important consideration in the NNU. Measures which may reduce numbers of blood samples being taken and the incidence include diagnostic testing based on individual neonate condition rather than routine testing, micro sample laboratory techniques, non-invasive monitoring methods and documentation of blood sample volumes collected.

MANAGEMENT OF ANAEMIA OF PREMATURITY

In preterm babies, optimal nutrition (e.g. iron supplementation) should be provided and patients monitored for signs of anaemia. Nurses also have a vital role in observing the neonate for progressive anaemia, both clinically and by analysis of blood Hb and PCV levels. Blood sampling should be limited to essential testing and micro techniques should be used to minimise blood loss due to phlebotomy.

The following management strategies of anaemia of prematurity (AOP) are used in NNUs in the UK:

- *Iron supplementation* Iron content at birth is lower in preterm neonates than in term neonates, and the iron stores are often depleted by 2–3 months of age. As a result, iron supplementation is recommended from 2 weeks of age until 6–12 months of age (British Association of Perinatal Medicine, 2023). Neonates who receive iron-fortified formula or breastmilk fortifiers containing sufficient iron need less additional supplementation than those who are exclusively breastfed.
- *Transfusion therapy* RBC transfusion is the most rapidly effective treatment for AOP. This is usually performed when anaemia is associated with clinical signs or is thought to compromise adequate oxygen delivery. Up to 80% of extremely premature neonates and around half of neonates born at less than 32 weeks' gestation may need at least one blood transfusion (Chaudhary et al., 2022).

Clinical decisions to transfuse neonates need to be made carefully, considering the associated risks. There has been a move from liberal use of blood transfusions to tolerance of lower Hb levels following findings of the PINT, ETTNO and TOP trials. Transfusion thresholds should be restrictive and taking into consideration haematocrit and clinical status of the neonate (Chaudhary et al., 2022). Usually, the transfusion volume is 15–20mL/kg, administered over 2–4 hours. Nurses are responsible for checking the blood product, setting up the transfusion, monitoring the baby and recording according to local policy. Transfusion is a temporary measure and has the disadvantages of further inhibiting erythropoiesis, as well as being associated with risks of transmitted infection, transfusion-associated NEC, graft versus host disease and toxic effects of anticoagulants and preservatives. To minimise these risks, blood is screened for many of the known organisms, including hepatitis B and C, human immunodeficiency virus (HIV) and cytomegalovirus (CMV). Irradiation of blood products prevents transfusion-associated graft versus host disease, which results from a potentially fatal incompatibility between recipient and donor cells. This rare condition is said to be more likely when the recipient receives blood from multiple donors, and the use of smaller packs of irradiated blood produced from one donor, stored for as long as possible, may help to prevent this (Jacquot et al., 2024).

> **ACTIVITY**
>
> The WHEAT trial, a multi-centre study examining whether withholding enteral feeds during blood transfusions resulted in a reduced incidence of NEC following blood transfusions, was due to conclude at the end of December 2025 – results are pending. Look up this trial and consider what the aims and focus of the study are.

- *Erythropoiesis-stimulating agents* Erythropoietin is a glycoprotein which regulates the production rate of RBC. Studies in the United States of America (USA) and the UK have demonstrated that erythropoiesis-stimulating agents (ESAs) including recombinant erythropoietin, are effective in raising Hb levels and maintaining haematocrit levels during the normal phase of anaemia in the preterm neonate, as well as reducing rates of intraventricular haemorrhage, periventricular leukomalacia, NEC and donor exposure, but there is a lack of clear guidance from available evidence. ESAs have also been proposed as neuroprotective agents that reduce poor long-term neurodevelopment outcome. Treatment with ESAs is usually commenced when neonates are stable, receiving enteral feeds and can tolerate iron supplementation (McKinney et al., 2020).

Pathological anaemia

Feto-maternal transfusion, twin-to-twin transfusion, obstetric difficulties and internal haemorrhage are causes of acute neonatal blood loss or haemorrhage. Chronic anaemia may be associated with RBC destruction and haemolysis secondary to maternal-fetal blood group incompatibilities as well as acquired or congenital defects of red blood cells. Neonatal haemolysis is most commonly caused by G6PD deficiency and less commonly with isoimmunisation, as seen in ABO and Rh incompatibilities. Haemolysis may occur as a result of bacterial sepsis and viral infections and drug ingestion (maternal or direct administration of the drug to the newborn). Other rare causes of RBC haemolysis are thalassaemia and hereditary spherocytosis (McKinney et al., 2020).

NEONATAL WHITE CELL ABNORMALITIES

Neutropenia is the low count of neutrophils, a subtype of white blood cells crucial for fighting bacterial infection. It is a commonly diagnosed condition in premature and sick neonates, seen in 6–8% of neonates on the NNU. The most common causes include infection/inflammation, maternal hypertension/pre-eclampsia, isoimmune neutropenia, maternal medication and other stressors, such as respiratory distress syndrome. Unless there is an underlying genetic cause, neutropenia is usually transient (McKinney et al., 2020).

While neutrophilia, an abnormally high white cell count, is relatively common in the immediate neonatal period secondary to the stressor of birth, when this is severe (a white cell count of >50,000) it is classified as a leukemoid reaction. This has been described in the extremely preterm population, usually in association with chorioamnionitis. Affected neonates often experience higher morbidity and mortality, though only a limited number of cases have been reported in the literature (Terry et al., 2023).

Transient abnormal myelopoiesis, the abnormal hyperproduction of white cells, is a temporary leukaemic syndrome which occurs in neonates with Down's syndrome and may progress to myeloid leukaemia by preschool age in up to 20% of affected neonates (Roberts, 2022).

NURSING CARE OF NEONATES WITH HAEMATOLOGICAL DISORDERS

Monitoring neonates with signs and symptoms of a haematological condition is a key nursing intervention. Neonatal nurses should be familiar with normal blood values and be able to identify any concerns or abnormalities that may indicate a haematological condition. Blood sampling that is safe and timely is also a key component in good haematological care which can be advocated by the neonatal nurse. This should be done as part of a neonate's holistic assessment in line with observation of clinical signs and associated changes in monitoring parameters. A summary of key areas of nursing assessment and care for each of the conditions in this chapter is outlined in Table 17.5.

TABLE 17.5 NURSING CARE IN NEONATAL HAEMATOLOGICAL CONDITIONS

Condition	*Nursing management*
Jaundice (hyperbilirubinaemia)	■ Clinical observation for presence of hyperbilirubinaemia, e.g. yellow skin and sclerae. ■ Bilirubin monitoring via transcutaneous or blood sampling methods. ■ Plotting bilirubin on threshold graph over time. ■ Eye protection, temperature monitoring, hydration and parental reassurance are essential during treatment.
Polycythaemia	■ Clinical observation for presence of polycythaemia-plethoric appearance/cyanosis, tachypnoea. ■ PCV monitoring – be aware that the blood sampling site and perfusion of the sampling site may impact values; free-flowing venous sample is preferred. ■ Nursing care focuses on maintaining hydration, monitoring glucose and preparing for partial exchange transfusion if required.
Coagulation abnormalities 1 – bleeding disorders (VKDB, thrombocytopenia, DIC)	■ Observe for signs of bleeding – via urine, bowel, stomach, bruises, at line insertion sites, abnormal bruising, petechiae, purpura, and intracranial haemorrhage. ■ Observe for signs such as poor feeding, pallor, poor weight gain, tachypnoea and lethargy. ■ Be familiar with normal clotting values and haemoglobin/platelet levels. ■ Coagulation monitoring. ■ Priorities include frequent observations, supporting circulation, liaising closely with medical team and sensitive communication with families about the seriousness of the condition.
Coagulation abnormalities 2 – thrombosis	■ Careful assessment and meticulous line care is essential in the prevention of thromboses and other serious complications. Venous access should be initiated only when necessary. ■ The nurse caring for the neonate with venous or arterial thrombosis should carefully assess the affected limb and be aware of subtle changes in perfusion or patient status that could occur because of clot extension or embolism.
Anaemia	■ Clinical observation for presence of anaemia – pallor, changes to oxygenation, lethargy, apnoea. ■ Haemoglobin monitoring and knowledge of normal values. ■ Supportive care includes oxygenation, transfusion if needed and explaining to parents why their baby may appear 'tired' or pale.
White cell disorders	■ Often linked to infection; nurses should monitor temperature, feeding tolerance and general wellbeing. ■ Provide infection-control measures, support antibiotic administration and explain to parents why blood counts are being checked frequently.

PRACTICE POINTS

Effective communication with parents is essential when managing neonatal haematological disorders. Providing clear explanations of blood results, treatments and potential complications helps reduce anxiety and promotes shared decision-making. Encouraging parental involvement in routine care, where safe, strengthens confidence and supports family integrated care, even during periods of clinical uncertainty.

Understanding the pathophysiology, signs and symptoms and basics of treatment is important in providing appropriate care in the NNU. This also ensures that healthcare professionals are in possession of the necessary information to support parents appropriately. The nurse has an important role in supporting families and, in the context of this chapter, answering questions about any haematological condition as they may struggle with not only the care of a new baby, but one with haematological problems.

Chapter takeaways

- Jaundice is very common in neonates, caused by excess bilirubin from red cell breakdown. Management includes phototherapy, IVIG for haemolytic disease and exchange transfusion in severe cases. Conjugated hyperbilirubinaemia always has a pathological underlying cause.
- Anaemia can result from haemolysis (Rh/ABO incompatibility, G6PD deficiency), blood loss or bone marrow suppression. It presents with pallor, lethargy and poor feeding; treatment may involve transfusion and addressing the underlying cause.
- Polycythaemia is an excess of red blood cells leading to increased blood viscosity. This can result in hypoglycaemia, respiratory distress and thrombosis risk. Affected neonates are managed with hydration and, in severe cases, partial exchange transfusion.
- Vitamin K deficiency bleeding (haemorrhagic disease of the newborn) results from immature clotting factor synthesis and can cause serious bleeding. This can be prevented by routine vitamin K administration at birth.
- Disseminated intravascular coagulation may follow sepsis, hypoxia or trauma. It causes widespread clotting and bleeding, requiring urgent supportive care and treatment of the underlying trigger.
- Thrombocytopenia may be due to maternal conditions, infection or immune-mediated destruction. Neonates are at risk of bleeding; platelet transfusion may be required.

- Though less common, neonatal white cell disorders such as leukopenia or leukocytosis can signal infection, immune dysfunction or congenital marrow problems. Management focuses on treating infection and monitoring immune function.

CASE STUDY

CASE STUDIES

Case study 1: The neonate with jaundice on day 1 of life

Amy was born at 37 weeks' gestation, birthweight 2.4kg, second child to parents Bob and Karen. She has developed hyperbilirubinaemia on day 1 of life and is transferred to the special care unit for observation and investigation. She looks visibly jaundiced.

Q.1. What type of jaundice is Amy presenting with and what are the potential causes?
Q.2. Can you explain the pathophysiology of this type of jaundice?
Q.3. What other types of jaundice are there and what is the associated physiology?
Q.4. What management and nursing care does this neonate require?
Q.5. What information do you require from the parents and what do you need to explain to them?

Case study 2: The neonate with abnormal blood results

Hassan is a 6-day-old premature neonate born at 29 weeks' gestation who has been very unstable in his first few days of life and continues to show a fluctuating oxygen requirement, metabolic acidosis, possible signs of infection. He has umbilical catheters in situ and is fully monitored. His blood results show a low haemoglobin, prolonged clotting time and a low level of platelets.

Q.1. What possible conditions is Hassan presenting with here and what are the underlying reasons for these blood results?
Q.2. What is the associated management and nursing care of this neonate in relation to theses specific findings?
Q.3. How would you explain this to his parents to reassure them?

Case study 3: The neonate who has a high red cell load

CASE STUDY

Tomos is a 35 weeks' gestation neonate with intrauterine growth restriction who is 1 day old. His blood results show he has a high packed cell volume (PCV) of > 65% and is experiencing respiratory distress at present, grunting and tachypnoea.

Q.1. What condition is Tomos presenting with here and what could be the potential underlying reasons for this blood result?
Q.2. What is the appropriate management and nursing care of this neonate?
Q.3. What is the associated risk with this condition and how would you explain this to parents to reassure them?

For suggested answer guides to the questions posed in these case studies, please refer to the web-based companion site specific to this chapter. See www.routledge.com/cw/petty

References

Ardell, S., Offringa, M., Ovelman, C., & Soll, R. (2018). Prophylactic vitamin K for the prevention of vitamin K deficiency bleeding in preterm neonates. *Cochrane Database of Systematic Reviews*, *2*, Article CD008342. https://doi.org/10.1002/14651858.CD008342.pub2

Bhutani, V. K., Wong, R. J., Turkewitz, D., Rauch, D. A., Mowitz, M. F., Barfield, W. D., & Committee on Fetus and Newborn. (2024). Phototherapy to prevent severe neonatal hyperbilirubinemia in the newborn neonate 35 or more weeks of gestation: Technical report. *Pediatrics*, *154*(3), 1–13.

British Association of Perinatal Medicine. (2023). *Early postnatal care of the moderate-late preterm neonate. A framework for practice.* Retrieved January 1, 2026, from https://www.bapm.org/resources/framework-early-postnatal-care-of-the-moderate-late-preterm-neonate

Chaudhary, N., Jassar, R., & Singh, R. (2022). Neonatal anemia. *Newborn*, *1*(3), 263–270.

Cremer, R. J., Perryman, P. W., & Richards, D. H. (1958). Influence of light on the hyperbilirubinæmia of neonates. *The Lancet*, *271*(7030), 1094–1097. https://doi.org/10.1016/S0140-6736(58)91849-X

Estcourt, L. J. (2019). Platelet transfusion thresholds in premature neonates (PlaNeT-2 trial). *Transfusion Medicine*, *29*(1), 20–22. https://doi.org/10.1111/tme.12587

Fair, F., Furness, A., Higginbottom, G., Oddie, S., & Soltani, H. (2024). Understanding stakeholder perspectives on Apgar score, cyanosis and identifying jaundice in ethnic minority neonates. *PLoS ONE*, *19*(10), e0311977. https://doi.org/10.1371/journal.pone.0311977

Furness, A., Fair, F., Higginbottom, G., Oddie, S., & Soltani, H. (2024). A review of the current policies and guidance regarding Apgar scoring and the detection of jaundice and cyanosis concerning Black, Asian and ethnic minority neonates. *BMC Pediatrics*, *24*(1), 198. https://doi.org/10.1186/s12887-024-04692-4

Jacquot, C., Mo, D. Y., & Webb, J. (2024). Blood component therapy for the neonate. In R. J. Martin, A. A. Fanaroff & M. C. Walsh (Eds.), *Fanaroff and Martin's neonatal-perinatal medicine: Diseases of the fetus and neonate* (12th ed., pp. 1572–1596). Elsevier.

Kamath-Rayne, B. D., Froese, P. A., & Thilo, E. H. (2020). Neonatal hyperbilirubinemia. In S. L. Gardner, B. S. Carter, M. E. Hines & J. A. Hernandez (Eds.), *Merenstein & Gardner's handbook of neonatal intensive care: An interprofessional approach* (9th ed., pp. 662–691). Elsevier.

Kollamparambil, T. G., Carroll, W., & Rayaroth, D. K. (2024). Neonatal anaemia. *Paediatrics and Child Health*, *34*(5), 154–159.

McKinney, C., Boulden Warren, B., & Harvey, S. (2020). Newborn hematology. In S. L. Gardner, B. S. Carter, M. E. Hines & J. A. Hernandez (Eds.), *Merenstein & Gardner's handbook of neonatal intensive care: An interprofessional approach* (9th ed., pp 623–661). Elsevier.

Mitra, S., & Rennie, J. (2017). Neonatal jaundice: Aetiology, diagnosis and treatment. *British Journal of Hospital Medicine*, *78*(12), 699–704.

National Institute for Health and Care Excellence. (2023a). *Jaundice in newborn babies under 28 days (CG98)*. NICE.

National Institute for Health and Care Excellence. (2023b). *2023 exceptional surveillance of jaundice in newborn babies under 28 days (NICE guideline CG98)*. NICE.

Noureldein, M., Mupanemunda, G., McDermott, H., Pettit, K., & Mupanemunda, R. (2021). Home phototherapy for neonatal jaundice in the UK: A single-centre retrospective service evaluation and parental survey. *BMJ Paediatrics Open*, *5*(1), e001027. https://doi.org/10.1136/bmjpo-2021-001027

Okwundu, C. I., Uthman, O. A., Suresh, G., Smith, J., Wiysonge, C. S., & Bhutani, V. K. (2017). Transcutaneous bilirubinometry versus total serum bilirubin measurement for newborns. *Cochrane Database of Systematic Reviews*. https://doi.org/10.1002/14651858.CD012660

Paediatric Formulary Committee. (2024). *BNF for children 2024–2025*. BMJ Group, Pharmaceutical Press and RCPCH Publications.

Roberts, I. (2022). Leukemogenesis in neonates and young children with trisomy 21. *Hematology*, *2022*(1), 1–8. Retrieved November 9, 2025, from https://doi.org/10.1182/hematology.2022000395

Sirachainan, N., Komvilaisak, P., Van Ommen, C. H., Revel-Vilk, S., Ohga, S., Zia, A., Ochiai, M., Takahashi, D., Suga, S., Labarque, V., Amankwah, E. K., Souvanlasy, B., Betensky, M., Chan, A. K., Chuansumrit, A., Goldenberg, N., & Rajpurkar, M. (2025). International perspectives on vitamin K deficiency bleeding in neonates: A cross-sectional questionnaire-based survey. *Pediatric Blood & Cancer*, *72*(10), e31889. https://doi.org/10.1002/pbc.31889

Terry, C., Kane, D., Eogan, M., McCallion, N., Doyle, E., & Drew, R. (2023). Retrospective analysis of leukemoid reactions in extremely preterm neonates in a tertiary NICU from 2018–2021. *The Journal of Maternal-Fetal & Neonatal Medicine*, *36*(2), 2225115. Retrieved November 9, 2025, from https://doi.org/10.1080/14767058.2023.2225115

World Health Organization. (2022). *WHO recommendations on maternal and newborn care for a positive postnatal experience*. World Health Organization.

18 MANAGEMENT OF NEONATAL FLUID AND ELECTROLYTE BALANCE

Natalie Anders

CONTENTS

DOI: 10.4324/9781003591405-22

GUIDANCE ON HOW TO ENHANCE PERSONAL LEARNING FROM THIS CHAPTER

Key points covered in this chapter

- The physiological principles underpinning fluid and electrolyte balance in neonates.
- Common causes and clinical consequences of fluid and electrolyte imbalances in neonatal care.
- Nursing management strategies, including assessment and monitoring of fluid and electrolyte status in neonates.

Reflection

Reading through the chapter, you are encouraged to engage with the key points and related literature in an enquiring way. Ask these questions:

- How can I recognise and respond to signs of fluid depletion or overload in neonates?
- Why is fluid and electrolyte management particularly complex in neonatal care?
- How and why do fluid requirements vary with gestational age and clinical condition?
- How does fluid management relate to nutrition and other aspects of neonatal care?

Implications for nursing care

- Finally: how will this chapter help you to understand and apply fluid and electrolyte balance in neonatal care? Consider how this knowledge will support your ability to assess, monitor and manage fluids safely, and how it contributes to delivering holistic, individualised family integrated care.

INTRODUCTION AND BACKGROUND

This chapter aims to emphasise the key elements of fluid and electrolyte balance, enabling nurses to anticipate problems, assess the adequacy of renal function and subsequently develop appropriate fluid management strategies as part of a multidisciplinary team (MDT) for infants in neonatal care (National Health Service (NHS) England, 2024). Fluid and electrolyte therapies are crucial in managing preterm and term infants admitted to the neonatal unit (NNU). A comprehensive understanding of these therapies enables neonatal nurses to effectively administer fluid therapy and monitor fluid balance, ensuring optimal care to improve short- and long-term outcomes. Disturbances in fluid and electrolyte balance increase the risk of morbidities such as bronchopulmonary dysplasia (BPD), patent ductus arteriosus (PDA), intraventricular haemorrhage (IVH) and necrotising enterocolitis (NEC; Bollaboina et al., 2023). Restriction of fluids can unintentionally reduce nutritional intake, potentially hindering growth and adversely affecting neurodevelopmental outcomes in neonates. Neonatal fluid and electrolyte management is complex and dynamic, requiring careful consideration of physiological, environmental, gestational and iatrogenic factors.

PHYSIOLOGICAL BASIS OF FLUID AND ELECTROLYTE BALANCE

Water and electrolytes are fundamental to physiological stability at all stages of life. In preterm infants, homeostasis is often compromised due to renal immaturity or altered function. In term infants, underlying conditions such as hypoxia or sepsis can further disrupt this balance. These challenges may be compounded by the administration of nephrotoxic drugs. Fluid and electrolyte imbalances in the neonatal period can lead to significant morbidity if not detected and managed early.

Understanding the vital role and function of the kidneys is essential before considering potential problems for the infant in the NNU. The kidneys are major determinants of blood composition and play a crucial role in maintaining homeostasis. Nephrogenesis, the formation of nephrons, initiates around the 9th to 10th week of gestation. Between the late second and third trimesters (approximately 18 to 32 weeks), there is a significant increase in nephron production. By 32 to 36 weeks of gestation, nephrogenesis is considered complete with each kidney containing around 1,000,000 nephrons (Rosenblum et al., 2017). In preterm infants, nephrogenesis may continue postnatally, with development extending up to 40 days postpartum with anatomical abnormalities occurring at any stage. Factors such as low birthweight, small size for gestational age (GA), and prematurity can reduce the number of nephrons, potentially leading to long-term renal implications (Low Birth Weight and Nephron Number Working Group, 2017). An infant born at 24 weeks' gestation may not complete nephrogenesis until 10–12 weeks postnatally. At 24 weeks, the kidney measures 2.5 cm and grows to 4.5 cm at term. The adult kidney size of around 6 cm is reached postnatally through elongation of the proximal renal tubules and loops of Henle. While maturation of renal function is usually complete by 2 years of age, extremely preterm infants may continue to show reduced renal function later in life. Kidney and nephron anatomy can be seen in Figures 18.1 and 18.2.

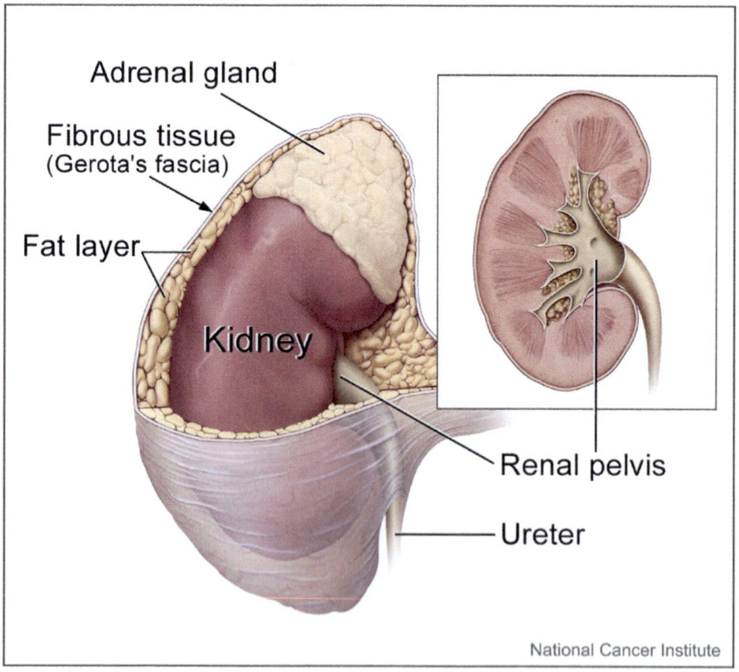

Figure 18.1 Renal anatomy (Source: Alan Hoofring, Creative Commons)

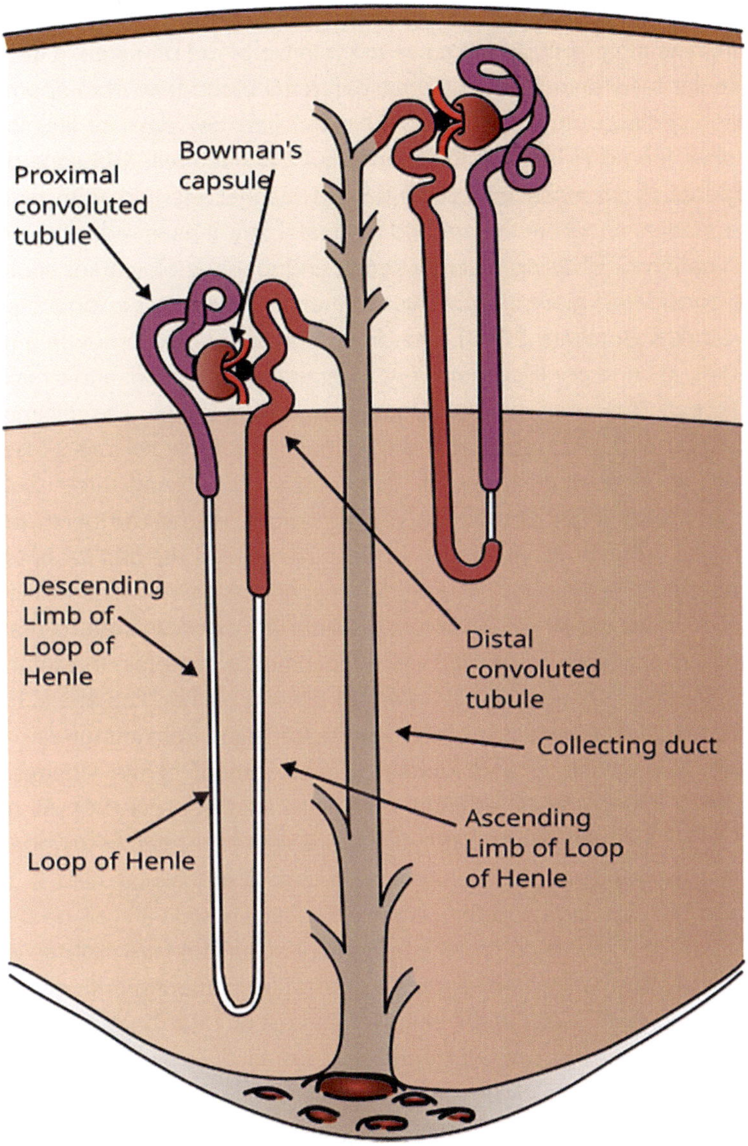

Figure 18.2 Nephron anatomy (Source: Holly Fischer, Creative Commons)

The maintenance of body water homeostasis relies on the kidneys' ability to control water loss by regulating urine production. Urine production begins with the process of glomerular filtration. As blood flows through the afferent arteriole into the glomerulus, non-selective filtration occurs, allowing fluid and **solutes** to pass through the capillary membrane into Bowman's capsule. The rate of filtration is influenced by various factors, with the most important being hydrostatic pressure (Polin et al., 2021).

In neonates, the **glomerular filtration rate** (GFR) is lower than in adults. GFR increases after birth due to a rise in systemic blood pressure, a decrease in renal vascular resistance and an increase in renal blood flow from approximately 4% of the cardiac output to 10%. Within the first few days of life, this gradually reaches the adult level of approximately 25% (Iacobelli & Guignard, 2021). GFR appears to increase in a programmed manner starting from at least 26 weeks' gestation, and from the second postnatal day, it rises regardless of GA at birth. Estimating GFR using a single serum endogenous biomarker such as creatinine is considered more clinically useful than the alternative exogenous marker (Muhari-Stark & Burckart, 2018). The preterm infant should produce a minimum of 25–60mL of urine per kilogram every 24 hours, which can rise to a maximum of 300mL/kg per 24 hours with acute increases in fluid intake. The minimum value on day 1 (0.51mL/kg/hr) represents the lowest acceptable volume, as below this level solute accumulation will occur. Between days two and three, 2–3mL/kg/hour is acceptable; infants producing a lower volume warrant further investigation as a matter of urgency. Most infants (95%) pass urine in the first 24 hours of life. Approximately 21% will pass urine at delivery, and as this may be missed or not recorded, it is advisable for the neonatal nurse to communicate to the professional who was present at the delivery of the infant to ascertain this information.

Physiological changes in neonates are dynamic rather than static. Following birth, several adaptive processes facilitate the transition from intrauterine to extrauterine life. The structural and functional development of the kidneys plays a crucial role in this postnatal adaptation (Saint-Faust et al., 2014). All neonates continue to adapt postnatally. Body fluids are split into specific compartments: the extracellular and intracellular compartments. Extracellular fluid is found in plasma and the circulatory system, while intracellular fluids are inside the body's cells. Both compartments control the movement of fluid and electrolytes within the body. Changes to the intracellular and extracellular compartments occur 12–48 hours following birth. After birth, the percentage of total body water gradually decreases, primarily because of decreasing extracellular fluid. Intracellular fluid proportionately increases postnatally.

Initial adaptations to total body water, which includes both the intracellular and extracellular compartments, occur to meet the newborn's elevated metabolic demands, maintain body temperature, and support growth (Avery et al., 2021). In the early postnatal period, a full-term infant typically loses 5–10% of their birthweight, while a preterm infant may experience a loss of 10–15% within the first week of life. For critically ill, extremely premature neonates, third space loss can occur. This refers to fluid shifting from the extracellular compartment into the interstitial spaces (the areas between the skin and fascia). This shift reduces circulating blood volume, which can lead to hypotension and **oedema**, necessitating senior medical advice and management (Fanaroff & Martin, 2020).

FLUID AND ELECTROLYTE MANAGEMENT

Fluid and electrolyte imbalances are common, and many neonates admitted to a NNU will require intravenous (IV) fluids during their hospital stay. Infants, particularly those who are of low birthweight or premature, experience higher rates of water loss due to increased skin permeability and a larger surface to body weight ratio (Table 18.1). Insensible water losses (IWL) are not readily measured, approximately 70% are lost through the skin and 30% via the respiratory tract. In extremely premature infants, the IWL increases. There are many factors which contribute to an increase (see Table 18.2) or reduction in IWL.

Maintaining normothermia is essential to minimise heat losses through radiation, conduction, convection, and evaporative losses, as these factors contribute to adverse outcomes in neonates (Gardner et al., 2020). The management of thermal stability is further discussed in Chapter 13.

> **THINK POINT**
>
> Reflect on the role of the wider MDT in managing neonatal fluid and electrolyte balance. How do professionals such as nurses, doctors, dietitians, pharmacists and speech and language therapists contribute to care? Why is collaborative input essential for safe, individualised management, and how is this reflected in practice on your unit?

FLUID REQUIREMENTS

Fluid requirements are calculated on the infant's birthweight until the current weight surpasses it, provided the gain is not attributed to fluid overload or oedema (NHS Greater Glasgow & Clyde (NHSGGC) and Scottish Perinatal Network,

TABLE 18.1 INSENSIBLE WATER LOSSES ACCORDING TO BIRTHWEIGHT

Birthweight	*IWL (mL/kg/day)*
<1000 grams	60–80
1000–1500 grams	40–60
>1500 grams	20

TABLE 18.2 CIRCUMSTANCES THAT LEAD TO INCREASED INSENSIBLE WATER LOSS

Causes of increased IWL	*Strategies to reduce IWL*
At delivery ■ Increased environmental temperature ■ Radiant heat sources (e.g. Resuscitaire®) ■ Extremely low birthweight infants (large surface area to body weight ratio, less subcutaneous fat) ■ Low GA.	At delivery ■ Placing preterm infants in polyethylene bags/wraps ■ Reduced staff traffic ■ Closed doors and windows ■ Ambient temperature 24–25°C ■ Covering the baby during transportation.
NNU ■ Heated mattresses ■ Forced convection, radiation, evaporation, conduction – draughts, open windows and doors ■ Hyperthermia ■ Tachypnoea ■ Surgical malformations (neural tube defects, gastroschisis, exomphalos – this is part of the rationale to cover such lesions with cling film) ■ Phototherapy ■ Frequent opening of incubator doors ■ Crying ■ Increased motor activity.	Following admission to NNU ■ High ambient humidity incubator ■ Humidified gases ■ Double-walled incubator ■ Minimal handling ■ Reduce staff traffic ■ Respiratory support with humidification ■ Good skin care.

2021). During the first few days of life, both sodium and water needs are relatively low due to natural extracellular fluid contraction and immature renal function and should only be increased after the onset of postnatal **diuresis** (Weaver et al., 2023). For preterm infants, the estimated fluid requirement to support growth ranges from 120–150 mL/kg/day. However, in the immediate postnatal period, prior to diuresis, a reduced volume is generally appropriate, often beginning at approximately 60mL/kg/day in a well-humidified environment. Careful regulation of fluid intake is necessary to meet physiological needs while preventing both dehydration and fluid overload. Some infants may require a more rapid increase in fluid volumes, such as very preterm neonates experiencing high insensible losses in environments where these losses are not sufficiently minimised. Term infants who have experienced perinatal asphyxia often require a more cautious approach and may undergo fluid restriction due to the risk of complications, as resultant multi-organ dysfunction heightens susceptibility to complications from fluid shifts and overload. Cerebral oedema caused by fluid overload can increase intracranial pressure and worsen neurological outcomes. Pulmonary oedema, in combination with congestive heart failure, myocardial dysfunction, and poor peripheral perfusion, impairs gas exchange and often necessitates increased respiratory and inotropic support. Fluid overload may also mask **oliguria**, complicate the management of acute kidney injury (AKI), and cause electrolyte imbalances such as dilutional **hyponatraemia**, increasing the risk of seizures and further cerebral oedema. Gastrointestinal complications such as NEC may also arise from intestinal oedema and impaired perfusion (Fanaroff & Martin, 2020).

When calculating an infant's fluid requirements, several factors must be considered, including current weight, clinical condition, underlying pathology, urine output, ongoing fluid losses, and blood chemistry. Significant fluid shifts occur in the first 48 hours of postnatal life as the neonate transitions from intrauterine to extrauterine fluid balance. For neonates who are preterm, critically ill, or otherwise compromised, fluid and electrolyte management must be tailored to individual needs due to altered physiology and increased risk of imbalance (Segar & Jetton, 2024). It is essential to carefully account for additional fluids administered via flushes used for IV medications and arterial line sampling, as these volumes are often inadvertently excluded from fluid balance records. In extremely preterm or fluid-restricted infants, the cumulative volume of such flushes can constitute a substantial portion of the prescribed daily fluid intake (mL/kg/day), which may have significant implications for fluid management and clinical outcomes.

THINK POINT

Consider a critically ill infant you have nursed in NNU who required multiple infusions, including an arterial line and several intravenous antibiotics. Reflect on the cumulative volume of additional fluids administered through flushes used for fluid changes, antibiotic administration, and arterial line flushes following blood sampling. Is this additional fluid accurately documented in the infant's fluid balance chart? What potential impact might this unrecorded fluid have on the infant's overall fluid status and clinical outcomes?

An adjusted fluid and electrolyte strategy may be required for neonates with specific conditions, including:

- Neonatal encephalopathy
- Hypoxic-ischaemic encephalopathy
  - likely renal compromise and oedema
  - decrease fluid volume to reduce the risks of cerebral oedema

- Renal conditions
- Acute kidney injury
- Cardiac conditions
- High IWL (especially neonates <28 weeks)
- Ascites
- Hypoglycaemia
  - may require a higher fluid volume and/or glucose concentration to normalise blood glucose
- Hyperglycaemia
  - may require a decrease in glucose concentration or fluid volume to normalise blood glucose
- Postoperative.

Key considerations before prescribing or administering intravenous fluids and electrolytes:

- Clinical history of the neonate's previous 24 hours to provide a basis for the following 24-hour fluid and electrolyte regime
- Physical examination
  - clinical condition
  - general wellbeing
- Cardiovascular system
  - heart rate, blood pressure
  - capillary refill time
  - oedema
- Weight trend
- Signs of dehydration
  - skin turgor
  - moist mucous membranes
  - fontanelles soft and flat, not sunken
- Fluid balance (input/output)
  - weigh all nappies
  - urine evaluation – output and specific gravity
  - gastric, chest drain losses etc.
  - stool
- Neurological assessment
  - good tone
  - activity
- Assessment of current fluids, maintenance and additional infusions
  - assess patency of all intravenous lines
  - fluid prescriptions

- Review laboratory results
  - full blood count, serum urea, electrolytes, creatinine, glucose, urinary electrolyte concentrations
- Blood gas
  - acidosis, alkalosis, base excess and lactate

The principles of fluid and electrolyte balance are to optimise nutrition by achieving an appropriate equilibrium that maintains normoglycaemia, prevents dehydration, fluid overload, and major electrolyte disturbances, and provides sufficient calories to prevent ketosis, support growth and maintain homeostasis.

Calculation of required daily fluid intake follows the formula outlined in Box 18.1, with an example in Box 18.2.

BOX 18.1 FLUID INTAKE CALCULATION

(weight (kg) × volume per day) ÷ 24 = hourly input

BOX 18.2 EXAMPLE OF A FLUID INTAKE CALCULATION

Olatayo was born today at 24 weeks' gestation at a birthweight of 600g. He requires 90mL/kg/day of 10% glucose. What is his hourly rate of IV glucose?

Answer:

(0.6 × 90) ÷ 24 = 2.25mL/hour

Birthweight is usually regained by 7–10 days in term infants, longer in preterm infants. Guidance regarding routine maintenance fluid intake per day varies across the United Kingdom (UK), differentiating infants either according to weight or GA. An example can be seen in Table 18.3, but readers are advised to refer to their local guidelines.

Depending on the neonatal age, gestation, birthweight and clinical condition, 10% glucose is the IV fluid of choice if the criteria for parenteral nutrition (PN) are not met, until full enteral feeds are established. Potassium and sodium are not required in the first 48 hours, as neonates have a low GFR (thus producing small quantities of urine), and are therefore unable to tolerate additional sodium, as this

TABLE 18.3 MAINTENANCE INTRAVENOUS FLUID REGIMES – EXAMPLE OF A UK NNU GUIDELINE

Infant specifics	*At risk of hypoglycaemia/large IWL*	*Other babies*
Day 1	90 mL/kg/day	75 mL/kg/day
Day 2	105 mL/kg/day	90 mL/kg/day
Day 3	120 mL/kg/day	105 mL/kg/day
Day 4	135 mL/kg/day	120 mL/kg/day
Day 5	150 mL/kg/day	135 mL/kg/day
Day 6	165 mL/kg/day	150 mL/kg/day
Day 7	165–180 mL/kg/day	150–165 mL/kg/day

(NHSGGC, 2021)

TABLE 18.4 PROBLEMS ASSOCIATED WITH FLUID IMBALANCE

Too much fluid will contribute to	*Too little fluid will contribute to*
■ Over-hydration	■ Under-hydration
■ Hyponatraemia	■ Hypernatraemia
■ Peripheral and pulmonary oedema	■ Hypovolaemia and hypotension
■ Pulmonary haemorrhage	■ Worsening jaundice
■ Increased respiratory illness	■ Metabolic acidosis
■ Symptomatic PDA	■ Low cardiac preload and impaired function
■ Heart failure	■ Impaired renal function and urine output
■ Hyperglycaemia	
■ Impaired renal function and urine output	

can cause fluid retention). After 48 hours, GFR increases with a corresponding diuresis, so that thereafter electrolytes can be added to the maintenance fluids. Rigorous surveillance of urea and electrolytes should be closely monitored 8–12 hourly. The extremely premature neonate's electrolytes and weight may fluctuate within a given 24-hour period. Adjustments must be tailored accordingly to maintain normal thresholds. PN should be initiated within 8 hours in all infants that meet the criteria: gestation <31 weeks, if enteral feeding is insufficient within the first 72 hours, infants with congenital gastrointestinal disorders or critically ill that will not establish adequate feeds, or if feeds are interrupted and not likely to recommence within 48–72 hours (National Institute for Health and Care Excellence (NICE), 2020). See Chapter 19 for further details on PN.

The problems associated with fluid imbalance are outlined in Table 18.4.

In accordance with laboratory guidelines for fluid and electrolyte therapies, IV fluids may be increased in addition to normal requirements based on postnatal age in the presence of;

- Increased weight loss (>2–3% per day, or a cumulative loss of more than 5–10% in term neonates and up to 15% in preterm neonates in the first week of life)
- Increased serum sodium (Na^+ >150 mmol/L)
- Increased **specific gravity** (>1.020) or urine **osmolality** (400mOsm/L)
- Decreased urine output (<1mL/kg/hr over 24 hours).

Conversely, IV fluids may need to be restricted in the presence of;

- Decreased weight loss (<1%/day or avoiding weight loss altogether)
- Decreased sodium content in the presence of weight gain (Na^+ <130mmol/L)
- Decreased urine specific gravity (1.005) or urine osmolality (<100mOsm/L; Ågren et al., 2022).

ELECTROLYTE REQUIREMENTS

Sodium

Sodium (Na^+)
Normal value 135–145mmol/L
Daily requirement varies 1–8mmol/kg/day
Average 2–4mmol/kg/day
Usually not required in the first 48 hours of life

Sodium is an electrolyte for neonatal growth and neurological health. Prolonged deficiency is associated with poor weight gain, neurodevelopmental delays, and hearing impairments, with extremely preterm infants having higher rates of growth failure (Araya et al., 2023). Sodium is the major **cation** in extracellular fluid and is vital for the regulation of circulating blood volume as well as weight gain and tissue growth. There is a lack of consensus for the assessment of total body sodium content in newborns. Evidence supporting sodium supplementation protocols based on adult models is limited and not validated in neonatal populations. In term newborns, the kidneys are relatively mature and capable of efficiently filtering and reabsorbing sodium. Approximately 9% of the infant's total oxygen consumption is dedicated to the energy-dependent process of reabsorbing sodium and water from the nephron into circulation. Due to the high concentration gradient of sodium, it is the first ion to move from the filtrate in the tubular lumen to the tubular epithelial cell. A normal physiological negative balance of sodium and water has been found to occur in healthy newborn infants during the first few days of life.

Preterm infants have an immature renal system with a limited capacity to excrete and reabsorb sodium, placing them at risk of early **hypernatraemia**, primarily due to high transepidermal water loss (TEWL) and inadequate renal sodium reabsorption. They are also vulnerable to late-onset hyponatraemia as a result of ongoing urinary sodium losses and insufficient dietary sodium intake. Reported risk factors for hyponatraemia in neonates include extreme prematurity coupled with a birthweight of less than 1 kg, the use of unfortified breastmilk, and the administration of loop **diuretics** or non-steroidal anti-inflammatory drugs (Pace et al., 2025). The introduction and benefits of enteral feeds will be explored in Chapter 19. In sick preterm infants, early intake of sodium is unnecessary and possibly harmful, and should be avoided until the physiological postnatal diuresis and extracellular fluid contraction have occurred, which typically coincides with a 6% loss of birthweight. Thereafter, normal maintenance requirements are 2–4mmol/kg/day. Sick infants' requirements, however, will vary according to several factors, and this requires careful clinical assessment prior to supplementation. The serum sodium level should be measured 8-hourly in the acutely sick infant. Reasons for sodium imbalances are shown in Table 18.5, while Box 18.3 outlines the calculation for the correction of a sodium deficit.

TABLE 18.5 CAUSES OF SODIUM IMBALANCE (ADAPTED FROM MODI, 2012)

Hyponatraemia	*Hypernatraemia*
■ Excess maternal fluid intake during labour/delivery ■ Excess renal loss (particularly very preterm) ■ Insufficient replacement ■ Sodium-poor intravenous therapy ■ Expressed breastmilk with low sodium fortifiers Medication ■ Diuretics (especially loop diuretics) ■ Xanthines (i.e. caffeine) Inappropriate ADH secretion Excess sodium losses ■ Diarrhoea, gastric, pleural, CSF ■ Salt-losing congenital adrenal hyperplasia (17 hydroxyprogesterone deficiency) ■ Adrenocortical failure ■ Acute tubular necrosis ■ Barter's syndrome (associated with hypokalaemia) ■ Haemolysis ■ Hyperlipidaemia	■ Excess IWL (particularly very preterm) ■ Insufficient fluid replacement ■ While under phototherapy or radiant heaters ■ Diarrhoea ■ Glycosuria causing osmotic diuresis ■ Drugs or PN/fluids containing excessive sodium

HYPONATRAEMIA

Low sodium levels are often evident at birth, reflecting the maternal serum sodium concentrations during pregnancy and delivery (Pace et al., 2025). Hyponatraemia occurring within the first postnatal week in neonates may arise from either water retention or renal sodium wasting; however, there remains ongoing debate regarding the predominant underlying mechanism, particularly in preterm infants (Durrani et al., 2022). **Inappropriate antidiuretic hormone** secretion (IADH) is frequently implicated as the factor responsible for hyponatraemia. Elevated levels of antidiuretic hormone (ADH) are frequently observed in conjunction with hyponatraemia; this elevation may represent a physiological response by the infant to conserve water and maintain circulating blood volume, despite the resultant reduction in plasma osmolality. It is likely that in these situations, secretion of ADH is physiologically appropriate. This differentiation is important, as a true case of IADH requires restriction of fluids, whereas in physiological adaptation due to low circulating volume an increase of fluid volume and sodium may be what is necessary. Irrespective of the underlying cause of hyponatraemia, maintaining an appropriate positive sodium balance and correcting deficits where needed (Box 18.3), is essential as prolonged sodium deficiency has been linked to impaired skeletal growth, suboptimal tissue development and adverse neurodevelopmental outcomes in preterm infants (Araya et al., 2023).

BOX 18.3 CALCULATION FOR CORRECTING A SODIUM DEFICIT

To calculate an infant's sodium deficit, the following formula is used:

$$0.7 \times \text{body weight (kg)} \times (140 - \text{serum sodium}) = \text{sodium deficit}$$

To correct the deficit, aim to replace two-thirds of this within 24 hours, while concurrently monitoring plasma and urine electrolytes at least daily, to determine subsequent replacement. Where the sodium deficit is due to inappropriate ADH secretion, fluids are restricted along with sodium replacement.

HYPERNATRAEMIA

A rising serum sodium (>145mmol/L) in extremely low birthweight (ELBW) neonates warrants prompt senior clinical review and may necessitate an increase in maintenance fluids by 10–30 mL/kg/day to prevent further hypernatraemia. Hypernatraemia usually presents in the very preterm infant secondary to TEWL or inadvertent sodium load from sources such as saline infusions for arterial lines, IV flushes following drugs, or sodium bicarbonate infusions. In moderate hypernatraemia (serum level of up to 155mmol/L), sodium supplements should generally be withheld, and appropriate fluid replacement should correct the imbalance. At higher levels (Na^+ >155mmol/L), the rate of sodium correction should not exceed a decrease of 10 mmol/L per 24 hours. Rapid falls in sodium concentration can precipitate cerebral oedema and convulsions. Judicious additional sodium may be required, while the fall in plasma sodium is carefully monitored.

Potassium

Potassium (K^+)
Normal value at 0–7days is 3.5–5.5/mmol/L
At 8–24 days 3.4–6.0mmol/L
Usually not required in the first 48 hours of life
Daily requirement 1–2 mmol/kg/day

Potassium is the principal intracellular cation and is required for maintenance of the intracellular fluid volume. Potassium reabsorption, which occurs mainly in the **distal** tubule, is mediated by aldosterone, which regulates the sodium-potassium-pump to maintain cellular electroneutrality. Renal regulation of potassium is linked to systemic acid-base balance. During metabolic alkalosis, the kidneys increase potassium excretion in exchange for intracellular bicarbonate retention, often resulting in **hypokalaemia**. Conversely, metabolic acidosis promotes potassium retention as hydrogen ions are exchanged for potassium in the renal tubules, leading to elevated plasma potassium levels. In infants requiring parenteral fluids, potassium supplementation should commence when urine output is adequate, providing that the plasma level is not elevated. Serum potassium levels should be measured 8-hourly in the acutely sick infant. Causes for potassium imbalances are shown in Table 18.6.

HYPOKALAEMIA

It has been found that extreme variations in the plasma concentration of potassium can occur in neonates, both above and below the normal range of 3.8–5.0mmol/L, indicating rapid changes between the intracellular and extracellular compartments. A deficiency invariably involves an excessive loss via either the intestinal or renal routes, both, or a lack of appropriate supplementation.

Potassium supplementation is typically initiated on the third postnatal day at a dosage of 1–2 mmol/kg/day, contingent upon adequate urine output (greater than 1 mL/kg/hr) and normal plasma potassium levels. Appropriate replacement

TABLE 18.6 CAUSES OF POTASSIUM IMBALANCE

Hypokalaemia	*Hyperkalaemia*
Insufficient replacement	Tissue damage
Excess losses	Excessive bruising
■ Renal	Nephrotoxic drugs
■ polyuric states	Renal impairment/failure:
■ chronic diuretics	■ Acute tubular necrosis
■ renal tubular acidosis	■ Renal vein thrombosis
■ Bartter's syndrome (with hyponatraemia)	■ Congenital chronic renal failure
■ Medication	■ Rhabdomyolysis
■ salbutamol	
■ insulin	
Hyperaldosteronism	
Alkalosis	
Gastrointestinal causes	
■ Gastric aspiration	
■ Vomiting	
■ Stoma losses	
■ Diarrhoea	

therapy should be guided by ongoing loss assessments and close monitoring of serum potassium concentrations (Moss, 2022).

HYPERKALAEMIA

A potassium (K^+) level >6.5mmol/L is commonly associated with impaired renal excretion or may arise secondary to conditions such as metabolic acidosis, severe infection, extensive tissue injury or ischaemia (Yu et al., 2019). Potassium supplementation must be omitted when **hyperkalaemia** is detected until levels normalise. Spurious hyperkalaemia can also be reported following haemolysis of blood cells during sampling. Capillary potassium values are generally higher than arterial potassium values, so low potassium on a capillary sample indicates significantly lower arterial potassium values. Hyperkalaemia can be an early indicator of congenital adrenal hyperplasia in neonates. True hyperkalaemia is extremely serious and due to the risk of life-threatening cardiac arrhythmias, necessitating prompt intervention. All potassium supplementation or drugs containing potassium must be stopped, and continuous electrocardiographic (ECG) monitoring should be initiated to detect arrhythmias. While arrhythmias are uncommon at potassium levels below 7.5 mmol/L, persistent hyperkalaemia may precipitate ventricular tachycardia, fibrillation or asystole (Paediatric Formulary Committee,

2024). Senior clinical input should be obtained immediately. There are several drug therapies to reduce the levels of potassium in the short term.

Calcium gluconate may be infused slowly to counteract the excitatory effects of potassium on the myocardium. Due to the risk of severe tissue injury from extravasation, calcium gluconate administration is preferable via a central venous line; if administered peripherally, the infusion site requires meticulous observation (Royal College of Nursing (RCN), 2016). Rectal calcium resonium works in the colon by exchanging calcium for potassium, binding potassium for excretion in the stool and lowering serum potassium levels over time: however, its use is contraindicated in neonates at risk of NEC. Other interventions include sodium bicarbonate infusion (4.2% solution over 5–10 minutes), glucose and insulin solutions (with concurrent careful blood glucose monitoring) or salbutamol, all of which promote the intracellular shift of potassium (Yu et al., 2019). In neonates with severe or persistent hyperkalaemia unresponsive to medical management, exchange transfusion or renal replacement therapies such as peritoneal dialysis or continuous hemofiltration may be required. Further details on drug therapies to normalise elevated potassium levels can be found in the web-based resources.

Chloride

Chloride (Cl^-)
Normal value 96–110mmol/L
Average requirement 2–4mmol/kg/day

Chloride is an **anion** abundant in extracellular fluid. **Hypochloraemia** may result from increased losses from gastric aspiration due to obstruction, or surgery leading to metabolic alkalosis. **Hyperchloraemia** can occur in infants who are hypernatraemic or receiving parenteral nutrition, where it is associated with metabolic acidosis. Although elevated chloride levels can affect acid–base balance, they are not independently associated with adverse neurological outcomes. Premature neonates are particularly susceptible to electrolyte imbalances due to immature renal function and an increased vulnerability to fluid volume shifts, with chloride homeostasis closely linked to sodium balance, impacting acid-base regulation and overall neonatal stability.

Calcium and phosphate

Calcium (Ca^{2+})
Normal value 1.8–2.9mmol/L
Calcium is bound to serum albumin, and thus monitored in conjunction

Phosphate (PO_4^{3-})
Normal values at day 2–3 are 1.8–3.0mmol/L
From day 21 1.7–2.6mmol/L
Requirements vary depending on GA, co-morbidities and type of enteral feeds
Raised alkaline phosphatase levels +/- hypercalcaemia in the presence of hypophosphatemia may be indicative of developing metabolic bone disease

Calcium and phosphate are essential minerals required for normal growth, development and bone mineralisation. Prolonged imbalances are associated with metabolic bone disease, which the preterm population is particularly at risk of (please see companion website for further details). Serum ionised calcium is considered the most accurate indicator of the body's calcium status, as it more precisely reflects the physiologically active and bioavailable fraction of total calcium (Vuralli, 2019). **Hypocalcaemia** in the newborn is defined as Ca^{2+} <2mmol/L in term infants and <1.75mmol/L in preterm infants. Clinical manifestations normally become apparent with an ionised calcium <0.75mmol/L. Calcium and phosphate are actively transported across the placenta to the fetus, resulting in higher fetal calcium levels compared to the mother, which supports fetal bone mineralisation (Moore et al., 2019). Perinatal asphyxia can also lead to a fall in calcium levels due to altered cell metabolism and phosphorus release, with alkalosis either from alkali therapy or over-ventilation, reducing the ionised serum calcium levels further. Clinical manifestations of hypocalcaemia are predominantly neurological, including tremors, twitching, irritability, laryngospasm, high-pitched crying, apnoea and seizures. Treatment involves administering intravenous calcium gluconate, typically 2 mL/kg of a 10% solution over 10 minutes (Paediatric Formulary Committee, 2024). Due to the risk of serious cardiac complications such as bradycardia and asystole if infused too rapidly, this administration must be closely monitored with continuous ECG surveillance. Calcium infusions are ideally delivered via a central line to minimise the risk of severe extravasation injury; if a peripheral line must be used, vigilant observation of the infusion site is essential.

Magnesium

Magnesium (Mg^{2+})
Normal value 0.7–1.0mmol/L
Daily requirement varies

Magnesium, along with phosphorous and calcium is the major cation in a newborn. Magnesium, primarily stored in the bones, plays a critical role in numerous physiological processes, including bone matrix formation, nerve conduction, muscle and cardiac function, as well as DNA and RNA synthesis. As an essential intracellular cation, magnesium also stabilises cell membranes. Complex homeostatic mechanisms regulate magnesium, calcium and phosphate via the kidney, bone and intestine to ensure parathyroid function and synthesis of vitamin D. In preterm infants, serum magnesium levels can fluctuate significantly during the first week of life, impacted by factors such as maternal health, neonatal renal perfusion and GFR. Infants with surgical conditions may have large losses of magnesium via stomas and thus require careful monitoring. Magnesium administration via injection, infusion, parenteral nutrition, formula and human breastmilk contribute to normal levels (Rigo et al., 2017). Magnesium is primarily excreted via the kidneys.

PRACTICE POINT

Family integrated care is vital for improving long-term outcomes in neonatal units, with safe, developmentally appropriate positioning as a key element. Infants on IV fluids often have multiple access points and monitoring lines, which can complicate positioning and skin-to-skin care. Consider how you would safely position such infants and how you could involve physiotherapists and occupational therapists to optimise care.

GLUCOSE REQUIREMENTS

Normal value 2.6–6.0mmol/L
Daily requirement varies (6–8mg/kg/minute)
Requirements may be increased in the presence of persistent hypoglycaemia
The usual requirement for glucose in a newborn is 4–8mg/kg/minute.

Glucose homeostasis

Monitoring blood glucose levels both at admission and throughout the neonatal period is an essential nursing responsibility to prevent adverse outcomes associated with glucose instability. It is therefore important for neonatal nurses to understand the physiological and clinical factors influencing glucose homeostasis in newborns. Prematurity significantly reduces **glycogen** and fat reserves, thereby increasing vulnerability to **hypoglycaemia**. At birth, the neonate transitions from an intrauterine **anabolic** state reliant on maternal glucose supply to an independent postnatal catabolic metabolism. While all neonates are at risk of glucose fluctuations, the risk is particularly heightened in those requiring admission to NNUs due to illness or prematurity (McKinlay et al., 2015).

Glucose is the main substrate required by the body to produce adenosine triphosphate (ATP), often described as the 'energy currency' of the cell (Berg et al., 2019). After birth, the infant has to regulate their own glucose metabolism to meet energy demands. Survival depends on metabolic pathways such as glycogenolysis, the breakdown of stored glycogen into glucose, and gluconeogenesis, which synthesises glucose from non-carbohydrate precursors like alanine derived from skeletal muscle. Additionally, it is also recognised that **ketone bodies** and **lactate** are also metabolised by the fetal and neonatal brain as an energy source. However, this pathway is often compromised in infants admitted to NNU, particularly preterm or growth-restricted infants and those who have experienced hypoxic insults.

The ability of the renal tubules to reabsorb glucose is decreased in the preterm infant and increases towards term. Consequently, preterm neonates exhibit a lower renal threshold for glucose conservation, making glycosuria a relatively common finding. When glycosuria occurs alongside hyperglycaemia, it can lead to osmotic diuresis, resulting in increased water loss due to elevated urinary solute concentration. This is unlikely to occur unless blood glucose levels exceed 12mmol/L.

This may be adjusted on an individual basis, as some infants require a higher percentage of glucose concentration to maintain normal plasma glucose levels. Table 18.7 shows glucose delivery based on standard glucose solutions. A neonate who persistently requires 10mg/kg/minute of glucose and above requires senior medical review. Box 18.4 shows the formula used to calculate an infant's glucose requirement.

TABLE 18.7 RATES OF INTRAVENOUS GLUCOSE IN MG/KG/MINUTE FROM STANDARD GLUCOSE CONCENTRATIONS

Infusion rate (ml/kg/day)	*10% glucose*	*12.5 % glucose*	*15% glucose*	*20% glucose*
60	4 mg/kg/min	5 mg/kg/min	6 mg/kg/min	8 mg/kg/min
75	5 mg/kg/min	7 mg/kg/min	8 mg/kg/min	11 mg/kg/min
90	6 mg/kg/min	8 mg/kg/min	9 mg/kg/min	13 mg/kg/min
120	8 mg/kg/min	10 mg/kg/min	13 mg/kg/min	17 mg/kg/min
150	10 mg/kg/min	13 mg/kg/min	16 mg/kg/min	21 mg/kg/min

BOX 18.4 GLUCOSE DELIVERY CALCULATION

(% glucose × hourly rate) ÷ (weight(kg) × 6)
= glucose load (mg/kg/minute)

HYPOGLYCAEMIA

The definition of neonatal hypoglycaemia remains controversial, with no universally accepted threshold. Blood glucose levels below 2.6 mmol/L are commonly used to indicate hypoglycaemia, though this cut-off is debated due to limited supporting evidence (Harding et al., 2017; Giouleka et al., 2023). Due to variability among national guidelines, clinical decisions should consider risk factors and symptoms, not just numerical values. Many healthy neonates experience transient hypoglycaemia as part of their normal physiological adaptation to extra-uterine life. This occurs due to the sudden discontinuation of placental glucose supply and typically results in a temporary drop in blood glucose levels (BGL), reaching its lowest point between 1 and 2 hours after birth, with levels as low as 1.6 mmol/L (30 mg/dL) in the first 4 hours (Harding et al., 2017). This early hypoglycaemia is usually asymptomatic and self-limiting, with glucose levels gradually rising to 2.5–4.4 mmol/L by 6 hours of age as a result of endogenous glucose production and the mobilisation of alternative energy sources, such as ketone bodies. Neonatal hypoglycaemia may manifest through both autonomic activation (including tachycardia, sweating, tremors, pallor, and hypothermia), reflecting sympathetic nervous system stimulation and neuroglycopaenic symptoms such as lethargy, poor feeding, seizures, hypotonia, and apnoea, reflecting impaired cerebral glucose (Kliegman et al., 2020). In recognition of this uncertainty, 'operational thresholds' for neonatal hypoglycaemia at which intervention should be considered have been suggested as: a single measurement of blood glucose < 1 mmol/L, a persistently low blood glucose < 2 mmol/L in an asymptomatic baby, and a single measurement of < 2.5 mmol/L in a baby with signs potentially attributable to hypoglycaemia (British Association of Perinatal Medicine (BAPM), 2024).

Close surveillance, early identification, and the instigation of prophylactic measures for the prevention of hypoglycaemia in the high-risk population constitute by far the best management strategy. Reasons for hypoglycaemia can be seen in Table 18.8. Treatment of hypoglycaemia will be according to individual unit guidelines, including commencement of early feeding, either enterally or IV with 10% glucose. This should be sufficient for most infants but may include a glucose bolus of 2.5ml/kg if the blood glucose does not respond to feeds or IV fluids. Buccal administration of 40% glucose gel can be used in infants over 32 weeks gestation who have a safe swallow and no contraindications to oral

TABLE 18.8 INFANTS AT RISK OF HYPOGLYCAEMIA

Infant group	*Mechanism*	*Expected duration*
Decreased stores		
Preterm	Decreased stores of glycogen and fat Enteral feed intolerance Fluid (caloric) restriction Impaired hormonal responses	Transient
Intrauterine growth restriction	Decreased stores of glycogen and fat Impaired hormonal responses	Transient
Inborn errors of metabolism	Glycogen storage disease Enzyme deficiencies impairing glycogenolysis and gluconeogenesis	Prolonged
Increased utilisation		
Perinatal hypoxia	Anaerobic cellular metabolism exhausting stores	Transient
Sepsis	Increased metabolic rate	Transient
Hypothermia	Increased metabolic rate and brown fat metabolism	
Infant of diabetic mother	Hyperinsulinaemia	Transient
Beckwith–Wiedemann syndrome	Hyperinsulinaemia from islet hyperplasia	Prolonged
Erythroblastosis fetalis	Hyperinsulinaemia from islet hyperplasia	Transient
Exchange transfusion	Excess insulin secretion due to glucose level in stored blood	Transient
Islet cell dysplasias	Hyperinsulinaemia	Prolonged
Other causes		
Iatrogenic	Malfunctioned intravenous access abruptly reducing supply Glucose infusion via UVC if tip is close to the coeliac axis	Transient
Maternal drugs	β-receptor antagonists (e.g. labetalol)	Transient

feeding, either in the absence of IV access or alongside a feeding plan, when blood glucose levels are between 1.0 and 1.9 mmol/L (BAPM, 2024).

If higher concentrations are required to maintain blood glucose levels, the infusion must be administered via a central venous line in order to prevent vessel damage, extravasation injury and scarring (RCN, 2016). Vigilant observation of the infusion site and infusion pump pressures must be undertaken. Hypoglycaemia resistant to high glucose infusions are usually secondary to hyperinsulinaemia. For infants with proven hyperinsulinaemia, drug therapies need to be instigated under regular liaison with the local endocrine team. Close frequent monitoring of fluid and electrolyte therapies is paramount to highlight changes to the infant's condition (NICE, 2020).

A newborn with persistent hypoglycaemia (<2 mmol/L on three or more occasions in the first 48 hours), severe hypoglycaemia (<1 mmol/L at any time), or signs of acute neurological dysfunction with blood glucose (<2.5 mmol/L) should undergo first-line investigations during the hypoglycaemic episode, after discussion with a consultant, including evaluation for early-onset sepsis, laboratory blood glucose with paired insulin and C-peptide (requested urgently), free fatty acids, beta-hydroxybutyrate, blood gases with lactate, cortisol, growth hormone, and ammonia.

Due to the neonatal brain's reliance on glucose for metabolic function, prolonged or recurrent hypoglycaemia, particularly in the early neonatal period, may result in neuronal energy failure, especially in regions such as the visual cortex and frontal lobes, contributing to long-term neurodevelopmental impairments including deficits in executive function, visual-motor integration, psychomotor development, and academic performance in later childhood (McKinlay et al., 2015; Wickström et al., 2018). Any neonate with a low blood sugar who is demonstrating seizure activity warrants urgent IV glucose treatment.

HYPERGLYCAEMIA

While **hyperglycaemia** is commonly defined as a true blood glucose concentration above 8 mmol/L, the safe upper limit in preterm infants remains unclear; however, many units adopt a higher treatment threshold, typically initiating intervention after two confirmed blood glucose readings of ≥12 mmol/L. Many NNUs manage hyperglycaemia by reducing glucose infusion; however, this approach can significantly limit calorie intake. Insulin therapy is effective in controlling hyperglycaemia, although international guidelines recommend cautious use. Maintaining strict normoglycaemia (<8 mmol/L) with insulin is linked to a high risk of hypoglycaemia. Nevertheless, insulin treatment can offer important growth benefits and potentially reduce mortality. These advantages may still be realised by using higher treatment thresholds (e.g. 12 mmol/L), which carry a lower risk of hypoglycaemia.

Reasons for hyperglycaemia in the infant can be seen in Table 18.9. Hyperglycaemia is more common in extremely preterm neonates receiving PN, particularly in those weighing less than 1 kg and in infants with intrauterine growth restriction (IUGR; Boscarino et al., 2021). It typically develops within the first week of life and peaks by the second week, with some infants experiencing recurrent episodes. The underlying causes are believed to involve pancreatic β-cell dysfunction resulting in immature insulin secretion, combined with insulin resistance due to immature liver function.

TABLE 18.9 INFANTS AT RISK OF HYPERGLYCAEMIA

Infant group	*Mechanism*	*Expected duration*
ELBW infants	High intravenous glucose concentration Immature insulin and regulatory mechanisms	Transient
Medication	E.g. methylxanthines, caffeine citrate, corticosteroids	Transient
Infants undergoing surgery	Release of stress-related hormones Infusion of high glucose-containing solutions Transfusion of blood with high glucose levels	Transient
Neonatal diabetes mellitus	Decreased insulin production	Prolonged

Hyperglycemia is associated with a higher incidence of IVH, and ultimately increased mortality if serum osmolality is increased due to high glucose levels. It must be remembered that hyperglycaemia without a significant change in infused glucose concentration may be an indicator of infection and should be investigated. Glycosuria accompanying hyperglycaemia may lead to **osmotic diuresis**, in which water loss occurs due to elevated urinary solute concentration. This can result in dehydration and electrolyte imbalances, such as hypernatraemia, particularly in very LBW infants, who have a lower renal threshold for glucose. While osmotic diuresis is uncommon at blood glucose levels below 12 mmol/L, reducing the glucose concentration in intravenous fluids is often sufficient to lower blood glucose. However, this approach may compromise the delivery of glucose needed to support optimal growth.

ASSESSMENT AND MONITORING OF FLUID AND ELECTROLYTE BALANCE

Neonatal nurses must ensure vigilant monitoring, documentation, and management of all intravenous therapies in line with national guidelines, with any unexpected changes in the infant's condition promptly escalated to senior medical and/or nursing staff for review (NICE, 2020).

Fluid balance

Accurate recording and monitoring of fluid balance in neonatal intensive care is fundamental to guiding clinical management (NHS England, 2024). This responsibility primarily lies with the nurse caring for the infant as part of regular observations. Imbalances or errors in fluid balance can lead to serious clinical deterioration or impair recovery, emphasising the need for precision equivalent to any other vital sign monitoring. While digital programmes are increasingly replacing traditional fluid balance charts, systematically documenting input and output remains essential for assessing individual fluid needs and guiding therapeutic interventions. Acknowledging the increasing use of digital technologies to track observations and fluid management in neonates, the nurse retains primary responsibility for verifying the accuracy and reliability of these recorded values.

Accurate measurement of body weight

Monitoring fluid balance includes accurate measurement of body weight, as weight closely correlates with total body water content during the early postnatal period. Regular weight assessment is required to guide fluid management and rehydration. While infants in intensive care are physiologically unstable and warrant minimal handling, weighing is an important marker for fluid balance and should be undertaken daily in most instances. Handling preterm infants for weighing introduces certain risks such as accidental extubation, thermoregulatory instability, and potentially brief disconnection from assisted ventilation, which must be carefully balanced against the clinical benefits of accurate weight measurement (European Standards of Care for Newborn Health, 2018). Many modern incubators include built-in scales that allow for in-bed weighing, reducing handling risks. Although these scales may be slightly less precise than external scales, when used consistently at the same time daily and under controlled conditions they reliably track weight trends. To further enhance safety, two-person weighing, where a staff member or parent assists while the infant is swaddled, can help minimise stress and reduce the risk of complications such as physiological instability. This approach is supported by evidence showing that swaddled weighing significantly lowers behavioural and physiological stress in preterm infants (Vicente-Perez et al., 2023).

Measurement of urine volume

Accurate measurement of urine output is vital as it provides insight into both fluid balance and renal perfusion in neonates (NICE, 2020). The volume voided can be estimated in several ways. Weighed nappies provide the simplest method and provide a degree of accuracy assuming the relative humidity is greater than 40%. However, evaporation of urine into the environment, or further damping of the nappy by incubator humidity may create spurious results. Commercially available adhesive bags may be used, but fixation and retention without leakage can be a problem. Additionally, when the bag is removed, significant epidermal stripping can occur. Urine output should be in the region of 1 mL/kg/hour on day 1, rising to >2–3mL/kg/hour subsequently. Urinary catheters can be used for accurate fluid balance monitoring but carry risks such as urinary tract infections, urethral trauma, discomfort, catheter blockage, false passage formation, bladder irritation, and potential long-term urological complications, making careful aseptic technique and gentle handling essential to minimise harm.

Urinalysis

Urinalysis is a valuable procedure nurses undertake very early in their clinical practice experience and remains vital for detecting renal compromise and early kidney disease. Only a small urine volume is needed for effective screening; placing a cotton wool ball in the infant's nappy and aspirating it with a syringe is sufficient. Minimising unnecessary use of adhesives, such as those from urinary collection bags, helps prevent skin trauma associated with adhesive devices in neonates (Allen et al., 2023).

- ***Specific gravity*** is an underused, non-invasive marker of renal concentrating ability and hydration status, though its interpretation must consider the developmental immaturity of neonatal kidneys. As the ability to concentrate urine is limited, the maximum specific gravity is usually 1.015 to 1.020, but the minimum may be as low as 1.001 to 1.005. As other factors such as glucose and protein can alter specific gravity, osmolality measurement of both blood and urine should be undertaken and compared if concentrating ability is in question. Urine osmolality determines movement of water into and out of the plasma. Typical neonatal urine osmolality ranges from 75 to 300 mOsm/kg, though term infants may reach 600–700 mOsm/kg under stress. Healthy infants should be able to adjust urine excretion with daily fluid intake 90–200mL/kg when sodium is constant. A preterm infant has a limited ability to concentrate urine beyond approximately 500 mOsm/kg, due to immature tubular function. A specific gravity of 1.020–1.030 typically corresponds to an osmolality of around 400 mOsm/L; however, this is less reliable in neonates due to low solute load and immature renal function (Modi, 2012).
- ***Urine pH*** is an indicator of the kidneys' ability to regulate acid-base balance through the excretion of hydrogen ions. In neonates, urine is generally more alkaline at birth, with a typical pH around 6.0, reflecting immature renal tubular function. Most term infants develop the capacity to acidify urine to a pH of ≤5.5 within the first 1–2 weeks of life, as renal function matures. In extreme prematurity, urinary bicarbonate losses may be high, increasing the pH to 7.0 or above.

- ***Glycosuria*** This is the presence of glucose in the urine that occurs when blood glucose levels exceed the renal threshold. This results in osmotic diuresis, which increases the risk of dehydration. Urine dipstick testing offers a rapid and practical method to detect glycosuria in neonates (Kliegman et al., 2020).
- ***Proteinuria*** This is frequently seen in small amounts and is related to GA. In neonates, normal urinary protein excretion is higher than in older children and can reach levels up to 300mg/m^2/24hrs; values in excess of this may indicate a pathology and warrant medical review (Kliegman et al., 2020).
- ***Haematuria*** or the presence of blood in the urine, is abnormal in neonates and often indicative of underlying renal injury or pathology. Potential causes include birth asphyxia related renal damage, arterial emboli stemming from umbilical arterial catheterisation, renal vein thrombosis, coagulopathies, and congenital anomalies such as renal cystic disease or urinary tract obstruction. Again, senior medical review is justified where haematuria is present.

ACID-BASE BALANCE

Acid-base balance is the tightly regulated process that maintains a stable pH in the body, which is vital for normal physiological function. This balance is maintained through a complex synergy of the lungs, kidneys, and brain, preventing excessive acidity (acidosis) or alkalinity (alkalosis). The kidneys contribute to maintaining homeostasis by regulating acid-base balance through the reabsorption and secretion of bicarbonate ions (HCO_3^-) within the nephron, responding to the concentration of hydrogen ions in the plasma. There are many pathologies, including renal disease, which may contribute to metabolic acidosis or alkalosis. Metabolic acidosis occurs when bicarbonate ions are low, causing a corresponding reduction in blood pH. Sodium bicarbonate is frequently administered to neonates to correct metabolic acidosis; however, its efficacy and safety are debated, as although it can quickly raise blood pH there is limited evidence of improved clinical outcomes and it carries associated risks such as cerebral blood flow fluctuations, heightened intraventricular haemorrhage risk (particularly in preterm infants), electrolyte disturbances, and tissue damage if improperly managed. A metabolic alkalosis occurs when bicarbonate levels are raised, causing a corresponding rise in pH.

The correlation of respiratory and metabolic components and resulting changes observable during blood gas analysis is further explored in Chapter 14.

ACUTE KIDNEY INJURY

AKI is characterised by a sudden decline in GFR, leading to the accumulation of creatinine and other waste products, disrupted fluid balance, and impaired

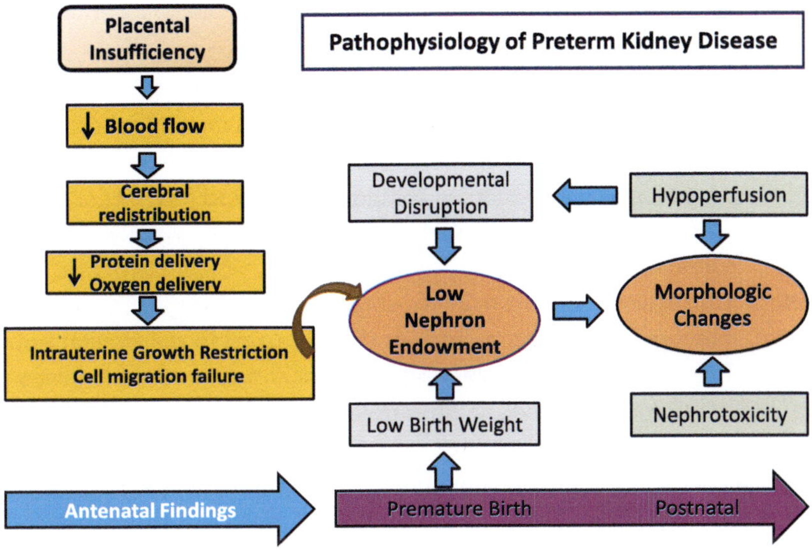

Figure 18.3 Pathophysiology of preterm kidney disease

electrolyte homeostasis. Clinically, reduced urine output (oliguria <0.5 mL/kg/hour), hypertension, signs of fluid overload or dehydration, and possible seizure activity are red-flag indicators suggestive of AKI. Neonates are particularly susceptible to AKI due to factors related to their immature renal physiology, including perinatal hypoxic-ischaemic events, prolonged resuscitation and acidosis, congenital malformations, episodes of hypotension, sepsis, and exposure to nephrotoxic medications (Jetton et al., 2017). The pathophysiology of kidney disease as applicable to the preterm infant can be seen in Figure 18.3.

Investigations

When AKI is suspected in a neonate, a structured assessment should be undertaken to identify the cause and guide early intervention.

Clinical history, examination and investigations are as follows;

- Review the infant's clinical history, including perinatal events, exposure to nephrotoxic drugs, hypotension, or sepsis.
- During physical examination:
  - Palpate the bladder to eliminate acute urinary retention, which may occur following hypoxic-ischaemic events or in infants receiving morphine infusions.
  - Assess circulatory status to evaluate the adequacy of renal perfusion, including:

    - Blood pressure
    - Capillary refill time
    - Core-periphery temperature gap
- Renal ultrasound is recommended to assess renal anatomy and urinary tract abnormalities.
- Paired blood and urine samples should be collected for:
    - Serum and urine electrolytes
    - Creatinine and urea
    - Urinalysis to identify markers of renal pathology
    - Fractional excretion of sodium (FeNa), used to distinguish between: Pre-renal AKI: $Fe_{Na} < 2.5\%$ (reflects sodium and water conservation) and intrarenal failure: $Fe_{Na} > 2.5\%$ (reflects tubular injury; see Table 18.10).

(Fe_{Na}) is calculated from the sodium and creatinine concentrations of serum and spot urine samples (Box 18.5).

Indices of renal failure are summarised in Table 18.10.

BOX 18.5 CALCULATION OF FRACTIONAL SODIUM EXCRETION

$$Fe_{Na} = (\text{urine sodium} \div \text{serum sodium}) \times (\text{serum sodium} \div \text{urine sodium}) \times 100$$

In low perfusion states, the kidneys conserve sodium and water, resulting in Fe_{Na} of less than 2.5%. In contrast, Fe_{Na} above 2.5% suggests intrarenal (tubular) injury as the cause of oliguria. However, this test is less reliable in very LBW

TABLE 18.10 INDICES OF RENAL FAILURE IN INFANTS

	Pre-renal failure	*Intrarenal failure*
Urine sodium	Low (<10mmol/L)	High (>20mmol/l)
Urine urea	High	Low
Urine creatinine	High	Low
Urine specific gravity	High (>1025)	Low (approx. 1010)
Urine osmolality	High (>500mOsm/kg)	Low (approx. 300mOsm/kg)
Fractional Na^+ excretion	Low (<1%)	High (>2.5–3.0%)
Urea: plasma creatinine	High (>40)	Low

infants, where Fe_{Na} can be as high as 15% due to immature renal function. Historically, 'fluid challenges' were used to assess renal perfusion. However, due to the associated risks of fluid overload, current practice has shifted towards individualised assessment and tailored fluid management. Improving urine output now focuses on enhancing kidney perfusion through optimised cardiac output, blood pressure support and, when appropriate, the use of diuretics (Weaver et al., 2023). As furosemide has a half-life of up to 8 hours in term infants and up to 24 hours in preterm babies, repeated or high doses are not advised due to the risk of ototoxicity and nephrotoxicity (Jetton et al., 2017).

ACTIVITY

Clinical decisions about neonatal nutrition and fluid management are presently guided by evaluating vital signs, monitoring fluid balance, tracking weight changes, analysing biochemical markers, and performing physical examinations. Investigate the potential of bioelectrical impedance analysis (BIA) as a non-invasive technique for assessing body composition in newborns, and consider how its use might impact nursing care, as well as the wellbeing of neonates and their families.

Management of acute kidney injury

The primary goal in managing neonatal AKI is to maintain fluid, electrolyte and acid-base homeostasis by supporting impaired renal function (Jetton et al., 2017). Approaches include:

- Discontinuing nephrotoxic drugs and adjusting dosing schedules of renally excreted medications guided by drug assays.
- Careful fluid balance including daily weights, meticulous input and output accounting for flushes, IWL and gastrointestinal losses.
- Cumulative as well as daily fluid balance, ensuring replacement in depleted infants, and use of diuretics in those overloaded.
- Methylxanthines – theophylline has been shown to prevent AKI in term infants following hypoxic-ischaemic perinatal events; while the use of caffeine in the preterm population is associated with a lower incidence of AKI (Starr et al., 2021).
- Ongoing management includes daily weights and frequent monitoring of urea, creatinine, and electrolytes. If AKI fails to improve or there are fluid overload, metabolic acidosis, hyperkalaemia, or neurological symptoms, dialysis should be considered, and early referral to a paediatric nephrologist is advised.

The Neonatal Kidney Collaborative, established in 2014, has significantly advanced research into neonatal AKI, particularly through the multinational AWAKEN study, which highlighted both the high incidence and the serious consequences of AKI in neonates (Jetton et al., 2017). This large prospective study revealed that AKI occurs in approximately 30% of high-risk neonates and is independently associated with increased mortality and prolonged hospital stay. These findings have challenged the earlier assumption that neonatal AKI was a transient issue with minimal long-term impact. More recent research confirms that survivors of neonatal AKI are at increased risk of chronic kidney disease, hypertension and neurodevelopmental impairment, emphasising the need for long-term surveillance and early intervention (Hessey et al., 2018).

Irreversible kidney disease requiring dialysis is rare in the neonate. Although the need for dialysis is relatively rare, there is a very high incidence of co-morbidity, and this affects survival, which for those on dialysis is about 80% at 5 years (Rees, 2017). Peritoneal dialysis (PD) is generally regarded as the optimal dialysis modality for neonates. PD allows for the slow removal of fluid and solutes while avoiding hemodynamic instability and is a relatively safe, simple and effective procedure. Nursing management of an infant undergoing PD is described in detail in the relevant section of the companion website.

Chapter takeaways

- Fluid and electrolyte homeostasis is vital to the short- and long-term outcomes of neonates, especially those born preterm or renally compromised.
- Advancements in technology and physiological understanding have improved the ability to manage fluid and electrolyte disturbances effectively.
- Neonates, especially preterm and low birthweight infants, are highly vulnerable to fluid and electrolyte imbalances due to immature renal function, high insensible water loss, and transitional physiological changes after birth. Management must be dynamic and patient specific.
- Accurate fluid calculations and vigilant assessment are essential, factoring in birthweight, postnatal age, clinical condition, weight trends, urine output and laboratory results. Maintenance needs must be carefully adjusted to prevent dehydration, fluid overload, and associated complications.
- A multi-professional approach is critical, involving nurses, neonatologists, dietitians, and pharmacists to ensure individualised, safe and evidence-based care, particularly when initiating IV fluids, electrolyte replacement, or PN.
- Clear communication with parents about fluid therapy is crucial to support informed involvement in care decisions, especially when IV therapy, feeding plans or long-term nutritional strategies are being implemented.

CASE STUDY

CASE STUDIES

Case study 1: Assessment and monitoring of fluid balance

Alice has twelve months' neonatal experience; she is providing nursing care for Amir today. Amir was born at 25 weeks' gestation and he is 20 hours old. His birthweight is 650g. His mum, Shara, has received a complete course of antenatal steroids 48 hours ago due to preterm labour. Shara has been well in her pregnancy.

Currently Amir's situation is as follows:

- Ventilated but stable
- Has lines in situ – a double lumen umbilical venous catheter and an umbilical arterial line. All vascular access is patent
- Receiving humidity at 90%
- Incubator temperature set at 38.5°C
- T1 37.3°C and T2 36.8°C – temperatures are stable
- HR 145, RR 60, BP 50/33mmHg, SpO_2 93%
- Electrolytes – sodium 137mmol/L, potassium 3.8mmol/L, glucose 4.8mmol/L
- 120mL/kg/day 10% glucose and maintenance parenteral nutrition. Amir is receiving trophic feeds 0.5mL 2 hourly
- Skin – his skin feels sticky and warm to touch
- Activity – he is flexed and appears comfortable

Q.1. Which aspects of Amir's clinical history indicate a need for close monitoring of his fluid balance, and why?

Q.2. Describe the methods you would use to accurately monitor fluid balance in Amir's care.

Q.3. What measures can be taken to minimise heat and insensible water loss in preterm neonates like Amir?

Q.4. Outline the clinical observations you would undertake hourly and explain why these are important for fluid and electrolyte management.

Case study 2: The infant who is volume-depleted

Finlay has just been repatriated to his local neonatal unit after a period in a Neonatal Intensive Care Unit where he was transferred for stabilisation and respiratory management on day 1 of life. He was born at 28+6 weeks'

CASE STUDY

gestation and is now 2 weeks old. Finlay has been slow to establish enteral feeds, receiving PN and 2mL/hr breastmilk via an orogastric tube, and is on high flow oxygen. His intravenous central line continues to alarm high pressure and is not infusing the correct volume of fluid per hour. He had a cannula for his repatriation, but this is no longer patent. His gastric aspirates are milky and larger than previously noted. On assessment, it is noted that he looks 'dry,' and Finlay's parents comment that he does not look right, particularly his skin colour.

Q.1. What key information would you require to accurately assess Finlay's fluid balance, and why is each element important?
Q.2. What clinical signs and symptoms would you expect if he is fluid-depleted?
Q.3. Describe the fluid management and nursing care priorities for Finlay, and explain the rationale for each.
Q.4. What information and support should be provided to Finlay's parents regarding his fluid management and overall care?

Case study 3: The infant with fluid imbalance

Saskia, a term infant, was admitted to the neonatal unit at birth following prolonged resuscitation and was diagnosed with meconium aspiration syndrome and hypoxic-ischaemic encephalopathy. She is currently undergoing therapeutic hypothermia and requires high levels of oxygen and ventilatory support. During the ward round, Saskia's father notes that she appears more swollen than the day before. A chest X-ray reveals a diffuse white-out in both lungs, indicating a change from previous imaging.

Q.1. How might Saskia's underlying conditions and current treatment contribute to her oedema and respiratory findings?
Q.2. Can you explain the physiology behind this picture?
Q.3. What are the key considerations for Saskia's fluid management, and what specific nursing interventions would support her care?
Q.4. How would you explain Saskia's current condition and treatment to her parents in a clear and compassionate way?

For suggested answer guides to the questions posed in these case studies, please refer to the web-based companion site specific to this chapter. See www.routledge.com/cw/petty

References

Ågren, J., Segar, J. L., Söderström, F., & Bell, E. F. (2022). Fluid management considerations in extremely preterm infants born at 22–24 weeks of gestation. *Seminars in Perinatology*, *46*(1), 151541. https://doi.org/10.1016/j.semperi.2021.151541

Allen, A., Zana-Taïeb, E., & Group of Reflection and Evaluation of the Environment of Newborns (GREEN) of the French Neonatology Society. (2023). Recommendations for use of adhesives on hospitalized newborns: A systematic review of the literature. *Archives de Pédiatrie*, *30*(7), 486–492.

Araya, B. R., Ziegler, A. A., Grobe, C. C., Grobe, J. L., & Segar, J. L. (2023). Sodium and growth in preterm infants: A review. *Newborn* (Clarksville), *2*(2), 142–147.

Avery, G. B., First, L. R., & Hartenstein, A. (2021). *Neonatology: Pathophysiology and management of the newborn* (8th ed.). Lippincott Williams & Wilkins.

Berg, J. M., Tymoczko, J. L., Gatto, G. J., & Stryer, L. (2019). *Biochemistry* (9th ed.). W. H. Freeman and Company.

Bollaboina, S. K. Y., Urakurva, A. K., Kamsetti, S., & Kotha, R. (2023). A systematic review: Is early fluid restriction in preterm neonates going to prevent bronchopulmonary dysplasia? *Cureus*, *15*(12), e50805. https://doi.org/10.7759/cureus.50805

Boscarino, G., Conti, M. G., Gasparini, C., Onestà, E., Faccioli, F., Dito, L., Regoli, D., Spalice, A., Parisi, P., & Terrin, G. (2021). Neonatal hyperglycemia related to parenteral nutrition affects long-term neurodevelopment in preterm newborn: A prospective cohort study. *Nutrients*, *13*(6), 1930.

British Association of Perinatal Medicine. (2024). *Identification and management of neonatal hypoglycaemia in the full-term infant (Birth to 72 hours)*. Retrieved July 23, 2025, from https://www.bapm.org/resources/identification-and-management-of-neonatal-hypoglycaemia-in-the-full-term-infant-birth-72-hours

Durrani, N. U. R., Imam, A. A., & Soni, N. (2022). Hypernatremia in newborns: A practical approach to management. *Biomedicine Hub*, 7(2), 55–69.

European Standards of Care for Newborn Health. (2018). *Weighing*. European Foundation for the Care of Newborn Infants. Retrieved August 27, 2025, from https://newborn-health-standards.org/standards/standards-english/care-procedures/weighing/

Fanaroff, S., & Martin, R. (2020). *Neonatal-perinatal medicine: Diseases of the fetus and infant* (11th ed.). Elsevier.

Gardner, S. L., Carter, B. S., Enzman-Hines, M. I., & Niermeyer, S. (Eds.). (2020). *Merenstein & Gardner's handbook of neonatal intensive care: An interprofessional approach* (9th ed.). Elsevier.

Giouleka, S., Gkiouleka, M., Tsakiridis, I., Daniilidou, A., Mamopoulos, A., Athanasiadis, A., & Dagklis, T. (2023.) Diagnosis and management of neonatal hypoglycemia: A comprehensive review of guidelines. *Children*, *10*(7), 1220.

Harding, J. E., Harris, D. L., Hegarty, J. E., Alsweiler, J. M., & McKinlay, C. J. (2017). An emerging evidence base for the management of neonatal hypoglycaemia. *Early Human Development*, *104*, 51–56.

Hessey, E., Morissette, G., Lacroix, J., Perreault, S., Samuel, S., Dorais, M., Jouvet, P., Lafrance, J. P., LeLorier, J., Phan, V., Palijan, A., Pizzi, M., Roy, L., & Zappitelli, M. (2018). Long-term mortality after acute kidney injury in the pediatric ICU. *Hospital Pediatrics*, *8*(5), 260–268.

Iacobelli, S., & Guignard, J. P. (2021). Maturation of glomerular filtration rate in neonates and infants: An overview. *Pediatric Nephrology*, *36*(6), 1439–1446.

Jetton, J. G., Boohaker, L. J., Sethi, S. K., Wazir, S., Rohatgi, S., Soranno, D. E., Chishti, A. S., Woroniecki, R., Mammen, C., Swanson, J. R., Sridhar, S., Wong, C. S., Kupferman, J. C., Griffin, R. L., & Askenazi, D. J. (2017). Incidence and outcomes of neonatal acute kidney injury (AWAKEN): A multicentre, multinational, observational cohort study. *The Lancet Child & Adolescent Health*, *1*(3), 184–194.

Kliegman, R., St. Geme, J., Blum, N., Shah, B., Tasker, R., & Wilson, N. (Eds.). (2020). *Nelson textbook of pediatrics* (21st ed.). Elsevier.

Low Birth Weight and Nephron Number Working Group. (2017). The impact of kidney development on the life course: A consensus document for action. *Nephron*, *136*(1), 3–49.

McKinlay, C. J. D., Alsweiler, J. M., Ansell, J. M., Anstice, N. S., Chase, J. G., Gamble, G. D., Harris, D. L., Jacobs, R. J., Jiang, Y., Paudel, N., Signal, M., Thompson, B., Wouldes, T. A., Yu, T. Y., Harding, J. E., & CHYLD Study Group. (2015). Neonatal glycemia and neurodevelopmental outcomes at 2 years. *New England Journal of Medicine*, *373*(16), 1507–1518.

Modi, N. (2012). Fluid and electrolyte balance. In J. M. Rennie (Ed.), *Rennie and Roberton's textbook of neonatology* (5th ed., pp. 331–343). Churchill Livingstone Elsevier.

Moore, K. L., Persaud, T. V. N., & Torchia, M. G. (2019). *The developing human: Clinically oriented embryology* (11th ed.). Elsevier.

Moss, C. R. (2022). Fluid and electrolyte management in the neonate: Potassium and phosphorus. *Neonatal Network*, *41*(4), 211–218.

Muhari-Stark, E., & Burckart, G. J. (2018). Glomerular filtration rate estimation formulas for pediatric and neonatal use. *Journal of Pediatric Pharmacology and Therapeutics*, *23*(6), 424–431.

National Institute for Health and Care Excellence. (2020). *Intravenous fluid therapy in children and young people in hospital (Guideline NG29)*. NICE. https://www.nice.org.uk/guidance/ng29

NHS England. (2024). *National standards for neonatal qualified in specialty (QIS) education*. Retrieved May 29, 2025, from https://www.england.nhs.uk/long-read/national-standards-for-neonatal-qualified-in-specialty-qis-education/

NHS Greater Glasgow & Clyde and Scottish Perinatal Network. (2021). *Parenteral feeding and fluid requirements in preterm and term infants: clinical guideline*. NHS Greater Glasgow & Clyde & SPN. Retrieved July 30, 2025, from https://clinicalguidelines.scot.nhs.uk/ggc-paediatric-guidelines/ggc-paediatric-guidelines/neonatology/parenteral-feeding-of-preterm-and-term-infant/ Available via NHS clinical guidance portal

Pace, M., van Sas, S., Salaets, T., Laenen, A., Raaijmakers, A., & Allegaert, K. (2025). Hypo- and hypernatremia in extremely low birth weight infants in the first 10 days of life: A review. *Children (Basel)*, *12*(2), 231.

Paediatric Formulary Committee. (2024). *BNF for children: 2024–2025 edition*. BMJ Group, Pharmaceutical Press and RCPCH Publications.

Polin, R. A., Abman, S. H., Rowitch, D. H., & Benitz, W. E. (2021). *Fetal and neonatal physiology* (6th ed.). Elsevier.

Rees, L. (2017). Renal replacement therapies in neonates: Issues and ethics. *Seminars in Fetal and Neonatal Medicine*, *22*(2), 104–108.

Rigo, J., Pieltain, C., Christmann, V., Bonsante, F., Moltu, S. J., Iacobelli, S., & Marret, S. (2017). Serum magnesium levels in preterm infants are higher than adult levels: A systematic literature review and meta-analysis. *Nutrients*, *9*(10), 1125.

Rosenblum, S., Pal, A., & Reidy, K. (2017). Renal development in the fetus and premature infant. *Seminars in Fetal and Neonatal Medicine*, *22*(2), 58–66.

Royal College of Nursing. (2016). *Standards for infusion therapy* (4th ed.). RCN Publishing. Retrieved July 30, 2025, from https://www.rcn.org.uk/professional-development/publications/pub-007326

Saint-Faust, M., Boubred, F., & Simeoni, U. (2014). Renal development and neonatal adaptation. *American Journal of Perinatology*, *31*(9), 773–780.

Segar, J. L., & Jetton, J. G. (2024). Fluid and electrolyte management in the neonate and what can go wrong. *Current Opinion in Pediatrics*, *36*(2), 198–203.

Starr, M. C., Charlton, J. R., Guillet, R., Reidy, K., Tipple, T. E., Jetton, J. G., Kent, A. L., Abitbol, C. L., Ambalavanan, N., Mhanna, M. J., Askenazi, D. J., Selewski, D. T., & Harer, M. W. (2021). Advances in neonatal acute kidney injury. *Pediatrics*, *148*(5), e2021051220. https://doi.org/10.1542/peds.2021-051220

Vicente-Perez, S., Robleda, G., Gich, I., Nolla, T., Ponce-Taylor, J., Verd, S., & Ginovart, G. (2023). Physiological responses and behavioural organization of very low birth weight infants during swaddled versus traditional weighing. *Nursing Open*, *10*(10), 6896–6902.

Vuralli, D. (2019). Clinical approach to hypocalcemia in newborn period and infancy: Who should be treated? *International Journal of Pediatrics*, *2019*, Article 4318075. https://doi.org/10.1155/2019/4318075

Weaver, L. J., Travers, C. P., Ambalavanan, N., & Askenazi, D. (2023). Neonatal fluid overload – Ignorance is no longer bliss. *Pediatric Nephrology*, *38*(1), 47–60.

Wickström, R., Skiöld, B., Petersson, G., Stephansson, O., & Altman, M. (2018). Moderate neonatal hypoglycemia and adverse neurological development at 2–6 years of age. *European Journal of Epidemiology*, *33*(10), 1011–1020.

Yu, A. S. L., Chertow, G. M., Luyckx, V. A., Marsden, P. A., Skorecki, K., & Taal, M. W. (Eds.). (2019). *Brenner and Rector's the kidney* (11th ed.). Elsevier.

19 NUTRITION AND FEEDING MANAGEMENT IN THE NEONATAL UNIT

Rebecca Murphy, Alexandra Connolly, and Lynette Forsythe

CONTENTS

DOI: 10.4324/9781003591405-23

GUIDANCE ON HOW TO ENHANCE PERSONAL LEARNING FROM THIS CHAPTER

Key points covered in this chapter

- Nutritional requirements, assessment, nutrition and growth monitoring in the neonatal unit.
- Feeding development and cue-based feeding for the infant in the neonatal unit.
- Family integrated multidisciplinary nutrition and feeding management of neonates.

Reflection

Reading through the chapter, you are encouraged to engage with the key points and related literature in an enquiring way. Ask these questions:

- Why is early nutrition important? Why are nutritional status and all anthropometry measurements necessary, not just weight checks?
- How is nutrition and feeding managed within your unit, and is this there a joint multidisciplinary approach?
- Can you think of how you currently support nutrition and feeding in your unit and what you could improve on?
- How can you support parents to develop the infant-parent feeding relationship on the neonatal unit?

Implications for nursing care

- Finally: this chapter should facilitate your understanding of best practice for nutrition and feeding management. Consider how you can contribute to the nutrition and feeding management in your neonatal unit in your country and what this means for the individual neonates you look after on a day-to-day basis. How can you support the family and infant on their feeding journey during their neonatal stay and following discharge?

INTRODUCTION AND BACKGROUND

Nutritional and feeding management on the neonatal unit has evolved over the last decade as neonatal care has become more holistic and family integrated. As developmental care has become more embedded within neonatal practice, there has been a universal shift to consider both short-term and long-term outcomes within nutritional and feeding management with the aim of optimising neurodevelopment (Mustapha et al., 2024).

The nutritional needs of preterm infants differ significantly from those of term infants. As survival rates continue to improve, especially among extremely preterm infants born at 22–24 weeks' gestation, neonatal teams are increasingly managing complex nutritional and feeding challenges. In response, the multidisciplinary team (MDT), working in partnership with families, strives to meet each infant's individual nutritional requirements and to optimise feeding strategies from birth to support growth and long-term outcomes (Murphy et al., 2021).

This chapter provides a standardised clinical approach to nutrition and growth in preterm and sick infants. It is beyond its scope to discuss nutritional requirements or specific nutrients in-depth. These topics are readily available in a range of reference materials. The reader is encouraged to not only consider the feeding differences of premature and/or sick infants but also their role in supporting the family and the feeding journey. An understanding of the development and function of the gastrointestinal tract is vital for professionals to understand the initiation of enteral feeds. Optimal nutrition and growth and long-term outcomes are dependent on the assessment, implementation and regular monitoring of parenteral and enteral nutrition.

SUPPORTING THE FEEDING RELATIONSHIP

The bond between a mother and her infant begins during pregnancy, as she creates images and ideas of what being a new parent is going to be like (Phillips, 2024).

For parents who experience admission to a neonatal unit (NNU), this is interrupted and replaced with a different reality. The shock of having a preterm birth or unwell infant can cause significant stress and have lasting effects on a mothers emotional and mental health, impacting early bonding between the parent and infant.

Feeding is one of the earliest acts of caregiving for the new parent and is how they begin to form their relationship with their infant and create their parental identity. Parents on the NNU will be experiencing a very different beginning from that which they imagined, and this can cause disconnect. How this is experienced may vary on how early their baby was born, the medical complexities the infant and parents are faced with and their own internal capacity. In this respect, the loss of the first breastfeed or bottle feed straight after birth can be emotionally challenging (Palmér & Ericson, 2019).

Maternal-infant separation can further contribute to feelings of disconnection (Wang et al., 2021). The Neonatal nurse and wider team play an integral role in supporting parents to understand their role in their baby's feeding development from the very beginning of the neonatal journey. Whether that is through expressing milk, holding their baby for tube feeds or understanding the transition from tube to suck feeding, this caregiving can help build closeness and confidence as they become aware of the positive impact this can have on their baby's development.

FEEDING DEVELOPMENT *IN UTERO*

Each infant is born with predetermined feeding skills including, sucking, rooting and swallowing. *In utero*, the fetus is exposed to a variety of sensory experiences, which serve to further prepare the baby for suck-feeding at birth. Amongst the earliest sense to develop is the chemosensory system which facilitates the perception of taste and smell in utero. From approximately 30 weeks' gestation, fetuses can discriminate odorous molecules present in amniotic fluid (Sarnat et al., 2017). Both term and preterm infants have demonstrated a preference for the smell of their mother's amniotic fluid (Ustun et al., 2023). Early taste and smell opportunities can help with calming the baby, attenuation of pain, maternal recognition and bonding (Boesveldt & Parma, 2021) and orientation to the breast, therefore supporting breastfeeding success.

Auditory experiences *in utero* also enhance the infant's sensory and emotional development. The womb provides opportunity to hear maternal voice. A preference for the mother's voice has been noted as early as the third trimester (Sullivan et al., 2011). Maternal voice exposure can support postnatal bonding. Although neonatal hospitalisation may result in physical separation from their parents, continued exposure to their parents' voices has been shown to have positive effects on feeding, cognitive and neurobehavioral development (Provenzi et al., 2018).

Feeding reflexes, present at birth, enable effective feeding. Rooting and swallowing begins around 10–14 weeks' gestation and by 20 weeks, rhythmical sucking has developed with observations of fetuses opening and closing their mouths at regular intervals.

The second and third trimesters of pregnancy are the time of anatomical and functional development of the gastrointestinal tract. When infants are born prematurely, particularly less than 28 weeks, the immaturity of the digestive and absorptive processes and of GI motility present feeding challenges to establish enteral nutrition and meet nutritional requirements. The presence of early infant gut microbiome is an important regulator of many developing functions and can influence the risk for some conditions such as late onset sepsis and necrotising enterocolitis (NEC). Early enteral feeding with human milk remains an important determinant of the gut microbiome (Indrio et al., 2022). Congenital gastrointestinal abnormalities such as oesophageal atresia, malformation of the small and large intestines including gastroschisis or Hirschsprung's disease limit the ability to establish enteral feeds.

AIMS OF NUTRITION MANAGEMENT IN NEONATAL CARE

Standardised approaches to nutrition and feeding management implemented by the MDT within NNUs are now well recognised to improve outcomes such as reduced clinical variation, reduced cost, quicker achievement of full enteral feeds, reduced duration of parenteral nutrition (PN), increased rates of breastfeeding, reduced length of hospital admission, reduced rates of NEC and improved growth and neurodevelopment (Bala et al., 2024). The aims can be summarised as follows:

- Achievement of growth and nutrient accretion similar to intrauterine rates
- Meeting the nutritional requirements of the preterm infant
- Preventing feeding-related morbidities
- Optimising long-term outcomes including neurodevelopmental outcomes

Details of the multidisciplinary feeding team are outlined in the web-based companion of the book.

NUTRITIONAL REQUIREMENTS

Preterm infants are at increased risk of developing significant cumulative nutritional deficits due to negligible energy stores, delays in establishing nutrition

TABLE 19.1 SUMMARY OF PRETERM ENTERAL NUTRITIONAL REQUIREMENTS (EMBLETON ET AL., 2023)

Nutrient	*Preterm Infant*
Energy (kcal/kg)	115–140 (- 160)
Protein (g/kg)	3.5–4.0 (– 4.5)
Sodium (mmol/kg)	3.0–5.0 (– 8.0)
Calcium (mmol/kg)	3.0–5.0
Phosphorus (mmol/kg)	2.2–3.7
Vitamin A (µg/kg)	400–1000
Vitamin D (µg)	10–17.5/kg/day
Iron (mg)	2.0–3.0 (– 6.0)

support and increased nutritional requirements (Bala et al., 2024). They have limited stores of nutrients as accretion occurs predominantly in the last trimester of pregnancy and consequently a limited capacity to tolerate starvation, especially if coupled with metabolic demands imposed by illness (Tesser et al., 2025). Requirements are influenced by both prenatal factors such as intrauterine growth restriction and postnatal illnesses such as sepsis, stress, surgery and bronchopulmonary dysplasia (BPD). Nutrition support during the first hours of life is based on fluid maintenance, glucose homeostasis and normal serum electrolytes. Evidence-based estimations (Table 19.1) published by the European Society for Paediatric Gastroenterology, Hepatology and Nutrition (ESPGHAN) form the basis of enteral nutritional requirements for preterm infants (Embleton et al., 2023). PN requirements have been published by National Institute of Health and Care Excellence (NICE, 2020) and ESPGHAN (Mihatsch et al., 2018).

PARENTERAL NUTRITION

PN is the cornerstone of neonatal nutritional care in premature and sick infants. It may be required for a period between birth and establishing enteral feeds. PN provides macronutrients, electrolytes, minerals, vitamins and trace elements. Premature infants are born with low nutritional reserves and an immature gut and are unable to digest sufficient milk to meet their nutritional requirements. Whilst enteral feeds are being established and in more mature infants with gastrointestinal malformation or impairment, PN is integral to the nutritional management. In some cases, PN is the sole source of nutrition depending on underlying diagnosis.

Almost all preterm infants less than 31 weeks will require PN, the duration of which is determined by gestation, birthweight and other concurrent morbidities.

A central venous catheter is required for longer term delivery of PN, most commonly in the NNU setting a peripherally inserted central catheter (PICC).

PRACTICE POINT

Parenteral nutrition should be given to all infants (NICE, 2020):

- Born before 31+0 weeks
- Born at or after 31+0 weeks if sufficient progress is not made with enteral feeding in the first 72 hours after birth
- Preterm and term infants who are unlikely to establish sufficient enteral feeds, for example, infants with a congenital gastrointestinal disorder or critical illness such as sepsis
- Preterm infants where enteral feeds have been stopped and it is unlikely they will be restarted within 48 hours or enteral feeds have been stopped for more than 24 hours and there is unlikely to be sufficient progress with enteral feeds within a further 48 hours
- Term infants on enteral feeds if enteral feeds have been stopped and it is unlikely they will be restarted within 72 hours or enteral feeds have been stopped for more than 48 hours and there is unlikely to be sufficient progress with enteral feeds within a further 48 hours

PN should be started as soon as possible after birth and ideally within 8 hours, especially in very preterm infants if the indications for PN are met. Standardised PN formulations are recommended due to being immediately available and appropriate for most infants (NICE, 2020). Standardised PN can help reduce prescribing and administration errors. There is limited evidence to the benefits on the long-term neurodevelopmental outcomes on specific PN macronutrient content; however, optimisation of nutritional care through adequate macronutrient intakes immediately after birth may positively improve growth and neurodevelopmental outcomes (Tesser et al., 2025). Enteral feeds are introduced when the infant is clinically stable according to a standardised local enteral feeding policy and PN volume is reduced. The total nutritional intake from parenteral and enteral nutrition, infant's tolerance of enteral feeds and the balance between nutritional intake and the risk of catheter-related infection should be considered when weaning PN. Earlier breastmilk fortification has been more recently recommended to avoid undernutrition during the transition phase of parenteral to enteral feeds (Embleton et al., 2023).

Local policy on routine biochemical monitoring is important. Close monitoring of blood glucose, blood pH, potassium, chloride and calcium levels is required for all infants on PN, and the frequency will depend on the stability of the infant. In addition to this, serum triglycerides, serum phosphate, liver function tests and iron status will also need to be monitored.

Complications associated with PN include electrolyte imbalances, central line associated bloodstream infections, extravasation, thrombosis and PN associated liver disease. Therefore, although PN is an integral part of nutritional care, it is vital to commence and advance enteral feeds at the earliest opportunity.

ENTERAL NUTRITION

Standardised enteral feeding protocols are recommended within NNUs and are usually categorised into high, medium and low risk. Enteral feeds tend to commence as **trophic** feeds or **minimal enteral feeds** which are defined as initial milk feeds of up to 1 mL/kg/hr, preparing the gut for subsequent advancement of enteral feeds. Benefits include stimulating **peristalsis**, immunomodulatory effects and growth and maturation of the gut mucosa.

It remains unclear whether continuing trophic feeds for several days has any advantage when compared to initial, early progressive feeding. However, early advancing of feeds in extremely, very preterm and low birthweight (LBW) infants supports gut development and the transition from parenteral to enteral nutrition. Trophic feeds can therefore be given for up to 7 days; they are not intended to contribute to the nutritional intake and are not included in total fluid volumes. Infants should be assessed daily for tolerance and consideration of advancing feeds.

There is also no clear evidence that slow advancement of feeds in very LBW infants reduces the risk of NEC. A pragmatic approach to the rate of feed advancement in the high-risk group of infants must be considered in addition to caution taken when advancing feeds in the medium risk group. Reaching full enteral feeds faster results in earlier discontinuation of PN and removal of vascular catheters, resulting in a reduced risk of sepsis and fewer catheter-related complications (Oddie et al., 2021).

Feeds should be given as 1–2 hourly bolus gravity feeds for both initiation and advancing enteral feeds. Giving bolus feeds allows for better establishment of beneficial intestinal hormones such as gastrin and enteroglucagon which encourage gut development and motility, as well as encouraging intestinal secretions (Bala et al., 2024). Parents should feel empowered and take an active role in enteral feeding, being able to feel that they are feeding their baby. Early involvement of parents in feeding and ward rounds as part of family integrated care (FiCare) can decrease the risk of readmission and reduce the length of hospital stay.

Breastmilk

Mother's own breastmilk (MOM) is the preferred feed choice for all infants and is associated with short- and long-term benefits. Lower mortality rates, lower rates of sepsis and NEC, improved neurodevelopmental outcomes, lower rates of BPD, retinopathy of prematurity and fewer hospital admissions are reported in infants receiving MOM (Taylor et al., 2022). Human milk (HM) is vital to aid gut maturity in extreme preterm infants, promote gut flora, prevent infection by bacteria and viruses and support the growth and adaptation of the gastro-intestinal (GI) tract along with promoting the growth of beneficial bacteria (British Association of Perinatal Medicine (BAPM), 2020).

Recent practice of **buccal colostrum**, 0.1–0.2mL of colostrum delivered into the buccal mucosa, provides the infant a positive oral experience even they are not yet ready for enteral feeds.

HM meets the nutritional needs of a term infant (Figure 19.1); however, HM alone will not meet the higher nutritional requirements for preterm infants especially the very- and extremely LBW infants. Human milk fortification (HMF) with a multicomponent supplement is therefore recommended in this population. Multicomponent fortifier contains protein, calcium, phosphate, vitamins A and D, zinc and other trace elements to support growth and bone mineralisation. HMF may be appropriate for discharge and there is a rising emergence of this practice to support establishing breastfeeding and maintaining appropriate growth once home.

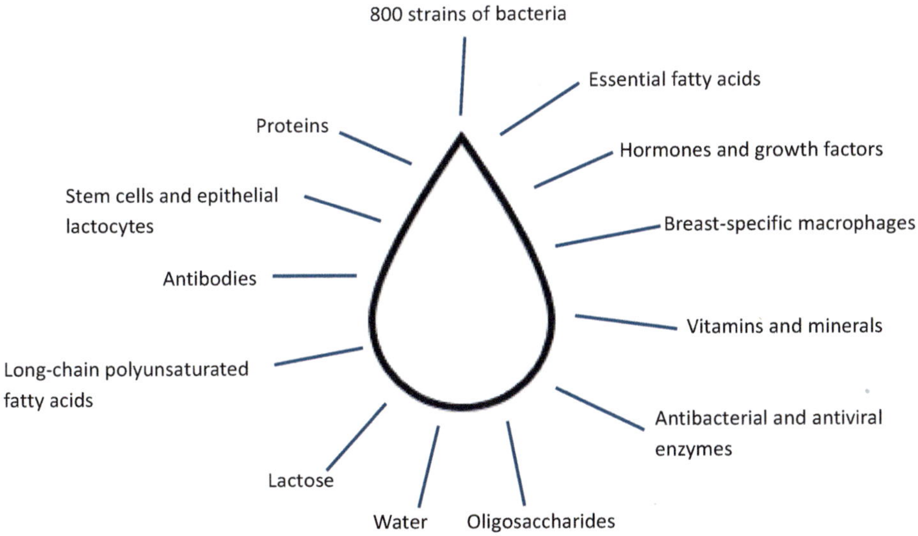

Figure 19.1 Components of breastmilk

DONOR EXPRESSED BREASTMILK

If MOM is unavailable or insufficient to meet an infant's nutritional requirements, donor expressed breastmilk (DEBM) may be used as the preferred alternative, particularly for infants at high risk of NEC. DEBM is associated with a lower incidence of NEC compared with preterm formula (Quigley et al., 2019; BAPM, 2023). Despite this, practice regarding DEBM use varies considerably between neonatal units. Although BAPM has outlined clinical criteria for when DEBM should be considered, guidance regarding the optimal duration of its use remains undefined. DEBM can be fortified in the same way as MOM to support adequate growth. Ongoing research is needed to better inform evidence-based use of DEBM in preterm infants.

Preterm infant formula

If the infant no longer meets criteria for DEBM when MOM is insufficient or unavailable, preterm infant formulas are available as an alternative. These formulas are nutrient-enriched to support the growth and developmental needs of preterm infants; however, they lack the bioactive components and immunological factors naturally present in HM, which are considered beneficial in reducing the risk of NEC. Nutrient-enriched post-discharge formulas (NEPDF) are also available and can be prescribed after discharge. Nonetheless, NEPDFs were developed from limited evidence, and their routine use is becoming less supported in practice due to the absence of robust data demonstrating clear benefit.

Probiotics

The use of probiotics has become more widespread in neonatal care. Much of the research suggests there may be benefits to reduce morbidity and mortality by reducing the rates of NEC and sepsis in the preterm population. Only a limited number of strains have shown preliminary potential effectiveness, and there is currently insufficient high-quality evidence to recommend one probiotic over the other of those available (Sharif et al., 2020).

METHODS OF FEEDING

Enteral feeding is commenced using a tube for neonates, passed either via the nose, nasogastric tube (NGT), or the mouth, orogastric tube (OGT). Orogastric tubes are most appropriately used in the smaller neonate if on non-invasive respiratory support. Checking for correct placement and position of NGT and OGT is vital to avoid aspiration (material entering the airway, below the level of the vocal cords), and is confirmed by pH testing of the aspirate. Gravity or bolus feed is the most common method of gastric tube feeding on the NNU using an open syringe with the plunger removed. Parents should be encouraged to carry out tube feeds.

Assessing feed tolerance in infants with a NGT or OGT in situ remains challenging, particularly when relying on routine measurement of **gastric residual volumes** (GRVs). This practice typically involves aspirating the stomach contents to evaluate the volume and appearance of the gastric aspirate. Significant variation exists both nationally and internationally in how GRVs are measured and managed. Importantly, changes in the volume or colour of aspirates may reflect gastrointestinal immaturity rather than true feed intolerance or early signs of necrotising enterocolitis (NEC), making interpretation difficult and potentially leading to unnecessary interruptions in enteral feeding.

> The neoGASTRIC trial is a large multicentre randomised controlled study in the UK and Australia investigating whether avoiding routine GRV measurement in preterm infants helps them reach full enteral feeds sooner without increasing the risk of necrotising enterocolitis (NIHR, 2022).

Gastrostomy tube feeds are occasionally considered when longer-term enteral feeding is indicated. Where a gastrostomy is formed feeds should be started as small bolus feeds as these infants may have a very small stomach. Nasojejunal (NJ) feeds allow for feeding directly into the jejunum and may be used in severe cases of gastro-oesophageal reflux disease (GORD). NJ tubes are difficult to place and to maintain in position. Feeding directly into the jejunum can cause dumping syndrome due to the rapid delivery of a hyperosmolar feed, therefore feeds are always delivered continuously via a pump. Post gastrointestinal surgery for conditions such as oesophageal atresia, a **trans-anastomotic tube** (TAT) may be required, through which continuous pump feeds are administered.

SUCKING, SWALLOWING, BREATHING COORDINATION

Sucking is a complex process that involves both positive and negative pressure mechanisms. Positive pressure, or compression, occurs when the infant applies pressure to the breast or bottle nipple with the tongue pushing up against the hard palate, forcing milk out. Negative pressure, or suction, is generated as the infant creates a seal around the nipple using the lips, tongue and palate. The downward movement of the jaw expands the oral cavity, creating negative pressure that draws milk into the oropharynx (Lau, 2015).

While compression alone can be used for bottle feeding, without suction it is not as efficient and often leads to fatigue. Successful breastfeeding requires both compression and suction, though predominately relies on suction, for effective milk transfer (Geddes & Sakalidis, 2015). Once milk transfer is achieved the infant will use their tongue to propel the bolus (milk) to the back of their mouth ready for swallowing. Anatomical abnormalities such as cleft palate or **micrognathia** can impact sucking efficiency. Similarly, infants with neurological impairment including hypoxic-ischaemic encephalopathy or neuromuscular conditions like spinal muscular atrophy may present with hyper- or hypotonia. These tone abnormalities can affect the strength of intraoral pressure needed for effective suction.

If typically developing, the infant will trigger a swallow as the bolus reaches the pharynx. This process can be impacted by existing co-morbidities with sensory and/or motor impairment. There are three mechanisms protecting the airway when the swallow is triggered: vocal cords close; the **epiglottis** folds over the airway; and swallow apnoea occurs (this is when breathing stops momentarily). Catch up breaths to compensate for the reduction in respiration during the sucking bursts occur in the pauses. In infants with respiratory compromise, particularly those with BPD, the repeated interruption of breathing during feeding can place additional strain on an already vulnerable respiratory system. This increased effort may lead to fatigue and respiratory instability, reducing effective gas exchange and resulting in episodes of oxygen desaturation. Reduced intake and fatigue are common clinical indicators that suck feeding may be exceeding an infant's capacity.

Oral motor control and coordination of the suck-swallow-breathe (SSB) sequence are fundamental for effective oral feeding (Lau, 2016). Approximately 80% of premature infants experience challenges with oral feeding during their stay in the NNU (Lau, 2016). From around 34 weeks' gestation SSB for effective coordination begins to emerge and will continue to mature towards term (Harding et al., 2018). However, this is highly individual for each infant and will be impacted by existing co-morbidities. Development of effective feeding depends on neurological maturity and may take time to be fully established. Because of the symbiotic relationship between infant and mothers, parents who wish to breastfeed may start their feeding journey earlier than bottle-fed infants, so that it is commonly seen that infants may start having their first attempts at the breast from 32 weeks or earlier.

Bottle feeding uses a different technique to breastfeeding and can present challenges for the preterm infant. Breastfeeding is only possible in keeping with a baby's developmental maturity and readiness. However, when bottle feeding the preterm or medically unwell infant, it is possible to override their cues, as the automatic sucking reflex in isolation may be wrongly interpreted as a sign of interest, maturity and skill.

When the infant is able to coordinate the SSB, milk is able to travel without risk of aspiration. Delay and dysfunction may lead to oral feeding disruption impacting swallow safety and/or efficiency (Lau, 2015).

Nutritive sucking patterns

Ross (2021) outlines five distinct nutritive sucking patterns used to characterise an infant's feeding behaviour:

- Obligatory: Infant fails to stop and breathe and needs the caregiver to intervene.
- Alternating: The infant alternates between breathing and sucking bursts without assistance from the feeder. The baby does not attempt to breathe during the sucking burst; consequently, sucking bursts are between 2 and 5 sucks.
- Intermittent: An infant takes breaths intermittently during the sucking bursts. The breaths happen irregularly. Because the infant is taking some small breaths within the sucking burst, the sucking burst may be longer than 5 sucks.
- Coordinated: The infant coordinates breathing fully within the sucking burst. SSB ratio may be 2:1:1 or 1:1:1. With regular small breaths within the sucking burst, the burst can lengthen to as much as 10–30 SSBs per burst, followed by a breathing break. SSB pattern is consistent.
- Integrated: An infant uses a coordinated breathing pattern and can begin socially interacting with the feeder while maintaining their coordination and stamina.

GROWTH MONITORING

Appropriate nutrition can be estimated by anthropometry measurements. Growth is not linear and is characterised by growth spurts and stagnation, making interpretation of measurements difficult. Growth assessments should include serial measurements for weight, length and head circumference. These need to be assessed with realistic goals along with consideration of the neonate's genetic potential, prenatal influences, nutritional adequacy and systemic illnesses (Fenton et al., 2022; see Figure 19.2). Evidence indicates that higher-quality nutritional intake in preterm infants promotes greater lean mass accretion, which in turn is positively associated with improved head growth and enhanced neurodevelopmental outcomes (Fenton et al., 2024).

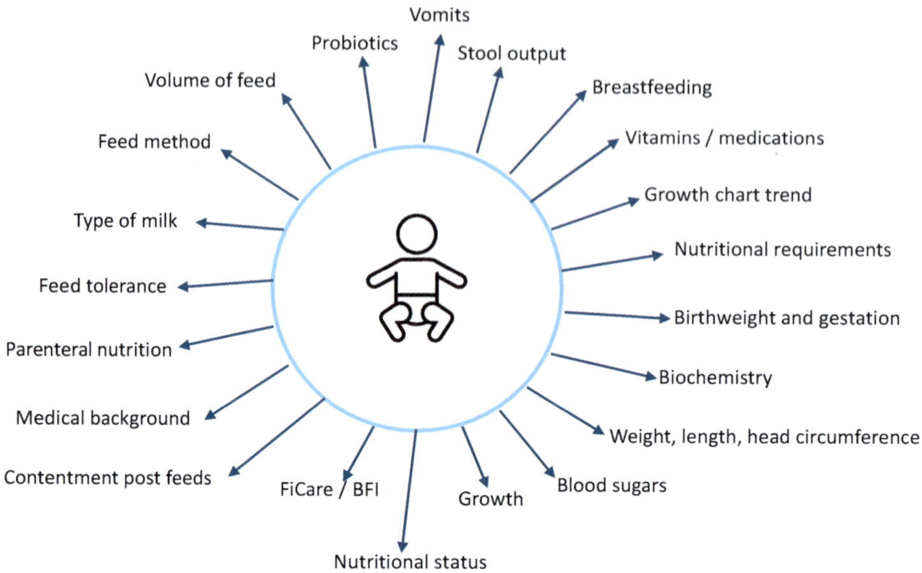

Figure 19.2 Multifactorial nutritional assessment

Intrauterine growth rate (15–20g/kg/day) is the most used and accepted standard for preterm growth, but is difficult to achieve in practice. Preterm infants should grow, after early postnatal weight loss, similar to the fetus and then term-born infants. Approximately 30g/day weight gain is expected in term infants. High-risk neonates need individualised nutrition and growth assessments and avoidance of the term 'growth failure' (Fenton et al., 2024).

Recommendations suggest to aim for weight, length and head circumference growth patterns to be maintained approximately parallel to growth chart curves. Accelerated growth in preterm infants should be avoided. There are various charts currently used in practice to help determine an infant's growth; these should be chosen for the appropriate clinical, demographic, ethnic and socioeconomic similarities of the population. The use of Z-scores (standard deviations) has been recommended and is becoming more widely used clinically to assess growth patterns.

Weight fluctuations can be seen if the weight is checked before or after urination and defecation, changes in fluid and nutrition intakes and diuretic or other medication use. It is therefore important to assess growth over several days. Length is now recognised as a required assessment for nutritional status as it reflects lean tissue mass and is unaffected by hydration status. Length is more challenging to measure accurately and consistently, especially in periods of medical instability. It is helpful to have serial measurements over a period of time. The most accurate measurement is a two-person technique (one of whom should be a parent) using a length board to ensure that the top of the head and the feet (with straight legs) are the measurement points. Head circumference measurements are essential for monitoring neurological health and potential neurodevelopmental concerns. Optimal head growth is seen with appropriate nutrition and absence of any neonatal morbidities. The practicalities of weighing and measuring a neonate can be a concern for nurses. A local unit guideline is required to achieve consistency, especially in intensive care, as the neonate may have splints, drains and multiple lines to consider.

Recommended frequency of anthropometry measurements – ideally carried out with parents

- Measure head circumference weekly
- Measure weight daily in intensive care where fluid balance management is critical, then less frequently, at least twice weekly when more stable
- Measure length weekly

CO-MORBIDITIES AND IMPACT ON FEEDING

An infant's ability to transition from tube to oral feeding may be influenced by anatomical, physiological, neurological, respiratory and developmental factors, either individually or in combination. Infants born at less than 28 weeks' gestation often experience significant delays in both the initiation and progression of enteral and suck feeds in the context of feeding readiness. This may lead to prolonged hospitalisation. Additionally, neonates with underlying morbidities (see Figure 19.3 and Table 19.2) are at increased risk for delayed achievement of full suck feeding due to compromised coordination, endurance and overall feeding efficiency (Kamity et al., 2021).

FEEDING DURING NON-INVASIVE RESPIRATORY SUPPORT

Infant's requiring non-invasive respiratory support have impaired respiration and increased work of breathing at baseline. This impacts their ability to co-ordinate airway closure during suck feeding placing them at increased risk of laryngeal penetration and/or aspiration (Lau, 2015). Beyond the risks associated with impaired breathing-swallowing coordination, is the impact of respiratory support on the swallow and airway protection. As the significance of this is unknown some clinicians choose to delay the introduction of oral feeding until the infant no longer requires this. However, delaying feeding has been associated with potential medical and neurodevelopmental consequences, such as prolonged hospital stay, persistent feeding disorders and impaired infant-parent attachment and bonding (Lau, 2016; Lainwala et al., 2020; Canning et al., 2021).

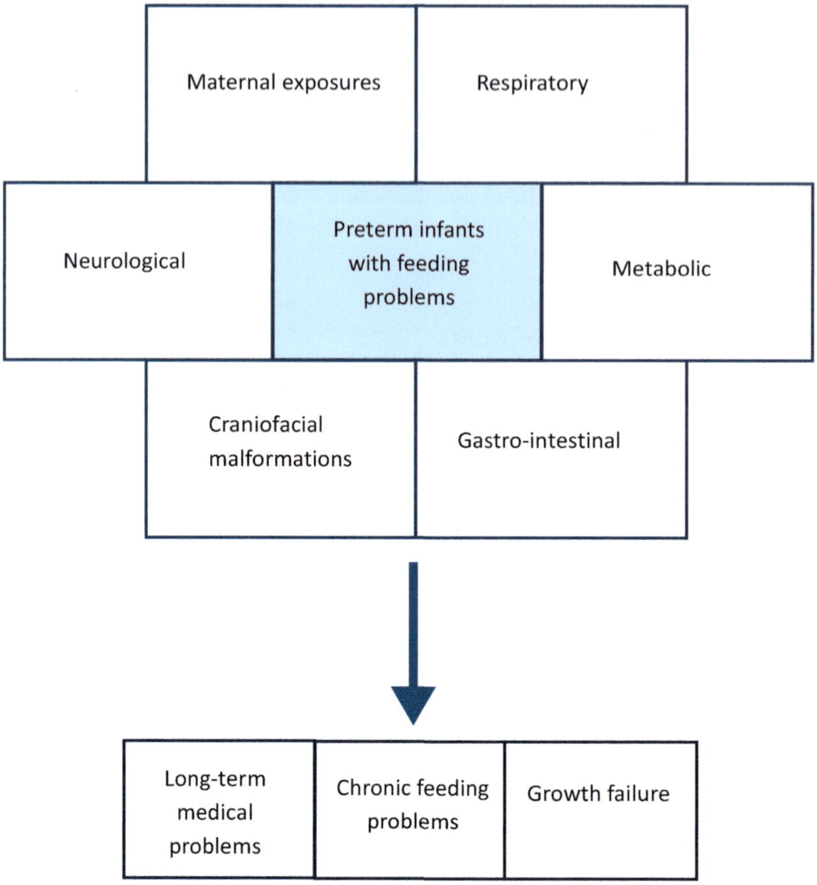

Figure 19.3 Underlying conditions leading to increased risk of feeding difficulties (adapted from Kamity et al., 2021)

GASTRO-OESOPHAGEAL REFLUX

Difficulties with digestion and gut motility are commonly seen in preterm infants due to gut immaturity but are often asymptomatic. Desaturations, bradycardias and irritability post feed may be due to immaturity and can be wrongly attributed to gastro-oesophageal reflux disease (GORD). Allied health professionals are integral to supporting both parents and neonatal team members to recognise what is normal baby behaviour versus what is pathological.

GORD, when identified can lead to oedema of the mucosal tissue, which can result in narrowing of the airway lumen and increase resistance within the respiratory tract (McDonnell et al., 2020). It can contribute to a range of clinical symptoms across multiple systems. Gastrointestinal symptoms may include spitting,

TABLE 19.2 RISK FACTORS FOR FEEDING DIFFICULTIES IN NEONATES

Risk factor	*Associated conditions*	*Potential impact*
Prematurity	Extreme prematurity, very LBW	Immature neurodevelopment, requirement for ventilation, immature gut.
Neurological	Hypoxic-ischaemic encephalopathy (stages II and III), intraventricular haemorrhage (grades III and IV), periventricular haemorrhage	Absent or weak suck, poor latch, hyper/hypotonia, impact on swallow/co-ordination.
Respiratory	Long periods of intubation, non-invasive respiratory support modalities or low flow nasal cannula oxygen, BPD	Endurance difficulties – fatigue, GORD, negative experiences around the face and mouth.
Cardiac	Congenital abnormalities	Endurance difficulties, increased incidence of aspiration post Patent Ductus Arteriosus ligation, Aortic Arch Reconstruction and Norwood Procedure if recurrent laryngeal nerve is damaged during surgery, increasing the incidence of vocal cord palsy.
Structural	Cleft lip and/or palate, laryngeal cleft, laryngomalacia, tracheo-oesophageal fistula, micrognathia	Poor latch, reduced intraoral pressure with cleft palate impacting milk transfer/efficiency. Potential respiratory compromise affecting suck, swallow, breath coordination. Risk of aspiration with laryngeal cleft and/or tracheo-oesphageal fistula.
Gastrointestinal	NEC, oesophageal atresia, GORD	Long periods of nil by mouth if surgery required, tolerance issues. GORD is associated with oral aversion.
Genetic	Trisomy 21, Pierre-Robin sequence, neuromuscular conditions, e.g. spinal muscular atrophy	Individual to each condition (e.g. difference in tone, impact on SSB coordination.

regurgitation and abdominal distention. Aerodigestive symptoms could present as swallowing or feeding difficulties, along with sneezing, coughing, wheezing and stridor. Cardiorespiratory involvement may lead to bradycardia, tachycardia, apnoea, tachypnoea, increased respiratory effort and oxygen desaturations. In addition, somatosensory symptoms such as irritability, back arching, straining, crying and grimacing are commonly observed in affected neonates.

Non-pharmacological strategies for managing GORD in the NNU reflect the principles of developmental care. Positioning and stress reduction using interventions such as skin-to-skin contact, gentle massage, supportive paced tube feeding, **non-nutritive sucking (NNS)**, protection of sleep and support for breastfeeding can alleviate GORD symptoms (NICE, 2019).

There is paucity of evidence regarding diagnosis and management of GORD in the NNU. When unrecognised or inadequately treated, it can contribute to the development of feeding difficulties, dysphagia and oral aversion (Grossbauer et al., 2023), potentially prolonging hospitalisation and negatively impacting the parent–infant feeding relationship.

THINK POINT

- What type of infant populations do you see on your neonatal unit?
- What are some of the feeding difficulties you have encountered?

SUPPORTING THE FEEDING JOURNEY

The final transition from tube to suck feeding represents a significant developmental period for preterm infants, many of whom will have completed a critical part of their feeding development in the NNU with extended periods of intravenous or tube feeding before they are medically and developmentally ready to begin suck feeding. During this time, the neonatal team play an integral role in facilitating the parent-infant feeding relationship.

Parents should be actively supported to participate in their baby's care, as this involvement strengthens parent–infant attachment and contributes positively to the infant's feeding development. Models of care commonly implemented within NNUs, such as the UNICEF Baby Friendly Initiative (BFI), developmental care approaches and FiCare, provide structured frameworks that promote and guide best practice in parental engagement. Figure 19.4 highlights examples of developmental care strategies to support the parent-infant relationship and feeding skill development. These include

- Skin-to-skin (kangaroo care) to support physiological stability, facilitate early feeding behaviours, improve infant weight-gain, enhance parent-baby bonding and improve infant sleep
- Positive smell opportunities to promote infants' sensory and emotional development by maintaining a fragrance-free unit, minimise exposure to

toxic odours and exposing babies to their parents' scent e.g. by using scent cloths

- Supportive early feeding strategies such as offering pacifiers, parents' clean finger or a gloved finger for non-nutritive sucking practice, providing mouth cares using MOM, positioning infants with hands-to-mouth and using cue-based feeding approaches
- Auditory protection to facilitate early feeding, language development and overall neurodevelopment by minimising sounds to support physiological stability and maintaining average sound levels of 45 dB. Comforting crying babies as quickly as possible and exposing babies to parental voice.

Multidisciplinary discussions with parents ensure that the infant's development, including feeding development, is considered throughout their neonatal journey and collaborative decision-making is established between parents and professionals. When the baby begins to demonstrate feeding readiness, collaborative decision-making helps to supports the transition from tube feeding to breast- or bottle feeding. Well timed, sensitive discussions regarding feeding intentions are essential to this.

Breastfeeding is widely recognised as one of the most effective public health interventions for reducing the risk of many common causes of infant morbidity and mortality. It supports optimal child development, health and wellbeing across the life course (World Health Organization, 2025). Consequently, breastmilk is considered the optimal method of feeding for all infants, including those born preterm or medically unwell. Within the United Kingdom (UK), NNUs work towards

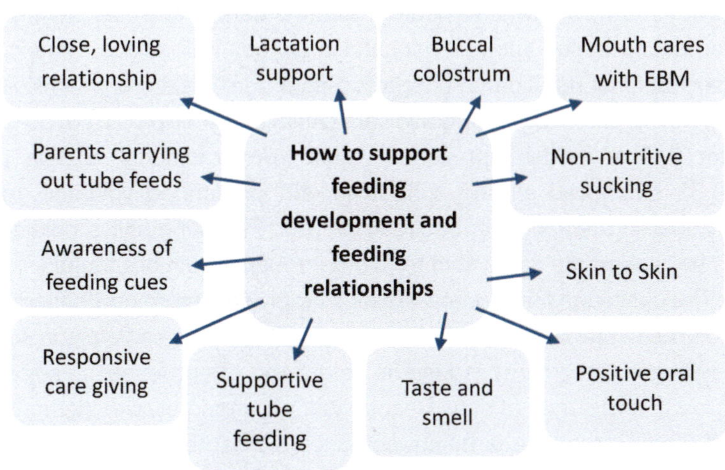

Figure 19.4 Caregiver activities that support the parent-infant relationship and feeding development (Imperial College NHS Trust, n.d.)

UNICEF BFI accreditation in recognition of the importance of protecting, promoting and supporting breastfeeding.

For parents or caregivers who choose to bottle-feed, or for those who are unable to breastfeed, the BFI provides clear guidance on how staff can support alternative feeding choices while still ensuring that breastfeeding and the use of breastmilk are protected and promoted for other families within the unit. Delivering this support sensitively, particularly during a period that may be emotionally and psychologically traumatic for parents, is a nuanced skill and one that services do not always achieve consistently (Palmér & Ericson, 2019). For this reason, it is recommended that neonatal units seek input from their psychology or perinatal mental health teams to ensure that communication and support are provided in ways that acknowledge and respond to parents' emotional needs.

CUE-BASED FEEDING

The terms *cue-based*, *infant-driven* and *attuned feeding* are used in the literature to describe an approach in which the infant's behavioural cues guide the initiation, pace and cessation of breast or bottle feeding (Tandberg et al., 2025). When adopting **cue-based feeding** practice, breast-, bottle- and tube feeding should be led by the infant, with caregivers observing and responding to signs of readiness and engagement. This supports physiological stability (McFadden et al., 2021; Samane et al., 2022) promotes positive early feeding experiences and strengthens the parent–infant relationship (Thomas et al., 2021).

Over the last twenty years, in line with increased awareness and a significant body of evidence in support of neuroprotective care, there has been a gradual shift towards cue-based care in neonatal practice. Within this context, feeding practice and optimal nutrition is recognised as a core measure in achieving family integrated, developmentally supportive care (Altimier & Phillips, 2016) as discussed in Chapter 7. This model represents a shift from traditional feeding practices (Table 19.3), structured around schedules and prescribed volumes, towards a more individualised relationship-based approach. Parenting styles outside of neonatal care have seen the same shift from strict routines to more flexible, responsive methods. The challenge for neonatal teams in applying a more cue-based approach to date, could be attributed to limited and low-quality evidence (Watson & McGuire, 2016) resulting in uncertainty around its safety and effectiveness in key measures such as growth and length of stay. Despite this, emerging studies demonstrate this method of feeding practice is being increasingly adopted worldwide (McFadden et al., 2021, Tandberg et al., 2025). Moving forward, neonatal teams must consider their approach in feeding their neonatal population aspiring towards care that is both cue-based and relationship based (Samane et al., 2022).

TABLE 19.3 COMPARISON OF THE TRADITIONAL METHOD OF FEEDING VERSUS CUE-BASED FEEDING PRACTICE

Traditional method	*Cue based method*
Scheduled (time-based, decided by caregiver)	Feeding is responsive to the infant's behavioural and physiological cues
Volume is predetermined by caregiver	Volume taken is guided by the infant's cues. Focus is on the quality of the feed rather than the volume
Fixed times for feeding	Infant's cues guide the readiness for feeding and progression of suck feeding
Routine/schedule-based care	Neurodevelopmental care that aligns with developmental care principles
Caregiver offers breast at scheduled feed times. Feed limited by specified length of time	Caregiver offers the breast when the infant shows hunger cues (rooting, sucking motions). The infant controls the pace and duration
Caregiver offers a prescribed volume by bottle at scheduled times	Caregiver offers the bottle/breast when the infant shows hunger cues. Caregiver uses infants' cues to determine when the pause or stop the feed

THINK POINTS

- Does the neonatal unit that you work on have a more traditional or cue-based approach to feeding?
- If more traditional, what steps could the neonatal unit that you work on take to becoming more cue-based?

It is acknowledged that a fully cue-based approach, requires a culture shift amongst the MDT. Neonatal teams may need to collaboratively review the evidence and develop a practical, individualised implementation plan for their unit. In the UK, Scotland were the first nation to introduce cue-based feeding as standard practice in their NNU (McFadden et al., 2021).

When neonatal teams support and empower parents to observe and respond to their baby's cues from admission, the transition to cue-based feeding may be more intuitive and less overwhelming. Parents will have time to learn about their baby and build their confidence (Tandberg et al., 2025). Anecdotally, parents, particularly those of extremely preterm infants, or term babies who have been critically unwell, often spend prolonged periods in intensive care, where the focus is understandably on medical stability and growth. In these highly medicalised settings, conversations frequently focus on volumes, schedules and treatment. Introducing cue-based language once suck feeding begins may be too late in the parents' journey and the transition from a number-based to a behaviour-based approach may be hard to rapidly adjust to. Early use of this concept from admission, can help build parental confidence and enable them to develop their connection with their baby. Preterm infants are at risk of accelerated weight gain and higher rates of childhood obesity if infant feeding cues are overridden. Interventions that support responsive feeding practice are required to establish healthy growth trajectories (Ou-Yang et al., 2020).

When bottle feeding, parents and caregivers should be actively encouraged to carry out most feeds whenever possible (UNICEF UK, 2016) It is not uncommon for parents to feel that neonatal professionals are the experts or to be uncertain about their role in bottle- and/or tube feeding, particularly as it can be delegated in their absence. However, time spent learning how their baby feeds, what cues to look for and which strategies best support their baby's feeding is just as important for bottle- and tube feeding as it is for breastfeeding. This parental role in bottle feeding may need to be clearly explained and reinforced, even to experienced parents, especially in the unfamiliar context of neonatal care. In cases where parents are caring for multiple children or live at a distance from the unit, it may be necessary for nurses to support bottle- and/or tube feeds. Nonetheless, every opportunity should be taken to empower and involve parents in this aspect of care to promote confidence, consistency and connection.

INITIATING SUCK FEEDING

Decision-making regarding when to start suck feeding is multi-factorial and should take place in the context of multidisciplinary discussion with parents at the heart. Levels of provision can make this challenging if MDT members, such as the speech and language therapist, are not available when needed; this should be the aim of all neonatal teams. Factors that influence decisions will include medical history, enteral feeding progression, the infant's neurobehaviour, respiratory status and the parents' feeding intention (Bedroni, 2023). Parents who breastfeed may have earlier opportunities to begin this journey than parents who choose to bottle feed, based on the infant-led, physiologically and developmentally supportive nature of breastfeeding (Harting et al., 2025).

FEEDING READINESS

Feeding readiness refers to the observable signs an infant displays, such as physiological stability and behavioural engagement, that indicate neurodevelopmental readiness to feed. Assessment of feeding readiness should occur before each feed, recognising that an infant's ability to feed can vary from one feed to the next and within a single feeding session. It is the responsibility of the caregiver to observe these cues and determine whether to proceed with feeding. Nurses play a pivotal role in supporting parents to recognise and interpret signs of feeding readiness. This skill is often developed through hands-on experience which develops over time.

Using feeding readiness tools or algorithms to support team decision-making can be helpful. Using a structured tool may guide identification cues in a more consistent way (Pados et al., 2021). There is limited validation, inconsistent inter-rater reliability and a lack of consensus with current tools used. Any tool used must be agreed by the MDT, ensuring it fits well within the processes of the unit, taking into account multiple factors.

Feeding readiness observations:

- Stable respiratory rate
- Maintains oxygen saturations during gentle handling
- Maintains stable heart rate
- Transitions readily to a quiet alert state
- Showing feeding readiness signs (e.g. rooting in response to touch around the mouth)
- Maintains a quiet alert state whilst licking, nuzzling or sucking non-nutritively on the breast or on a pacifier

Disengagement cues

The terms *disengagement*, *stress*, *avoidance* and *stop cues* (see Table 19.4) are often used interchangeably in the literature to describe signals that indicate an infant is becoming overwhelmed, disorganised or needs to pause (Als et al., 1986). These cues may be observed during handling, interaction or feeding and are an important part of understanding an infant's communication and capacity for engagement.

For parents, recognising disengagement can be particularly valuable during the transition to suck feeding, as they help guide responsive, infant-led care. Parents who have received cot-side coaching from the neonatal team, particularly in the context of cue-based care, are more likely to be familiar with these terms and confident in identifying them in their own baby. Supporting parents to observe and respond to disengagement cues not only protects the infant's neurodevelopmental wellbeing but also strengthens the parent–infant relationship through attuned, sensitive caregiving.

It is important to support parents in understanding that sucking is a reflex, triggered involuntarily when the infant's palate is stimulated. As such, the presence

TABLE 19.4 SIGNS OF DISENGAGEMENT DURING INFANT FEEDING

Autonomic	*Motor*	*State*
Respiratory rate	Limbs tensed or extended	Sudden loss of alertness
Heart rate	Jerky movements	Sudden fuss or cry
SpO_2 levels (desaturations)	Flaccidity of trunk, neck, face, extremities	Sudden onset of sleepiness
Colour change	Arching	Frowns, grimaces
Hiccoughs	Variable tone	Sudden fatigue or weak state
Vomiting	Tongue extensions	Irritability
		Shift to hyperalert, panicked or worried face

of sucking alone is not a reliable indicator of feeding readiness or interest. True feeding readiness involves a broader range of behavioural and physiological signs, both before and during the feed. These cues reflect the infant's active participation, engagement and underlying neurodevelopmental maturity.

SUPPORTIVE STRATEGIES FOR SUCK FEEDING

In addition to reading and responding to the infant's cues, caregivers should approach each feed using developmentally supportive strategies, including awareness of optimal positioning, flow rate and both external and co-regulated pacing techniques. These approaches are essential for supporting the infant's physiological stability and feeding success, particularly during the early stages of suck feeding (see Box 19.1). As the infant shows increasing neurodevelopmental maturity and feeding competence, support can be gradually reduced, allowing the baby to assume greater control and self-regulation during feeds.

BOX 19.1 CAREGIVER INTERVENTIONS FOR SUPPORTIVE BOTTLE-FEEDING

- Developmental care and supportive feeding environment
- Modifying flow rate using slow flow teats
- Providing elevated side-lying position
- Co-regulated pacing

- Behavioural state support
- Supportive swaddling

Caregiver interventions for supportive breastfeeding

- Skin to skin to support wakefulness, feeding cues and lactation
- Developmental care and supportive feeding environment
- Supportive swaddling
- Expressing to reduce flow
- Positioning using gravity to reduce the flow (e.g. laid-back nursing)

PREPARING FOR HOME

When care has been holistic, multidisciplinary (Figure 19.5) and collaborative within a FiCare framework, the journey towards home is already well supported and planned for. Parents will have been gradually developing confidence and skills to care for their baby once home. As infants develop feeding competence,

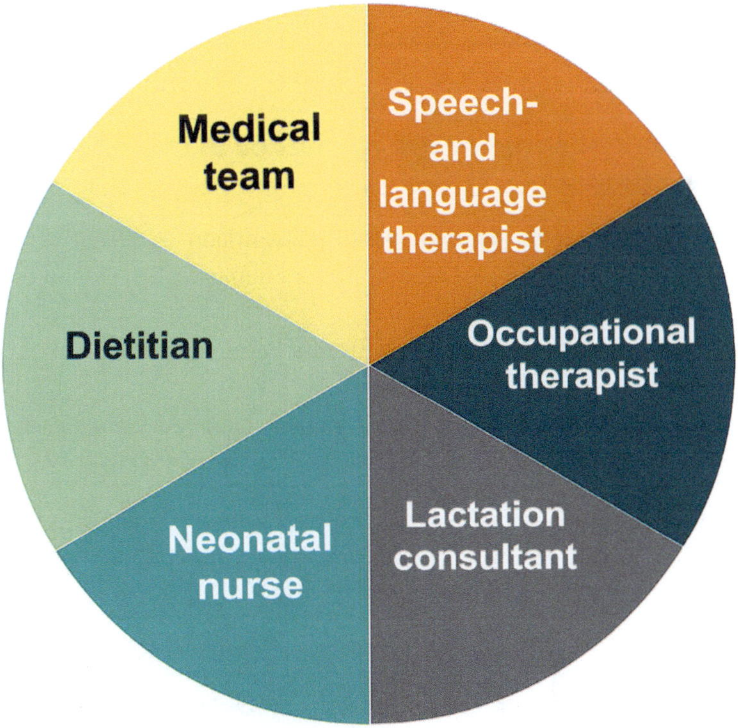

Figure 19.5 The multidisciplinary feeding team

supporting families to understand responsive feeding is essential. BFI describe responsive feeding as feeding that goes beyond hunger cues and focuses on love, comfort and connection. Mothers are encouraged to offer the breast in response to their baby's cues or their own comfort.

In this respect, cue-based feeding lays the foundations for this, attuning to their baby's signs and responding sensitively, rather than feeding to a schedule with target volumes. BFI note that bottle feeding although cue-based and responsive when carried out by a parent sensitive to the infant's needs, may not be able to be truly responsive due to the risk of overfeeding.

Rooming in facilities are integral to supporting the transition to home and providing experience of caring for their baby out of the view of the neonatal team. When the infant can sustain their body temperature, feed independently without the NGT and gain weight, they will be ready to go home. On some NNU, discharge home with a NGT in situ can facilitate this to take place earlier. The outreach team or discharge planning nurse are key in supporting a smooth transition (BAPM, 2025). In some services around the country, allied health professionals are also part of the outreach service. Models of provision are being redesigned to demonstrate the value added to families with the added support of these services, ensuring a safe and seamless discharge home (see Chapter 3 for more details).

ACTIVITIES

Take a look at some of the resources in the reference list for this chapter

- NICE guidance on Neonatal parenteral nutrition (2020)
- BAPM framework – The Use of Donor Human Milk in Neonates (2023)
- ESPGHAN Enteral Nutrition in Preterm Infants (Embleton et al., 2023)
- RCSLT Speech and Language Therapy in Neonatal Care: Feeding and Non-Invasive Respiratory Support Position Paper (2023)

Observe an infant on your neonatal unit shortly before their feed, are they showing any of the following feeding cues (see *https://metronorth.health.qld.gov.au/rbwh/wp-content/uploads/sites/2/2017/07/10239.pdf*; Queens land Health, 2024)?

Watch the following webinar on how to support infant communication: Exploring the importance of infant communication: Building stronger foundations for language development (https://player.vimeo.com/video/986478255)

Think points

When families ask for guidance while their preterm infant is on parenteral nutrition, what advice do you offer to help them support the transition to milk feeds?

Chapter takeaways

- Early nutrition is fundamental for preterm and unwell infants, supporting survival, growth and long-term neurodevelopment. A standardised MDT-led approach helps reduce variation in care and improves outcomes. Optimal nutrition, feeding and growth have a positive impact on parent-infant bonding, neurodevelopment, length of stay and long-term outcomes.
- Parenteral and enteral nutrition work together to meet the high metabolic needs of preterm infants, especially while gut maturity develops. Early initiation of enteral feeds, preferably with mother's own milk, supports gut function and reduces complications.
- Human milk is the optimal first feed, providing immunological, developmental and protective benefits, including reduced NEC and sepsis. For very preterm infants, fortification is essential to meet increased nutritional requirements.
- Cue-based feeding is now recognised as best practice, shifting away from volume-driven or time-scheduled approaches. This method focuses on the infant's behavioural cues to guide readiness, pacing and stopping, supporting neuroprotection and positive feeding experiences.
- Feeding development and suck–swallow–breathe coordination mature over time, often emerging around 34 weeks but influenced by co-morbidities. Supportive strategies, such as paced feeding, optimal positioning and non-nutritive sucking, promote safety and efficiency.
- Growth monitoring must include weight, length and head circumference, using serial measurements and Z-scores to assess trends rather than single values. Appropriate nutrition improves lean mass accretion, head growth and later neurodevelopment.
- Co-morbidities such as prematurity, respiratory disease, neurological conditions or structural anomalies significantly affect feeding skills and readiness. Individualised assessment, multidisciplinary planning and parental involvement are essential to manage these complexities.
- FiCare is central to successful feeding outcomes. Supporting parental involvement from birth, through skin-to-skin, participation in tube feeds and early cue-based interactions, strengthens bonding and prepares families for discharge.

CASE STUDY

CASE STUDIES

Case study 1: Supporting the establishment of breastfeeding in the neonatal unit

Carter was born at 23 weeks' gestation. His birthweight was 550g, which was on the 25th centile. Carter commenced parenteral nutrition at birth. Enteral feeds commenced with Mum's own breastmilk. Feeds stopped and restarted a few times due to tolerance concerns in the early days. PN was discontinued at 27 weeks gestation and Carter was on full feeds of MOM. Carter required oxygen support for all his neonatal admission. He was weaned onto low flow oxygen requiring this for discharge. Carter's mother had a good supply of expressed breastmilk and her preference was to breastfeed. Carter was struggling to gain weight appropriately and his weight was now below the 2nd centile.

Q.1. Why is it important to start early enteral feeding with mother's own milk?

Q.2. What are the risk factors that will have impacted Carter establishing enteral feeds?

Q.3. What considerations can you think of in Carter's transition onto enteral feeds from parenteral nutrition?

Q.4. How could you have improved nutritional intake earlier to avoid poor weight gain?

Q.5. How would you support transitioning to breastfeeding while achieving appropriate growth?

Case study 2: Transition to oral feeding in a preterm infant

Priya is the mother of Aarya, who was born prematurely at 28 weeks' gestation and is now 38 weeks corrected age. Aarya is Priya's third child. Having successfully breastfed her two older children, Priya has established a good milk supply and expresses a strong desire to exclusively breastfeed Aarya. Currently, breastfeeding is progressing well, supported by nasogastric top-ups of fortified mother's own milk. During the ward round, the clinical team raises the possibility of introducing bottle feeds to support more efficient oral intake and potentially facilitate an earlier discharge from the NNU.

Q.1. What are the key benefits of breastmilk and breastfeeding for preterm infants?

Q.2. How can the MDT best support this mother in achieving her feeding goals?

Q.3. Which evidence-based tools and resources can guide the team?

Q.4. What are the potential barriers to establishing exclusive breastfeeding in the neonatal unit?

Case study 3: Assessment of feeding readiness

Femi is a surviving twin, son of Olu. He was born at 23 weeks' gestation and is now 38 weeks old. Femi's respiratory support has been weaned, and the MDT feel he is stable from a medical perspective. Olu has been receiving support to provide cue-based care from the very beginning of his journey. She is confident in recognising his signs of contentment (approach cues) and signs of stress (disengagement cues). This has been reinforced by the neonatal team including the cotside nurses and therapy teams. She expressed her milk when Femi was born but has struggled with her supply. It is likely that he will be fed by a combination of breast and bottle.

Q.1. Other than physiological/respiratory stability, what other signs of feeding readiness and development should the team be supporting Olu to look out for?

Q.2. What kind of caregiving activities can support Olu to identify signs of feeding readiness?

Q.3. Which supportive strategies (breast and bottle) will support Olu and Femi to get off to the best start when he starts to suck feed?

For suggested answer guides to the questions posed in these case studies, please refer to the web-based companion site specific to this chapter. See www.routledge.com/cw/petty

References

Als, H., Lester, B. M., Brazelton, T. B., & Click, S. B. (1986). Toward a research instrument for the assessment of preterm infants' behaviour (APIB). In H. E. Fitzgerald, B. M. Lester, & M. W. Yogman (Eds.), *Theory and research in behavioral pediatrics* (pp. 35–63). Plenum Press.

Altimier, L., & Phillips, R. (2016). The Neonatal Integrative Developmental Care Model: Advanced clinical applications of the seven core measures for neuroprotective family-centered developmental care. *Newborn and Infant Nursing Reviews*, *16*(4), 230–244. https://doi.org/10.1053/j.nainr.2016.09.030.

Bala, F. E., McGrattan, K. E., Valentine, C. J., & Jadcherla, S. R. (2024). A narrative review of strategies to optimize nutrition, feeding, and growth among preterm-born infants: Implications for practice. *Advances in Nutrition*, *15*(11), 100305.

Bedroni, M. (2023). Breastfeeding preterm infants as the initial oral feeding: An integrative review. *Journal of Neonatal Nursing*, *29*(2), 267–272.

Boesveldt, S., & Parma, V. (2021). The importance of the olfactory system in human well-being, through nutrition and social behavior. *Cell and Tissue Research*, *383*(1), 559–567.

British Association of Perinatal Medicine. (2020). *Optimising early maternal breast milk for preterm infants: A BAPM quality improvement toolkit*. Retrieved June 2, 2025, from https://www.bapm.org/pages/196-maternal-breast-milk-toolkit

British Association of Perinatal Medicine. (2023). *The use of donor human milk in neonates: A BAPM framework for practice*. Retrieved June 2, 2025, from https://www.bapm.org/resources/the-use-of-donor-human-milk-in-neonates

British Association of Perinatal Medicine (BAPM). (2025). Neonatal outreach service: A BAPM framework for practice. *Resources*. Retrieved June 2, 2025, from https://www.bapm.org/resources/neonatal-outreach-service

Canning, A., Clarke, S., Thorning, S., Chauhan, M., & Weir, K. A. (2021). Oral feeding for infants and children receiving nasal continuous positive airway pressure and high flow nasal cannula: A systematic review. *BMC Pediatrics*, *21*, 125.

Embleton, N. D., Jennifer Moltu, S., Lapillonne, A., Van Den Akker, C. H. P., Carnielli, V., Fusch, C., Gerasimidis, K., Van Goudoever, J. B., Haiden, N., Iacobelli, S., Johnson, M. J., Meyer, S., Mihatsch, W., De Pipaon, M. S., Rigo, J., Zachariassen, G., Bronsky, J., Indrio, F., Köglmeier, J., . . . Domellöf, M. (2023). Enteral nutrition in preterm infants: A position paper from the ESPGHAN Committee on Nutrition and invited experts. *Journal of Pediatric Gastroenterology and Nutrition*, *176*(2), 248–268.

Fenton, T. R., Dai, S., Lalari, V., & Alshaikh, B. (2022). Neonatal and preterm infant growth assessment. *Clinics in Perinatology*, *49*(2), 295–311.

Fenton, T. R., Merlino Barr, S., Elmrayed, S., & Alshaikh, B. (2024). Expected and desirable preterm and small infant growth patterns. *Advances in Nutrition*, *15*(6), 100220.

Geddes, D. T., & Sakalidis, V. S. (2015). Breastfeeding: How do they do it? Infant sucking, swallowing and breathing. *Infant*, *11*(5), 146–150.

Grossbauer, A., Mnatsakanian, A., Costeloe, A., & Thottam, P. J. (2023). The effects of untreated reflux on the incidence of dysphagia, oral aversion, and feeding difficulty in the NICU population. *International Journal of Pediatric Otorhinolaryngology*, *174*(111734).

Harding, C., Cockerill, H., Cane, C., & Law, J. (2018). Using non-nutritive sucking to support feeding development for premature infants: A commentary on approaches and current practice. *Journal of Pediatric Rehabilitation Medicine*, *11*(3), 147–152. https://doi.org/10.3233/PRM-170442

Harting, K. M., Singer, D., & Heiter, J. (2025). Optimizing breastfeeding for hospitalized newborns: A narrative review of midwifery-led interventions. *European Journal of Midwifery*, *9*. https://doi.org/10.18332/ejm/200341

Indrio, F., Neu, J., Pettoello-Mantovani, M., Marchese, F., Martini, S., Salatto, A., & Aceti, A. (2022). Development of the gastrointestinal tract in newborns as a challenge for an appropriate nutrition: A narrative review. *Nutrients*, *14*(7), 1405.

Imperial College NHS Tryust. (n.d.). *Supporting feeding development and feeding relationships [figure]*. Unpublished educational material.

Kamity, R., Kapavarapu, P. K., & Chandel, A. (2021). Feeding problems and long-term outcomes in preterm infants – a systematic approach to evaluation and management. *Children*, *8*(12), 1158.

Lainwala, S., Kosyakova, N., Power, K., Hussain, N., Moore, J. E., Hagadorn, J. I., & Brownell, E. A. (2020). Delayed achievement of oral feedings is associated with adverse neurodevelopmental outcomes at 18 to 26 months follow-up in preterm infants. *American Journal of Perinatology*, 37(5), 483–490.

Lau, C. (2015). Development of suck and swallow mechanisms in infants. *Annals of Nutrition and Metabolism*, *66*(Suppl. 5), 7–14.

Lau, C. (2016). Development of infant oral feeding skills: What do we know? *American Journal of Clinical Nutrition*, *103*(2), 616S–621S. https://doi.org/10.3945/ajcn.115.109603

McDonnell, M. J., Hunt, E. B., Ward, C., Pearson, J. P., O'Toole, D., Laffey, J. G., Murphy, D. M., & Rutherford, R. M. (2020). Current therapies for gastro-oesophageal reflux in the setting of chronic lung disease: State of the art review. *ERJ Open Research*, *6*(4), 00190–2019.

McFadden, A., Fitzpatrick, B., Shinwell, S., Tosh, K., Donnan, P, Wallace, L. M., Wallace, L., Johnson, E., Macgillivray, S., & Gavine, A. (2021). Cue-based versus scheduled feeding for preterm infants transitioning from tube to oral feeding: The Cubs mixed-methods feasibility study. *Health Technology Assessment*, *25*(74), 1–146.

Mihatsch, W. A., Braegger, C., Bronsky, J., Cai, W., Campoy, C., Carnielli, V., Darmaun, D., Desci, T., Domellöf, M., Embleton, N., Fewtrell, M., Mis, N. F., Franz, A., Goulet, O., Hartman, C., Susan, H., Hojsak, I., Iacobelli, S., Jochum, F., . . . Yan, W. (2018). Espghan/Espen/ESPR/CSPEN guidelines on pediatric parenteral nutrition. *Clinical Nutrition*, *37*(6), 2303–2305.

Murphy, R., Harding, C., Aloysius, A., Sweeting, M., & Crossley, S. (2021). Developments in allied health professionals' role in UK neonatal units: A speech and language therapy perspective. *Infant*, *17*(4), 157–161.

Mustapha, M., Blair, H., Leake, N., Johnson, V., van den Akker, C. H. P., & Embleton, N. D. (2024). The evolution of nutritional care in preterm infants with a focus on the extreme preterm infant. *Journal of Human Nutrition and Dietetics*, *38*(1).

National Institute for Health and Care Excellence. (2019). *Gastro-oesophageal reflux disease in children and young people: Diagnosis and management*. Retrieved September 16, 2025, from https://www.nice.org.uk/guidance/ng1

National Institute for Health and Care Excellence. (2020). *Neonatal parenteral nutrition guideline*. Retrieved September 16, 2025, from www.nice.org.uk/guidance/ng154

National Institute for Health Research (NIHR). (2022). *The neoGASTRIC trial: Avoiding routine gastric residual volume measurement in neonatal critical care: A multicentre randomised controlled trial*. Retrieved September 16, 2025, from https://www.npeu.ox.ac.uk/neogastric

Oddie, S. J., Young, L., & McGuire, W. (2021). Slow advancement of enteral feed volumes to prevent necrotising enterocolitis in very low birth weight infants. *Cochrane Database of Systematic Reviews*, *8*(8).

Ou-Yang, M., Sun, Y., Liebowitz, M., Chen, C., Fang, M., Dai, W., Chuang, T., & Chen, J. (2020). Accelerated weight gain, prematurity, and the risk of childhood obesity: A meta-analysis and systematic review. *PLoS ONE*, *15*(5), e0232238.

Pados, B. F., Hill, R. R., Yamasaki, J. T., Litt, J. S., & Lee, C. S. (2021). Prevalence of problematic feeding in young children born prematurely: A meta-analysis. *BMC Pediatrics*, *21*, 1–15.

Palmér, L., & Ericson, J. (2019). A qualitative study on the breastfeeding experience of mothers of preterm infants in the first 12 months after birth. *International Breastfeeding Journal*, *14*, 1–8.

Phillips, R. (2024). Bonding and attachment with baby in the womb or in the neonatal intensive care unit: The critical role of early emotional connections. *Critical Care Nursing Clinics of North America*, *36*(2), 157–165.

Provenzi, L., Broso, S., & Montirosso, R. (2018). Do mothers sound good? A systematic review of the effects of maternal voice exposure on preterm infants' development. *Neuroscience & Biobehavioral Reviews*, *88*, 42–50.

Quigley, M., Embleton, N. D., & McGuire, W. (2019). Formula versus donor breast milk for feeding preterm or low birth weight infants. *Cochrane Database of Systematic Reviews*, 7, CD002971.

Ross, E. (2021). BROSS: Nutritive sucking patterns. *Member Resources*. Retrieved June 2, 2025, from https://www.feedingfundamentals.com/

Royal College of Speech and Language Therapists. (2023). *Speech and language therapy in neonatal care: Feeding and non-invasive respiratory support*. Retrieved June 2, 2025, from https://www.rcslt.org/wp-content/uploads/2023/03/Neonatal-care-position-paper-2023.pdf

Samane, S., Yadollah, Z. P., Marzieh, H., Karimollah, H., Reza, Z. M., Afsaneh, A., & Als, H. (2022). Cue-based feeding and short-term health outcomes of premature infants in newborn intensive care units: A non-randomized trial. *BMC Pediatrics*, *22*(1), 23.

Sarnat, H. B., Flores-Sarnat, L., & Wei, X. (2017). Olfactory development, part 1: Function, from fetal perception to adult wine-tasting. *Journal of Child Neurology*, *32*(6), 566–578.

Sharif, S., Meader, N., Oddie, S. J., Rojas-Reyes, M. X., & McGuire, W. (2020). Probiotics to prevent necrotising enterocolitis in very preterm or very low birth weight infants. *Cochrane Database of Systematic Reviews*, *10*.

State of Queensland (Queensland Health). (2024, February). *Baby feeding cues (signs) term* (Version 6.1, CPN/840). Metro North Health, Women's & Newborn Services, Royal Brisbane & Women's Hospital. Retrieved September 17, 2025, from https://metronorth.health.qld.gov.au/rbwh/wp-content/uploads/sites/2/2017/07/10239.pdf

Sullivan, R., Perry, R., Sloan, A., Kleinhaus, K., & Burtchen, N. (2011). Infant bonding and attachment to the caregiver: Insights from basic and clinical science. *Clinics in Perinatology*, *38*(4), 643.

Tandberg, B. S., Grundt, H., Maastrup, R., Aloysius, A., Nagy, L., & Flacking, R. (2025). Practices supporting cue-based breastfeeding of preterm infants in neonatal intensive care units across Europe. *International Breastfeeding Journal*, *20*(1), 2.

Taylor, S. N., Fenton, T. R., Groh-Wargo, S., Gura, K., Martin, C. R., Griffin, I. J., Rozga, M., & Moloney, L. (2022). Exclusive maternal milk compared with exclusive formula on growth and health outcomes in very-low-birthweight preterm infants: Phase II of the Pre-B Project and an Evidence Analysis Center systematic review. *Frontiers in Pediatrics*, *9*, 793311.

Tesser, F., Meneghelli, M., Martino, D., Pegoraro, L., Pelosi, M. S., Sebellin, S., & Verlato, G. (2025). Early optimal parenteral nutrition during NICU stay and neurodevelopmental outcomes in very preterm infants: State of the art. *Nutrients*, *17*(2), 232.

Thomas, T., Goodman, R., Jacob, A., & Grabher, D. (2021). Implementation of cue-based feeding to improve preterm infant feeding outcomes and promote parents' involvement. *Journal of Obstetric, Gynecologic & Neonatal Nursing*, *50*(3), 328–339.

Unicef UK Baby Friendly Initiative. (2016). *Guide to bottle feeding: Responding to your baby's cues and fostering relationship building*. UNICEF UK Baby Friendly Initiative. Retrieved September 16, 2025, from https://www.unicef.org.uk/babyfriendly/baby-friendly-resources/bottle-feeding-resources/guide-to-bottle-feeding/

Ustun, B., Covey, J., & Reissland, N. (2023). Chemosensory continuity from prenatal to postnatal life in humans: a systematic review and meta-analysis. *PLOS ONE*, *18*(3), e0283314.

Wang, L., Ma, J., Meng, H., & Zhou, J. (2021). Mothers' experiences of neonatal intensive care: A systematic review and implications for clinical practice. *World Journal of Clinical Cases*, *9*(24), 7062.

Watson, J., & McGuire, W. (2016). Responsive versus scheduled feeding for preterm infants. *Cochrane Database of Systematic Reviews*, *8*.

World Health Organization. (2025). *Optimal duration of breastfeeding*. Retrieved September 16, 2025 from https://www.who.int/tools/elena/review-summaries/exclusive-breastfeeding-optimal-duration-of-exclusive-breastfeeding

20 NEONATAL INFECTION

Lisa Kaiser

CONTENTS

DOI: 10.4324/9781003591405-24

GUIDANCE ON HOW TO ENHANCE PERSONAL LEARNING FROM THIS CHAPTER

Key points covered in this chapter

- The nature of immunity and how this predisposes the high-risk neonate to infection.
- The types and presentations of infection in the neonatal period.
- The signs of infection and the nurse's role in recognising and managing it in the neonatal unit.

Reflection

Reading through the chapter, you are encouraged to engage with the key points and related literature in an enquiring way. Ask these questions:

- Have you seen infection presenting in the neonates in your care, and what challenges does this pose for the infant and family?
- What are the current evidence base and guidelines relating to neonatal infection?
- What are the key nursing care responsibilities in relation to infection control in the neonatal unit?

Implications for nursing care

- Finally: how will this chapter enable you to consider the implications of what you learn for your nursing care relating to neonatal infection, assessment and nursing care?

INTRODUCTION AND BACKGROUND

Infection in the newborn period continues to drive mortality and serious morbidity worldwide. While **early onset infection** (EOI) has fallen in many high-income settings following intrapartum antibiotic prophylaxis and improved management of membrane rupture, **late onset infection** (LOI) has risen proportionally as survival of extremely preterm and extremely low birthweight (LBW) infants has improved. These infants are especially vulnerable because of immunological immaturity, prolonged hospitalisation, exposure to invasive devices, parenteral nutrition, and repeated antibiotic courses (Dong & Speer, 2015; Johnson et al., 2021). **Sepsis**, life-threatening organ dysfunction caused by a dysregulated host response to infection (National Institute for Health and Care Excellence (NICE), 2016), remains a rare but devastating complication. Without prompt recognition and treatment, infection can progress rapidly to septic shock, meningitis, multi-organ failure, and death.

This chapter will review the current evidence regarding neonatal susceptibility to, and acquisition of infection, the organisms commonly implicated and investigation and treatment modalities. It aims to support the neonatal nurse's ability to identify and manage infection in neonates.

NEONATAL IMMUNITY

The neonatal immune system is complete but functionally immature. Two complementary arms, **innate and acquired immunity** (see Table 20.1), work together to identify, contain, and eliminate pathogens. Innate defences (skin and mucosal barriers; **phagocytes** (Figure 20.1) such as **macrophages**, neutrophils, and monocytes; complement; acute-phase proteins; cytokines) provide rapid, non-specific protection. However, neonatal phagocytes migrate less effectively to infection sites, have reduced **opsonisation** and killing, and **inflammatory signalling** is blunted in very preterm infants.

Acquired (adaptive) immunity, humoral and cell-mediated, relies on antigen-specific responses. Placental **immunoglobulin** (IgG) transfer peaks in the third trimester; consequently, extremely preterm infants have very low IgG at birth and limited immunological memory. B-cells produce immunoglobulins (IgM as early responders; IgG crosses the placenta), while T-cells coordinate and execute cellular responses against intracellular pathogens. In both preterm and term infants, mucosal immunity is underdeveloped: epithelial barriers are more permeable, secretory IgA is low, and the gut **microbiome** is immature or perturbed by

TABLE 20.1 TYPES OF IMMUNITY

Innate immunity	*Acquired immunity*
■ Present from birth	■ Antigen-specific
■ Not antigen-specific	■ Enhanced response to subsequent exposure
■ Same response to repeated exposure	■ Has memory
■ Has no memory	■ Uses cellular and humoral components
■ Uses cellular and molecular components	■ Works in conjunction with innate immunity
■ Works in conjunction with acquired immunity	

(adapted from Delves & Roitt, 2000)

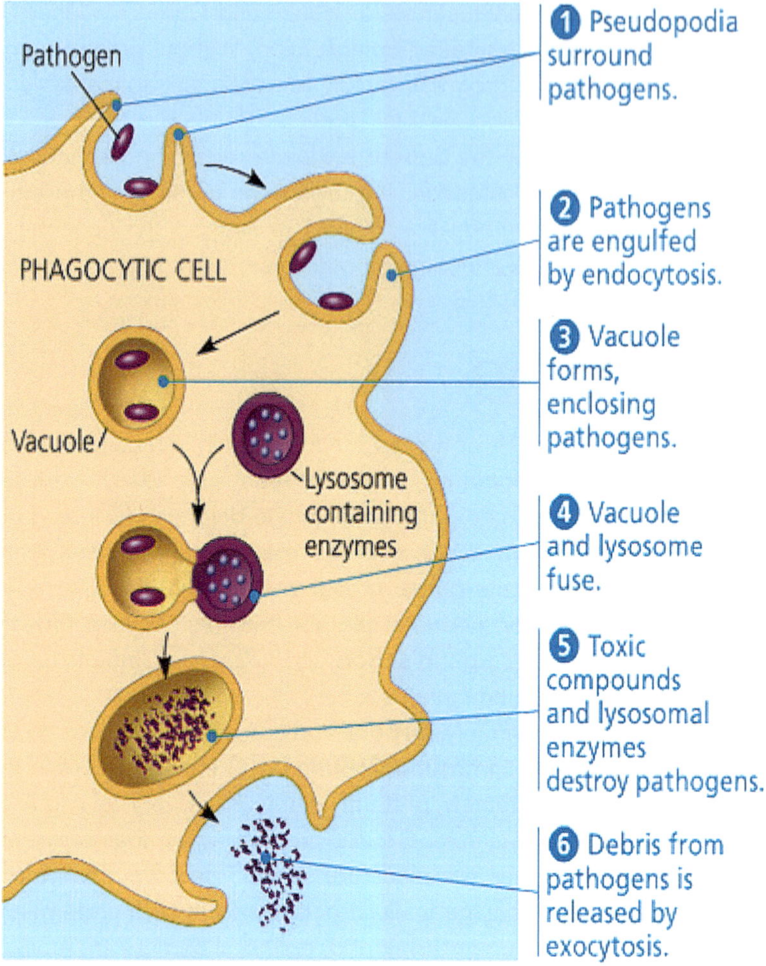

Figure 20.1 Phagocytosis (Source: Creative Commons)

necessary clinical interventions. Collectively, these features increase susceptibility to infection and partially explain the atypical or subtle clinical presentations seen in neonatal sepsis. Table 20.2 details differences in the immune response of preterm infants. See the web-based companion for more detail on immunity.

NEONATAL INFECTION

Significant mortality and morbidity are associated with neonatal infection, particularly in the preterm and LBW population (Fox et al., 2017; Cailes et al., 2018a). Infections causing sepsis, meningitis, or pneumonia contributed directly to around

TABLE 20.2 IMMUNE DEFICIENCIES IN PRETERM INFANTS

Immunity aspect	*Preterm neonate*	*Consequence*
Non-specific immunity	Phagocytes functional but less effective migration to infection site	Slow response to infection
Specific immunity	Develops during fetal life, but T- and B-cells are immature Low number of 'surveillance' T-cells Poor cytokine production of T-cells Very low levels of immunoglobulins (IgG antibodies virtually absent in extremely preterm infants)	Inefficient primary immune response, which means increased susceptibility to infection

(adapted from Melville & Moss, 2013)

0·6 million neonatal deaths worldwide in 2016, and indirectly to many more, through resultant preterm birth and neonatal encephalopathy (Seale & Agarwal, 2018).

Across the world, surveillance networks have been set up to document the incidence of neonatal infections, associated pathogens, and their resistance patterns. Among their objectives are the comparison and optimisation of clinical practice and antibiotic regimes (Cailes et al., 2015). In the United Kingdom (UK), 30 neonatal units (NNUs) throughout the country have been contributing data on infection to the Neonatal Infection Surveillance Network (NeonIN) since 2004. In the USA, there are the Centers for Disease Control and Prevention Active Bacterial Core surveillance and Neonatal Research Network; and internationally, over 1,200 hospitals contribute to the Vermont Oxford Network. In low-and middle-income countries (LMICs), data acquisition is more challenging due to regional variation in reporting (Sands et al., 2022). Broadly speaking, high-income countries (HICs; including the UK and other European countries, Australia and the USA) worldwide experience very similar infection rates, yet in LMICs; (China, African countries, South America, Asia, and the Middle East) these are much higher, reflecting resource constraints, reporting differences, and structural challenges to infection prevention and control (Cailes et al., 2018a; Sands et al., 2022; Flannery et al., 2025).

Infection in the neonate is typically described as EOI or LOI. Depending on definition, EOI occurs within 48–72 hours of life, and its mode of acquisition is described as 'vertical'; i.e., transplacental or ascending vaginal infection.

LOI arises after 48–72 hours from birth and is most commonly a 'horizontal' or healthcare-acquired (nosocomial) infection (Fox et al., 2017).

Early onset infection

The overall incidence of EOI in the UK decreased significantly between 2005 and 2015. Nearly half of all infants affected were born >37 weeks and weighed >2500g (Cailes et al., 2018a). The USA experienced a vast reduction of group B streptococcus (GBS) EOI since the introduction of intrapartum prophylaxis 1996, but over the past 10 years EOI rates appear to have plateaued. Globally, the rates of EOI affecting infants >34 GA in HICs such as Australia, the USA, Canada, and some European countries range from 0.17–0.7/1000 live births (LB; Flannery et al., 2025). LMICs, including China, African countries, and the Middle East, showed greater variation, with (likely partially under-) reported rates ranging from 9.7–21/1000 LB; South America reported an incidence of around 1.3–1.7/1000, and South Asia had the highest rates at 77/1000 LB (Sands et al., 2022).

The pathogens most commonly associated with EOI are GBS (43% in the UK; 33% in the USA) and *Escherichia coli* (18% in the UK; 28% in the US; Cailes et al., 2018a; Flannery et al., 2025). This is different to LMICs, where gram negative bacteria are prevalent (Sands et al., 2022). *Listeria monocytogenes* infection, which is increasingly rare, will also usually present in the early postnatal period (Mukherjee & Ryan, 2024).

Risk factors associated with EOI are outlined in Box 20.1.

BOX 20.1 RISK FACTORS FOR EARLY ONSET INFECTION

- Suspected or confirmed infection in another baby in the case of a multiple pregnancy (red flag risk factor).
- Invasive group B streptococcal infection in a previous baby or maternal group B streptococcal colonisation, bacteriuria or infection in the current pregnancy.
- Preterm birth following spontaneous labour (before 37 weeks' gestation).
- Confirmed rupture of membranes for more than 18 hours in a preterm birth.
- Confirmed prelabour rupture of membranes at term for more than 24 hours before the onset of labour.
- Intrapartum fever higher than 38°C if there is suspected or confirmed bacterial infection.
- Clinical diagnosis of chorioamnionitis.

(adapted from NICE, 2021)

PATHOGENS IN EARLY ONSET INFECTION

- *S. agalactiae*, more commonly referred to as GBS, colonises the bowel flora of approximately 18% of pregnant women worldwide, with regional variations and lower prevalence in Southern and Eastern Asia according to a recent systematic review (Russell et al., 2017). Carriers can be identified via rectal and vaginal swabs or urine samples. The Royal College of Obstetricians and Gynaecologists (RCOG) has produced a guideline with the aim of preventing GBS EOI by offering antibiotic prophylaxis in labour to any woman who is a known GBS carrier, who had a previous baby with GBS infection, or who goes into preterm labour (Hughes et al., 2017; Williams, 2018). Routine screening for GBS is not advocated in the UK due to a lack of evidence that it would be beneficial (UK National Screening Committee, 2017), despite the rates of infants developing invasive GBS infection having risen in the UK and Ireland over the past two decades (Hughes et al., 2017; Reynolds et al., 2019). This will be reviewed in line with the publication of ongoing research, expected in late spring 2026 (Daniels et al., 2026). In the USA and Australia, the introduction of universal screening guidelines has shown a subsequent decrease of GBS disease (Yanni et al., 2023; Mukherjee & Ryan, 2024).

  A review of the global impact of GBS identified that it resulted in up to 3.5million preterm births, 90,000 infant deaths and 10,000 children with long term disability in 2015. Just over half of estimated cases, and two thirds of infant deaths, were found to be in Africa (Seale et al., 2017). In the US, GBS disease affects more Black and ethnic minorities, thought to be due to a combination of inequalities in the healthcare system and, in the case of GBS, a higher incidence of colonisation in Black pregnant women (Flannery et al., 2025). A vaccine for administration to mothers in pregnancy is currently under development. This is projected to reduce annual infant deaths from GBS by up to 13,000 infants, and GBS-related preterm births by up to 44,000 worldwide (varying numbers according to region; World Health Organization (WHO), 2021). It is hoped that the vaccine will replace intrapartum antibiotic prophylaxis (Flannery et al., 2025).

  GBS infection, which most frequently presents as congenital pneumonia or bacteraemia, can also manifest as meningitis or bone/joint infections. Mortality rates are reported around 5–15% in the UK, and <2–20% in the US, with preterm infants worse affected (Fox et al., 2017; Mukherjee & Ryan, 2024). Most infants with GBS disease will display signs of infection within 12 hours of life (Fox et al., 2017), which is why this is recommended as a minimum observation period for infants born to GBS-colonised mothers (NICE, 2021).

- *E. coli* is one of the family of gram-negative (see Figure 20.2) *Enterobacterales*, which can survive under both aerobic and anaerobic conditions and predominantly reside in the gut. Gram-negative infections result in high morbidity and mortality in newborn infants. There are increasing cases of *E.coli* known

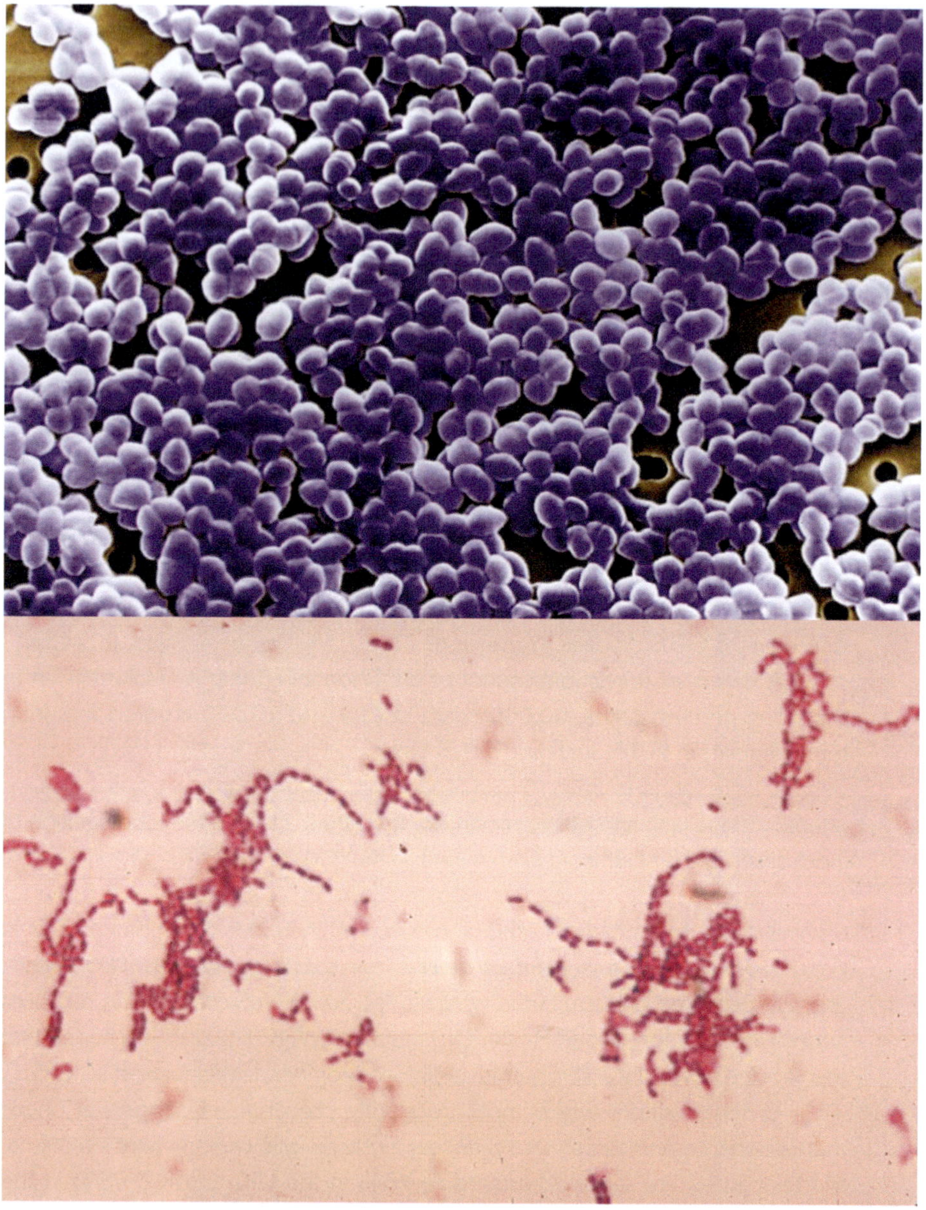

Figure 20.2 Gram-positive (top) and gram-negative organisms (Source: Creative Commons)

to produce extended-spectrum β-lactamases (ESBL), enzymes which can deactivate antibiotics from the penicillin and cephalosporin groups, making their treatment a potential challenge (Hoffman et al., 2024). Rates of *E. coli* EOI have been rising in the USA, so the introduction of vaccines currently in development are anticipated (Flannery et al., 2025).

- *L. monocytogenes* is transmitted through certain foods, particularly dairy products and some meat varieties, and predominantly affects pregnant women and their babies. When early pregnancy is affected, this is highly associated with spontaneous abortion or poor prognosis for the surviving infant. In later pregnancy, listeriosis can result in fetal death and preterm birth. Meconium-stained liquor is present in many cases. The majority of *L. monocytogenes* infections are transplacentally or perinatally acquired and thus present early and similarly to GBS with pneumonia, bacteraemia, meningitis, and focal infections, with a mortality rate of over 50%. A later onset of listeriosis more commonly presents with meningitis and is fatal in approximately 25% of cases (Mukherjee & Ryan, 2024).

TREATMENT OF EARLY ONSET INFECTION

Because of their susceptibility to perinatally and nosocomially acquired infection, newborn infants are often empirically prescribed antibiotics for presumed sepsis pending culture results to avoid acute deterioration. It has been suggested that the number of infants treated for suspected EOI without microbiological evidence of infection is between 6 and 16 times higher than those with positive blood cultures (Klingenberg et al., 2018). Implementation of the Kaiser-Permanente sepsis risk calculator (SRC) has led to significant reduction (ranging from 50–80%) of empirical antibiotic use and subsequently length of stay in a number of neonatal networks across the UK (Goel et al., 2020; van Hasselt et al., 2021; Ziprin et al., 2021). This tool has been endorsed by NICE, provided implementation is accompanied by prospective audit (2021); however, there has also been call for caution (British Association of Perinatal Medicine (BAPM), 2024).

ACTIVITY

Access the Neonatal Sepsis Calculator (https://neonatalsepsiscalculator.kaiserpermanente.org/) and, using an incidence of 0.5/1000, experiment with different values for each predictor, to see how these impact the score.

BOX 20.2 NEW DEVELOPMENTS

Artificial intelligence (AI) can support the early detection of neonatal sepsis by recognising subtle physiological patterns that may signal rising risk before clinical signs become obvious. When built and validated carefully, these systems can prompt timely bedside assessment, giving clinicians an early warning that a baby's condition may be changing. Crucially, AI does not replace clinical judgement; instead, it complements nursing and medical expertise by highlighting when closer observation or intervention may be needed. When thoughtfully implemented, AI-assisted sepsis alerts have the potential to enhance safety and improve outcomes for vulnerable infants (Sullivan et al., 2023).

Initially, broad-spectrum cover is prescribed, which is usually dependent on local policies and the unit flora, changing to specific antibiotics when dictated by the culture and sensitivity results. While this is accepted as the most appropriate and safe practice for the infant, administration of broad-spectrum agents for empirical treatment of presumed sepsis is highly implicated in antimicrobial resistance, which is an increasing problem worldwide. In the UK, antimicrobial stewardship programmes are aiming to address this issue. These suggest after broad-spectrum cover has been commenced, focusing antibiotic treatment to the narrowest spectrum possible, ensuring appropriate route of administration and dose, and limiting the duration to the shortest necessary course (UK Health Security Agency (UKHSA), 2023a). In line with these principles, NICE (2021) has devised a guideline to inform decisions about the treatment of EOI (see Table 20.3), though antibiotic regimens may vary in different NNUs, with wholly different agents used in other HICs (Ericson, 2023; Mukherjee & Ryan, 2024).

TABLE 20.3 ANTIBIOTICS FOR PREVENTION AND TREATMENT OF EARLY-ONSET INFECTION

Antibiotic	*Clinical Scenario*
Benzylpenicillin and gentamicin	Suspected EOI, GBS meningitis (but amend benzylpenicillin dose)
Benzylpenicillin, gentamicin, and gram-negative cover, e.g. cefotaxime	Gram-negative bacteraemia
Cefotaxime	Gram-negative meningitis
Amoxicillin and cefotaxime	Meningitis, pathogen unknown, or gram-positive (in the latter case also seek expert microbiology advice
Amoxicillin and gentamicin	*Listeria* bacteraemia/meningitis

(adapted from NICE, 2021)

The recommendation is that antibiotics should be stopped at the earliest opportunity (usually 36 hours) once negative blood cultures have been obtained. A 7-day course is suggested for infants with positive blood cultures or with a strong suspicion of infection, and a minimum of 14 days' treatment for proven meningitis (NICE, 2021).

Penicillins: These antimicrobials belong to the group of β-lactam antibiotics, which have bactericidal action by interfering with the synthesis of the bacterial cell wall. They are safe to use in neonates. Some pathogens, particularly some gram-negative bacteria and *Staphylococcus aureus* (S. aureus), have evolved resistance to penicillin antibiotics by producing β-lactamases.

- *Benzylpenicillin*, also known as penicillin G, is effective for GBS, with enhanced permeation of inflamed meninges in combination with gentamicin.
- *Amoxicillin* and *ampicillin* extend gram-negative coverage and are first-line for *Listeria* infection (Ainsworth, 2020).

Aminoglycoside antibiotics: Antimicrobials from the aminoglycoside group have both bactericidal actions, by damaging the bacterial cell membrane, and bacteriostatic (inhibition of bacterial reproduction) action. Their potential to have nephrotoxic and **ototoxic** effects necessitate drug level monitoring. Extended dosing frequency was suggested to reduce the likelihood of toxic trough levels (Rao et al., 2016).

- *Gentamicin* is effective against a number of gram-negative pathogens such as *Pseudomonas aeruginosa* and microbes from the *Enterobacterales* but also coagulase-negative staphylococci (CoNS) and *S. aureus*, so that it is commonly used in LOI as well as EOI (Ainsworth, 2020).

BOX 20.3 EXCITING NEW DEVELOPMENT

The PALOH UK study is investigating the feasibility of point of care testing for a genetic variant associated with non-dose related hearing loss following the administration of aminoglycosides (McDermott et al., 2021).

Cephalosporins: Cephalosporin antibiotics belong to the group of β-lactam antimicrobials and are thus bactericidal. They provide good cover against gram-positive and gram-negative organisms and are not affected by the β-lactamases produced by staphylococci. These antibiotics are used both in EOI and LOI.

- *Cefotaxime* is effective in a number of organisms affecting neonates, apart from *Pseudomonas* and *Listeria.* It has good CSF penetration, but problems associated with its use include the occurrence of secondary fungal infections and the emergence of pathogens producing ESBL (Ericson, 2023).
- *Ceftazidime* provides good gram-negative cover and is additionally suitable for treating *Pseudomonas* (Ainsworth, 2020).

Late onset infection

Improved survival rates of extremely preterm and very LBW infants have led to an increase in LOI incidence. The strong association between low gestational age (GA) and birthweight with LOI is supported by NeonIN findings that over 90% of cases in the UK occur in infants of <32 weeks GA (Cailes et al., 2018a). Worldwide, there are an estimated 1.3–3.9 million annual cases of sepsis in the neonatal period (WHO, 2020). Factors apart from prematurity and immunological immaturity predisposing to LOI are prolonged hospitalisation, resulting in exposure to a multitude of hospital staff, nosocomial pathogens, and potentially contaminated equipment, missed opportunities for early enteral breastmilk administration and protracted use of parenteral nutrition, which necessitates the presence of indwelling central venous catheters (CVC), and other invasive apparatus, such as endotracheal tubes (ETTs). A more recent area of research interest, the gut microbiome, is a further factor predisposing the preterm population to infection: first, its immaturity resulting in reduced immune function, and, second, the microbiome can constitute a source of infection due to imbalances, partly exacerbated by antibiotic treatment (Ericson et al., 2025; McGann et al., 2025). Further issues facing LMICs include potential problems with water supply, overcrowding, high patient-to-nurse ratios, and reuse of single-use equipment, amongst others (Johnson et al., 2021).

It follows that a significant role in the management of LOI may be preventative strategies, and indeed the introduction of such is thought to have resulted in a decreasing trend of LOI (Cailes et al., 2018a).

PREVENTION OF LATE ONSET INFECTION

- *Early introduction of breastmilk* Development of normal gut flora is impaired in infants admitted to the NNU, due to exposure to both broad-spectrum antibiotics and a range of bacteria with the potential of pathogenicity. It has been demonstrated that commencing early trophic feeds of breastmilk has a positive impact on evolving neonatal gut flora, with a protective effect from necrotising enterocolitis (NEC) as well as sepsis (Schüller et al., 2018; McGann et al., 2025). While the administration of probiotics to preterm infants is becoming more widespread in the UK, currently available evidence is at odds whether there is a resultant reduction in LOI (Rao et al., 2016; Sharif et al., 2023).

- *CVC care* Recognition of an association between increased incidence of LOI and the presence of a CVC has led to a number of attempts to reduce CVC-related infection (Shane et al., 2017). Trials have addressed a number of strategies, including prophylactic antibiotics with CVCs (Inglis & Davies, 2005; Inglis et al., 2007; Jardine et al., 2008), antimicrobial dressings (Lai et al., 2016), early vs. expectant removal of CVCs (Gordon et al., 2017), antimicrobial-impregnated catheters (Gilbert et al., 2019; Klemme et al., 2020) among others. These have not yet shown any significant difference in the incidence of LOI compared to controls. A study from Italy reported a positive impact on LOI rates with the use of silver zeolite-impregnated UVCs (Bertini et al., 2013), but this is currently not endorsed in the UK due to questions about study quality and transferability of results (NICE, 2021). It appears that the most effective strategies in the reduction of CVC-associated infection remain care bundles involving aspects such as hand hygiene, barrier precautions, and adequate catheter care (Payne et al., 2018; Pharande et al., 2018; Aleem et al., 2020).

PRACTICE POINT

After reading the above, consider whether your unit has previously faced infection control/prevention challenges. Which measures particularly made a difference?

- *Immuno-supportive treatment* With awareness that the preterm immune system is immature, several methods of supportive therapy have been examined, but none have demonstrated any benefit in the treatment or prevention of LOI. These include the administration of intravenous immunoglobulin; Granulocyte-Macrophage Colony-Stimulating Factor; granulocyte transfusions; antioxidants such as selenium, melatonin, and vitamin A; and glutamine (Schüller et al., 2018).

PATHOGENS IN LATE ONSET INFECTION

The vast majority of LOI is caused by bacteria – gram-positive bacteria in HICs, and gram-negative bacteria in LMICs; however, in cases where blood cultures remain negative, fungi and viruses ought to be considered causative organisms (Coggins & Glaser, 2022; Ericson et al., 2025).

Gram-positive pathogens

- *Coagulase-negative Staphylococci (CoNS)* account for a third to half of LOI cases globally (Cailes et al., 2018b; Ericson et al., 2025). Species such as *S. epidermidis*, *S. haemolyticus*, and *S. hominis* colonise skin and mucosa and are readily transmitted via hands. Biofilm production facilitates adherence to plastics (e.g. CVCs) and confers antimicrobial tolerance (Dong et al., 2018). Over recent years, the UKHSA has been monitoring a type of *S. capitis*, exclusive to NNUs, where it has contributed to outbreaks (UKHSA, 2023b). This has highlighted the need for standardisation in vancomycin administration, as widespread utilisation of this antibiotic appears to have driven this (Harvey et al., 2023). Definitive diagnosis of CoNS bacteraemia can be challenging, as contamination of blood cultures can trigger a falsely positive result. This is, however, of great importance both due to the fact that it is associated with significant mortality and adverse neurodevelopmental outcome in preterm infants and in the interest of antimicrobial stewardship and prevention of resistance (Dong et al., 2018; Ericson et al., 2025).
- *S. aureus* This staphylococcus can cause EOI but was associated with 31% of gram-positive LOI cases in UK NNUs, with 23% incidence reported from the Vermont Oxford Network (Cailes et al., 2018a; Flannery et al., 2022). It can lead to a variety of presentations, including bacteraemia, soft tissue infections such as staphylococcal scalded skin syndrome and omphalitis, pneumonia, meningitis, endocarditis, and osteomyelitis. Initially susceptible to penicillin antimicrobials, treatment can be a potential challenge, as *S. aureus* strains have evolved increasing virulence and resistance, such as methicillin resistance (Mukherjee & Ryan, 2024).
- *Enterococci* such as *E. faecalis* and *E. faecium* are intestinal commensals that can cause both EOI and LOI when translocated. The former usually presents as mild respiratory illness, whereas LOI is associated with acute clinical deterioration (Dobson & Baker, 1990).
- *Gram-negative pathogens* Infections produced by gram-negative bacteria (see Table 20.4) globally make up between 15 and 45% of LOI, remain a significant cause of mortality and are associated with prolonged hospital stay and adverse neurodevelopmental outcomes in the neonatal population (Cailes et al., 2018a; Flannery et al., 2022). Gram-negative pathogens are mostly associated with bacteraemia but also meningitis and pneumonia. They contain endotoxins which, when released, can result in septic shock. Many produce ESBL or are resistant to carbapenems (CRE), and resistance is much more an issue among this group of pathogens compared to those commonly associated with EOI (Kent et al., 2016; Cailes et al., 2018b; Flannery et al., 2022).

TABLE 20.4 GRAM-NEGATIVE PATHOGENS CAUSING NEONATAL SEPSIS AND THEIR TRANSMISSION PATHWAYS

Pathogen	*Naturally occurring*	*Transmission*
E. coli *Klebsiella spp.* *Enterobacter spp.* *Citrobacter spp.* *Salmonella spp.* *Morganella morganii*	Gut colonisation	Translocation
Neisseria spp.	Mucosal colonisation	Translocation
Pseudomonas aeruginosa *Acinetobacter* *Serratia marcescens*	Water reservoirs	Healthcare staff

(adapted from Kent et al., 2016)

- *Fungi* Invasive candidiasis accounts for roughly 10% of LOI in some high-income countries and remains an important cause of mortality and neurodevelopmental impairment (Cailes et al., 2018a; Kilpatrick et al., 2022; Kaufman & Mukhopadhyay, 2025). Risk factors include extreme prematurity, broad-spectrum antibiotics, prolonged CVC use, parenteral nutrition (especially lipids), ventilation, fungal colonisation, antacid and steroid use, and mucosal barrier immaturity (Kaufman & Mukhopadhyay, 2025). Some centres employ antifungal prophylaxis (e.g. fluconazole) in the highest-risk infants; while prophylaxis reduces the incidence of invasive fungal infection, it does not necessarily improve mortality and can drive resistance (Austin et al., 2015; Cleminson et al., 2015). When treating proven fungal sepsis, courses of 14–21 days or until cultures are clear (Fox et al., 2017; Kaufman & Mukhopadhyay, 2025).

A number of antifungal agents are available:

- *Fluconazole* is fungistatic and convenient orally but prone to resistance.
- *Amphotericin B* (preferably liposomal formulations) is fungicidal with strong activity and limited resistance. Resistance is rarely seen, and it is preferable particularly if fluconazole was used prophylactically.
- *Flucytosine* is associated with rapid development of resistance but advocated in combination with amphotericin in cases where sterile body sites such as CSF, kidneys and retina are involved.

- *Echinocandins:* The latest class of antifungal agents has not been widely researched in the neonatal population. Resistance is rarely seen (Fox et al., 2017; Kilpatrick et al., 2022).

TREATMENT OF BACTERIAL LATE ONSET INFECTION

Please note, this section applies to UK practice – treatment regimens are different in various countries across the world based on causative organisms, antibiotic susceptibility/resistance patterns, availability, etc.

Penicillins

- *Flucloxacillin* belongs to the group of anti-staphylococcal penicillins which are very effective against *S. aureus*, but not most CoNS, *Enterococci* and enteric gram-negative bacteria (Ainsworth, 2020). In UK NNUs, flucloxacillin in combination with gentamicin often constitutes first-line antibiotic choice in suspected LOI, which provides good coverage of many causative organisms except CoNS (Fox et al., 2017).
- *Piperacillin with Tazobactam* Piperacillin alone has good activity against *Pseudomonas aeruginosa* and *Enterococci but* does not provide coverage for organisms producing β-lactamases or ESBL. It has therefore been combined with tazobactam, which is a β-lactamase inhibitor. Given its broad spectrum, resistance is an issue, which is why it needs to be utilised with caution (Ainsworth, 2020).
- *Amoxicillin* see p. 593.
- *Cephalosporins* (see p. 593) may be indicated in meningitis due to better tissue penetration (Fox et al., 2017).
- *Aminoglycosides*; see p. 593.
- *Glycopeptide antibiotics* Due to their effectiveness against CoNS, which are the most common causative organisms of LOI, glycopeptide antimicrobials are among the most frequently used antibiotics in the treatment of LOI. Their spectrum of activity means they are bactericidal only to *Enterococci and* otherwise have bacteriostatic action.
    - *Vancomycin* was predominantly developed for the treatment of staphylococcal infections and remains important in infections secondary to MRSA. Issues associated with drug reactions ('red man syndrome'), ototoxicity and nephrotoxicity are circumvented with considerations around administration, such as infusion over 30–60 minutes or continuously, and drug level monitoring. Emergence of vancomycin-resistant enterococci (VRE) and MRSA means empiric use of vancomycin should be avoided and its usage limited to infants who are seriously ill, particularly in the presence of a CVC (Cailes et al., 2015; Ainsworth, 2020).

  - *Teicoplanin* may be considered a good alternative to vancomycin, as it provides coverage of a similar spectrum of pathogens but is not as nephrotoxic or ototoxic (Ainsworth, 2020).
- *Metronidazole* has excellent activity against gram-negative bacteria and should be used if there is a high index of suspicion for NEC (Fox et al., 2017; NICE, 2021).
- *Meropenem* is part of the broad-spectrum Carbapenem antimicrobials, which provide excellent cover for many gram-positive and gram-negative pathogens. Meropenem has good CSF penetration (Fox et al., 2017).

  Carbapenems are strongly associated with emerging resistance among a multitude of pathogens, including those producing metallo-β-lactamase for which there is hardly any effective antimicrobial treatment. Therefore, empiric treatment with meropenem should be avoided (Ainsworth, 2020).

Viral infections

A number of viruses can affect infants in the neonatal period. These are mostly vertically transmitted, though postnatal infection can also occur. Those most likely to be encountered in the UK are briefly discussed in this section, which is by no means exhaustive.

For many years practitioners have referred to the TORCH (**To**xoplasma, **R**ubella, **C**ytomegalovirus, and **H**erpes Simplex) group of pathogens when signs were indicative of congenital viral infection. It is, however, now understood that some of these infections are acquired perinatally rather than antenatally. And, as some of the viruses associated with this group can be excluded based on clinical presentation or maternal serology, sending investigations for a TORCH screen is no longer recommended. Other viruses which can present in the neonatal period are syphilis, zika virus, varicella zoster virus, hepatitis B and C, parvovirus B19, human immunodeficiency virus (HIV), and enteroviruses.

The presentation associated with each pathogen varies, but common signs seen in affected infants are growth restriction, a petechial rash, jaundice, hepatosplenomegaly, and sometimes thrombocytopaenia. Some infections can be associated with severe systemic illness (Fox et al., 2017).

- *Toxoplasmosis* Maternal infection usually occurs as a result of exposure to cat faeces or through handling raw meat and can be silent or accompanied by mild flu-like symptoms. If the infection is transmitted to the fetus (usually transplacentally), outcomes are generally poor with a mortality of approximately 25%, or deafness, congenital cataracts, intracranial calcifications, and hydrocephalus. Treatment, if continued for a year, has been associated with significant improvement in outcomes; this consists of pyrimethamine, sulfadiazine, and folinic acid (Fox et al., 2017).

- *Varicella zoster virus (VZV; chickenpox)* This highly contagious virus is part of the herpesvirus family and may be antenatally, perinatally, or postnatally acquired. Depending on disease onset, varicella can result in congenital problems such as limb and eye abnormalities and CNS damage (neonatal varicella syndrome) or devastating systemic illness. Based on maternal onset of the illness, treatment is with zoster immunoglobulin +/− systemic acyclovir. Vaccination is now widespread in HICs (Desai et al., 2024).
- *Rubella* The incidence of rubella is now extremely low thanks to routine vaccination. Transmission to the fetus occurs transplacentally, frequently results in abortion and is associated with multiple congenital anomalies, particularly if it occurs before the third trimester of pregnancy. Apart from the common signs named above, these can include congenital cataracts or glaucoma, sensorineural deafness, congenital heart disease, microcephaly, and developmental delay. There is no treatment other than supportive management. Like with VZV, barrier precautions need to be considered (Kabani & Kimberlin, 2023).
- *Cytomegalovirus (CMV)* Maternal infection can be primary or recurrent, with more serious implications for the fetus in primary infection, particularly if the infection occurs earlier in gestation. Apart from growth restriction, jaundice, and thrombocytopaenia, CMV infection may otherwise be silent in the neonate and if untreated can lead to progressive sensorineural hearing loss and developmental delay.

  Acquisition can be postnatal as well as vertical, for example through CMV-positive breastmilk (Stark et al., 2025). Treatment is with ganciclovir or valganciclovir for 6 months. There is suggestion that universal screening is warranted and indeed has been implemented in some states of the USA (Permar & Salvatore, 2023). Furthermore, vaccines are currently in development (Plotkin & Boppana, 2019).
- *Herpes simplex virus (HSV)* Transmission of HSV can be transplacentally (rarely), postnatally, nosocomially, or from family members, but the vast majority of cases occur perinatally via passage through an infected birth canal. Illness severity varies from superficial skin lesions only to disseminated systemic/central nervous system disease requiring intensive care, and its onset can be delayed (day 10–14). Treatment is with systemic acyclovir, which has been shown to successfully treat the condition and prevent long term sequelae. Preventative obstetric practices such as maternal oral acyclovir prophylaxis late in pregnancy and delivery via elective caesarean section seek to eliminate perinatal transmission of HSV (Kabani & Kimberlin, 2023).

- *Human immunodeficiency virus (HIV)* The most common route of HIV infection in infants is through mother-to-child-transmission, with the risk directly related to maternal viral load and illness severity. Transmission rates in untreated women range from 15–45%. Since the implementation of WHO recommendations, the proportion of pregnant and lactating women receiving antiretroviral treatment (ART) has risen globally from 44% in 2010 to 82% in 2022 (WHO, 2025). In recent years in the UK, as across many other European countries, breastfeeding is no longer discouraged for HIV-positive mothers, following findings from the PROMISE study (Flynn et al., 2018); however, differences in practice and recommendations remain, emphasising the importance of disseminating accurate information (Fernandes et al., 2025).
- *Respiratory syncytial virus (RSV)* This is the leading respiratory infection in infants, with most children infected by age 2 and many experiencing reinfection. Although often mild, RSV can cause severe bronchiolitis and pneumonia, particularly in premature infants, those with chronic lung disease, congenital heart disease, or immunodeficiency. Hospital outbreaks are common because the virus spreads easily through direct contact, droplets, and contaminated surfaces, and it can survive for hours on clothing and equipment. Early RSV infection is linked to a higher risk of recurrent wheeze and later asthma. Management is largely supportive, with oxygen, hydration, and careful monitoring. Prevention focuses on infection control, hand hygiene, and targeted prophylaxis for high-risk infants throughout the RSV season (Desai et al., 2024). In the UK, palivizumab was utilised until 2025; however, nirsevimab is now preferentially administered, as it offers more prolonged protection and requires only a single injection per season (UKHSA, 2025).

Please refer to the companion website for details about zika virus and SARS-CoV-2.

VACCINATION

Vaccines work by creating active immunity and establishing immunological memory, allowing the immune system to recognise an infection later and respond quickly to prevent or lessen disease. Even when antibodies are not detectable, memory responses may still be present. Traditional vaccines use whole pathogens that are either inactivated or live-attenuated, or they use specific components such as toxins, viral-like particles, or subunit proteins. More recent approaches use recombinant viral vectors to deliver antigens, either replicating (similar to live vaccines) or non-replicating (more like inactivated vaccines). The newest technologies use the pathogen's genetic code itself, enabling the host cell to produce the antigen internally, which then triggers an immune response (UKHSA, 2021). In the UK, the immunisation schedule is regularly updated, so that nurses functioning as administrators or prescribers, medical professionals, and pharmacists need to ensure in a multidisciplinary effort that the most recent programme is followed.

SIGNS OF NEONATAL INFECTION

Neonatal infection frequently presents with subtle, non-specific changes. Skilled nursing assessment is fundamental: early recognition and escalation are vital given the speed at which infants may deteriorate. Patterns often evolve rapidly, and single signs cannot reliably differentiate infection from other conditions; a composite view of cardiorespiratory status, temperature, behaviour, feeding, and skin findings is necessary.

- *Respiratory signs:* Tachypnoea, grunting, recession, and apnoea may signal EOI (including congenital pneumonia) or non-infectious respiratory conditions (e.g. respiratory distress syndrome). Chest radiography may show overlapping features (Crowley, 2024). Pulse oximetry screening can identify hypoxia early even in apparently well term infants, prompting further evaluation (Ewer et al., 2024). Respiratory instability from GBS is partly mediated by thromboxane A2–driven pulmonary vasoconstriction; LOI/meningitis may depress the respiratory centre, increase ventilator requirements, or trigger apnoea (Mukherjee & Ryan, 2024).
- *Thermal signs:* Temperature instability is a useful early marker, especially in the first three days (>90% specificity). Preterm infants more often present with hypothermia; most babies with a fever are term infants. In LOI, hypothermia, hyperthermia, or labile temperature may occur. A widening toe-to-core gradient (>2°C) suggests vasoconstriction and poor perfusion in sepsis. Environmental causes must be excluded before attributing temperature changes to infection (Stocker et al., 2023).
- *Cardiovascular signs:* Tachycardia, hypotension, and prolonged capillary refill time (>2 seconds) reflect compromised cardiac output or peripheral vasoconstriction. Emerging analytics of heart-rate characteristics show promise for early detection, but bedside clinical assessment remains central and broadly available. Perfusion trends, blood pressure, lactate, and urine output should be reassessed frequently as status can change quickly (Stocker et al., 2023).

- *Skin signs:* Skin findings are varied and must be interpreted in context. Pallor or cutis marmorata indicates poor perfusion (Stocker et al., 2023); a generalised petechial rash may reflect congenital viral infection or disseminated intravascular coagulation – both warrant urgent evaluation. Omphalitis presents with umbilical erythema and purulent discharge, requiring prompt treatment to forestall systemic spread. Jaundice is common in newborns and less strongly correlated with sepsis than previously thought. Depending on the causative organism, rashes and skin lesions can have characteristic appearances; more information on these can be found on the companion website (Mukherjee & Ryan, 2024).
- *Gastrointestinal signs:* Distension and ileus are a common and important sign of sepsis and need to be differentiated from intestinal obstruction or NEC, all of which may present similarly with poor feed tolerance and bile-stained gastric aspirates. The latter may be early signs of sepsis in an infant who has previously tolerated enteral feeds (Stocker et al., 2023).
- *Neurological signs:* Lethargy, irritability or 'not handling' well occurs in approximately half of the number of infants with sepsis and should always be further investigated. Meningitis may be heralded by increasing irritability, lethargy, hypo- or hypertonia, and seizures activity (Stocker et al., 2023; Mukherjee & Ryan, 2024).

THINK POINT

- Have you looked after a baby before who developed an infection?
- What were the first signs/changes in observations you noticed?
- What were the signs the parents noticed?

INVESTIGATIONS

If the decision for antibiotic treatment has been made based on a baby's risk factors for infection or clinical concerns, a number of investigations, generally still known as a septic screen (though this term is becoming outmoded), have to be carried out before therapy is instigated. These will subsequently guide antibiotic choice and duration of treatment as well as aid prognosis of the illness course. The aim is for the first dose of antibiotics to be administered within an hour from the decision to treat (NICE, 2021).

Baseline investigations for both EOI and LOI include a blood culture and C-reactive protein (CRP) measurement. A lumbar puncture is advisable where there is strong suspicion of infection or there are signs of meningitis; and only if there is evidence of localised skin or eye infections, appropriate swabs (NICE, 2021). Depending on the circumstances and signs present, investigations such as placental swabs (EOI only), chest or abdominal X-rays, urine culture, microbial investigations of ETT/nasopharyngeal secretions, ETT, or central venous catheter tips should also be considered (Fox et al., 2017).

- *Blood culture:* Despite ongoing evaluations of alternative methods, blood culture remains the gold standard diagnostic tool for neonatal sepsis. This is discussed in detail in Chapter 23.
- *CSF culture:* NICE guidelines suggest taking CSF samples in case of signs of meningitis or otherwise strong clinical suspicion of infection (NICE, 2021). Please refer to Chapter 23 for details about CSF analysis.
- *Urine culture:* Urinary tract infections (UTIs) are predominantly LOIs. Routine urine culture in suspected EOI is not recommended, and more recently UK guidelines have been updated to suggest they are not routinely performed as part of a LOI screen in NNU inpatients (NICE, 2021). The collection method of urine cultures is of importance: 'bag specimens' will only exclude a UTI if clear but not be of diagnostic value in a true UTI due to high contamination rates. Collection via suprapubic aspiration or catheterisation are preferable (Fox et al., 2017).
- *Surface swabs, gastric aspirate, and endotracheal aspirate:* Cultures from these sites will identify colonisation, which is not necessarily an indication of invasive infection. Management and antimicrobial therapy therefore need to be guided by other investigations and the baby's clinical status rather than these results alone, and they no longer routinely constitute part of septic screens (NICE, 2021).
- *Molecular markers:* Studies evaluating the hundreds of molecular markers used to diagnose infection have not demonstrated sufficient precision, either on their own or in various combinations. This is in part because many of them can become deranged in response to other conditions than infection. Nonetheless, in the absence of an effective alternative, and given the time it takes to obtain blood culture results, they are widely used by clinicians to guide the commencement and cessation of antibiotic treatment (Stocker et al., 2023; Mukherjee & Ryan, 2024).
    - *Cell count:* Overall, cell count has not been shown to be of significant value in the detection of neonatal infection (Hornik et al., 2012a, 2012b), and the full blood count does, in fact, not form part of the recommended investigations in the most recent version of the NICE guideline (NICE, 2021).
        - *White cell count (WCC)* This has been suggested to be of limited value in the diagnosis of infection, as the normal range is wide,

dependent on gestational and postnatal age, and can be raised in conditions other than sepsis, such as hypoxic-ischaemic encephalopathy (HIE) and neonatal seizures. High WCC may be indicative of LOI, whereas leukopenia can occur in either EOI or LOI.

  - *Neutrophil count* A low neutrophil count in early postnatal life may be associated with infection, but more often due to causes such as growth restriction or pregnancy-induced hypertension and pre-eclampsia. LOI commonly results in high neutrophil count, but neutropenia has also been associated with NEC. An abnormal I:T (immature: total neutrophil) ratio and evidence of toxic granulation on the blood film are reasonably sensitive indicators of infection (Hornik et al., 2012a, 2012b).
  - *Platelets* Neonates can be thrombocytopenic for the same non-infective reasons they can be neutropenic, or due to HIE in early life. Infective causes of thrombocytopenia include congenital or acquired viral as well as bacterial infections (Mukherjee & Ryan, 2024).
- *Other molecular markers*
  - *CRP* measurement is recommended when antibiotic therapy is commenced, with elevated levels being indicative of infection (NICE, 2021). CRP levels also rise in NEC, meconium aspiration, HIE, and following surgery. Whether it is a sensitive enough predictor for infection in isolation is doubtful, but its value in monitoring the course of infection and infant response to therapy is recognised and widely used (Mukherjee & Ryan, 2024).
  - *Procalcitonin* This infection marker has superseded CRP measurements in some UK hospitals, and there is evidence that it can facilitate shorter antibiotic duration compared to CRP in EOI.
  - *Cytokines* These include interleukin (IL) 1, IL-6, IL-8, and tumour necrosis factor α, amongst others. However, even though there is suggestion of their usefulness, evidence available to date does not currently support their routine use in clinical practice, due to various limitations (Stocker et al., 2023).
  - *Polymerase chain reaction (PCR)* This technique, in which certain DNA sequences are amplified, has become widely used in the UK, at least for CSF samples (NICE, 2021). It has been suggested that it may detect pathogens where blood cultures have been negative (Oeser et al., 2020). When routinely performed on CSF, PCR has much improved detection of HSV; it has also become the gold standard for detection of VZV in vesicular fluid and CMV in saliva or urine in some HICs (Desai et al., 2024).

- *Radiology:* A chest X-ray should be performed in infants with suspected infection, particularly if associated respiratory signs are present. Depending on clinical presentation, an abdominal X-ray should furthermore be considered, which may be helpful in the exclusion of NEC or other surgical causes of clinical abdominal concerns (Fox et al., 2017). See Chapter 23 for further details.

THE NURSE'S ROLE IN NEONATAL INFECTION

Due to the potential sequelae of neonatal infection, it is of high importance that nurses have an awareness of potential risk factors and are able to recognise signs of infection in an infant as early as possible, so that appropriate treatment is commenced, and complications avoided. The neonatal nurse, as the baby's advocate in partnership with the parents, is ideally placed to pick up on subtle clinical and behavioural changes and communicate these to the medical members of the multidisciplinary team.

However, the prevention of infection must be among the first concerns in providing neonatal care, and there are a number of ways in which nurses can lead on this. The appropriate cleaning and disinfection, particularly of shared and multiple use equipment, is, sadly, still predominantly instigated and monitored by members of the nursing team. This aspect, alongside regular cleaning of incubators, contributes greatly to reducing pathogen transmission and avoiding outbreaks of multi drug resistant organisms (Johnson et al., 2021; UKHSA, 2022).

The prevention of CVC-related LOI has been broadly discussed in relation to reducing sepsis rates through the introduction of care bundles (Payne et al., 2018). More specifically, exemplary CVC care is predominantly the responsibility of the nurse caring for the infant with indwelling lines, and good practice in this area has been associated with a reduction in infection rates. This consists of regular review of the insertion site including dressing integrity, as well as the ongoing need for the line and, if deemed no longer required, its prompt removal, as well as the utilisation of aseptic techniques when manipulation of the catheter hub is necessary (Payne et al., 2018; Johnson et al., 2021).

Asepsis is furthermore practiced in the preparation of IV fluids and medication. In the UK, multi-dose vials and sharing of IV solution bags for infusion preparation are no longer common practice but may still be a necessity in lower resource settings (Johnson et al., 2021).

Family integrated care has been associated with reduced infection rates and mortality (BAPM, 2021; Johnson et al., 2021), and the neonatal nurse is heavily involved in the facilitation of this. More specifically, kangaroo care through its positive impact on the neonatal microbiome is an important protective factor (McGann et al., 2025) and an easy intervention to encourage.

The cornerstone of infection prevention, however, remains good hand hygiene, which the expert neonatal nurse does not only practice, but also promotes by fulfilling monitoring and educational functions among the multidisciplinary team, parents and visitors (Payne et al., 2018; Johnson et al., 2021).

Chapter takeaways

- Neonatal infection remains a major cause of mortality and long-term morbidity, particularly among preterm, very low birthweight, and extremely low birthweight infants. Improvements in survival have shifted the burden toward LOI, which is strongly associated with adverse neurodevelopmental outcomes, prolonged hospitalisation, and increased healthcare costs.
- The neonatal immune system is functionally immature at birth, with deficiencies in both innate and acquired immunity. Preterm infants are especially vulnerable due to limited transplacental transfer of maternal IgG, ineffective mucosal barriers, impaired phagocyte function, and reduced cytokine responses, all of which compromise the ability to contain infection.
- Early onset infection and late onset infection differ in timing, transmission pathways, and causative organisms. EOI is usually vertically acquired and most commonly caused by GBS and *E. coli*, whereas LOI is predominantly healthcare-associated and linked to invasive devices, prolonged parenteral nutrition, and exposure to nosocomial pathogens.
- Clinical signs of neonatal infection are often subtle, non-specific, and rapidly evolving, requiring expert nursing assessment and continuous vigilance. Changes in respiratory status, temperature instability, cardiovascular compromise, feeding intolerance, neurological behaviour, or skin appearance may represent early indicators of sepsis.
- Diagnosis of neonatal infection relies on a combination of clinical judgement and targeted investigations, as no single laboratory test can reliably confirm or exclude infection. Blood culture remains the diagnostic gold standard, while inflammatory markers and molecular techniques are used to support treatment decisions and guide antibiotic duration.
- Empirical antibiotic therapy is frequently initiated to prevent rapid deterioration, but a significant proportion of treated infants have no microbiological evidence of infection. Decision-support tools, early review of culture results, and timely cessation of antibiotics are essential components of antimicrobial stewardship in neonatal care.
- Prevention of late onset infection is a central component of neonatal nursing practice. Effective strategies include strict hand hygiene, meticulous central venous catheter care, environmental cleaning, early use of breastmilk,

promotion of kangaroo care, and family integrated care models, all of which contribute to reduced infection rates.

- Neonatal nurses play a pivotal role in infection prevention, early recognition, and management, acting as advocates for the infant and family. Through skilled observation, leadership in infection control practices, timely escalation of concerns, and family education, nurses directly influence outcomes for vulnerable neonates.

CASE STUDY

CASE STUDIES

Case study 1: Early onset infection in a term neonate

Kanlaya is a term baby born vaginally to a second-time mother after 42 hours' rupture of the membranes. She was admitted to the NNU as she developed severe respiratory distress in the delivery room and commenced on CPAP, requiring 35–40% oxygen to maintain normal saturations. She continues to have significant subcostal recession and is noted to be grunting, which worsens with handling.

Following admission, Kanlaya was started on benzylpenicillin and gentamicin following a partial septic screen, and she is nil by mouth on IV fluids. Kanlaya's chest X-ray shows bilateral 'ground glass' consolidation.

After 2 hours her blood gases still show a respiratory acidosis, her oxygen requirements are climbing, and her work of breathing is worsening. Her blood results show a raised WCC, and her initial CRP is 27mg/L.

Q.1. What is Kanlaya's diagnosis likely to be? Can you think of a pathogen which typically presents like this?
Q.2. Do you think Kanlaya's condition is likely to improve over the next few hours?
Q.3. What other supportive treatment may be required in this case?
Q.4. Which other investigations may need to be considered here?

Case study 2: The extremely preterm NICU resident

Harry is a 39-day-old baby born at 24^{+6} weeks. He now weighs 984grams. He is currently stable on high flow 6L/minute in 28–34% oxygen and on a combination of nasogastric feeds of maternal breastmilk and parenteral nutrition through a CVC, as he had multiple episodes of abdominal and feed tolerance concerns in his early weeks. This was inserted when he was a week old.

CASE STUDY

Q.1. What measures can you take to help prevent Harry developing CVC-related infection?
Q.2. Which changes in his observations would make you concerned that he may be infected?
Q.3. Is there anything you would like to discuss with the medical team on Harry's ward round this morning?

Case study 3: Unexpected admission from the postnatal ward

Baby Tariq, a term baby boy, is admitted to the NNU from the postnatal ward at 2 hours of age following an episode of sudden transient cyanosis. On assessment, the midwife heard respiratory grunting and his breathing rate had become more rapid, with his colour looking pale and mottled.

Q.1. What do you think is going on here, and what risk factors would you need to consider in relation to his birth, delivery, and details about his mother's health?
Q.2. What nursing assessment would he require?
Q.3. What would you explain to the parents and how would they be supported at this time?

For suggested answer guides to the questions posed in these case studies, please refer to the web-based companion site specific to this chapter. See www.routledge.com/cw/petty

References

Ainsworth, M. (2020). *Neonatal formulary: Drug use in pregnancy and the first year of life* (8th ed.). Oxford University Press.

Aleem, S., Wohlfarth, M., Cotten, M., & Greenberg, R. G. (2020). Infection control and other stewardship strategies in late onset sepsis, necrotizing enterocolitis, and localized infection in the neonatal intensive care unit. *Journal of Paediatrics and Child Health*, *54*(12), 1314–1320.

Austin, N., Cleminson, J., Darlow, B. A., & McGuire, W. (2015). Prophylactic oral/topical non-absorbed antifungal agents to prevent invasive fungal infection in very low birth weight infants. *Cochrane Database of Systematic Reviews*, *10*, Article CD003478. https://doi.org/10.1002/14651858.CD003478.pub5

Bertini, G., Elia, S., Ceciarini, F., & Dani, C. (2013). Reduction of catheter-related bloodstream infections in preterm infants by the use of catheters with the AgION antimicrobial system. *Early Human Development*, *89*(1), 21–25.

British Association of Perinatal Medicine. (2021). *Family integrated care. A framework for practice.* British Association of Perinatal Medicine. Retrieved April 24, 2025, from https://www.bapm.org/resources/ficare-framework-for-practice

British Association of Perinatal Medicine. (2024). *Safety alert: Using the KP risk calculator/NICE categorical framework with the NEWTT2 tool.* Retrieved March 20, 2025, from https://www.bapm.org/articles/safety-alert-using-the-kp-risk-calculator-nice-categorical-framework-with-the-newtt2-tool

Cailes, B., Kortsalioudaki, C., Buttery, J., Pattnayak, S., Greenough, A., Matthes, J., Bedford Russell, A., Kennea, N., & Heath, P. T. (2018a). Epidemiology of UK neonatal infections: The neonIN infection surveillance network. *Archives of Disease in Childhood: Fetal and Neonatal Edition*, *103*(6), F547–F553.

Cailes, B., Kortsalioudaki, C., Buttery, J., Pattnayak, S., Greenough, A., Matthes, J., Bedford Russell, A., Kennea, N., & Heath, P. T. (2018b). Antimicrobial resistance in UK neonatal units: Neonin infection surveillance network. *Archives of Disease in Childhood: Fetal and Neonatal Edition*, *103*(5), F474–F478.

Cailes, B., Vergnano, S., Kortsalioudaki, C., Heath, P., & Sharland, M. (2015). The current and future roles of neonatal infection surveillance programmes in combating antimicrobial resistance. *Early Human Development*, *91*(11), 613–618.

Coggins, S. A., & Glaser, K. (2022). Updates in late-onset sepsis: Risk assessment, therapy, and outcomes. *NeoReviews*, *23*(11), 738–755. https://doi.org/10.1542/neo.23-10-e738

Crowley, M. A. (2024). Spectrum of neonatal respiratory disorders. In R. J. Martin, A. A. Fanaroff & M. Walsh (Eds.), *Fanaroff and Martin's neonatal-perinatal medicine: Diseases of the fetus and infant* (12th ed., pp. 1271–1303). Elsevier.

Daniels, J. P., Walker, K. F., Bradshaw, L., Dorling, J., Ohja, S., Gray, J., Thornton, J. G., Plumb, J., Petrou, S., Ayers, S., Mitchell, E., Downe, S., Grace, N., Cooper, T., Plachcinski, R., Moore, S., Jones, A.-M., Harrison, E., Brooks, J., . . . Moody, S. (2026). Universal maternal testing for group B streptococcus in late pregnancy: Process outcomes and alongside qualitative study for the GBS3 trial. *Early Human Development*, *213*, 106442. https://doi.org/10.1016/j.earlhumdev.2025.106442

Delves, P. J., & Roitt, I. M. (2000). The immune system. First of two parts. *New England Journal of Medicine*, *343*(1), 37–49.

Desai, A. P., Lim, P. P. C., Olajumoke Ogundare, M., & Gonzalez, B. E. (2024). Viral infections in the neonate. In R. J. Martin, A. A. Fanaroff & M. Walsh (Eds.), *Fanaroff and Martin's neonatal-perinatal medicine: Diseases of the fetus and infant* (12th ed., pp. 917–978). Elsevier.

Dobson, S. R. M., & Baker, C. J. (1990). Enterococcal sepsis in neonates: Features by age at onset and occurrence of focal infection. *Pediatrics*, *85*(2), 165–171. https://doi.org/10.1542/peds.85.2.165

Dong, Y., & Speer, C. P. (2015). Late-onset neonatal sepsis: Recent developments. *Archives of Disease in Childhood: Fetal and Neonatal Edition*, *100*(3), F257– F263.

Dong, Y., Speer, C. P., & Glaser, K. (2018). Beyond sepsis: Staphylococcus epidermidis is an underestimated but significant contributor to neonatal morbidity. *Virulence*, *9*(1), 621–633. https://doi.org/10.1080/21505594.2017.1419117

Ericson, J. E. (2023). Empiric therapy for neonatal sepsis. In W. E. Benitz, J. L. Wynn, P. B. Smith & R. A. Polin (Eds.), *Neonatology questions and controversies: Infectious disease, immunology and pharmacology* (2nd ed., pp. 15–24). Elsevier.

Ericson, J. E., Agthe, A. G., & Weitkamp, J.-H. (2025). Late-onset sepsis: Epidemiology, microbiology, and controversies in practice. *Clinics in Perinatology*, *52*(1), 33–45.

Ewer, A. K., Edi-Osagie, N., & Adams, E. (2024). Newborn pulse oximetry screening: Time for equity in the UK? *The Lancet*, *403*(10438), 1732–1734. https://doi.org/10.1016/S0140-6736(24)00417-3

Fernandes, G., Chappell, E., Goetghebuer, T., Kahlert, C. R., Ansone, S., Bernardi, S., Castelli Gattinara, G., Chiappini, E., Dollfus, C., Frange, P., Freyne, B., Galli, L., Giacomet, V., Grisaru-Soen, G., Königs, C., Lyall, H., Marczynska, M., Mardarescu, M., Naver, L., . . . & Bamford, A. (2025). HIV postnatal prophylaxis and infant feeding policies vary across Europe: Results of a penta survey. *HIV Medicine*, *26*(2), 207–217.

Flannery, D. D., Chiotos, K., Gerber, J. S., & Puopolo, K. M. (2022). Neonatal multidrug-resistant gram-negative infection: Epidemiology, mechanisms of resistance, and management. *Pediatric Research*, *91*(2), 380–391. https://doi.org/10.1038/s41390-021-01745-7

Flannery, D. D., Ramachandran, V., & Schrag, S. J. (2025). Neonatal early-onset sepsis. *Clinics in Perinatology*, *52*(1), 15–31. Retrieved May 23, 2025, from https://linkinghub.elsevier.com/retrieve/pii/S0095510824001027

Flynn, P. M., Taha, T. E., Cababasay, M., Fowler, M. G., Mofenson, L. M., Owor, M., Fiscus, S., Stranix-Chibanda, L., Coutsoudis, A., Gnanashanmugam, D., Chakhtoura, N., McCarthy, K., Mukuzunga, C., Makanani, B., Moodley, D., Nematadzira, T., Kusakara, B., Patil, S., Vhembo, T., . . . the PROMISE Study Team. (2018). Prevention of HIV-1 transmission through breastfeeding: Efficacy and safety of maternal antiretroviral therapy versus infant nevirapine prophylaxis for duration of breastfeeding in HIV-1-infected women with high CD4 cell count (IMPAACT PROMISE): A randomized, open-label, clinical trial. *Journal of Acquired Immune Deficiency Syndromes*, 77(4), 383–392.

Fox, G., Hoque, N., & Watts, T. (2017). *Oxford handbook of neonatology* (2nd ed.). Oxford University Press.

Gilbert, R., Brown, M., Rainford, N., Donohue, C., Fraser, C., Sinha, A., Dorling, J., Gray, J., McGuire, W., Gamble, C., Oddie, S. J., & PREVAIL Trial Team. (2019). Antimicrobial-impregnated central venous catheters for prevention of neonatal bloodstream infection (PREVAIL): An open-label, parallel-group, pragmatic, randomised controlled trial. *Lancet Child Adolesc Health*, *3*(6), 381–390. https://doi.org/10.1016/S2352-4642(19)30114-2

Goel, N., Shrestha, S., Smith, R., Mehta, A., Ketty, M., Muxworthy, H., Abelian, A., Kirupaalar, V., Saeed, S., Jain, S., Asokkumar, A., Natti, M., Barnard, I., Pitchaikani, P. K., & Banerjee, S. (2020). Screening for early onset neonatal sepsis: NICE guidance-based practice versus projected application of the Kaiser Permanente sepsis risk calculator in the UK population. *Archives of Disease in Childhood – Fetal and Neonatal Edition*, *105*(2), 118–122. Retrieved May 24, 2025, from https://doi.org/10.1136/archdischild-2018-316777

Gordon, A., Greenhalgh, M., & McGuire, W. (2017). Early planned removal of umbilical venous catheters to prevent infection in newborn infants. *Cochrane Database of Systematic Reviews*, *10*, Article CD012142. https://doi.org/10.1002/14651858.CD012142.pub2

Harvey, E. J., Ashiru-Oredope, D., Hill, L. F., Demirjian, A., Paranthaman, K., Jauneikaite, E., Wan, Y., Hope, R., Robb, A., Thorn, L., Fleming, P., Pichon, B., Ready, D., Elsayed, M., Felgate, H., Moore, G., Pattnayak, S., Ali, S., Gasiorowski, T., . . . & Patel, B. (2023). Need for standardized vancomycin dosing for coagulase-negative staphylococci in hospitalized infants. *Clinical Microbiology and Infection*, *29*(1), 10–12.

Hoffman, A., Satyavolu, S., Muhanna, D., Malay, S., Raffay, T., Windau, A., Ransom, E. M., & Mukherjee, D. (2024). Predictors of mortality and severe illness from Escherichia coli sepsis in neonates. *Journal of Perinatology*, *44*(12), 1816–1821. Retrieved May 24, 2025, from https://www.nature.com/articles/s41372-024-02117-9

Hornik, C. P., Benjamin, D. K., Becker, K. C., Benjamin, D. K., Li, J., Clark, R. H., Cohen-Wolkowiez, M., & Smith, P. B. (2012a). Use of the complete blood cell count in early-onset neonatal sepsis. *Pediatric Infectious Disease Journal*, *31*(8), 799–802.

Hornik, C. P., Benjamin, D. K., Becker, K. C., Benjamin, D. K., Li, J., Clark, R. H., Cohen-Wolkowiez, M., & Smith, P. B. (2012b). Use of the complete blood cell count in late-onset neonatal sepsis. *Pediatric Infectious Disease Journal*, *31*(8), 803–807.

Hughes, R. G., Brocklehurst, P., Steer, P. J., Heath, P., & Stenson, B. M. On behalf of the Royal College of Obstetricians and Gynaecologists. (2017). Prevention of early-onset neonatal group B streptococcal disease. Green-top guideline no. 36. *British Journal of Obstetrics and Gynaecology*, *124*(12), e280–e305.

Inglis, G. D. T., & Davies, M. W. (2005). Prophylactic antibiotics to reduce morbidity and mortality in neonates with umbilical venous catheters. *Cochrane Database of Systematic Reviews*, *4*, Article CD005251. https://doi.org/10.1002/14651858.CD005251.pub2

Inglis, G. D. T., Jardine, L. A., & Davies, M. W. (2007). Prophylactic antibiotics to reduce morbidity and mortality in neonates with umbilical artery catheters. *Cochrane Database of Systematic Reviews*, *4*, Article CD004697. https://doi.org/10.1002/14651858.CD004697.pub3

Jardine, L. A., Inglis, G. D. T., & Davies, M. W. (2008). Prophylactic systemic antibiotics to reduce morbidity and mortality in neonates with central venous catheters. *Cochrane Database of Systematic Reviews*, *1*, Article CD006179. https://doi.org/10.1002/14651858.CD006179.pub2

Johnson, J., Akinboyo, I. C., & Schaffzin, J. K. (2021). Infection prevention in the neonatal intensive care unit. *Clinics in Perinatology*, *48*(2), 413–429. Retrieved May 23, 2025, from https://linkinghub.elsevier.com/retrieve/pii/S0095510821000245

Kabani, N., & Kimberlin, D. W. (2023). Neonatal herpes simplex virus infection. In W. E. Benitz, J. L. Wynn, P. B. Smith & R. A. Polin (Eds.), *Neonatology questions and controversies: Infectious disease, immunology and pharmacology* (2nd ed., pp. 35–42). Elsevier.

Kaufman, D. A., & Mukhopadhyay, S. (2025). Neonatal invasive fungal infections. *Clinics in Perinatology*, *52*(1), 47–66. https://doi.org/10.1016/j.clp.2024.10.004

Kent, A., Kortsalioudaki, C., Monahan, I. M., Bielicki, J., Planche, T. D., Heath, P. T., & Sharland, M. (2016). Neonatal gram-negative infections, antibiotic susceptibility and clinical outcome: An observational study. *Archives of Disease in Childhood: Fetal and Neonatal Edition*, *101*(6), F507– F512.

Kilpatrick, R., Scarrow, E., Hornik, C., & Greenberg, R. G. (2022). Neonatal invasive candidiasis: Updates on clinical management and prevention. *The Lancet Child & Adolescent Health*, *6*(1), 60–70.

Klemme, M., Staffler, A., De Maio, N., Lauseker, M., Schubert, S., Innocenti, P., Wurster, T. M., Foerster, K., Herber-Jonat, S., Mittal, R., Messner, H., & Flemmer, A. W. (2020). Use of impregnated catheters to decrease colonization rates in neonates – A randomized controlled pilot trial. *Journal of Neonatal-Perinatal Medicine*, *13*(2), 231–237. Retrieved July 18, 2025, from https://doi.org/10.3233/NPM-190273

Klingenberg, C., Kornelisse, R. F., Buonocore, G., Maier, R. F., & Stocker, M. (2018). Culture-negative early-onset neonatal sepsis – At the crossroad between efficient sepsis care and antimicrobial stewardship. *Frontiers in Pediatrics*, *6*, 285. Retrieved May 24, 2025, from https://www.frontiersin.org/article/10.3389/fped.2018.00285/full

Lai, N., Taylor, J. E., Tan, K., Choo, Y., Ahmad Kamar, A., & Muhamad, N. (2016). Antimicrobial dressings for the prevention of catheter-related infections in newborn infants with central venous catheters. *Cochrane Database of Systematic Reviews*, *3*, Article CD011082. https://doi.org/10.1002/14651858.CD011082.pub2

McDermott, J. H., Mahood, R., Stoddard, D., Mahaveer, A., Turner, M. A., Corry, R., Garlick, J., Miele, G., Ainsworth, S., Kemp, L., Bruce, I., Body, R., Ulph, F., Macleod, R., Harvey, K., Booth, N., Roberts, P., Wilson, P., & Newman, W. G. (2021). Pharmacogenetics to Avoid Loss of Hearing (Paloh) trial: A protocol for a prospective observational implementation trial. *BMJ Open*, *11*(6), e044457. https://doi.org/10.1136/bmjopen-2020-044457

McGann, C., Phyu, R., Bittinger, K., & Mukhopadhyay, S. (2025). Role of the microbiome in neonatal infection. *Clinics in Perinatology*, *52*(1), 147–166. Retrieved July 18, 2025, from https://linkinghub.elsevier.com/retrieve/pii/S0095510824001106

Melville, J. M., & Moss, T. J. M. (2013). The immune consequences of preterm birth. *Frontiers in Neuroscience*, 7. Retrieved May 23, 2025, from http://journal.frontiersin.org/article/10.3389/fnins.2013.00079/abstract

Mukherjee, D., & Ryan, R. M. (2024). Postnatal bacterial infections. In R. J. Martin, A. A. Fanaroff & M. Walsh (Eds.), *Fanaroff and Martin's neonatal-perinatal medicine: Diseases of the fetus and infant* (12th ed., pp. 857–880). Elsevier.

National Institute for Health and Care Excellence. (2016). *Sepsis: Recognition, diagnosis and early management*. NICE.

National Institute for Health and Care Excellence. (2021). *Neonatal infection: Antibiotics for prevention and treatment*. NICE Guideline NG195. NICE.

Oeser, C., Pond, M., Butcher, P., Bedford Russell, A., Henneke, P., Laing, K., Planche, T., Heath, P. T., & Harris, K. (2020). PCR for the detection of pathogens in neonatal early onset sepsis. *PLoS ONE*, *15*(1), e0226817. https://doi.org/10.1371/journal.pone.0226817

Payne, V., Hall, M., Prieto, J., & Johnson, M. (2018). Care bundles to reduce central line-associated bloodstream infections in the neonatal unit: A systematic review and meta-analysis. *Archives of Disease in Childhood – Fetal and Neonatal Edition*, *103*(5), F422–F429. Retrieved May 23, 2025, from https://fn.bmj.com/lookup/doi/10.1136/archdischild-2017-313362

Permar, S. R., & Salvatore, C. M. (2023). When and how to treat neonatal CMV infection. In W. E. Benitz, J. L. Wynn, P. B. Smith & R. A. Polin (Eds.), *Neonatology questions and controversies: Infectious disease, immunology and pharmacology* (2nd ed., pp. 25–34). Elsevier.

Pharande, P., Lindrea, K. B., Smyth, J., Evans, M., Lui, K., & Bolisetty, S. (2018). Trends in late-onset sepsis in a neonatal intensive care unit following implementation of infection control bundle: A 15-year audit. *Journal of Paediatrics and Child Health*, *54*(12), 1314–1320.

Plotkin, S. A., & Boppana, S. B. (2019). Vaccination against the human cytomegalovirus. *Vaccine*, *37*(50), 7437–7442.

Rao, S. C., Srinivasjois, R., & Moon, K. (2016). One dose per day compared to multiple doses per day of gentamicin for treatment of suspected or proven sepsis in neonates. *Cochrane Database of Systematic Reviews*, *12*(12), CD005091. https://doi.org/10.1002/14651858.CD005091.pub4

Reynolds, A. J., Campbell, R., Doherty, L., Boyle, M., Kaptai, G., Chalker, V., Lindsay, D., Smith, A., Davies, E., Jones, C. E., & Heath, P. T. (2019). Group B streptococcal disease in UK and Irish infants younger than 90 days, 201–15: A prospective surveillance study. *The Lancet Infectious Diseases*, *19*(1), 83–90. https://https://doi.org/10.1016/S1473-3099(18)30555-3

Russell, N. J., Seale, A. C., O'Driscoll, M., O'Sullivan, C., Bianchi-Jassir, F., Gonzalez-Guarin, J., Lawn, J. E., Baker, C. J., Bartlett, L., Cutland, C., Gravett, M. G., Heath, P. T., Le Doare, K., Madhi, S. A., Rubens, C. E., Schrag, S., Sobanjo-Ter Meulen, A., Vekemans, J., Saha, S. K., & Ip, M., GBS Maternal Colonization Investigator Group. (2017). Maternal colonization with group B streptococcus and serotype distribution worldwide: Systematic review and meta-analyses. *Clinical Infectious Diseases*, *65*(suppl_2), S100–S111. Retrieved May 23, 2025, from https://academic.oup.com/cid/article/65/suppl_2/S100/4589589

Sands, K., Spiller, O. B., Thomson, K., Portal, E. A., Iregbu, K. C., & Walsh, T. R. (2022). Early-onset neonatal sepsis in low- and middle-income countries: Current challenges and future opportunities. *Infection and Drug Resistance*, *15*, 933–946. Retrieved May 23, 2025, from https://www.dovepress.com/early-onset-neonatal-sepsis-in-low-and-middle-income-countries-curren-peer-reviewed-fulltext-article-IDR

Schüller, S. S., Kramer, B. W., Villamor, E., Spittler, A., Berger, A., & Levy, O. (2018). Immunomodulation to prevent or treat neonatal sepsis: Past, present, and future. *Frontiers in Pediatrics*, *6*, 199. https://doi.org/10.3389/fped.2018.00199

Seale, A. C., & Agarwal, R. (2018). Improving management of neonatal infections. *The Lancet*, *392*(10142), 100–102.

Seale, A. C., Bianchi-Jassir, F., Russell, N. J., Kohli-Lynch, M., Tann, C. J., Hall, J., Madrid, L., Blencowe, H., Cousens, S., Baker, C. J., Bartlett, L., Cutland, C., Gravett, M. J., Heath, P. T., Ip, M., Le Doare, K., Madhi, S. A., Rubens, C. E., Saha, S. K., . . ., & Lawn, J. E. (2017). Estimates of the burden of group B streptococcal disease worldwide for pregnant women, stillbirths, and children. *Clinical Infectious Diseases*, *65*(suppl_2), S200–S219. Retrieved May 24, 2025, from https://academic.oup.com/cid/article/65/suppl_2/S200/4589594

Shane, A. L., Sánchez, P. J., & Stoll, B. J. (2017). Neonatal sepsis. *The Lancet*, *390*, 1770–1780.

Sharif, S., Meader, N., Oddie, S. J., Rojas-Reyes, M. X., & McGuire, W. (2023). Probiotics to prevent necrotising enterocolitis in very preterm or very low birth weight infants. *Cochrane Database of Systematic Reviews*, *2023*(7). https://doi.org/10.1002/14651858.CD005496.pub6

Stark, A., Crooks, C. M., Permar, S. R., & Dew Weimer, K. E. (2025). Neonatal cytomegalovirus infection. *Clinics in Perinatology*, *52*(1), 115–132.

Stocker, M., Fillistorf, L., & Giannoni, E. (2023). Clinical and molecular markers to assist decision-making in neonatal sepsis. In W. E. Benitz, J. L. Wynn, P. B. Smith & R. A. Polin (Eds.), *Neonatology questions and controversies: Infectious disease, immunology and pharmacology* (2nd ed., pp. 243–257). Elsevier.

Sullivan, B. A., Kausch, S. L., & Fairchild, K. D. (2023). Artificial and human intelligence for early identification of neonatal sepsis. *Pediatric Research*, *93*(2), 350–356. https://doi.org/10.1038/s41390-022-02274-7

UK Health Security Agency. (2021). Immunity and how vaccines work: The green book (chap. 1). In M. Ramsay (Ed.), *Immunisation against infectious disease*. https://assets.publishing.service.gov.uk/media/5ff49153d3bf7f65de80157d/Greenbook_chapter_1_Jan21.pdf

UK Health Security Agency. (2022). *Good IPC practice for the cleaning and handling of incubators and other equipment in neonatal units*. UK Health Security Agency. Retrieved April 24, 2025, from https://www.gov.uk/government/publications/infection-prevention-and-control-incubators-on-neonatal-units/good-ipc-practice-for-the-cleaning-and-handling-of-incubators-and-other-equipment-in-neonatal-units

UK Health Security Agency. (2023a). *Start smart then focus: Antimicrobial stewardship toolkit for inpatient care settings*. UK Health Security Agency. Retrieved March 20, 2025, from https://www.gov.uk/government/publications/antimicrobial-stewardship-start-smart-then-focus/start-smart-then-focus-antimicrobial-stewardship-toolkit-for-inpatient-care-settings

UK Health Security Agency. (2023b). *Staphylococcus capitis: guidance, data and analysis: Findings from a 2021 to 2022 incident response by the UK Health Security Agency to Staphylococcus Capitis in UK neonatal units*. UK Health Security Agency. Retrieved March 24, 2025, from https://www.gov.uk/government/collections/staphylococcus-capitis-guidance-data-and-analysis

UK Health Security Agency. (2025). Respiratory syncytial virus: The green book (chap. 27a). In M. Ramsay (Ed.), *Immunisation against infectious disease*. Retrieved January 28, 2026 from https://assets.publishing.service.gov.uk/media/686fbfcf2557debd867cbf9d/Green_Book_Chapter27a_RSV_14July2025.pdf

UK National Screening Committee. (2017). *UK NSC group B streptococcus (GBS) recommendation*. Retrieved March 20, 2025, from legacyscreening.phe.org.uk/policydb_download.php?doc=688

van Hasselt, T. J., McDermott, H., Surana, P., Eltahir, R., Macaskill, L., Jain, R., McMullan, N., Slee, S., Jagga, M., Naseem, M., Alake, O., Cherry, C., Miguras, B., & Ewer, A. K. (2021). Impact of neonatal sepsis calculator in West Midlands (UK). *Archives of Disease in Childhood – Fetal and Neonatal Edition*, *106*(5), 568–569.

Williams, M. (2018). RCOG guidance: Early-onset neonatal GBS disease. *Prescriber*, *29*(1), 34–36.

World Health Organization. (2020). *Global report on the epidemiology and burden of sepsis. Current evidence, identifying gaps and future directions*. World Health Organization.

World Health Organization. (2021). *Group B Streptococcus vaccine: Policy and implementation issues* (1st ed.). World Health Organization.

World Health Organizaton. (2025). *Global HIV, hepatitis and STIs programmes. Pregnant and lactating women and girls*. Retrieved March 26, 2025, from https://www.who.int/teams/global-hiv-hepatitis-and-stis-programmes/populations/pregnant-and-lactating-women-and-girls

Yanni, M., Stark, M., Francis, L., Francis, J. R., McMillan, M., Baird, R., Heath, P. T., Gordon, A., Riccardione, J., Wilson, A., Lee, R., Chooi, K., Quinn, O.-P., & Marshall, H. S. (2023). Neonatal group B streptococcal infection in Australia: A case–control study. *Pediatric Infectious Disease Journal*, *42*(5), 429–435. Retrieved May 24, 2025, from https://journals.lww.com/10.1097/INF.0000000000003881

Ziprin, J., Ben-Sasi, K., Ferretti, L., Panagiotopoulou, E., Geer, D., Dominguez, S. F., Anthony, L., Naidu, H., Wong, A., Chow, L., & Tho-Calvi, S. (2021). 1226 The safe implementation of the kaiser permanente sepsis risk calculator in 4 neonatal units. *Abstracts* (pp. A282.1–A282). BMJ Publishing Group Ltd and Royal College of Paediatrics and Child Health. Retrieved May 24, 2025, from https://adc.bmj.com/lookup/doi/10.1136/archdischild-2021-rcpch.490

PART 4

PRACTICES AND PROCEDURES IN NEONATAL CARE

DOI: 10.4324/9781003591405-25

21 MEDICATION PRACTICE IN THE NEONATAL UNIT

Peter Venables

CONTENTS

DOI: 10.4324/9781003591405-26

GUIDANCE ON HOW TO ENHANCE PERSONAL LEARNING FROM THIS CHAPTER

Key points covered in this chapter

- Neonatal pharmacokinetics impacting on medication practice.
- The nurse's role in all important aspects of neonatal drug administration.
- The factors for consideration in relation to minimising risk and ensuring safety in neonates who require drugs.

Reflection

Reading through the chapter, you are encouraged to engage with the key points and related literature in an enquiring way. Ask these questions:

- Do you understand your role in relation to safe drug administration for infants in neonatal care?
- What are neonatal-specific considerations in this area of practice?
- Are you aware of the latest guidance relating to neonatal drugs and administration?

Implications for nursing care

- Finally: consider the implications of what you learn for your nursing care relating to neonatal medication practice.

INTRODUCTION AND BACKGROUND

The aim of medication therapy in the newborn is to administer a given drug at a given dose to achieve a desired therapeutic effect, with the minimum risk of toxicity. However, this is a complex issue, as neonates are a very diverse group comprising wide gestational and postnatal age and weight ranges, which requires individualised dosing with drugs that lack data for the neonatal population. There is great variability in how drugs act and how they exert their desired therapeutic effect in this population, what with maturational changes and illness, as well as interventions such as therapeutic hypothermia (TH; Ruggiero et al., 2019). In term and preterm neonates this knowledge and acute awareness is essential for effective, safe drug administration and also predictable drug responses.

The risks of toxicity are high, as demonstrated by numerous historical examples, and medication errors remain a major concern. It is estimated that approximately 65% of the drugs used in Neonatal Units (NNUs) are off-label and require dose optimisation before administration. However, drug therapy is vital in the contribution to improved neonatal outcomes, and decisions about the use of appropriate drugs should be tailored to the specific needs of neonates (Bansal et al., 2023). Having an understanding and appreciation of the complex relationships and interactions between drugs and the body enables neonatal nurses to improve care and reduce risks by being aware of the impact of drugs in these vulnerable patients. This chapter will provide a concise summary of the above pharmacological issues, relating them back to the basic principles and definitions of this discipline.

PHARMACODYNAMICS

Pharmacodynamics is a branch of pharmacology that explores how drugs affect the body by studying the mechanisms of drug action and the relationship between drug concentration and effect. It comprises various processes such as receptor binding, interactions and post-receptor effects; factors that are all crucial in optimising therapeutic treatment strategies (Ritter et al., 2024).

PHARMACOKINETICS

Pharmacokinetics (PK) is a category of pharmacology that relates to the administration of a drug into the body. The drug's effect is then determined by its **a**bsorption, **d**istribution, **m**etabolism and **e**xcretion (ADME; Ritter et al., 2024).

Effective and safe drug administration in neonates is based on current knowledge of the physiological characteristics of the infant and the PK profile of a given drug. In neonatology, PK principles observed in adult medicine cannot be extrapolated, as there is such variability within and between neonates secondary to varying gestational ages (GAs), but also rapid physiological and maturational changes (Van den Anker et al., 2018). The latter include alterations in body composition, fluid distribution, hepato-renal function and the expression of drug-metabolising enzymes. These components are outlined in Table 21.1. Underlying pathological processes such as infection, growth restriction and organ dysfunction, as well as some interventions inpatients of the NNU undergo, such as concomitant medication administration, surgery, TH or extracorporeal membrane

TABLE 21.1 NEONATAL PHARMACOKINETICS

Pharmacokinetic component	*Neonatal considerations*
Absorption of drugs	Decreased absorption: Oral route: increased gastric pH decreases bioavailability, delayed gastric emptying, decreased bile concentrations. Intramuscular route: decreased muscle mass results in variable absorption Increased absorption: Transdermal route: ■ Increased permeability ■ Increased surface area to weight
Distribution of drugs	Increased total body water: increased volume of distribution for water soluble drugs Decreased fat: increased plasma concentration for fat-soluble drugs Decreased plasma proteins and binding ability: increased plasma concentration of free drug Increased permeability of blood–brain barrier: increased uptake of unbound drugs to brain
Metabolism of drugs	Decreased phase 1 and 2 hepatic enzymes: decreased biotransformation of drugs This is exacerbated by: ■ Prematurity ■ Serious illness ■ Genetic variation ■ Interventions, i.e. therapeutic hypothermia
Excretion of drugs	Decreased glomerular filtration rate and tubular excretion: ■ Decreased excretion of water-soluble drugs ■ Increased half-life for most drugs This is exacerbated by: ■ Prematurity ■ Serious illness ■ Drugs e.g. Aminoglycosides, ACE inhibitors, NSAIDs

oxygenation, are additional complicating factors (Allegaert et al., 2017; Van den Anker et al., 2018; Bansal et al., 2023).

Absorption of drugs

Absorption is the movement of a drug from its administration site into the bloodstream, and the route of administration determines its **bioavailability** (how available the drug is to the circulation). Intravenous (IV) drugs require no absorption and have 100% bioavailability (Ritter et al., 2024). The extent of enteral absorption of a drug is determined by gastric pH and the rate of gastric emptying. At birth, infants have a gastric pH that is near neutral and have immature acid secretion. Together, this results in decreased absorption of weakly acidic drugs such as phenobarbital and phenytoin. In preterm infants, this initially high pH is sustained for a prolonged period. With increasing maturity and postnatal age (PNA), the gastric pH decreases. Delayed gastric emptying in neonates allows more extensive absorption of some drugs because of greater diffusion through the stomach wall. Drugs normally absorbed through the small intestine will have delayed onset. Human milk appears to increase gastric transit time (Bennett, 2014; Bansal et al., 2023). Delayed gastric emptying is most apparent in preterm infants, those on high caloric feeds and in severe illness (Anderson, 2017).

Oral drugs such as propranolol, morphine and midazolam are absorbed in the small intestine after first being metabolised in the liver resulting in a drug with less predictable effects. Decreased secretion of bile acids, and the lack of flora in the gut at birth, reduces fat absorption. There is consequently decreased absorption of fat-soluble drugs such as vitamin A and D (Bansal et al., 2023). These factors result in a slow time to peak concentrations of orally administered drugs, and these effects are more pronounced in the most immature (Bennett, 2014). Gastro-oesophageal reflux disease (GORD) can also affect the absorption of oral drugs (Rossor et al., 2018).

Distribution of drugs

The process of distribution occurs after absorption and is the movement of the drug from the intravascular space to the extravascular compartments where it can be utilised (Bansal et al., 2023). It influences efficacy and duration of action.

VOLUME OF DISTRIBUTION

The volume in which the drug is distributed in the body is called the volume of distribution (V_D), and it depends on the amount of body water and fat components. Neonates have increased membrane permeability and have a higher proportion of total body water than children or adults; 80% at birth vs. 60% in adults, with preterm infants having up to 85% (Anderson, 2017). Because of this, neonates need higher doses per kg of weight for water-soluble drugs such as gentamicin, which is widely distributed throughout the body (i.e. has a large V_D) compared to older children (Ainsworth, 2020). The proportion of body water decreases rapidly over the first week, therefore the dose of water-soluble drugs, must be decreased to prevent toxicity (Bennett, 2014). It is important to note that **lipophilic** drugs (agents that have a high affinity for lipids and fats) have a relatively larger volume of distribution (Ritter et al., 2024).

The percentage of fat in neonates is much less than in adults, with a term baby having around 12% body fat, but a 1.5kg baby only 3%. Drugs which rely on redistribution to fat, such as fentanyl, will have a prolonged and higher plasma concentration (Anderson, 2017).

HALF-LIFE

Half-life ($t_{1/2}$) is the period of time required for a drug's concentration in the body's serum to be reduced by half. It depends on the V_D and the clearance or elimination of the drug. Half-life also determines the time a drug reaches a **steady state** and is used to ascertain appropriate drug dosing intervals (Bansal et al., 2023). This pharmacological concept can be demonstrated by the drug adenosine, which is used for supraventricular tachycardia. Adenosine has a half-life of less than 10 seconds. This means it must be given very quickly, before it is inactivated. It should, therefore, be administered intravenously via an upper limb, so it reaches the site of action, the sino-atrial node, where it exerts its effect by slowing conduction to the atrioventricular node. Other drugs including dobutamine, dopamine and noradrenaline have half-lives of around 5–10 minutes and need to be given by continuous infusion. In contrast, phenobarbital has a half-life of 2–4 days in newborns, and caffeine has an even longer half-life of 2.5–6 days (Ainsworth, 2020). With such long half-lives, these drugs are prescribed only once daily. Therefore, the longer the half-life, the longer the drug takes to be eliminated, and the less often it needs to be given (Ritter et al., 2024).

The changes in drug dosing with increasing PNA and improving renal function reflects the changes in half-life, and this can be demonstrated by the commonly used antibiotic cefotaxime. Its half-life is inversely related to GA. It is recommended the drug be given 12-hourly in the first 6 days, then 8-hourly between 7 and 20 days, then 6–8-hourly after this (Paediatric Formulary Committee, 2024).

STEADY STATE

'Steady state' is an important concept of PK. Administration of a large first dose (loading dose) results in steady state being rapidly reached, where the amount of the drug administered in each new dose equals the amount eliminated since the last dose. Generally, steady state is reached in approximately 5 half-lives of the drug (Ritter et al., 2024). With some medicines, such as caffeine and phenobarbital, the time taken for five half-lives to elapse would take too long, potentially causing significant delays in their therapeutic efficacy. In this case, a **loading dose** ensures that the desired effect is achieved more rapidly (Van den Anker & Allegaert, 2021; Bansal et al., 2023).

The subsequent smaller maintenance doses, determined by a drug's clearance and its half-life, are used to keep the drug plasma concentration at therapeutic levels (Ritter et al., 2024). Interval and dosage of maintenance doses are furthermore quantified with the aim of avoiding potential side effects (Bansal et al., 2023).

BLOOD–BRAIN BARRIER

The blood–brain barrier (BBB) mediates the transport of nutrients into, and toxic **metabolites** out of, the central nervous system (CNS). However, the BBB is more permeable in neonates compared to adults, and its integrity is reduced further by severe illness. This immaturity results in faster morphine uptake into the CNS and may be responsible for the increased sensitivity of the neonate to morphine (Anderson, 2017).

PLASMA PROTEIN BINDING

Protein binding affects the V_D of drugs and so how the drug is distributed throughout the body. Unbound drugs are able to exert their effect, whereas drugs bound to proteins cannot (Ritter et al., 2024). However, plasma proteins such as albumin are decreased in neonates, and they have less binding ability compared to adults. This lower protein binding of drugs means there is greater free drug concentration and therefore, greater drug effects (Anderson, 2017). This is predominantly relevant for medicines which are highly protein bound and have a narrow therapeutic range, such as phenytoin (Van den Anker et al., 2018).

Protein-bound drugs such as ceftriaxone can displace bilirubin from albumin, potentially increasing the risk of bilirubin-induced neurotoxicity (kernicterus), as unbound bilirubin crosses the BBB (Amin & Wang, 2018). The administration of sulphonamide antibiotics has been associated with a higher incidence of kernicterus, and it was later found that this was due to the marked ability of these drugs to displace bilirubin from albumin (Lee et al., 2023). Contrarily, hyperbilirubinemia reduces the binding of acidic drugs such as ampicillin, phenobarbital and phenytoin.

Preterm infants below 30 weeks' gestation are at higher risk of kernicterus at lower concentrations of bilirubin than term infants, because they have a decreased ability to bind bilirubin as well as lower albumin levels (Amin & Wang, 2018). Ibuprofen displaces bilirubin from albumin, but clinically significant displacement in preterm infants is unlikely if used at the recommended dosage and the serum albumin level is normal. Intralipids can also displace bilirubin, and evidence suggests that intake should be limited in babies under 28 weeks in the first week of life when unconjugated levels of bilirubin are high. Routine measurements of albumin levels in preterm infants below 34 weeks with elevated unconjugated bilirubin levels and consideration of treatment at lower bilirubin levels when other risk factors for bilirubin displacement, such as hypoxia, acidosis or sepsis are also present, have been recommended (Lee et al., 2023).

Metabolism of drugs

The liver is the main organ for the metabolism of drugs. Metabolism mainly occurs through hepatic enzymes transforming drugs to a water-soluble form for excretion in the urine or to render the drug inactive or weaker (Ritter et al., 2024). Hepatic enzymes metabolise drugs via phase 1 or phase 2 reactions, with both involving a variety of metabolic pathways. These all mature at different rates and are furthermore impacted by genetic and environmental components (Bansal et al., 2023).

PHASE 1 REACTIONS

Phase 1 reactions are important for the metabolic transformation (biotransformation) of most drugs and alter the structure of the drug by a variety of chemical reactions such as oxidation, reduction or hydroxylation (Ritter et al., 2024). An important group of enzymes involved in phase 1 reactions include the **cytochrome** P450 (CYP450) system, which is made up of a number of enzymes, although not all are present at birth, and their activity is reduced compared to adults. Individual enzymes mature at different rates, and the most important, CYP3A4 isoenzyme, metabolises more than 50% of all drugs. Its activity is very low in neonates and does not reach adult levels for several weeks (Bansal et al., 2023). For example, the clearance of midazolam is prolonged particularly in the preterm infant because of reduced CYP3A4 activity (Anderson, 2017). Some drugs, such as the antibiotic erythromycin, inhibit individual CYP enzymes, while others, including phenobarbital, dexamethasone and phenytoin, induce multiple enzymes (Bansal et al., 2023). Reduced phase 1 enzymes can also have paradoxical effects as demonstrated by the metabolism of paracetamol. Paracetamol normally breaks down to the toxic metabolite NAPQ1 which is excreted but will cause hepatotoxicity if produced in large amounts. However, neonates are less prone to liver toxicity from paracetamol overdose than older children and adults, because they have reduced levels of the phase 1 enzyme necessary to convert paracetamol to NAPQ1 (Anderson, 2017).

PHASE 2 REACTIONS

Phase 2 reactions (which include acetylation, methylation, glucuronidation and sulphation) are mediated by enzymes such as glutathione S-transferase and N-acetyltransferase. They convert lipid-soluble drugs to water-soluble compounds by conjugation (attachment) of the drug to a molecule, enabling it to be excreted by the kidneys. The different phase 2 reactions mature at variable rates, some quite slowly, and reach adult levels at around 2 years. Examples of the implications of this immaturity are demonstrated by a number of drugs. In the 1950s, the antimicrobial chloramphenicol was commonly used, until several infants presented with cardiovascular collapse and the so-called 'grey baby syndrome.' This was due to toxic levels of the drug because of a lack of a phase 2 enzyme, which normally metabolises chloramphenicol (Bansal et al., 2023). The phase 2 pathway that converts morphine to its metabolites (a process called glucuronidation) is also reduced in neonates, so clearance is lower, and the risk of toxicity is increased. There is a rapid increase in metabolism from 27 weeks' gestation, necessitating a corresponding increase in the dose to maintain sedation (Anderson, 2017).

OTHER FACTORS THAT AFFECT DRUG METABOLISM

Variation in genes involved in drug metabolism may result in increased or decreased drug metabolism. Certain genetic mutations have been linked to sensitivity to ototoxic aminoglycosides, and these individuals are at high risk of bilateral deafness if treated with aminoglycosides, even when therapeutic blood levels are normal (Ritter et al., 2024). CYP enzyme activity is reduced by serious illness, and this can decrease elimination of some drugs, resulting in accumulation and possible toxicity (Allegaert et al., 2017). Many drugs metabolised by liver enzymes are temperature-dependent, therefore TH can lead to a lack of action for some drugs and accumulation of others, so that usual drug doses may need to be adjusted (Ainsworth, 2020; Bansal et al., 2023).

The delayed clearance of some drugs has been seen with increased intra-abdominal pressure after exomphalos repair for example, and this is thought to be due to reduced hepatic blood flow from regions of CYP450 activity (Anderson, 2017).

Bacterial colonisation of the intestines has consequences too in terms of drug metabolism, as demonstrated with the excretion of digoxin by inactivation if this is altered or undergoes maturational changes (Pacifici, 2021).

THINK POINT

Ethnic background can influence pharmacokinetics because genetic variations affect how efficiently certain enzymes metabolise medications. A clear example is codeine, which relies on the CYP2D6 enzyme for conversion into its active form. Some populations have a higher proportion of *ultra-rapid metabolisers*, while others have more *poor metabolisers*, meaning the same dose can lead to either unexpectedly strong effects or very little therapeutic benefit. For neonatal nurses, this highlights why close observation of each infant's response is essential, even when dosing follows standard guidelines.

Excretion of drugs

The major pathway for drug excretion is via the kidneys. However, this is dependent on glomerular filtration rate (GFR), which is the rate at which blood is filtered through the kidney. GFR is around 30% of adult levels in the newborn and even lower in preterm infants. GFR is also reduced by serious illness and the use of drugs such as ibuprofen that cause hypoperfusion (Bansal et al., 2023). It increases over the first few weeks of life and reaches 50% of adult levels at 3 months, but takes longer in extremely preterm babies (Anderson, 2017). Nephron development is not complete until around 36 weeks gestational age (Bennett, 2014) and kidney tubules are also immature. Therefore, the half-life of many drugs is prolonged, as they require longer to be eliminated. As such, gentamicin dosing must reflect the changes in GFR and tubular maturity that occur with increasing gestational and postnatal age (Ainsworth, 2020). Conversely, the evolution of renal tubular transport mechanisms also influences the elimination of drugs as demonstrated by digoxin, which is extensively excreted within the tubular cell. Neonates therefore require higher doses of digoxin per kg body weight than adults (Pacifici, 2021). Hypothermia induces vasoconstriction, which reduces GFR and therefore, elimination of drugs requiring renal clearance. Since neonates requiring TH often already have renal impairment, dosages for drugs excreted via the kidney will require adjustment to prevent toxicity (Ainsworth, 2020). Other drugs with decreased clearance during TH include phenobarbital, which requires doses to be adjusted according to serum levels, and atracurium, which is titrated according to response (Paediatric Formulary Committee, 2024).

ACTIVITY

Choose one commonly used neonatal drug (e.g. gentamicin, caffeine or phenobarbital) and map out its pharmacokinetics in neonates; covering absorption, distribution, metabolism and excretion. Then, identify how nursing practice ensures safe administration and monitoring for that drug.

WHAT IS THE DIFFERENCE BETWEEN A DRUG AND A MEDICINE?

The terms 'drug' and 'medicine' are frequently used interchangeably in pharmacy practice, as their meanings often overlap. A drug is defined as a substance that affects the body's function, whether for therapeutic use or not; it is the active component responsible for producing the intended effect. In contrast, medicine refers to a formulated product that contains both the active substance and excipients designed for patient administration (Ritter et al., 2024).

ROUTES OF DRUG ADMINISTRATION

A drug's route of administration refers to the pathway through which it enters the body for diagnosis, prevention, treatment or cure of various diseases and disorders. To achieve its intended therapeutic effect, the drug must interact with organ tissues and cells, which requires appropriate administration. The available administration routes are broadly classified into local and systemic categories. The local route, being the simplest, delivers the drug directly to the site where its action is needed. When systemic absorption is required, drugs are commonly administered via two primary routes: enteral and parenteral. The chosen administration method significantly influences the drug's bioavailability, affecting both its onset and duration of effect (Ritter et al., 2024).

Selecting the appropriate administration route is determined by various factors, including convenience, the drug's characteristics (e.g. insulin is only effective through the parenteral route), pharmacokinetic properties (e.g. gastric pH, digestive enzymes and first pass metabolism), the patient's condition and the required onset of action. Administering drugs to neonates can present additional challenges (O'Brien et al., 2019; Bansal et al., 2023).

- *Buccal:* Drugs are absorbed through the **buccal** membrane in neonates, but this results in uneven absorption and inability to control the dosage (O'Brien et al., 2019). One drug that is very effective via this route is glucose gel, a quick-acting carbohydrate for the treatment of hypoglycaemia. It is massaged into the cheek's mucosa and is absorbed rapidly through the buccal membrane into the systemic circulation (Ainsworth, 2020).
- *Oral*: Once absorbed, oral drugs pass through the hepatic portal system and are metabolised in the liver before they reach the systemic circulation to exert their effects. This mechanism is called 'first pass metabolism'; most oral drugs undergo this. However, if this is extensive, the drug will have a lower concentration in the blood and therefore, lower bioavailability (O'Brien et al., 2019). Oral drugs have poor bioavailability in the newborn.

Caffeine is an exception as it is completely absorbed orally with almost no first pass metabolism (Ainsworth, 2020). Oral drugs are drawn up using enteral syringes and then administered into the mouth slowly while waiting for the baby to swallow or via a gastric tube. The practical problems associated with oral administration in newborns include vomiting after a dose and residual volumes of the drug remaining in gastric tubes if these are not fully flushed (Bennett, 2014).

- *Inhalation:* Inhaled budesonide, a corticosteroid, for the prevention of bronchopulmonary dysplasia (BPD) in extremely preterm newborns, had become popular in the late 2000s. However, a Cochrane review found no evidence that budesonide reduced BPD compared to systemic steroids, although there were fewer adverse effects (Shah et al., 2017). Numerous factors such as equipment used affect drug delivery into the lungs, and the amount of aerosol delivered can be less than 14% (Ainsworth, 2020).
- *Intratracheal*: The classic example of an intratracheally administrated drug is pulmonary surfactant. Surfactants include beractant (Survanta) or poractant alfa (Curosurf) and are used for preterm infants with surfactant-deficient lung disease (respiratory distress syndrome) and in those with meconium aspiration where surfactant is inactivated. In recent times, non-invasive techniques of surfactant administration have been incorporated in neonatal care. With the INSURE (**In**tubation – **Sur**factant – **E**xtubation) method, the baby is intubated, usually after a small dose of morphine or fentanyl and the dose injected into the endotracheal tube (ETT), followed by extubation. The tube used to inject the drug should not protrude beyond the end of the ETT, or only one lung will receive the surfactant. The now preferred technique of inserting a fine-bore tube through the vocal cords to administer surfactant while the baby remains on non-invasive respiratory support is known as LISA (**L**ess **I**nvasive **S**urfactant **A**dministration). In this scenario, surfactant is injected directly via the catheter which is then removed. Sedation is not always given with this technique (Niemarkt et al., 2017).
- *Percutaneous:* Percutaneous absorption of a drug is related to surface area and the thickness of the stratum corneum. Neonates, and in particular extremely preterm infants, have a high surface area to weight ratio and a thinner stratum corneum compared to older children and adults. This increase in water content and the high ratio between body surface and weight results in greater absorption through the skin into the systemic circulation and can result in toxicity (O'Brien et al., 2019). For example, the use of hexachlorophene in infant bathing products resulted in neurotoxicity and death in a number of infants in France and the United States in the 1970s (Bansal et al., 2023). More recently, iodine-containing skin cleansing

solutions have been associated with hypothyroidism in babies of less than 32 weeks (Aitken & Williams, 2014). Chlorhexidine skin disinfection prior to umbilical and central line placement in newborns under 32 weeks has been shown to result in chlorhexidine in the bloodstream of neonates, of which the long-term effects are not known. The other main risk is skin damage from contact dermatitis and burns (Neonatal and Paediatric Pharmacists Group (NPPG) and British Association of Perinatal Medicine (BAPM), 2024).

An example of topical administration that does work well is tetracaine gel (Ametop 4%), a local anaesthetic, recommended for use in neonates from one month old. The entire contents of the tube (1.5g) is applied to the skin 30 minutes prior to a procedure such as cannulation or lumbar puncture and an occlusive dressing applied. The gel should only be applied to a small area of skin (around 5cm by 5cm, and it must be wiped off before the procedure; Ainsworth, 2020).

- *Subcutaneous:* This is rarely used in neonates due to the lack of subcutaneous tissue and variable perfusion (Bansal et al., 2023).
- *Intramuscular:* This is used less commonly in neonates because they have little muscle mass and a poorer blood supply to muscle, making absorption unpredictable with variable times to the onset of action and peak concentrations. However, this slow absorption is ideal for vitamin K administration at birth, as it provides slow release over a few months, protecting the infant from haemorrhagic disease of the newborn (Bennett, 2014). Vaccines are given via the intramuscular (IM) route, as there is less tissue injury than in subcutaneous administration, and IM injections induce an immune response. However, this route of administration should not be used in babies who have a risk of bleeding i.e. those with thrombocytopaenia (Ainsworth, 2020). Absorption is also influenced by the pH, molecular weight and solubility of the actual drug e.g. water-soluble drugs have higher IM absorption in neonates (Ruggiero et al., 2019). The only safe site for IM administration in neonates is the anterior aspect of the quadriceps muscle, as the buttocks do not have enough muscle mass. The needle should be inserted well into the muscle and the plunger withdrawn to ensure a blood vessel has not been entered (Ainsworth, 2020).
- *Intravenous*: Although IV administration eliminates variables associated with other routes, the infusion of a drug via a lower limb vein or a low umbilical venous catheter can result in reduction of the active drug entering the circulation, because it is metabolised as it passes through the liver (Bansal et al., 2023). Other factors such as in-line filters can also affect IV delivery of a drug. These filters remove bacteria and endotoxins, but a drug can adhere to (be adsorbed by) the filter and delivery prevented until the filter is saturated. This is a well-known effect with insulin, where a filter should

not be used (National Health Service (NHS) Injectable Medicines Guide, 2025). Insulin can also adsorb to the IV tubing, so this needs to be primed with the insulin infusion solution to allow total adsorption into the lining. This is particularly important when the syringe and line are being changed, as the initial response determines the infusion rate, but inadequate preparation of a replacement set could destabilise the glucose level (Ainsworth, 2020; NHS Injectable Medicines Guide, 2025).

PRACTICE POINT

Managing multiple infusions in the NNU demands a high level of nursing precision, especially when working with limited access ports in unstable neonates. Nurses must continuously assess line compatibility to prevent precipitation or drug interactions, often relying on compatibility charts and pharmacy guidance to safely co-administer medications through shared lumens. Flow rates require meticulous calculation and monitoring, as even small deviations can lead to fluid overload or subtherapeutic dosing in these tiny patients. Infection control is paramount; each line break or manipulation increases the risk of central line-associated bloodstream infections, so nurses must balance the urgency of medication delivery with strict aseptic technique and minimal line access. This complexity is compounded by the need to prioritise infusions such as nutrition, antibiotics and vasoactive agents, often requiring creative solutions like Y-site configurations or staggered administration schedules to ensure safe and effective care.

- *Intraosseous:* The intraosseous (IO) route provides access to the systemic circulation via the bone marrow and can be used if access via an IV line or umbilical vein is not possible. The onset of action of drugs is the same as for those administered IV, and any drug or fluid which can be given IV can be administered via this route, including blood products. A dedicated IO needle is inserted into the upper tibia (see Figure 21.1), and correct placement is confirmed by aspiration of marrow. Other needles can be used, and there is an example of an 18-gauge butterfly needle placed in an oedematous preterm infant. Complications include osteomyelitis, bone fracture and extravasation, and the needle should be removed as soon as IV access is obtained (Scrivens et al., 2019).
- *Rectal:* Rectal absorption is variable in neonates, influenced by administration depth, and the enhanced expulsion reflex can make administration difficult (Bansal et al., 2023). Suppositories are often cut in half or even quarters, and as drug content is not evenly distributed in a suppository, the actual dose delivered will not be accurate (Ainsworth, 2020).

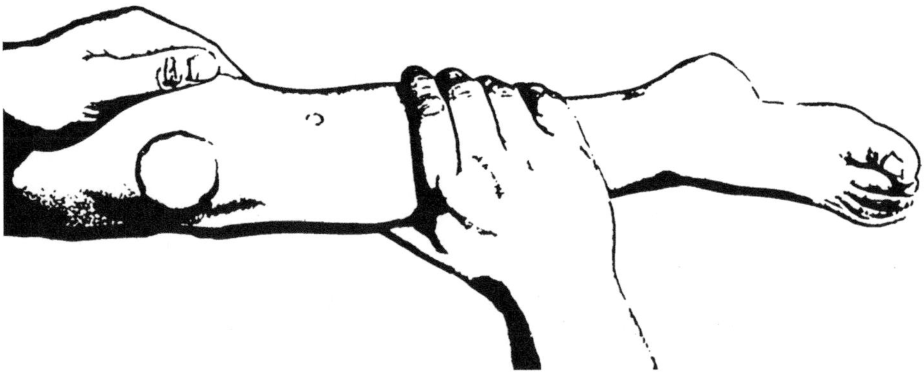

Figure 21.1 Site of intraosseous needle insertion (Source: Creative Commons)

THERAPEUTIC DRUG MONITORING

Therapeutic drug monitoring (TDM), the evaluation of drug concentrations in body fluids (usually plasma), is used during treatment to enhance and individualise drug efficacy, reduce toxicity or assist with diagnosis. This is especially necessary for drugs with a narrow therapeutic index, where the range between the therapeutic and toxic dose (i.e. where the drug is effective but not toxic), is narrow. TDM can be especially beneficial for neonates due to their underdeveloped liver and renal systems, which affect how they process medications. In these situations, the clinical benefits can be optimised while minimising toxicity or adverse effects by modifying either the dosage intervals or the dose itself. It is also valuable in cases where treatment response fails without a clear cause, allowing for necessary adjustments to the dosage regimen. Commonly encountered drugs in the NNU which require TDM include gentamicin, vancomycin, phenobarbital and digoxin. Typically, there are either peak or post dose levels that are reported by the laboratories. Peak (post-dose) levels are evaluated to monitor the efficacy of a drug and are taken after the dose is given. Trough (pre-dose) levels on the other hand are used to avoid toxicity from drug accumulation and are the levels of the drug in the body *before* the drug dose is administered. The most common drug monitored in neonates is the antibiotic gentamicin, with the development of ototoxicity and nephrotoxicity related to elevated trough levels (Pauwels & Allegaert, 2016). If the trough level is high, the drug dosing interval should be extended (Paediatric Formulary Committee, 2024).

EXCIPIENTS IN MEDICINE FORMULATIONS

An excipient is any component of a medicinal product that is not an active substance but required in the preparation of a drug. Excipients include preservatives, sweeteners, binders, fillers and solvents. They serve specific functions, such as enhancing the taste and texture of the medicine, facilitating its manufacturing process or improving the overall safety and efficacy of the product. However, certain excipients may be present in amounts that could potentially lead to adverse effects or harm in neonates (Ainsworth, 2020). Additionally, the off-label use of liquid formulations intended for adults or the administration of unlicensed medications introduces further excipient-related challenges for neonates (O'Brien et al., 2019).

While excipients have to be represented in a medicine's product information (Medicines and Healthcare Products Regulatory Agency, 2022), there is additional guidance for pharmacists and procurement teams, aiming to aid in the safe selection of neonatal drugs (NPPG, 2020). Nurses have agency in this complex area of neonatal drug administration by being vigilant about medicines which do not feature in their local formulary or are a different formulation than the usual product. In this case, close liaison with the neonatal pharmacist is important to maintain safe medicines management.

DRUG TOXICITY

Drug toxicity occurs if a drug's concentration exceeds its therapeutic range. This may be secondary to an unintentional or intentional overdose or because of drug accumulation. Practice examples in neonatology include severe hypoglycemia and/or death due to an overdose of insulin, excessive sedation to coma or death from an overdose of morphine. Neonates experience additional side effects of drugs due to direct toxicity on immature and developing organs (Bansal et al., 2023). Postnatal corticosteroids were introduced in the 1980s to prevent and treat BPD and they were targeted to preterm babies who could not be weaned off the ventilator. However, in the late 1990s their use fell out of favour after it was found that they doubled the risk of cerebral palsy, and subsequently decisions for their administration were made cautiously. Despite this, the neonatal specialty has remained interested in corticosteroids as a means to prevent BPD, and more recently the PREMILOC trial has shown that low-dose treatment regimens appear to be reasonably safe with regard to adverse neurodevelopmental outcomes (Trousson et al., 2023).

DRUGS AND BREASTFEEDING

All medications enter breastmilk to some degree, although in small amounts, and most are considered to be compatible with breastfeeding. However, there is a lack of data regarding the risks of adverse effects in infants. The presence and concentration of drug compounds in breastmilk depends upon factors such as how much of the drug binds to plasma proteins and how soluble the drug is in lipids. Highly lipid-soluble drugs such as diazepam and phenobarbital penetrate milk, as do low molecular weight drugs such as alcohol and amphetamines. The dose the infant receives depends upon the amount excreted into breastmilk, the volume of milk ingested and how fast the infant eliminates the substance (Berlin, 2022).

However, there are historical reports of clinical toxicity from some medications, particularly opioids. A 13-day-old breastfed infant died of morphine poisoning. The mother was taking codeine regularly for episiotomy pain, and when the infant became sleepy and was not feeding well, she froze the breastmilk, which was later found to contain high levels of morphine. Codeine is metabolised to morphine via the CYP450 pathway, and some individuals are ultra-rapid metabolisers, as this mother was found to be. Therefore, it is advised that codeine should be avoided in breastfeeding mothers considering that the frequency of ultra-metabolisers is common, particularly in individuals of African descent (Koren et al., 2006). For mothers on methadone for narcotic addiction, there is evidence that infants may benefit from breastfeeding by having less severe withdrawal symptoms than infants on formula (Berlin, 2022). The British National Formulary (BNF) identifies drugs for breastfeeding mothers which should be used with caution or are contraindicated. This and other breastfeeding references and databases, or medicine information helplines, of which many are available online or over the phone (e.g. the National Breastfeeding Helpline), should be consulted when offering advice to a breastfeeding mother. In many NNUs, there are now breastfeeding leads or champions (often with a neonatal nursing background) to support mothers. While the effect of medicines on breastmilk consists of a vast and complex knowledge base, anyone supporting breastfeeding individuals needs to have an awareness of this and the resources available.

BOX 21.1 THE ROLE OF FAMILY INTEGRATED CARE IN NEONATAL PHARMACY

- Almost a third of babies admitted to NNU are prescribed 3 or more medicines at discharge
- In preterm infants receiving medicines from their parents at home, a 66% administration error rate has been described
- Parents report both a lack of preparation for medicines administration at home before discharge, as well as a lack of support with managing their baby's medication afterwards and the significant stress this causes

- Neonatal nurses can provide invaluable input with educating parents about medication administration, as well as signposting them to available resources, such as the PADDINGToN medicines information booklet, co-designed by parents of NNU graduates (see web-based companion for link)

Adapted from Bracken et al. (2023)

UNLICENSED MEDICINES

Many studies have shown that neonates, in particular preterm infants, receive medications that are unlicensed (their use has not been approved for the indication for which it is administered) or those that are off-label (the indication has been approved, but not for the age, dose, frequency or route used; O'Brien et al., 2019). Unlicensed or off-label medicines use is associated with significant medication errors. However, they are used in most infants below 32 weeks' gestation (Krzyzaniak & Bajorek, 2016). The use of unlicensed drugs in neonatal care is well illustrated by the management of suspected GORD. Gastric acidity is an important defence against infection, and reducing this acidity in preterm infants can increase vulnerability to gastrointestinal and systemic complications. Histamine-2 receptor blockers such as ranitidine (now unavailable in the UK) lower gastric acidity and have been associated with an increased risk of necrotising enterocolitis (NEC). Historically, **prokinetic** agents such as domperidone, cisapride and metoclopramide were used to treat suspected GORD, but significant adverse effects led to their withdrawal from neonatal practice, and current guidance does not recommend the use of any prokinetic therapies (Vandenplas & Huysentruyt, 2024). Proton pump inhibitors (PPIs), including omeprazole, also suppress gastric acid secretion and carry similar risks, together with a heightened incidence of bloodstream infections (Lockyear et al., 2025). Despite their widespread use, evidence supporting the safety and efficacy of PPIs in preterm infants remains insufficient (Tighe et al., 2023; King et al., 2025). The OTTER trial is due to commence to evaluate omeprazole specifically in this population (National Institute for Health and Care Research, 2026).

While there is no recent data regarding the management of GORD in UK NNUs, a 2018 review showed persistent use of these unlicensed medications, with 53% of units administering ranitidine, 23% PPIs and 22% domperidone (Rossor et al., 2018). In contrast, use of PPIs and H2 blockers has been declining over the past decade in the United States (Lockyear et al., 2025).

In the UK, several regulatory bodies state that the responsibility of using unlicensed medicines lies with the prescriber, including independent and in some cases supplementary prescribers, who may be nurses (Paediatric Formulary Committee, 2024). Particular attention should be paid to the risks associated with using unlicensed medicines or using a licensed medicine off-label. These include adverse reactions; unknown product quality; conflicting product information or labelling (e.g. absence of information for some unlicensed medicines, information in a foreign language for unlicensed imports and potential confusion for patients or carers when the patient information leaflet is inconsistent with a medicine's off-label use). The British National Formulary for Children (BNFC) lists the licensing status of each drug in its monograph to aid prescribers in their decision-making.

MEDICATION ERRORS

Medication use in neonates is more complex than in any other group due to differences in weight, gestational and postnatal age requiring individualised dosing and their physical size and immaturity of body systems leaving a narrow margin of safety for error. Table 21.2 outlines medication errors in the NNU. The widespread use of unlicensed and off-label medications and limited access to neonatal-specific formulations also increases the risk of error, which can have serious consequences in such small, immature patients. A review of 20 articles on medication errors throughout the age spectrum found that up to 60% of incidents involved administration errors by nurses. Neonates are more prone to medication errors due to the increased need for calculations, dilutions, manipulations of medication and complex dosing instructions; also common were errors in administration times and administration of an extra dose. 47% of administration errors involved at least tenfold overdoses. One of the studies highlighted found that 31% of IV medications prescribed for neonates were at doses of less than one-tenth of a vial, increasing the risk from ten- to a hundredfold dosing errors. Medicines most commonly associated with dosing errors included IV formulations of morphine, furosemide, gentamicin, insulin and benzylpenicillin (Krzyzaniak & Bajorek, 2016).

The dead space of a needle and syringe may be sufficient to overdose a very small infant, as was found in the case of a neonate who developed arrhythmias due to a digoxin overdose. This was accounted for by the drug contained in the dead space of a 1mL syringe; the diluent was drawn up into the same syringe as the drug itself, which meant the infant received four times the amount of the drug prescribed (Bhambhani et al., 2005). Therefore, it is recommended to inject a drug directly into its diluent, so that the excess drug remains in the hub.

Administering drugs via the wrong route used to be a common problem because of identical Luer Lock connections in both peripheral and central lines and enteral feeding tubes, with reports of serious adverse effects. For example, a case report from Germany described a 6-week-old infant who was inadvertently given 5mL breastmilk via an IV line (Döring et al., 2014). Such wrong route errors were more prevalent in the UK before the introduction of specifically designed enteral lines and syringes fitted with connectors which were no longer compatible with IV lines (National Patient Safety Agency, 2007).

Other errors include administration to the wrong patient, the incidence of which one review found to be as high as 25%, mainly due to similar or identical names and confusion with babies of multiple births. One cause noted for this was that identification bracelets on wrists and ankles were often removed in order to place IV lines or to take blood samples and then not replaced, leading to risk of misidentification (Krzyzaniak & Bajorek, 2016).

Preventing medication errors

Medication errors are unavoidable but can be minimised by specific interventions. Electronic prescribing eliminates errors due to illegible handwriting and the rewriting of prescription charts. Educational intervention programmes providing practical teaching sessions, including skills sessions and simulation, for nurses and prescribers alike have been associated with a reduction in error rates (Sheiniz et al., 2025). Specialist pharmacists' activities include reviewing prescription charts, collaborating on formularies and guidelines as part of the MDT, providing advice on medications on ward rounds and implementing educational activities for staff, and their input has been associated with an improvement in medication error rates (Krzyzaniak & Bajorek, 2016; BAPM, 2025). Furthermore, the standardisation of prescribing and administration practices that comes with the use of a neonatal formulary has been associated with improved patient safety (Shaniv et al., 2023). Similarly, the availability of more specialist neonatal textbooks, continuing professional development modules and online resources like the NHS Injectable Medicines Guide (MEDUSA) and the BNFC can further reduce errors and enhance practice. Over the past decade the inception and development of smart pump technologies and drug libraries and collaborative projects on drug concentration calibration have standardised practice in NNUs and decreased errors such as incorrect rate and doses associated with IV therapy (NPPG and the Royal College of Paediatrics and Child Health, 2023).

The most likely contributor to improved error rates, however, is the adoption of a culture which not only incorporates all of the abovementioned measures, but closely monitors near misses, to identify systemic issues predisposing to medication errors (Sheiniz et al., 2025).

TABLE 21.2 MEDICATION ERRORS IN THE NEONATAL UNIT

Type of error	*Clinician involved*	*Causes of error*
Prescribing	Prescriber	Wrong administration route Incorrect placement of decimal point
Transcription	Prescriber	Wrong weight Wrong dosage Wrong unit, i.e. grams instead of milligrams
Dispensing	Pharmacist	Wrong labelling of drug Incorrect calculation, dose or dilution Delayed dispensing time
Administration	Nurse	Incorrect administration time Incorrect preparation and dilution Patient misidentification Administering additional dose of drug
Monitoring	Medical and nursing professionals	Incorrect interpretation of laboratory results Omission of therapeutic drug monitoring Missing symptoms of adverse events

NON-MEDICAL PRESCRIBING

Nurse independent prescribers (NIP) or non-medical prescribers (NMP) are able, after an appropriate educational programme, to prescribe any medicine for any medical condition, including the administration of scheduled and controlled drugs. However, they must work within their own level of professional competence and expertise (Paediatric Formulary Committee, 2024).

In neonatology, NIPs are often Advanced Neonatal Nurse Practitioners who commonly work autonomously in either a medical or nursing role or a combination of both. Their ability to prescribe has had demonstrable positive effects on the quality of patient care (Dunn & Pryor, 2023).

Chapter takeaways

- Neonatal pharmacokinetics differ greatly from adults due to immature organ systems, variable gestational ages and rapid developmental changes, making individualised dosing essential.
- Absorption of drugs in neonates is influenced by high gastric pH, delayed gastric emptying and immature bile secretion, which can reduce bioavailability of many oral medications.

- Distribution is affected by high total body water, low fat stores, reduced plasma proteins and increased blood–brain barrier permeability, all of which heighten drug sensitivity and toxicity risk.
- Drug metabolism is limited by immature hepatic enzymes, with phase 1 and phase 2 pathways maturing at different rates, leading to slower clearance and potential accumulation.
- Excretion is reduced due to immature renal function and low glomerular filtration rate, prolonging half-lives of many drugs and requiring careful dose adjustments.
- Routes of administration carry unique risks in neonates such as unpredictable absorption with oral, intramuscular or percutaneous routes, requiring careful selection and monitoring to minimise harm.
- The nurse's role is central in ensuring safe drug administration, monitoring for toxicity and adapting practice to neonatal-specific pharmacological challenges, as well as integrating families with their babies' pharmacological therapies.

CASE STUDY

CASE STUDIES

Case study 1: The preterm infant who has become unwell

Jonathan is a 25^{+2}-week baby who is now 3 weeks old. He has developed signs of NEC and has been prescribed cefotaxime 6-hourly IV and metronidazole IV as a loading dose, followed by a maintenance dose after 24 hours.

Q.1. Why is cefotaxime prescribed 6-hourly for this baby?
Q.2. How often would you expect it to be prescribed in a 1-day-old baby?
Q.3. Why does metronidazole need a loading dose and why is the next dose not given for 24 hours?
Q.4. What drugs would you consider for pain and stress management in line with any non-pharmacological strategies?

Jonathan becomes increasingly unwell and is intubated and ventilated. He is then started on dopamine and dobutamine infusions for hypotension.

Q.5. Why are some drugs given by continuous infusion?
Q.6. What factors predispose this baby to medication errors?
Q.7. What are the potential side effects of inotropes such as dopamine and dobutamine?

CASE STUDY

After a period of stabilisation, Jonathan improves and at the age of 5 weeks is being weaned from ventilation requirements. He is commenced on caffeine as part of this management.

Q.8. Why is caffeine given to the infant?

Case study 2: Medication during therapeutic hypothermia (TH)

Caroline is a 2-day-old term baby undergoing TH for hypoxic-ischaemic encephalopathy (HIE). She was commenced on gentamicin after birth but has now developed renal failure. She is also receiving phenobarbital, a morphine infusion and a dopamine infusion.

Q.1. How are the medications Caroline is on affected by TH?
Q.2. Does gentamicin dosage need amending and why?
Q.3. What are the potential side effects of morphine and phenobarbitone?

Case study 3: The late preterm infant with multiple issues

A new mother of a 35-week gestation baby girl called Petra (who is admitted to the neonatal unit with a low blood sugar and jaundice), wants to breastfeed but is concerned about the medication she is taking. Petra also develops an eye infection and thrush around the nappy area.

Q.1. What advice would you give to mum about breastfeeding, eye and skin care and how would this baby be managed?

For suggested answer guides to the questions posed in these case studies, please refer to the web-based companion site specific to this chapter. See www.routledge.com/cw/petty

References

Ainsworth, S. B. (Ed.). (2020). *Neonatal formulary 8: Drug use in pregnancy and the first year of life* (8th ed.). John Wiley & Sons.

Aitken, J., & Williams, F. L. (2014). A systematic review of thyroid dysfunction in preterm neonates exposed to topical iodine. *Archives of Disease in Childhood: Fetal and Neonatal Edition*, *99*(1), F21–F28.

Allegaert, K., Simons, S. H. P., Tibboel, D., Krekels, E. H., Knibbe, C. A., & Van den Anker, J. N. (2017). Non-maturational covariates for dynamic systems pharmacology models in neonates, infants, and children: Filling the gaps beyond developmental pharmacology. *European Journal of Pharmaceutical Sciences*, *109*(S), S27–S31.

Amin, S. B., & Wang, H. (2018). Bilirubin albumin binding and unbound unconjugated hyperbilirubinemia in premature infants. *The Journal of Pediatrics*, *192*, 47–52.

Anderson, B. J. (2017). Neonatal pharmacology. *Anaesthesia and Intensive Care Medicine*, *18*(2), 68–74.

Bansal, N., Momin. S., Bansal, R., Gurram Venkata, S. K. R., Ruser, L., & Yusuf, K. (2023). Pharmacokinetics of drugs: Newborn perspective. *Pediatric Medicine*, *7*, 19.

Bennett, S. (2014). Pharmacology in neonatal care: Prescribing considerations. *Nurse Prescribing*, *12*(2), 87–92.

Berlin, C. M. (2022). Medications and the breastfeeding mother. In D. Mattison & L.-A. Halbert (Eds.), *Clinical pharmacology during pregnancy* (2nd ed.). Academic Press.

Bhambhani, V., Beri, R. S., & Puliyel, J. M. (2005). Inadvertent overdosing of neonates as a result of the dead space of the syringe hub and needle. *Archives of Disease in Childhood: Fetal and Neonatal Edition*, *90*(*5*), F444–F445.

Bracken, L., Clark, J., Gill, A., O'Brien, F., Dewey, R., Barker, C., & Carter, B. (2023). "A hard-won capability": The experiences of parents managing their babies' medicines after discharge from a neonatal unit. *Frontiers in Communication*, *8*, 1204599. Retrieved July 17, 2025, from https://www.frontiersin.org/articles/10.3389/fcomm.2023.1204599/full

British Association of Perinatal Medicine. (2025). *Pharmacists*. Retrieved March 10, 2025, from https://www.bapm.org/pages/203-pharmacists

Döring, M., Brenner, B., Handgretinger, R., Hofbeck, M., & Kerst, G. (2014). Inadvertent intravenous administration of maternal breast milk in a six-week-old infant: A case report and review of the literature. *BMC Research Notes*, *7*(1), 17.

Dunn, J., & Pryor, C. (2023). Non-medical prescribing in nursing: The history and evolution of independent and supplementary prescribing. *British Journal of Nursing*, *32*(20), 1004–1008. https://doi.org/10.12968/bjon.2023.32.20.1004

King, E., Horn, D., Gluchowski, N., O'Reilly, D., Bruschettini, M., Cooper, C., & Soll, R. F. (2025). Safety and efficacy of proton pump inhibitors in preterm infants with gastroesophageal reflux disease. *Cochrane Database of Systematic Reviews*, *2025*(3). https://doi.org/10.1002/14651858.CD015127.pub2

Koren, G., Cairns, J., Chitayat, D., Gaedigk, A., & Leeder, S. J. (2006). Pharmacogenetics of morphine poisoning in a breastfed neonate of a codeine-prescribed mother. *The Lancet*, *368*(9536), 704.

Krzyzaniak, N., & Bajorek, B. (2016). Medication safety in neonatal care: A review of medication errors among neonates. *Therapeutic Advances in Drug Safety*, *7*(3), 102–119.

Lee, Z.-M., Chang, L.-S., Kuo, K.-C., Lin, M.-C., & Yu, H.-R. (2023). Impact of protein binding capacity and daily dosage of a drug on total serum bilirubin levels in susceptible infants. *Children*, *10*(6), 926. https://doi.org/10.3390/children10060926

Lockyear, C., Stark, A., Foote, H. P., Agyeman, A., Bouleqcha, M., Cohen, N., Matusevich, C., Pantsari, A., Wang, S., Rent, S., Malcolm, W., Tolia, V. N., Greenberg, R. G., & Aleem, S. (2025). Medical treatment of gastroesophageal reflux in the neonatal intensive care unit: Current practice. *Journal of Perinatology*, *45*(5), 616–621. https://doi.org/10.1038/s41372-025-02238-9

Medicines and Healthcare Products Regulatory Agency. (2022). *2022 edition of rules and guidance for pharmaceutical manufacturers and distributors – the orange guide*. Pharmaceutical Press.

National Health Service (NHS) Injectable Medicines Guide. (2025). *Injectable medicines guide (MEDUSA)*. Retrieved March 21, 2025, from http://medusa.wales.nhs.uk. Password controlled.

National Institute for Health and Care Research. (2026). *Omeprazole for treatment of term and preterm infants with gastro-oesophageal reflux (OTTER)*. Retrieved March 17, 2026, from https://www.fundingawards.nihr.ac.uk/award/NIHR165206

National Patient Safety Agency (NPSA). (2007). Promoting safer measurement and administration of liquid medicines via oral and other enteral routes. *Patient Safety Alert*, *19*, 1–12.

Neonatal and Paediatric Pharmacists Group. (2020). *NPPG excipient position statement.* Retrieved March 10, 2025, from Position-Statement-Liquid-Choice-V1-November-2020.pdf

Neonatal and Paediatric Pharmacists Group and British Association of Perinatal Medicine. (2024). *Chlorhexidine for skin cleansing in neonates. Position statement.* Retrieved October 14, 2025, from https://nppg.org.uk/wp-content/uploads/2024/12/Chlorhexidine-Position-Statement-V1a.pdf

Neonatal and Paediatric Pharmacists Group and the Royal College of Paediatrics and Child Health. (2023). *Standardising intravenous infusion concentrations for neonates and children in the UK* [Online]. Retrieved March 20, 2025, from https://www.rcpch.ac.uk/sites/default/files/2023-12/standard_infusions_feb_2023.pdf

Niemarkt, H. J., Hütten, M. C., & Kramer, B. W. (2017). Surfactant for respiratory distress syndrome: New ideas on a familiar drug with innovative applications. *Neonatology*, *111*(4), 408–414.

O'Brien, F., Clapham, D., Krysiak, K., Batchelor, H., Field, P., Caivano, G., Pertile, M., Nunn, A., & Tuleu, C. (2019). Making medicines baby size: The challenges in bridging the formulation gap in neonatal medicine. *International Journal of Molecular Sciences*, *20*(11), 2688. https://doi.org/10.3390/ijms20112688

Pacifici, G. M. (2021). Clinical pharmacology of digoxin in infants and children. *Clinical Medicine*, *3*(2), 1036.

Paediatric Formulary Committee. (2024). *BNF for children 2024–2025.* BMJ Group, Pharmaceutical Press and RCPCH Publications.

Pauwels, S., & Allegaert, K. (2016). Therapeutic drug monitoring in neonates. *Archives of Disease in Childhood*, *101*(4), 377–381.

Ritter, J. M., Flower, R., Henderson, G., Loke, K. Y., MacEwan, D., Robinson, E., & Fullerton, J. (Eds.). (2024). *Rang and Dale's pharmacology* (10th ed.). Elsevier.

Rossor, T., Andradi, G., Bhat, R., & Greenough, A. (2018). Investigation and management of gastro-oesophageal reflux in United Kingdom neonatal intensive care units. *Acta Paediatrica*, *107*(1), 48–51.

Ruggiero, A., Ariano, A., Triarico, S., Capozza, M. A., Ferrara, P., & Attinà, G. (2019). Neonatal pharmacology and clinical implications. *Drugs Context*, *8*, 212608.

Scrivens, A., Reynolds, P. R., Emery, F. E., Roberts, C. T., Polglase, G. R., Hooper, S. B., & Roehr, C. C. (2019). Use of intraosseous needles in neonates: A systematic review. *Neonatology*, *116*(4), 305–314. https://doi.org/10.1159/000502212

Shah, V. S., Ohlsson, A., Halliday, H. L., & Dunn, M. (2017). Early administration of inhaled corticosteroids for preventing chronic lung disease in very low birth weight preterm neonates. *Cochrane Database of Systematic Reviews*, *1*(1), CD001969. https://doi.org/10.1002/14651858.CD001969.pub4

Shaniv, D., Bolisetty, S., Young, T. E., Mangum, B., Ainsworth, S., Elbers, L., Schultz, P., Cucchi, M., De Wildt, S. N., Van Der Zanden, T. M., Caldwell, N., Smits, A., & Allegaert, K. (2023). Neonatal drug formularies – A global scope. *Children*, *10*, 848.

Sheiniz, G., McCallion, N., Allegaert, K., & O'Brien, F. (2025). Safeguarding drug safety in neonates: Addressing the impact of in-hospital medication administration errors through prevention and standardization. *Expert Opinion on Drug Safety*, 1–3. https://doi.org/10.1080/14740338.2025.2585069

Tighe, M. P., Andrews, E., Liddicoat, I., Afzal, N. A., Hayen, A., & Beattie, R. M. (2023). Pharmacological treatment of gastro-oesophageal reflux in children. *Cochrane Database of Systematic Reviews*, *2023*(8). https://doi.org/10.1002/14651858.CD008550.pub3

Trousson, C., Toumazi, A., Bourmaud, A., Biran, V., & Baud, O. (2023). Neurocognitive outcomes at age 5 years after prophylactic hydrocortisone in infants born extremely preterm.

Developmental Medicine & Child Neurology, *65*(7), 926–932. https://doi.org/10.1111/dmcn.15470

Van den Anker, J., & Allegaert, K. (2021). Considerations for drug dosing in premature infants. *Journal of Clinical Pharmacology*, *61*(S1), S141–S151.

Van den Anker, J., Reed, M. D., Allegaert, K., & Kearns, G. L. (2018). Developmental changes in pharmacokinetics and pharmacodynamics. *Journal of Clinical Pharmacology*, *58*, S10–S25.

Vandenplas, Y., & Huysentruyt, K. (2024). Gastroesophageal reflux disease in preterm infants: Unmet needs. *Expert Review of Gastroenterology & Hepatology*, *18*(9), 485–491. https://doi.org/10.1080/17474124.2024.2407116

22 NEONATAL SURGICAL CARE

Lisa Kaiser and Dr Ramon Fernandez

CONTENTS

DOI: 10.4324/9781003591405-27

GUIDANCE ON HOW TO ENHANCE PERSONAL LEARNING FROM THIS CHAPTER

Key points covered in this chapter

- An overview of surgical problems that present in the neonatal population.
- General management and nursing care of the surgical neonate in the pre-, peri- and post-operative periods.
- Common diagnoses, their underlying pathophysiology and clinical presentation.

Reflection

Reading through the chapter, you are encouraged to engage with the key points and related literature in an enquiring way. Ask these questions:

- Have you been involved in the care of infants with surgical problems? What were these and the underlying causes?
- How did these infants present?
- How were these infants managed?

Implications for nursing care

- Finally: How will this chapter enable you to approach the assessment, management and nursing care of neonates with surgical problems? Consider the implications of what you learn for your daily practice relating to this area.

INTRODUCTION AND BACKGROUND

Neonatal surgery and anaesthesia have evolved rapidly over the past 50 years, their success contributing to a reduction in neonatal mortality in high income countries (HICs). Sophisticated antenatal screening and fetal anomaly detection have led to a changing pattern of operable malformations, and the delivery of a baby with an undiagnosed major structural anomaly is now rare.

Regrettably, in many low- and middle-income countries, if surgery is even attempted, neonates face high mortality due to limited resources, lack of specialised anaesthesia and outdated beliefs about pain. Even with skilled intervention, poor post-operative care and inadequate facilities often lead to fatal outcomes, yet the urgent need for specialised neonatal surgical and anaesthesia services remains a low priority in these regions (Bösenberg, 2024).

This chapter will cover surgical issues commonly seen in the neonatal period, providing an insight into their causes and clinical presentation. General peri-operative and anaesthetic management will be discussed, with more detailed care considerations relating to individual conditions under their respective headings.

PRE-OPERATIVE MANAGEMENT

Antenatal considerations and delivery room management

With the development of high-resolution non-invasive fetal imaging, many congenital defects are being diagnosed earlier, and with this there has been an increase in fetal interventions. This can be seen in areas such as lower urinary tract obstruction, congenital diaphragmatic hernia (CDH), congenital pulmonary airway malformation (CPAM), spina bifida and myelomeningocele (Varthaliti et al., 2025).

Antenatal diagnosis of surgically correctable malformations will allow for *in utero* transfer and planned delivery in a specialist centre. Regionalisation secures optimal utilisation of resources and the expertise of the highly specialised multidisciplinary team (MDT), which is crucial to the peri-operative care and recovery of these babies. Parents should meet with the surgeon as soon as the diagnosis is made, ideally with the support of the fetal medicine team, where information about the anomaly, its short-term management and the possible long-term sequelae should be given (British Association of Perinatal Medicine (BAPM), 2024). Meeting professionals who will be involved in the baby's care, visiting the neonatal unit (NNU) and early receipt of specialist information booklets may help avoid long periods of uncertainty, especially when the diagnosis is made antenatally.

Following the birth of their baby, the parents need support in dealing with the information given to them. Informed consent stating the risks, benefits and nature of the procedure will be required from the parents in order for surgery to take place. In the United Kingdom (UK), consent is required from an individual with parental responsibility (usually present if married or named on the birth certificate). Other people able to give consent include a legally appointed guardian; the local authority if the child is on a care order; or a person named in a residence order in respect of the child (Department of Health, 2009). However, in emergency situations, treatment should proceed in the infant's best interests in accordance with UK legal and professional guidance. Local trust policies should be followed where there is uncertainty.

Multiple defects can be associated with chromosomal abnormalities. If a chromosomal anomaly is found in the fetus or neonate, the parents should be offered genetic counselling.

The timing and mode of delivery should be a joint decision between the obstetrician, the neonatal team and the surgeon. Although many conditions are managed with a natural birth, occasionally a caesarean section might be safer with an anomaly that causes size mismatch between the fetus and maternal pelvis (cephalopelvic disproportion). In infants with known congenital anomalies, appropriately skilled personnel should be present at the delivery. Consideration should be given to the availability of professionals with advanced airway skills depending on the expected congenital anomaly. The main goal on arrival of a baby into the NNU is expedient stabilisation. Skilful assessment and management pre-operatively will ensure minimal risk from anaesthesia and surgery.

Pre-operative assessment

A comprehensive pre-operative evaluation in neonates is essential to mitigate peri-operative risks, especially in those undergoing high-risk surgeries with co-morbidities.

Successful neonatal anaesthesia and surgery hinges on meticulous planning, interdisciplinary collaboration and individualised care tailored to each infant's unique physiology and clinical status.

- *Relevant history* Detailed maternal and family histories inform anaesthetic planning, especially in cases of inherited conditions like malignant hyperthermia. Gestational age (GA), birthweight and postnatal age also influence care.
- *Airway assessment and respiratory function* Assessment of respiratory function is a prerequisite for all surgical neonates, as urgent intervention may be required. Airway evaluation is vital, particularly in neonates with craniofacial anomalies or congenital syndromes, as intubation challenges can lead to rapid desaturation. Anatomical abnormalities or increasing abdominal distension may compromise ventilation, such as in the case of CDH, which is often associated with pulmonary hypertension due to lung hypoplasia. Additionally, some infants with surgical problems may be further compromised from surfactant deficiency or aspiration pneumonia. Pulmonary assessment should include imaging, ventilation history and increased work of breathing or pulmonary hypertension, especially in infants with bronchopulmonary dysplasia.
- *Cardiovascular considerations* Cardiac evaluation must identify congenital heart defects and shunt physiology, which affect oxygenation and fluid balance, so that **echocardiography** may be necessary. The current and recent need for inotropic support and blood products must be established (Macrae et al., 2021). Some infants will need fluid resuscitation pre-operatively; hypovolaemia can result from continuous loss of fluid from, for example, the exposed viscera in gastroschisis and exomphalos. Losses via the nasogastric tube (NGT) should be measured and may need replacement with electrolyte solutions, usually normal saline with potassium. A neonate's blood volume is approximately 80mL/kg body weight. A 2kg infant, therefore, has a circulating volume equivalent to the average loss during minor adult surgery. A full blood count, serum creatinine, urea and electrolytes, should be obtained pre-operatively and the need for a coagulation profile discussed with the surgeon and anaesthetist. Any requirements should be treated accordingly and necessary blood products made available for surgery. The neonate should have received vitamin K in the first few hours of life.
- *Fluids, nutritional and gastrointestinal considerations* Fluid and electrolyte balance is dependent upon fulfilling the maintenance requirements (insensible water losses, urine and stool), the replacement of ongoing losses and the correction of deficit losses due to fluid compartment shifts (third space losses). Fluid compartment shifts can be difficult to determine. The neonatal nurse's role, through observations of alterations in heart rate, urine output, capillary refill, blood pressure and core-to-peripheral temperature

difference, is crucial with regard to this. Laboratory tests form the mainstay of assessment: serum creatinine, urea and electrolytes, plasma osmolality, urine electrolytes and specific gravity and blood gas analysis. Adequate nutrition and hydration can be provided by glucose and electrolyte solutions and/or parenteral nutrition (PN). Intestinal obstruction and/or sepsis predispose the infant to increased gastric fluids which may consist of bile, gastric juices or blood. Gastric **decompression** is necessary to avoid vomiting and aspiration pneumonia; it will also reduce splinting of the diaphragm and aid ventilation. Gastric decompression is achieved with a correctly positioned gastric tube (naso- or oro-gastric), large enough to prevent blockage (8Fg or greater), left on continuous open drainage with gentle intermittent aspiration as directed by the surgeon. In preparation for surgery, if the infant is not already nil by mouth, he or she will have to be fasted for a period of time, as discussed with surgical and anaesthetic teams. Generally, breastmilk without fortifiers or formula can be offered up to four to six hours pre-operatively (Pilkington et al., 2024).

- *Metabolic requirements* Alterations in acid-base-balance can be caused by several factors. Respiratory acidosis results from inadequate ventilation, for example, in pulmonary hypoplasia secondary to CDH. Metabolic acidosis can occur when bicarbonate losses are increased or with poor tissue perfusion, tissue necrosis, infection, hypovolaemia and because of intestinal **fistula**s and necrotising enterocolitis (NEC). Glycogen is a carbohydrate stored in skeletal muscle and the liver and is metabolised when blood glucose falls outside the homeostatic range. Neonates have limited glycogen stores due to decreased availability of substrate *in utero* and therefore need a constant glucose intake. It is essential that glucose be administered and the blood glucose monitored frequently, maintaining a level of 2.6 (3.4 after the first 48–72 hours) – approximately 8mmol/L (Zhu et al., 2025).
- *Thermoregulation* Thermoregulation for the neonate, especially low birth weight (LBW) infants, can be a challenge. Infants requiring surgical intervention such as laparotomy, and those with anomalies like abdominal wall defects, are going to be at increased risk of temperature instability due to heat loss from exposed viscera. Temperature instability is associated with increased metabolic demands, leading to increased oxygen consumption, which may further compromise the cardiorespiratory system and ultimately contribute to mortality and morbidity (BAPM, 2024).
- *Neurological concerns* Neurological assessment is critical, as haemodynamic instability may affect cerebral perfusion, and conditions like intraventricular haemorrhage or hydrocephalus require tailored anaesthetic strategies.

- *Access requirements* Appropriate vascular access will depend upon the nature of the surgery. However, for major surgery at least two intravenous (IV) lines will be needed, including a central venous line (CVL). This is necessary to provide inotropic support and for prolonged venous access in the provision of PN. Arterial access should always be made available for major surgery and where significant blood loss is expected. Existing IV access and any prior difficulties must be reviewed. Umbilical vascular lines may obstruct the surgical field and require removal; otherwise their placement should be evaluated before use. Scalp veins and narrow lines like peripheral percutaneously inserted CVLs are less suitable for large boluses or viscous fluids such as blood products (Macrae et al., 2021).

PERI- AND INTRAOPERATIVE MANAGEMENT

Specific considerations for anaesthesia in neonates

Administering anaesthesia to neonates demands specialised knowledge of their unique anatomy, physiology and altered drug pharmacology, especially in preterm infants. As the youngest and most vulnerable patients, neonates face heightened perioperative risks, making the expertise of paediatric anaesthesiologists essential. All children in the UK should receive anaesthesia from paediatric-trained professionals to reduce complications, and often neonates undergo surgery in specialist tertiary centres (Royal College of Anaesthetists (RCoA), 2023). Unlike adults, neonates undergo rapid developmental changes, with immature organ systems and metabolic pathways that require tailored anaesthetic approaches.

While animal studies have raised concerns about anaesthetic-induced neurotoxicity, recent human trials suggest that brief, single exposures do not adversely affect long-term cognitive outcomes. Nevertheless, caution needs to be exercised with repeated or prolonged anaesthetic use in children under three. Ultimately, the benefits of anaesthesia – especially for urgent neonatal surgeries – often outweigh potential risks. Current evidence supports the safety of short anaesthetic exposures during early development, reinforcing the importance of careful risk-benefit assessment in neonatal care (Macrae et al., 2021) but with an understanding that preterm infants might be at an increased risk of neurotoxic effects of anaesthesia (Spaeth & Lam, 2024).

The operating environment

Depending on the procedure and condition of the infant, the most appropriate place for surgery may be the neonatal intensive care unit (NICU), if facilities allow, particularly where the additional risks of transfer to an operating theatre may adversely impact mortality and morbidity risks (BAPM, 2024). Box 22.1 details necessary operating room equipment, although the list is not exhaustive.

BOX 22.1 OPERATING ROOM EQUIPMENT

- Transport system (incubator/pod, ventilator and appropriate monitoring)
- Airway equipment (suction catheters, oral airways, face masks, breathing circuit, laryngoscope, tracheal tubes, stylet, ventilator and gases)
- Thermoregulation equipment (forced warm air delivery device, underbody warming blanket/gel warming mattress, circuit humidifier)
- Monitoring equipment (pulse oximeter, electrocardiography, blood pressure monitor, end-tidal CO_2, temperature probe, invasive monitoring of central venous pressure and/or arterial blood pressure if indicated, cerebral near-infrared spectroscopy (optional)
- Infusion devices (for both maintenance fluids and required drug infusions)
- Intravenous fluids and easily accessible blood products as required
- Medication (anaesthetic agents including opioids, neuromuscular blocking drugs and local anaesthetics, emergency drugs, vasoactive drugs)
- Documentation

Adapted from BAPM (2024) and Spaeth and Lam (2024)

Intraoperative care

Ventilation Lung-protective ventilation strategies, with careful monitoring of tidal volumes, should continue throughout surgery.

Cardiovascular support It is not uncommon for neonates to require blood product administration during surgery to correct anaemia, thrombocytopenia or coagulopathies. Administration thresholds tend to follow national guidance.

Fluid management The goal of intraoperative fluid replacement is maintenance of cardiovascular stability, organ perfusion whilst prevention of fluid overload. PN is not commonly continued intraoperatively (BAPM, 2024). There is a risk of hyponatraemia, particularly if hypotonic infusion solutions are used (Pilkington et al., 2024).

Thermoregulation Maintenance of stable temperatures can be a challenge within the operating theatre, so that heat loss mechanisms and preventative measures need to be considered even pre-operatively on the NNU and when transferring the neonate for surgery. The operating theatre needs to be warm (up to 28°C; RCoA, 2023) to provide a neutral thermal environment, with the additional use of radiant warmers, force air heating units, heated mattresses, humidified and warm inspired gases, warm solutions for cleansing and intraoperative irrigation and warm blood and intravenous solutions. The baby's core temperature should be maintained between 36.5 and 37.5°C (BAPM, 2024).

Anaesthetic agents

General anaesthesia is the cornerstone of neonatal surgical care in HICs, often supplemented by regional techniques for enhanced analgesia. Neonates require tailored anaesthetic management due to immature physiology and variable drug metabolism.

INHALATIONAL ANAESTHETICS

Inhalational agents such as sevoflurane and isoflurane are commonly used, with sevoflurane preferred for mask induction due to its non-irritant profile and rapid onset. Nitrous oxide may be used briefly during induction but is generally avoided in maintenance due to risks of bowel distension and hypoxia (Spaeth & Lam, 2024).

INTRAVENOUS AGENTS

These include propofol, ketamine and opioids. Propofol is used cautiously due to its vasodilatory effects and slower clearance in neonates. Ketamine is a potent analgesic, which also provides amnesia, and offers haemodynamic stability, but can lead to airway obstruction and apnoea. Fentanyl is widely used for its cardiovascular safety and potent analgesia, though dosing must be titrated carefully. Morphine is used post-operatively, while remifentanil may be suitable for short procedures due to its rapid metabolism (Spaeth & Lam, 2024).

> **Induction of anaesthesia** is typically intravenous in neonates, with mask induction reserved for stable infants. Rapid sequence induction is essential in case of a full stomach, using agents like propofol and rocuronium.

NEUROMUSCULAR BLOCKERS

Non-depolarising agents such as rocuronium, cisatracurium and vecuronium may be reversed with neostigmine with glycopyrrolate; sugammadex is used off-label in neonates for profound blockade reversal. Succinylcholine is a depolarising agent that is reserved for rapid sequence induction due to risks of hyperkalaemia, bradycardia and its potential association with malignant hyperthermia.

REGIONAL AND LOCAL ANAESTHESIA

Regional anaesthesia is increasingly used in neonates across UK centres, driven by concerns over general anaesthetic neurotoxicity. Techniques include local infiltration, fascial plane blocks, peripheral nerve blocks and neuraxial approaches. Most are performed alongside general anaesthesia to reduce intraoperative drug requirements and improve post-operative analgesia, though spinal or caudal blocks may be used alone in high-risk infants (Spaeth & Lam, 2024). Caudal anaesthesia is commonly used for lower abdominal and limb surgery, often with bupivacaine or ropivacaine. Epidural catheters, placed via caudal or direct lumbar/thoracic routes, allow continuous infusion and reduce opioid use. Spinal anaesthesia, typically with bupivacaine or tetracaine, is effective for short procedures like inguinal herniotomy. Local infiltration techniques are effective for minor procedures, but the risk of systemic toxicity warrants careful dosage calculation. Ultrasound guidance has improved safety and precision across all techniques (Macrae et al., 2021).

POST-OPERATIVE CARE

Management in the post-operative period mirrors pre-operative care in aiming to achieve and maintain physiological stability. Transport from the operating room must ensure thermal stability and airway protection. In addition, the factors listed in Box 22.2 require careful consideration.

BOX 22.2 GENERAL CONSIDERATIONS FOLLOWING MAJOR SURGERY

- Do not leave the operating rom until the baby is stable and a complete handover has taken place. A doctor/nurse practitioner and nurse experienced in the transfer of infants should be in attendance on the return journey to the NNU.
- Optimise sedation, analgesia and muscle relaxants (if required) for the return journey.
- Check baby's temperature and use additional heat aids as required for transfer.
- Prophylactic antibiotic administration within an hour of skin incision is associated with reduced incidence of surgical site infection. Whether a course of antibiotics is continued post-operatively depends on the underlying surgical condition and baby's clinical status (Pilkington et al., 2024).

Recovery from anaesthesia

Recovery from anaesthesia in neonates, particularly premature or critically ill infants, requires vigilant monitoring and supportive care. Extubation is often delayed in the sickest neonates due to prolonged drug clearance and immature respiratory control, necessitating continued NNU care. Neuromuscular blockade must be fully reversed, and hypothermia, common post-operatively, should be corrected to avoid delayed emergence. Indicators of readiness for extubation include rhythmic spontaneous breathing, adequate tone and signs of airway reflex return. Laryngospasm remains a risk during extubation, requiring readiness to reintubate. Premature infants are prone to post-operative apnoea, especially those under 60 weeks' post-conceptual age and may need prolonged (at least 12–24 hour) close monitoring after surgery. Anaemia may exacerbate apnoea risk.

Pain assessment and management are important aspects of immediate as well as intermediate term post-operative care. While opioid analgesics remain at the forefront of post-operative pain management, the use of paracetamol and non-steroidal anti-inflammatory drugs provides an acceptable adjunct, with a better side effect profile (Ohliger et al., 2021). Chapter 8 covers neonatal pain scales and pain management strategies in detail.

In UK neonatal practice, multidisciplinary coordination between anaesthetics, surgery and neonatal teams is essential to ensure safe recovery and early detection of complications (RCoA, 2023).

Return to the neonatal unit

The following aspects need to be closely coordinated during readmission to the NICU, during which the neonatal nurse has a central role:

- Before returning the baby to the incubator and connecting to the ventilator, check settings of both.
- Ensure ventilator settings are still appropriate when reconnecting. Check airway and position of endotracheal tube. Check blood gas and adjust ventilation accordingly.
- Reconnect all monitor leads and record hourly:
  - blood pressure
  - SpO_2
  - transcutaneous pO_2/pCO_2 (as indicated)
  - skin temperature – peripheral and core.
- Check infusion sites, then reconnect fluids.
- Adjust maintenance and arterial line fluids. Take into consideration any fluids given intraoperatively. Check surgical recommendations regarding maintenance fluids.

- Aspirate NGT according to surgical instructions and leave on free drainage. Record accurately and commence NG replacement of losses if necessary.
- Take a blood gas sample including glucose level, monitor according to results.
- Organise a chest X-ray if there is a chest drain in situ and following diaphragmatic hernia repair.
- Record urinary output – attach urine bag, weigh nappies or measure catheter output – aim for at least 1 mL/kg/hour after the first 24 hours.
- Take blood samples and check biochemical and haematological status.
- Position baby as comfortably as possible, developmentally appropriate, while responding to specific requirements of surgery.
- Assess, administer and evaluate pain relief.
- Carefully observe wounds, stomas etc., recording any losses and replacing as prescribed.
- Consult surgical instructions for care of any drains.
- Ensure parents are informed of the outcome of surgery and of the post-operative management plan.
- Encourage parental involvement in care as possible.

Table 22.5 (see p.40) outlines specific nursing considerations in general and related to the individual conditions explored in the following section

CONGENITAL SURGICAL CONDITIONS

Oesophageal atresia and tracheo-oesophageal fistula

The oesophagus and trachea have a common embryological origin. Initially they are fused, but a septal separation occurs by week 6; where this is not the case, this results in fistula formation. The oesophagus should re-canalise and become patent by week 10; failure to do this leads to atresia. Thus tracheo-oesophageal fistula (TOF) and oesophageal **atresia** (OA) can occur as separate entities, but more frequently occur concurrently (Gallagher et al., 2020; see Figure 22.1).

Associated anatomical features include a hypertrophied proximal oesophageal pouch; a result of fetal swallowing of amniotic fluid. If the pouch is not hypertrophied, a fistula should be suspected. Almost 50% of neonates with TOF/OA are thought to have coexisting anomalies such as VACTERL (**V**ertebral defects – **A**norectal malformations (ARM) – **C**ardiac defects – **TOF/OA** – **R**enal abnormalities – **L**imb abnormalities) and CHARGE (**C**oloboma – **H**eart defects – **A**tresia of the nasal choanae – **R**estricted growth/development – **G**enital/urinary anomalies – **E**ar abnormalities/deafness) syndromes (Gallagher et al., 2020).

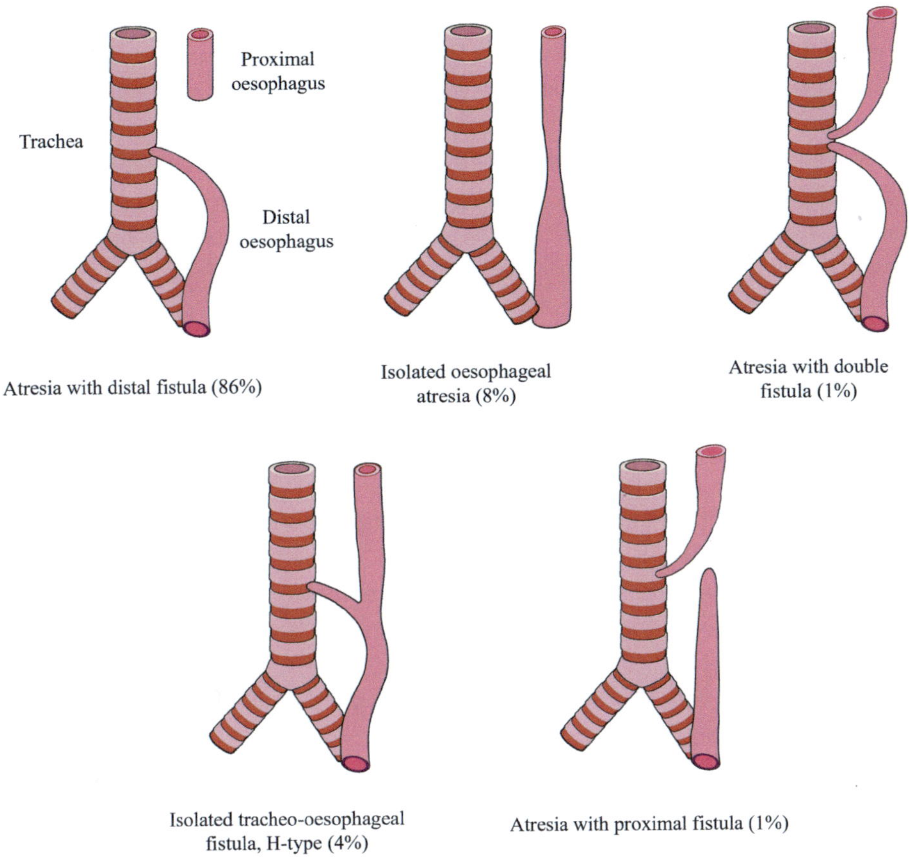

Figure 22.1 Types of tracheo-oesophageal fistula (Source: Jarrick Harris)

Diagnosis antenatally is challenging, and **polyhydramnios** may or may not be present. The anomaly may be diagnosed by antenatal ultrasound, where the inability to demonstrate a fetal stomach in the presence of normal or increased amniotic fluid is highly suggestive of OA (Hochart et al., 2015). However, if there is no antenatal diagnosis, symptoms will present in the early postnatal hours. The neonate will cough and choke on excessive saliva in the oropharynx and upper respiratory tract. If enteral feeds are offered, the oesophageal pouch will fill, followed by regurgitation and similar symptoms. Gastric contents can also reflux from the stomach through the fistula into the respiratory tract, presenting a danger of aspiration and pneumonitis. The abdomen will rapidly distend as the intestines fill with air.

Fetal magnetic resonance imaging (MRI) has been suggested to be of value in confirming the diagnosis when there is antenatal suspicion of OA (Hochart et al., 2015). The diagnosis of a proximal atresia is usually confirmed by passing a radio-opaque tube size 8–10Fg through a nostril until resistance is felt and by X-ray of the neck, chest and abdomen. The tube will sit in the oesophageal pouch or be coiled, if too small a tube is used. If there has been any suggestion of a possible fistula or atresia on the fetal **ultrasound scan** (USS), an attempt at passing a tube should be made soon after birth to confirm diagnosis. Although infants with an H-type fistula may have early signs of respiratory distress, aggravated by feeding orally, the diagnosis is not often confirmed in the early neonatal period and may not be diagnosed until adulthood (Suen, 2018).

Pre-operative care – key points:

- The neonate should be positioned with the head elevated at 45 degrees to prevent **aspiration** pneumonia
- A double lumen **Replogle tube** is placed in the upper pouch and connected to low-pressure continuous suction; this needs to be continuously observed to avoid this blocking with thick secretions (see Figure 22.2)
- Antacid administration to prevent pneumonitis secondary to reflux of stomach contents
- Endotracheal intubation is not routinely required prior to transfer in stable infants; however, airway management should be individualised. Positive pressure ventilation may lead to marked gastric distension via a **distal** fistula and should therefore be used cautiously in discussion with the surgical and anaesthetic teams.

Echocardiography should ideally take place prior to surgery, to identify any associated cardiac anomalies. In particular, the position of the aortic arch needs to be identified to

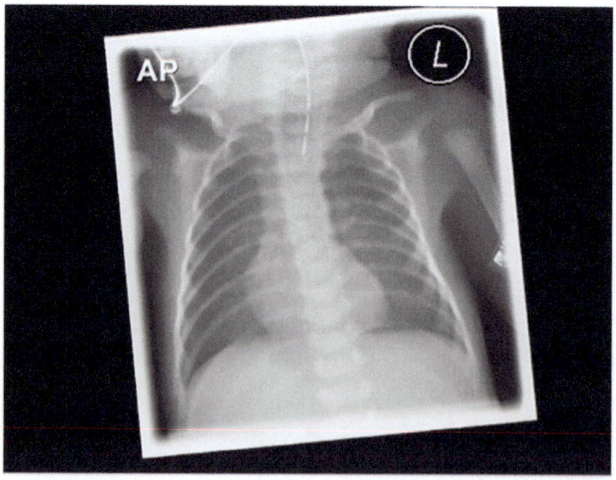

Figure 22.2 Replogle tube arrested in proximal oesophageal pouch (Source: Iain Yardley)

exclude a right-sided arch, as the OA/TOF repair via a thoracotomy is usually on the infant's right side. Other investigations to identify associated anomalies include renal and spinal USS, which can be undertaken once the baby is stable post-operatively.

The timing of the repair to the fistula and the establishment of oesophageal continuity, depends on the width of the oesophageal gap. Fistulae are usually repaired within hours of birth, with ideally end-to-end primary **anastomosis** of the oesophagus performed at the same time. More recently, repairs have been made via less invasive thoracoscopy.

If the gap is too long to allow for primary repair, this requires staged surgery allowing time for growth of the oesophagus. A delayed repair necessitates formation of a gastrostomy to allow for milk feeding. Currently, cervical oesophagostomies are only used in the context of severe chromosomal abnormalities or heart defects. Although the ideal oesophagus is the patient's own and every effort should be made towards oesophageal preservation, sometimes the gap never shortens to an operable length and it is necessary to perform a jejunal, gastric or colonic interposition. However, this is a huge undertaking with potential serious complications and should only be considered if the condition is otherwise irremediable (Gallagher et al., 2020). 'Sham feeding' is a technique by which any milk the baby obtains through oral feeding is simultaneously removed via a Replogle tube and subsequently administered via a gastrostomy. This can be employed while awaiting corrective surgery to maintain the sucking reflex and has been shown to reduce oral aversion and time to full oral feeds (Golonka & Hayashi, 2008).

Post-operative care – key points:

- The need for post-operative ventilatory support not only depends on the infant's respiratory status, but also the difficulty of the initial repair. If the anastomosis is under tension, muscle relaxants will be required and the baby nursed with the neck flexed for several days while healing takes place to avoid any possible tears at the anastomotic site.
- A chest drain or **retropleural** drain may have been inserted depending on the surgical approach and integrity of the pleura.
- A **transanastomotic tube** (TAT) will be in situ to minimise the potential for oesophageal stenosis and allow for early enteral feeding post-operatively. It is essential that the TAT is securely fixed and labelled, as unplanned removal can delay enteral feeding, and replacement of the TAT can seriously damage the surgical site.
- Mechanical and pharmacological management of reflux.

Complications of OA/TOF include:

- *Anastomotic stricture (in 30–50% of cases)* Feeding difficulties and vomiting, which may last for years, especially following tight repairs, are common and often relate to oesophageal **strictures.** The causes of strictures are multifactorial and include tension, reflux and anastomotic leaks. Frequent oesophageal dilatations may be necessary to enable normal eating and swallowing.

- *Gastro-oesophageal reflux* This is one of the most common long-term problems and is thought to be due to disordered oesophageal motility and the presence of a small-volume stomach. Treatment may involve non-invasive measures such as positioning, thickened feeds and prophylactic anti-reflux medication. However, recent studies have cast doubt over the efficacy of these medications and highlighted additional risks in their use with the LBW infant (Miyake et al., 2018).
- *Anastomotic leak* (in up to 20%) This can present as a tension pneumothorax, sepsis, mediastinitis and, if a chest drain is in situ, frothy saliva (Lee & Meeker, 2018). A minor leak will heal spontaneously, while a major leak will necessitate a chest drain, antibiotics or re-anastomosis. If a primary anastomosis has been performed, a contrast swallow may be requested to check for an anastomotic leak.
- *Tracheomalacia* This can be serious enough to progress to respiratory distress and causes the characteristic 'TOF cough' or 'seal bark' (Lee & Meeker, 2018). Severe cases of **tracheomalacia** may require aortopexy; fixation of the aorta to the sternum to maintain an adequate tracheal lumen. This pulls the aorta forward, which in turn pulls the anterior tracheal wall forward, preventing it from collapsing into the airway lumen.
- *Injured laryngeal nerve* This causes a hoarse voice due to vocal cord dysfunction.
- *Disordered peristalsis* This can contribute further to gastro-oesophageal reflux as well as constipation.
- *Recurrent fistulas* may occur and should be suspected in the child who develops frequent respiratory infections, with gagging, cyanosis and apnoea.

Parents should be given detailed information and advice about the long-term problems they may encounter. It may be useful to put them in contact with families of other children with OA/TOF and/or local support groups.

Early diagnosis, improved surgical techniques and sophisticated intensive care have positively influenced survival. Prognosis and quality of life is, however, significantly altered in association with presenting severity and other anomalies (Gallagher et al., 2020).

Intestinal obstruction

Signs of obstruction include bile-stained vomiting, abdominal distension, large gastric aspirates and delay or failure to pass meconium. Intestinal obstruction may be congenital and mechanical e.g. due to stenosis (narrowing), atresia (closure) or webs within the gastrointestinal (GI) tract; or functional e.g. meconium ileus due to cystic fibrosis or Hirschsprung's disease. Antenatal diagnosis of intestinal obstruction is usually identified on USS during the second to third trimester. The more distal the obstruction, the later in gestation the diagnosis is usually made, and the higher the likelihood of other anomalies. Fetal MRIs are now available, which can provide additional, more detailed information about the location of an obstruction, the presence of additional anomalies and anomalies previously difficult to identify, such as anorectal malformations (Lau et al., 2017).

There are three common causes of obstruction in the upper part of the GI tract and three in the lower part (Table 22.1) An abdominal X-ray may highlight the position of the obstruction, with the possible assistance of additional imaging studies such as contrast studies and MRI scans.

In general, the lower down the small intestine the defect, the later the presentation after birth. Irrespective of the cause, if obstruction is suspected, a size 8–10Fg oral or nasogastric tube (OGT or NGT) should be passed, aspirated regularly and left on free drainage. This will decompress the gut and prevent aspiration of GI contents. Intravenous therapy should be commenced and fluid and electrolyte imbalances corrected.

BOWEL ATRESIAS AND STENOSES

Stenosis or atresia (see Table 22.2) can affect any segment of the intestine, but most commonly affects the duodenum, followed by ileum, jejunum and colon.

The duodenum begins its development in the fourth week of gestation. Epithelial proliferation is so abundant that at 5 to 6 weeks there is temporary duodenal occlusion, and its failure to become recanalised by the end of the embryonic period (10 weeks) results in an obstruction. This obstruction varies from a simple membranous obstruction to a complete gap with two separate blind ends (duodenal atresia). Approximately 30% of patients with duodenal atresia have associated anomalies (vertebral, gastrointestinal, cardiac and renal anomalies), with up to 60% having Trisomy 21.

TABLE 22.1 CAUSES OF INTESTINAL OBSTRUCTION

Upper	*Lower*
Pyloric stenosis (usually several weeks after birth) Duodenal atresia Malrotation with volvulus	Meconium ileus (due to cystic fibrosis) Hirschsprung's disease Anorectal malformations (stenosis or atresia)

Jejunal, ileal and colonic atresias, on the other hand, are thought to be due to a localised intrauterine vascular accident with ischaemic necrosis of the bowel and subsequent reabsorption of the affected segment later in pregnancy and rarely have associated anomalies.

Presenting signs and symptoms vary depending on the site of obstruction:

- *Polyhydramnios* This is more commonly seen when the atresia affects more proximal regions of the intestine.
- *Small for gestation infant*
- *Vomiting* This tends to occur later in a more distal obstruction and tends to be bile stained (green), unless the atresia occurs before the ampulla of Vater (approximately 15% of duodenal atresias).
- *Abnormal abdominal appearance* Duodenal and jejunal atresia often coincide with a scaphoid appearance of the abdomen, whereas ileal and colonic atresia present with significant abdominal distension and visible bowel loops.
- *Passage of meconium* Depending on timing of the obstruction in pregnancy, meconium may be passed early on, followed by failure to open bowels. However, if the event occurs at an early gestational point, only mucus may be passed postnatally.
- *Abdominal X-ray indicative of obstruction* In the case of duodenal (and less overtly jejunal) atresia this is the classic 'double bubble' appearance (see Figure 22.3), caused by the presence of fluid in the stomach and duodenum proximal to the obstruction.

  Multiple dilated bowel loops are seen with more distal intestinal obstruction, usually in the absence of rectal gas. An upper gastrointestinal contrast study demonstrates obstruction by showing dilatation of the oesophagus, stomach or proximal duodenum with delayed or absent passage of contrast beyond the obstruction, sometimes with characteristic patterns such as a 'corkscrew' appearance in midgut volvulus or an abrupt cut-off in duodenal obstruction.

  A lower gastrointestinal contrast study (contrast enema) identifies distal obstruction by revealing a narrow distal segment with a proximal dilated bowel and a transition zone, as seen in conditions such as Hirschsprung's disease.

  Other findings can include a microcolon suggesting unused distal bowel in meconium ileus or distal atresia or filling defects within the colon caused by inspissated meconium.

Pre-operative care – key points:

- Gastric decompression
- Fluid resuscitation
- Correction of electrolyte disturbances
- IV antibiotics

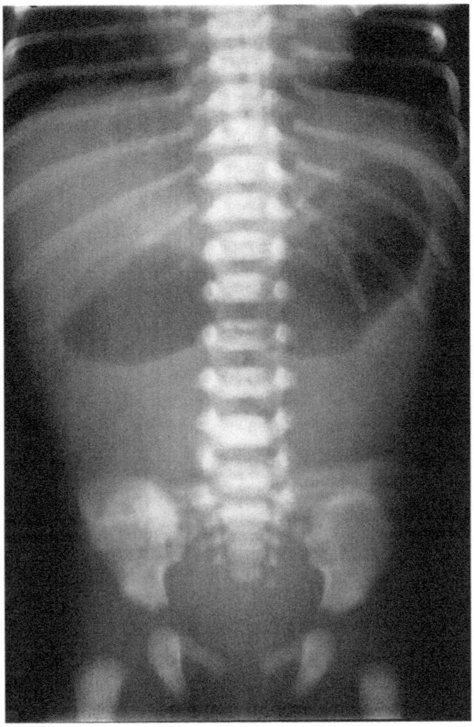

Figure 22.3 'Double bubble' indicating duodenal obstruction

Duodenoduodenostomy can be performed laparoscopically or as standard laparotomy, in a diamond-shaped fashion. Obstruction affecting other aspects of the intestine tend to be repaired as standard end-to-end anastomosis, but size discrepancy between the bowel sections proximal and distal to the atresia may necessitate formation of stomas, to allow for growth of the distal segment, if it is not possible to taper or cut the bowel section in such a way as to allow for primary anastomosis (Gallagher et al., 2020).

Post-operative care – key points:

- Continuing stomach decompression via a gastric tube
- Stoma care
- Replacement of stoma outputs – these will be particularly high in proximal obstructions – and correction of electrolyte imbalances
- Possibly refeeding stoma losses into the distal segment
- PN via a central line – this may be required for prolonged periods of time, as the return of bowel function can be slow

Generally, the long-term prognosis following the repair of intestinal obstruction is good, with sepsis and wound infections constituting the main potential issues in the early post-operative period (Gallagher et al., 2020).

TABLE 22.2 TYPES OF ATRESIAS

Type I	Mucosa and submucosa form a membrane
Type II	Bowel not joined, connected by fibrous cord
Type IIIa	No cord, V-shaped mesenteric defect, bowel variably shortened
Type IIIb	Large mesenteric defect, bowel significantly shortened. Also known as Christmas Tree or Apple Peel deformity due to appearance
Type IV	Multiple atresias of any combination, appearing as a string of sausages

(adapted from Gallagher et al., 2020)

MALROTATION WITH VOLVULUS

Development of the midgut results in rapid growth and physiological umbilical herniation during the sixth week of gestation. At 10 to 11 weeks, the gut begins a 270-degree counter-clockwise rotation around the superior mesenteric artery. The bowel destined to be the caecum re-enters the abdomen descending to the right iliac fossa, where fixation followed by closure of the abdomen occurs around the twelfth week. The duodenum with the duodenojejunal flexure (DJF) in the midline or to its left, and the proximal colon, are attached to the posterior abdominal wall. The small bowel is suspended posteriorly by **mesenteries** which carry blood, lymphatic vessels and nerves and extends from the DJF to the ileocaecal region.

Normally the mesentery has a broad base and cannot undergo **torsion**. **Malrotation** occurs when development is halted, and the caecum ends up adjacent to the duodenum. The mesenteries fail to become normally fixated, so the small intestines are suspended by a narrow stalk, which can twist into a volvulus, causing an acute obstruction. All bilious vomiting in the otherwise healthy term baby should arouse the suspicion of volvulus, which is a surgical emergency. An upper GI contrast study can confirm the diagnosis by showing the position of the DJF. As the volvulus continues to twist a few more degrees, the superior mesenteric artery becomes kinked and blood supply to the midgut becomes severely compromised leading to bowel ischaemia. Prompt surgical intervention is required to prevent bowel necrosis.

Pre-operative care – key points:

- Gastric decompression
- Fluid resuscitation
- Correction of acid-base-balance
- IV antibiotics (Gallagher et al., 2020)

Surgery involves untwisting the volvulus as soon as possible. Frequently Ladd's bands are found between the caecum and the peritoneum causing further obstruction by compressing the duodenum. These are divided, and the gut is mobilised and returned to the abdomen with the caecum on the left and the duodenum on the right, broadening the base of the mesentery, preventing the tendency to further twisting. Malrotation is thus changed into non-rotation (Ladd's procedure; Gallagher et al., 2020).

Commonly, an appendicectomy may be performed at the same time to minimise the future risk of a missed diagnosis of appendicitis, due to the position of the appendix now on the left. Recently there has been a move away from doing this routinely due to the immunological role of the appendix, so that the parents need to be made aware of this potential diagnostic difficulty (Lukish et al., 2022). Complications following malrotation include:

- Adhesive obstruction
- Short bowel syndrome
- Recurrent volvulus – higher risk with laparoscopic procedures vs laparotomy (Gallagher et al., 2020)

MECONIUM ILEUS

Meconium is a dark mucilaginous material that is a mixture of secretions of the maturing intestinal glands, ingested amniotic fluid and the debris of proliferative epithelial cells. It begins to fill the lower ileum and colon late in the fourth month of gestation and continues until the time of birth. Meconium ileus is caused by abnormal meconium blocking the terminal ileum and occurs in up to 25% of patients diagnosed with cystic fibrosis (CF). The neonate with meconium ileus will need to be further investigated to determine the diagnosis of this condition.

Within 48 hours of birth, the infant usually has abdominal distension and is vomiting bile. On examination, loops of gut may be visible or palpable, and meconium plugs may be passed following rectal examination. The abdominal X-ray shows dilated loops of bowel with a soap-bubble appearance of the bowel contents. Differential diagnosis includes Hirschsprung's disease (HD), ileal atresia and meconium plug syndrome. Perforation and meconium peritonitis may occur. Providing there is no evidence of this and the infant is stable, this obstruction can often be relieved with the hydroscopic action of a hyperosmolar enema (in term neonates). Adequate intravenous hydration is essential to avoid hypovolaemia, which could lead to shock. If enemas fail to relieve the obstruction or are contraindicated (as in preterm infants), surgery may be necessary. At laparotomy an incision is made into the bowel just above the obstruction and the abnormal meconium is washed out. A temporary de-functioning stoma may be formed (Gallagher et al., 2020).

Post-operative care – key points:

- Nasogastric decompression
- Parenteral nutrition
- Washouts of rectum or stomas
- Introduction of feeds once bowel functioning

HIRSCHSPRUNG'S DISEASE

Hirschsprung's disease (HD) is characterised by an absence of enteric ganglion cells in the submucosa of the distal bowel. These first appear in the developing oesophagus at five weeks and migrate down to the anorectal junction by 12 weeks. Their absence is attributed to the failure of migration, and the earlier the arrest of migration, the longer the affected segment of bowel. The **aganglionic** segment always includes the rectum, with the total colon affected in 10% of cases. This section is collapsed and non-peristaltic, causing functional intestinal obstruction. HD is the most common congenital bowel motility disorder, presenting in the first few days of life (Chhabra & Kenny, 2016). The neonate displays signs of distal intestinal obstruction: abdominal distension, (occasionally bile-stained) vomiting and delay or failure to pass meconium. Contrast studies show the aganglionic section to be contracted, with dilated proximal bowel. Gentle rectal examination may cause the explosive passage of meconium and flatus followed by normal bowel movements for a few days before signs of obstruction recur. Hirschsprung-associated enterocolitis, indicated by the presence of foul-smelling diarrhoea, abdominal distension, bile vomiting and potential perforation, may occur and is associated with a 50% mortality rate.

The diagnosis of HD is confirmed with suction biopsies of the colorectal mucosa.

Pre-operative care – key points:

- Nasogastric decompression
- Multiple daily rectal washouts as required. If these are successful in an otherwise well appearing infant, enteral feeds may be tolerated until the time of surgery
- Broad-spectrum IV antibiotics
- In those infants who have developed enterocolitis, fluid resuscitation and correction of electrolyte and acid-base imbalances are essential while the baby remains nil by mouth until surgery is performed on an emergency basis.

Surgery involves resection of the aganglionic bowel and a 'pull-through' procedure, although depending on the length of bowel affected, and in more unwell infants, a stoma may be fashioned and the pull-through carried out between 3 and 6 months after this.

Post-operative care – key points:

- Feeds may be introduced as soon as bowel function returns (usually after 24 to 48 hours) and built up gradually after this. Stools may be very frequent in the early post-operative period
- Meticulous perianal skin care
- Avoidance of manipulation of the area, such as introduction of temperature probes and suppositories, for 4 weeks post-operatively.

In the early post-operative period, wound dehiscence, anastomotic ischaemia and stricture may occur. Long-term complications include recurrent constipation, sometimes necessitating a colostomy, skin problems in the perianal area, enterocolitis and obstruction (Gallagher et al., 2020).

There is ongoing research with regard to stem cell therapy in HD; this promises to reestablish normal bowel function without the need for surgery and its associated long-term sequelae (Jevans et al., 2024).

MECONIUM PLUG SYNDROME

A distal obstruction is caused by firm meconium remaining in the colon, thought to be associated with immature ganglion cells. While it is not associated with CF, it has been linked to HD. Usually rectal irrigation or dilation resolves the condition, without a tendency for recurrence.

> **ACTIVITY**
>
> If you work in a NNU that does not care for surgical neonates, you may infrequently still be required to look after a baby with a stoma. Do you have resources locally to support families and staff with this?
>
> Have a look at this leaflet by stoma product supplier Hollister UK:
>
> https://www.hollister.co.uk/-/media/files/hollister-clinical-education/hollister-care-tip-pouchkins-premie-pouching-systems-all-01504.pdf (see web-based companion for a parent leaflet, which also contains lots of helpful information on everyday life with a stoma)

ANORECTAL MALFORMATIONS

Anorectal malformation (ARM) results from anomalous development of the urorectal septum, causing incomplete separation into urogenital and anorectal sections and an aberrant anal orifice. They present with a spectrum of anomalies, from minor malformations requiring minimal treatment, to a very sick infant with intestinal obstruction and complex life-limiting malformations. Anomalies of the upper urinary tract, cardiovascular system and spine are associated, as are atresias of the gastrointestinal tract and trisomy 21. Therefore, due to the high association with other anomalies, screening tools such as echocardiograms, renal and spinal USS need to be undertaken.

Complementary MRI studies are now providing valuable, reliable evaluation of ARM pre-operatively, but are not yet standard practice (Stafrace et al., 2022). Lesions are classified depending on whether the rectum ends superior or inferior to the puborectalis sling (see Figure 22.4). High lesions present as anorectal agenesis or rectal atresia, frequently associated with recto-urethral, -vestibular or -vaginal **fistulae**. Alternatively, low lesions are classified as anal agenesis, stenosis or an imperforate anus (which may be just a thin membrane through which meconium can be excreted). Low lesions are associated with anocutaneous fistulae and, in girls, an ectopic stenotic anus. Low lesions require division of fistula or anoplasty and may need frequent subsequent anal dilatations, but the prospects of long-term faecal continence are good. If the fistula can be dilated, the parents can be taught to perform this once or twice a day, as directed by the surgeon.

High lesions require formation of a stoma, anorectoplasty at several months of age, followed by anal dilatations and subsequent closure of stoma. Continence may remain a long-term problem. Urinary tract infections are common, especially with high lesions, and therefore, these babies are often given long-term prophylactic antibiotics (Gallagher et al., 2020).

Cloaca in females, where the bladder, rectum and genitalia have remained as one channel, represents a spectrum of defects. Depending on the ARM present, surgery required can vary significantly. Complex cloaca with a common channel above a certain length should be treated by a specialised team dedicated to these malformations (Bischoff, 2016). A team approach involving surgeons, urologists, nephrologists, gynaecologists, clinical nurse specialists and psychologists, will be needed in the long-term care of these children.

Post-operative care – key points:

- Following anorectoplasty of a low lesion, the focus is on skin care and regular dilation, commenced 2 weeks post-operatively and continued until approximately 6 months
- The more complex repair of a high lesion, after initial colostomy formation, is usually performed at 3 to 6 months of age, so that parents need to learn stoma care. The stoma is then closed 6 to 8 weeks after surgery.

A Foley catheter needs to remain in situ for up to two weeks in males, to allow for adequate bladder emptying.

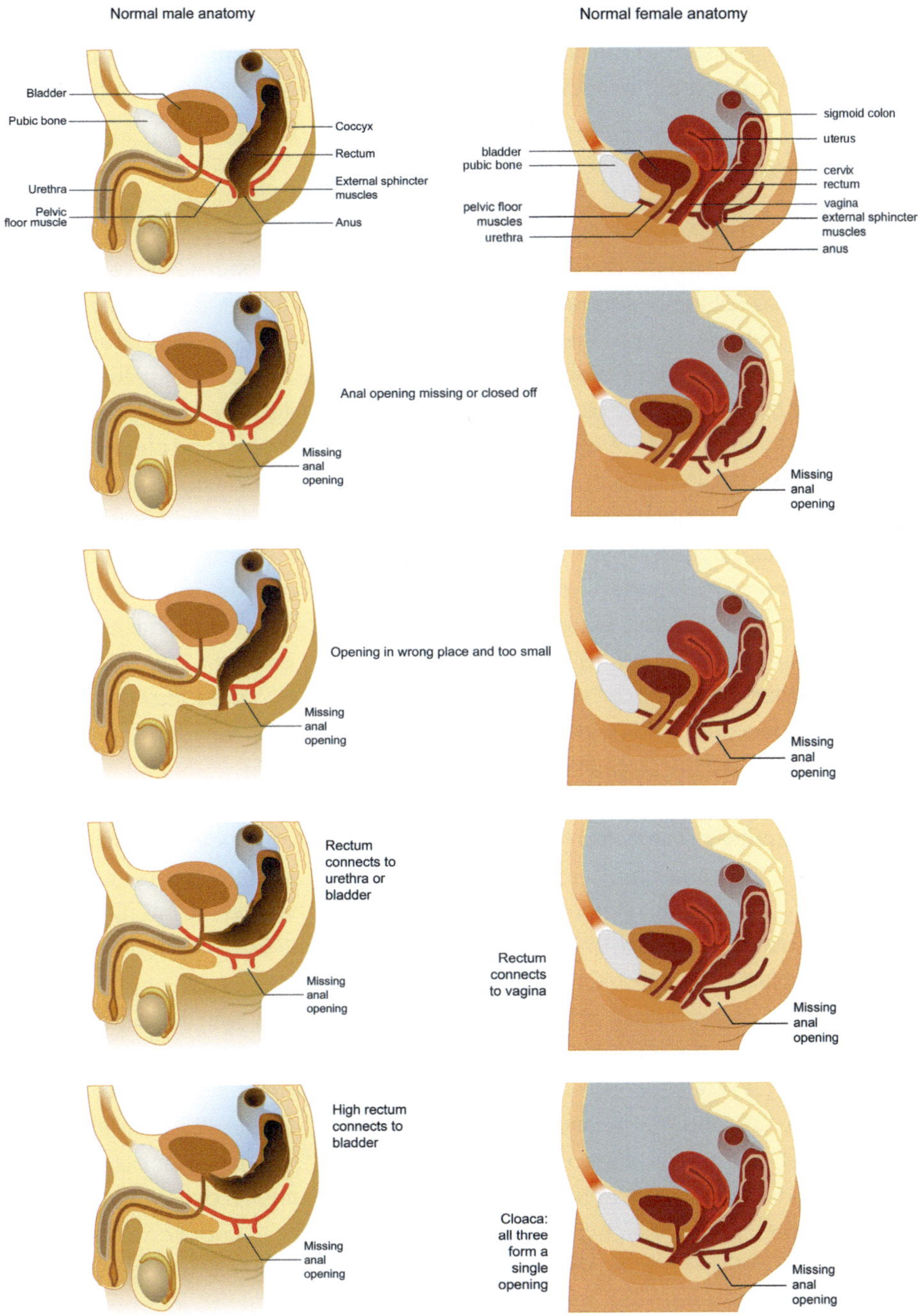

Figure 22.4 Types of anorectal malformation (Source: Jarrick Harris)

Apart from the risk of urinary tract infections, constipation in the low lesions and continence issues in the high lesions, sometimes necessitating formation of a permanent stoma, are the main long-term complications (Gallagher et al., 2020).

Congenital diaphragmatic hernia

During embryological development the thoracic and abdominal portions of the body cavity move freely until the diaphragm develops to separate them. CDH results from defective fusion of the pleuroperitoneal membrane when the intestines return by 11 weeks to the abdomen from the umbilical cord and allows the abdominal viscera to slip into the thorax. It is most commonly a posterolateral defect (95%), through the foramen of Bochdalek, but can also occur anteromedially, near the **xiphisternum** through the foramen of Morgagni. The resultant abnormal alveolar and pulmonary vascular development leads to pulmonary hypertension, which contributes to mortality and morbidity (Gallagher et al., 2020). The mortality rate worldwide between 2001 and 2012 was reported on average as 38%, varying from 11–55%, but decreasing over time. The overall mortality in the UK during this period was 36%. Higher rates were reported in countries where elective termination of pregnancy based on fetal anomaly was not permitted, with most deaths occurring between 2–6 days of age. Associated anomalies occur in 36% (Politis et al., 2021). These include chromosomal disorders and syndromes, cardiac defects, neural tube defects, genitourinary anomalies, cleft palate, omphalocele and oesophageal atresia.

Antenatal diagnosis can be made by USS as early as 12 weeks. For some neonates, however, it may not have been detected, so that they will present with respiratory distress soon after delivery. Some individuals may be asymptomatic and not diagnosed until later in infancy or childhood. The severity of CDH can be estimated using observed-to-expected lung-head ratios by ultrasound and total fetal lung volumes by MRI (Gallagher et al., 2020).

Clinical presentation includes a scaphoid abdomen with increased chest diameter, a shift in the trachea and cardiac impulse and decreased breath sounds, potentially with bowel sounds in the chest on the ipsilateral side. Radiologically, there is bowel in the thorax and an absent diaphragm (Figure 22.5). Malrotation may coexist. The main differential diagnosis is CPAM. Management is aimed at correcting the abnormality antenatally (rare) or ameliorating its devastating effects by preventing pulmonary hypertension postnatally. Fetal endoscopic tracheal occlusion (FETO), trapping fluid and thus stimulating pulmonary growth, has been recommended for fetuses with severe left-sided CDH to improve survival and reduce the need for extracorporeal membrane oxygenation (ECMO), but due to risks like preterm birth, it should only be performed at specialised fetal care centres. Careful patient selection and thorough parental counselling are essential before proceeding (Riddle et al., 2023).

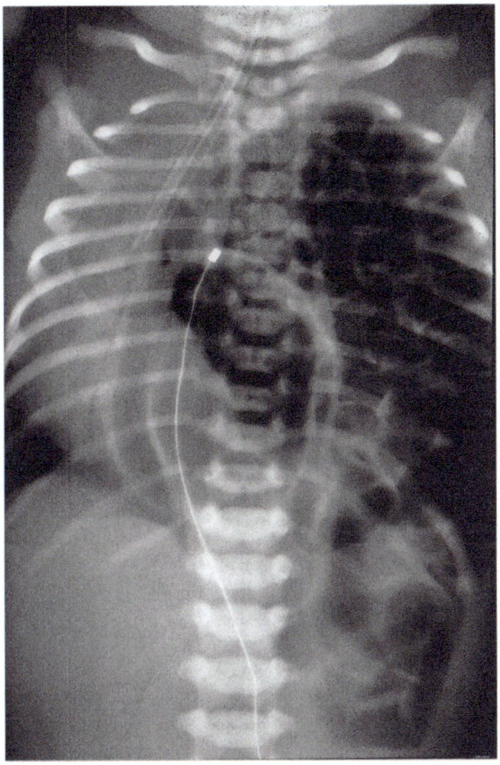

Figure 22.5 X-ray appearance of congenital diaphragmatic hernia

Pre-operative care – key points:

- At birth, it is important to avoid mask ventilation; if air is forced into the GI tract in the thorax, ventilation could be further compromised.
- Elective early intubation and consideration of muscle relaxants, even in the delivery room.
- GI decompression with a large bore NGT on continuous drainage with intermittent aspiration is of the utmost importance.
- Ventilation strategies to manage pulmonary hypertension, but with a focus on avoiding barotrauma/volutrauma. This may necessitate high frequency oscillatory ventilation and the use of inhaled nitric oxide.
- Ongoing sedation, pain control and neuromuscular blockade may need to be provided.
- Echocardiography within 48 hours to evaluate cardiac function and evidence of pulmonary hypertension.
- Haemodynamic support with administration of crystalloids, inotropic agents and hydrocortisone to treat poor perfusion to maintain urine output above

at least 1 mL/kg/hr and maintain blood pressure within normal range may all be required.

- Arterial access is crucial for determination of blood gas values.
- Life support in the form of ECMO may need to be considered in the management of the resulting pulmonary hypertension. Its role remains context-dependent. While some studies have not demonstrated a clear survival benefit at a population level, it is used as a rescue support in selected infants with severe disease, with outcomes influenced by case selection and centre expertise (The Canadian Congenital Diaphragmatic Hernia Collaborative (TCCDHC), 2018).

A delayed approach to surgical repair allows for adequate pre-operative stabilisation and has been shown to decrease mortality and morbidity. Surgery involves reduction of the viscera and repair of the defect, usually through a subcostal incision. For those defects not amenable to primary repair, a synthetic patch will be used. It may also be necessary to delay full abdominal closure, as the abdominal cavity can be too underdeveloped to accommodate its contents (Gallagher et al., 2020; see Figure 22.6 for an example of postoperative imaging).

Post-operative care – key points:

Initial post-operative care is not significantly different from pre-operative management.

- Avoidance of pulmonary hypertension and associated shunting. Ventilatory support can be weaned once the infant is stable with normalised blood gases.
- Pain control should be assessed, implemented and evaluated.
- Nutritional requirements will be provided by PN until the GI tract has recovered from the effects of surgery, analgesia and paralysis.

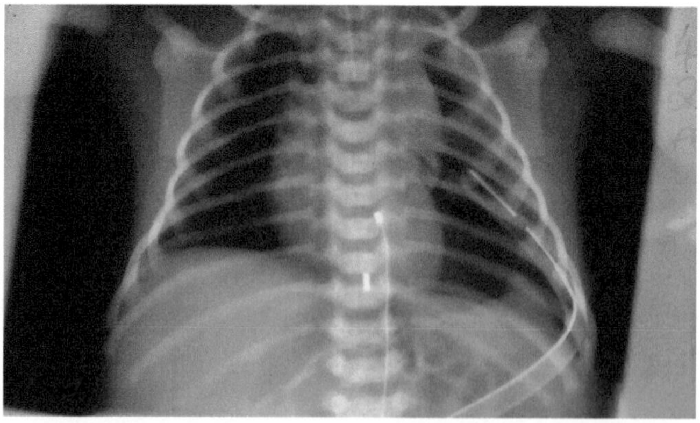

Figure 22.6 Chest radiograph following surgical repair of diaphragmatic hernia

Long-term complications include respiratory insufficiency, gastro-oesophageal reflux, failure to thrive, neurodevelopmental delay, behavioural problems, hearing loss, hernia recurrence and musculoskeletal deformities. Follow-up provided by a multidisciplinary team is essential in view of these associated long-term morbidities (Gallagher et al., 2020).

THINK POINT

Some of the surgical conditions presented in this chapter, and CDH in particular, require a high level of intensive care for a baby in critical condition. How could you promote family integrated care and facilitate healthy bonding within the physical constraints of the neonate's condition and the high demands on you as the nurse caring for the baby?

Abdominal wall defects

GASTROSCHISIS AND EXOMPHALOS

Gastroschisis and exomphalos, or omphalocele, two distinct conditions, are the most common congenital abdominal wall defects. The incidence of gastroschisis appears to be rising in HICs for reasons unknown, while the incidence of exomphalos has remained stable. The embryology of normal abdominal wall closure, and the sequence of events leading to umbilical and para-umbilical defects, are speculative.

The most popular description of exomphalos is a developmental arrest resulting in failure of the midgut to return to the abdominal cavity. The amount of herniated intestine varies from a small umbilical hernia-like lesion to a large anomaly containing the entire midgut and liver. Unless ruptured, it is covered with a sac consisting of peritoneum and amnion, the umbilical cord emerging from the caudal part. Eviscerated bowel in exomphalos is usually normal in appearance.

Gastroschisis is thought to be due to a vascular accident leading to incomplete closure of the anterior abdominal wall. There is no membrane covering the herniated bowel, which is usually to the right of the midline, and the cord is intact. The eviscerated bowel may be foreshortened, inflamed, thickened and matted with serosal peel due to prolonged amniotic fluid exposure. Up to 15% of infants with gastroschisis may also present with intestinal atresia (complex gastroschisis; Gallagher et al., 2020).

Accurate antenatal diagnosis can be made as early as 12 weeks of gestation, as an exomphalos in its sac is distinguishable from gastroschisis. Anomalies associated with gastroschisis are thought to be around 10%, whereas with exomphalos there is an association of chromosomal and genetic abnormalities such as trisomy 13, 18 and 21 in 50% of babies. Pentralogy of Cantrell,

Beckwith–Wiedemann syndrome and OEIS (**O**mphalocele – **E**xstrophy of the cloaca – **I**mperforate anus – **S**pinal defects) complex are widely discussed associated syndromes.

Vaginal birth has not been shown to result in damage to the bowel for infants with gastroschisis, whereas this is contraindicated in omphalocele if there is herniation of the liver present. If a baby with gastroschisis is noted to have signs indicative of inflammation on antenatal ultrasound, elective early delivery may be necessary. Table 22.3 details important aspects of care.

Surgery is not always necessary, and while primary closure is preferred, the intestines may be encased within a silo on the NNU. Mechanical ventilation with muscle relaxation may be required to aid the closure process. If a silo is used, it may remain in place for a period of 5 to 7 days, during which time the surgeons will gradually reduce the silo until full closure can take place. Pain control needs to be assessed, implemented and evaluated, and careful observation of the colour of the bowel within the silo is crucial.

Following any adjustments to the silo and immediately post closure, observations should be made for potential increased intra-abdominal pressure which can cause inferior vena cava compression and diaphragmatic splinting resulting in increasing respiratory requirements and haemodynamic compromise with cyanotic lower extremities and decreased renal perfusion causing renal dysfunction and metabolic acidosis. Surgical decompression may be required.

TABLE 22.3 CARING FOR A BABY WITH ABDOMINAL WALL DEFECT

Nursing consideration	*Details*
Heat loss prevention	Large heat loss from exposed bowel (gastroschisis) or through amnion (omphalocele).
Lesion protection	Cover immediately to prevent trauma (rupture of the sac in omphalocele), contamination and mesenteric traction.
Covering method	Cling film commonly used; bespoke bowel bag preferred for fluid retention and visibility.
Infant positioning	Place infant on right side to avoid mesenteric kinking.
Gastrointestinal decompression	Large-bore gastric tube on free drainage to decompress gut and prevent aspiration.
Respiratory support	Manage respiratory distress as needed. Avoid prolonged periods of non-invasive respiratory support to minimise gaseous bowel distension.
Imaging	Chest and abdominal X-rays to assess lungs, heart, diaphragm, bowel gas pattern and NGT position.

There will be decreased gastric motility and/or prolonged ileus which will delay enteral feeds. Therefore, central line insertion for the administration of PN is usually necessary (Gallagher et al., 2020). The commencement and time for tolerating full enteral feeds can vary significantly, reported at 9 to 14 days post-operatively depending on whether closure was primary or delayed, and generally tends to improve when feeding protocols are adhered to (Gilliam et al., 2021; Jyoti et al., 2024). NEC poses a considerable risk and therefore protective measures like the use of breastmilk should be promoted. This can be a very challenging time with the feeding regime subject to frequent changes due to dysmotility issues.

PRACTICE POINT

Neonates undergoing gastroschisis closure are at particular risk of abdominal compartment syndrome (ACS) due to reduced abdominal space and increased intra-abdominal pressure after returning the bowel.

Watch for *progressive abdominal distension, tense abdomen, rising ventilatory pressures, decreased urine output* and *systemic acidosis*. These may precede overt cardiovascular collapse.

Continuous observation of abdominal circumference, ventilatory parameters and urine output is critical. Nurses are often the first to detect subtle changes. Prompt escalation to the surgical and neonatal team is vital. Early recognition may lead to staged closure, silo adjustment or decompression to prevent catastrophic outcomes.

A large exomphalos containing centrally herniated liver poses challenges – the most significant being space limitations of the abdominal cavity and hypotension as well as impaired respiratory function from diaphragmatic splinting. In addition, the liver may exert pressure on the vena cava creating acute hepatic vascular outflow obstruction and renal compromise. If primary closure is not feasible, the defect may be left to develop an eschar (covering of slough) with the final repair at a later date; drying agents such as silver sulfadiazine may be used in the process. Granulation, epithelialisation and contraction of the sac size occur, allowing for reconstruction of the abdominal wall some months later. Enteral feeding does not normally pose as much of a challenge as with gastroschisis.

The prognosis of infants with abdominal wall defects is generally favourable unless there are significant concomitant abnormalities. Short term problems include dysmotility and risk of intestinal ischaemia and atresia. Morbidity in the long term is usually due to short gut syndrome or complications of long-term PN in gastroschisis. The process of closure for an omphalocele can be comparatively more complicated and carry a higher risk of compartment syndrome, but generally speaking, long-term prognosis is dependent on associated anomalies (Gallagher et al., 2020).

UMBILICAL HERNIA

This is due to a protrusion of a loop of bowel through the **linea alba** into a patent umbilicus. Unlike an omphalocele, it is covered by subcutaneous tissue and skin and distends during straining and crying. It is relatively common, with a higher incidence in infants of African American descent and babies born preterm. Complications are rare and include incarceration (where it cannot be returned to the abdominal cavity) and spontaneous rupture. Most defects up to 1 cm in size will close spontaneously by age 2, otherwise an umbilical hernia is generally repaired by the age of 5 years (Troullioud Lucas et al., 2023).

INGUINAL HERNIA

An inguinal hernia develops, often bilaterally, due to the **processus vaginalis** remaining patent after birth. It is one of the most common surgical conditions in infancy; the incidence increasing rapidly in preterm and small for GA infants, presumably precipitated by respiratory effort and positive pressure ventilation. It is more common in males, sometimes associated with undescended testes, and can be secondary to increased abdominal pressure with NEC and tight gastroschisis/ exomphalos repairs.

Presentation is a swelling in the groin, extending to the scrotum or the labia, and may only be visible while the infant is crying, feeding or straining to pass stool. The hernia can usually be reduced initially by gentle pressure, when it will return to the abdomen with a characteristic 'gurgle' (Ahmad & Greenaway, 2018). There is significant variability between hospitals worldwide with regard to timing of repair: while it remains reducible and asymptomatic, most centres delay definitive surgery until the preterm infant is ready for discharge. However, delayed repair has been associated with incarceration and bowel obstruction and early repair with a higher rate of post-operative respiratory complications and the need for reoperation. Hernia repair may be via open surgery or laparoscopic; again, each strategy has risks and benefits (Alquahtany et al., 2025).

Bowel ischaemia and ovarian or testicular atrophy can occur due to incarceration. Abdominal X-ray will show bowel, fluid levels and abdominal gas within the hernia. If the hernia strangulates, laparotomy and repair will be required. Resection and anastomosis may be necessary if the affected bowel is non-viable (Ahmad & Greenaway, 2018).

HYDROCELE

Occasionally the abdominal end of the processus vaginalis remains open but is too small to permit herniation of the intestine. Peritoneal fluid passes into it and forms a hydrocele; a painless collection of fluid around the testicle, presenting as a soft, non-tender, translucent swelling. Hydroceles are very common, usually resolve spontaneously by one year of age and are of no significance unless they become very large and tense, when a surgical opinion should be sought to avert torsion of the testes. Usually, hydroceles can be identified through transillumination of the scrotum, but, in case of any doubt, ultrasound provides a definitive diagnosis. Surgery, if required, consists of ligation of the inguinal canal (Radmayr et al., 2021).

Biliary atresia

Biliary atresia is a rare but severe neonatal condition marked by progressive inflammation and obstruction of the bile ducts, leading to liver fibrosis and cirrhosis. Affecting 1 in 5,000–20,000 newborns, its highest incidence is in Asia. Though its exact cause remains unknown, genetic susceptibility, environmental exposures and immune dysregulation are implicated. Diagnosis is challenging and typically confirmed via intraoperative cholangiography, but, in the absence of antenatal diagnosis via ultrasound, infants usually present with prolonged jaundice and pale stools. Early surgical intervention with Kasai portoenterostomy may restore bile flow, but many patients eventually require liver transplantation. Adjuvant therapies such as antibiotics, ursodeoxycholic acid, corticosteroids, are widely used but lack definitive evidence. Stem cell and tissue engineering therapies show promise in preclinical models but remain experimental.

Long-term complications include portal hypertension, cholangitis and cirrhosis. Nearly half of native liver survivors require transplantation by adulthood. Surveillance for hepatocellular carcinoma is essential. Growth and neurodevelopment are generally normal, though risks of malnutrition, bone disease and cognitive delays persist. Quality of life is reduced, especially in school-age children and adult women. Lifelong multidisciplinary follow-up is vital, with structured transition to adult care and holistic support addressing both medical and psychosocial needs (Tam et al., 2024).

Congenital pulmonary airway malformation

CPAM was previously known as congenital cystic adenomatoid malformation (CCAM) and is a developmental malformation of the lower respiratory tract. This is monitored on serial antenatal USS with the consideration of additional fetal MRI. Many lesions will regress in the third trimester; however, some lesions will progress to cause hydrops fetalis, a major prognostic factor. Antenatal management includes administration of steroids and minimally invasive procedures, such as drainage via a thoraco-amniotic shunt to alleviate the mass effect or even resection of the lesion. Postnatally, ultrasound or CT scan may be required for diagnosis as well as chest X-ray. Surgery is recommended if the baby is symptomatic with marked respiratory distress. While spontaneous regression has been described, current recommendations tend towards surgical removal even in asymptomatic cases, considering the low rate of complications intra- and postoperatively, being mindful of the increased risk of recurrent infections and malignancy with expectant management (Gallagher et al., 2020).

ACQUIRED SURGICAL CONDITIONS

Necrotising enterocolitis

NEC is a gastrointestinal inflammatory disease that can affect any part of the gastrointestinal tract, but those most frequently affected are the ileocaecal region, followed by the colon (Gallagher et al., 2020). It is associated with high mortality and morbidity, but particularly at risk are those babies born prematurely (before 32 weeks) and/or of LBW (less than 1500g). Among infants who develop severe NEC, mortality approaches 20–30% in very LBW infants and 40–50% in those weighing <1000g. In recent years, the prevalence of NEC in the most preterm population (22–24 weeks) appears to be declining secondary to feeding practices and likely also reduced use of antibiotics and antacids (Swanson et al., 2022). Its aetiology is incompletely understood with a multifactorial pathophysiology.

There appears to be a complex relationship between mucosal injury, infection and hyperosmolar enteral feeds:

Mucosal injury Hypoxia and systemic hypotension lead to sparing of the vital organs at the expense of the gut, which is vulnerable to hypoperfusion and ischaemic damage. Factors associated with hypoxic stress include prolonged rupture of membranes, placental abruption, poor condition at birth, respiratory distress syndrome and apnoea. Left-to-right shunting through a patent ductus arteriosus compromises blood flow to the gut, as does treatment to effect its closure (Gallagher et al., 2020).

Propensity for infection Due to their immature immune system, preterm infants are prone to entering an inflammatory state. Inflammation of the intestinal mucosa can render this more permeable, allowing for bacterial translocation in a population more at risk of infection due to indwelling central lines, prolonged ventilation and sometimes a delay in introducing enteral feeds. Furthermore, a dysbiotic, much less diverse microbiome in preterm infants contributes to reduced mucosal immunity. Whilst in milder cases of NEC signs and symptoms are limited to the gastrointestinal system, those more severely affected tend to be systemically unwell with positive blood cultures as in sepsis.

Enteral feeds The protective qualities of maternal or donor breastmilk over formula feeds have long been reported. In more recent years, growing evidence for the use of probiotics in high-risk infants has led to their widespread use in many countries (Duess et al., 2023). Since the 2010s there has been a distinct shift towards early introduction of enteral feeds, and there is a large evidence base demonstrating resultant reduced length of hospital stay and late onset infection. While commencing enteral feeds within 72 hours of birth does not reduce the incidence of NEC, this practice has not been shown to increase it (Chitale et al., 2022).

There is variance in the definition of the disease based on clinical signs and radiological findings both internationally and within the UK, which may arguably affect accurate reflection of NEC outcomes. The modified Bell Staging (see Table 22.4) is still the most commonly used tool worldwide (Patel et al., 2020). Its use as a diagnostic aid rather than a staging tool has, however, arguably contributed to the incorrect diagnosis of NEC in infants who may display some of the signs due to prematurity rather than pathology (Duess et al., 2023).

TABLE 22.4 MODIFIED BELL'S CLASSIFICATION

Stage	*Clinical findings*	*X-ray findings*	*GI findings*
IA	Apnoea and bradycardia, temperature instability, lethargy	Normal or bowel dilatation indicative of mild ileus	Increased gastric aspirates, vomiting, mild abdominal distension, occult blood in stool
IB	As above	As above	Bright red blood from rectum in addition to the above
IIA	As above	Bowel dilatation indicative of ileus, pneumatosis	As above, and absent bowel sounds, tenderness
IIB	Mild metabolic acidosis and mild thrombocytopenia in addition to the above	Widespread pneumatosis, ileus, ascites, portal venous gas	Abdominal cellulitis, right lower quadrant mass in addition to the above
IIIA	Acidosis, neutropenia, hypotension, coagulopathy in addition to the above	Definite ascites, in addition to the above, no free air	Generalised peritonitis, marked distension and tenderness
IIIB	As IIIA	Pneumoperitoneum	Same as stage IIIA

(adapted from Patel et al., 2020)

Abdominal X-ray can help confirm the diagnosis, showing distended and thickened loops suggestive of oedematous bowel. Pneumatosis intestinalis (the presence of gas within the bowel wall) can sometimes be seen confirming the diagnosis, although this can also present in other less severe bowel conditions. Serial films may reveal fixed, distended loops of bowel and an increasing 'white out' suggestive of free fluid (ascites). In the presence of perforation, **pneumoperitoneum** and gas in the portal vein may occur. Treatment for mild to moderate NEC is with antibiotics, intravenous nutrition and the suspension of enteral feeds with decompression via gastric tube for about 10 days. Sicker infants may require supplemental oxygen, analgesia and, in severe cases, full respiratory support, inotropes, fluid resuscitation and blood products, with operative intervention as a lifesaving measure.

Surgery is required when there is perforation or continued clinical deterioration. Laparotomy aims to preserve the maximum length of intestine while removing the necrotic bowel. The affected gut may be just an isolated perforation or a much larger area which is dilated and discoloured (see Figure 22.7), with denuded areas of mucosa, but still viable. Alternatively, there may be patchy, necrotic or totally disintegrated areas. If resection and anastomosis of the gut are not possible, formation of one or more stomas will be necessary. Stoma closure will be performed no earlier than after 6 to 8 weeks following contrast studies to ensure no strictures have formed (Gallagher et al., 2020).

Primary peritoneal drainage has been explored as an alternative to laparotomy but is not associated with improved mortality or neurodevelopmental outcomes,

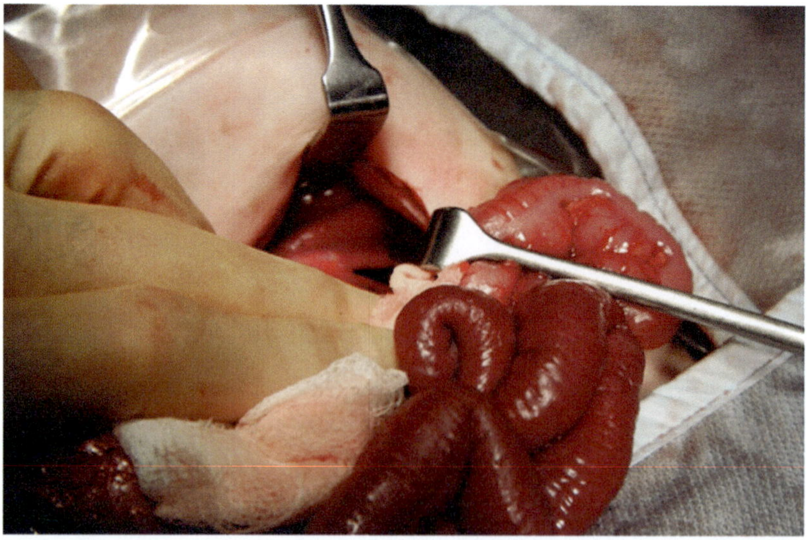

Figure 22.7 Ischaemic bowel identified at laparotomy (Source: Iain Yardley)

and many infants go on to still require surgery. Current guidelines recommend that the choice of management lies with the treatment centre, but suggests peritoneal drainage in order to stabilise infants who are too unwell for primary laparotomy (Hulscher et al., 2024).

Post-operatively, the stoma should be observed closely for deterioration in perfusion. There is a risk of recurrence of NEC, strictures and rarely the formation of fistulae. Malabsorption, failure to thrive and weight loss can be a problem post-operatively, and short gut syndrome may follow extensive resection (Gallagher et al., 2020). Enteral feeds should ideally recommence within seven days of surgery (Hulscher et al., 2024).

Despite improved survival rates, the aggressive form of the disease has not decreased and is still associated with significant rates of mortality and neurodevelopmental delay, including visual, cognitive and motor impairment (Duess et al., 2023).

Spontaneous bowel perforation

Spontaneous intestinal perforation (SIP) appears to have become more prevalent in extremely preterm infants over the past 15 years. It is diagnosed at laparotomy, where an isolated focal perforation is seen with the surrounding tissue of normal appearance. The ileum is the most commonly affected part of the bowel. Due to its similarities in clinical presentation, it can be confused with NEC. There are multiple associated factors, including LBW and the use of non-steroidal anti-inflammatory drugs, particularly if administered concurrently with steroids. Babies with SIP tend to be less likely develop severe illness. While mortality is noted to be significantly lower than that of NEC, long term outcomes are poor to a similar degree (Swanson et al., 2022).

Neonatal tumours

Neonatal tumours are rare, occurring in approximately 1 in 12,500 to 25,000 live births, and represent around 2% of all childhood cancers. Among the most frequently encountered are teratomas, cystic hygromas and neuroblastomas, each with distinct clinical implications.

Teratomas, particularly sacrococcygeal and cervical types, may be large and vascular, posing risks such as haemorrhage, dystocia or airway obstruction. Cervical teratomas often necessitate an EXIT procedure (see Box 22.3) at delivery to secure the airway before severing the umbilical cord.

Cystic hygromas, fluid-filled lymphatic malformations typically found in the neck, can similarly obstruct the airway and may require antenatal planning and postnatal intervention, including sclerotherapy or surgical excision.

Neuroblastomas, commonly arising in the adrenal glands, are notable for their potential to regress spontaneously, especially in infants under six months. Many are detected antenatally and present as stage I disease, often requiring only observation or surgical removal. Despite their generally benign or low-grade nature, neonatal tumours can be life-threatening due to their size, location or vascularity.

Histologically benign lesions may behave aggressively, and some embryonal tumours retain features of early development without full cellular differentiation. Advances in prenatal imaging have improved early detection, but survival outcomes remain variable. Genetic anomalies are present in a notable proportion of cases, and the underlying causes of tumour development in neonates continue to be a subject of active research (Gallagher et al., 2020).

BOX 22.3 EXIT PROCEDURE

The EXIT (*ex utero* intrapartum treatment) procedure is a specialised surgical delivery technique used when a fetus has a life-threatening airway obstruction or other congenital anomaly, allowing clinicians to secure the airway or perform urgent interventions while the baby remains supported by placental circulation (Gallagher et al., 2020).

Ovarian cyst

Ovarian cysts in fetuses and neonates are relatively common and identified on antenatal USS. They are thought to occur due to excessive stimulation of the fetal ovary by placental and maternal hormones. While many will regress, complications include haemorrhage, rupture, torsion, as well as vascular, urinary tract and intestinal obstruction. They should be followed up postnatally with an USS, and large or complex cysts may be laparoscopically removed (Laufer, 2024).

Testicular torsion

The neonatal testis may be prone to torsion because of its extreme mobility within the scrotum. On examination, the scrotum is non-translucent, swollen, firm and discoloured. USS with Doppler may be used to confirm diagnosis. The management is controversial and variable; however, immediate surgery is required, as, depending on the degree of torsion, complete atrophy of the testicle may occur within a few hours of the onset of symptoms (Radmayr et al., 2025).

FAMILY INTEGRATED CARE IN THE CONTEXT OF NEONATAL SURGERY AND ANAESTHESIA

The well-documented benefits of family integrated care (FiCare) extend also to the surgical neonate. Parental involvement should be maximised beyond mere partnership in decision-making. For instance, the positive impact of the presence of a calm parent during induction of anaesthesia has been well documented. Preparation of the parent for the physical changes they will witness their child undergo during this process is crucial, so as to avoid distress (Ohliger et al., 2021). Once the baby is in recovery, parents should be enabled to visit as soon as possible (RCoA, 2023). Both these measures are experienced as reassuring by parents (Gallagher et al., 2020).

The perceived loss of the parental role when an infant undergoes surgery can be counteracted somewhat by involving families at the earliest opportunity post-operatively in soothing their baby and supporting them in the acquisition of skills necessary for care activities such as gastric tube feeds, dressing changes and stoma care. Nursing care of the surgical neonate (see Table 22.5) must therefore encompass intensive family support. Adequate parental preparation, combined with the knowledge of possible post-operative complications, have been associated with a reduction in accessing healthcare facilities following discharge home (Gallagher et al., 2020; Pilkington et al., 2024).

TABLE 22.5 NURSING CARE OF THE SURGICAL NEONATE

Priority	*General nursing care*	*Condition-specific tasks*
Thermoregulation	Maintain neutral thermal environment; use warmed blankets/fluids; monitor core temp continuously.	**Abdominal wall defects**: Cover exposed viscera with warm, sterile, moist dressings pre-op; minimise heat loss.
Airway and ventilation	Position appropriately; monitor oxygen saturation and ventilatory pressures; anticipate airway difficulties post-op.	**CDH**: Avoid bag-mask ventilation pre-op; maintain gentle ventilation; monitor for pulmonary hypertension.
Haemodynamic stability	Continuous monitoring of HR, BP, perfusion; titrate fluids carefully; escalate changes promptly.	**NEC**: Watch for septic shock signs; support circulation with fluids/vasoactive agents as prescribed.
Fluid and electrolyte balance	Strict input/output measurements; monitor electrolytes; adjust IV fluids as prescribed.	**GI obstruction**: Maintain NGT on free drainage; replace losses with appropriate IV fluids; monitor for electrolyte imbalance.

TABLE 22.5 (Cont.)

Priority	*General nursing care*	*Condition-specific tasks*
Pain and comfort	Use neonatal pain scales; administer analgesia per protocol; provide non-pharmacological comfort (swaddling, buccal breastmilk, sucrose).	**Post abdominal surgery**: Balance analgesia with risk of ileus; monitor for escalating pain as a sign of complication.
Wound and line care	Maintain aseptic technique; inspect surgical site, drains, stomas; monitor for infection or leakage.	**Abdominal wall defects**: Monitor silo or closure site for tension, leakage or ischaemia; ensure secure line fixation.
Nutrition support	Initiate parenteral nutrition if enteral feeds delayed; transition carefully to NG/oral feeds; monitor tolerance.	**OA/TOF**: Delay oral feeds until repair integrity confirmed; monitor for aspiration; support with PN until safe enteral feeding.

Chapter takeaways

- Advances in antenatal imaging allow many congenital anomalies to be identified before birth, enabling planned delivery in specialist centres and early multidisciplinary involvement.
- Pre-operative stabilisation is critical. Careful assessment of airway, cardiovascular status, fluid balance and metabolic needs reduces perioperative risk. Neonates often require correction of hypovolaemia, electrolyte imbalance and glucose support before surgery.
- Surgical neonates, especially those with abdominal wall defects, are highly vulnerable to heat and fluid loss. Maintaining a neutral thermal environment is vital to reduce metabolic stress and improve outcomes.
- Neonates, particularly those born preterm, have unique physiology and immature drug metabolism. Paediatric-trained anaesthetists are essential, and strategies such as lung-protective ventilation and cautious drug titration underpin safe care.
- Intraoperative priorities include stability and monitoring. Continuous monitoring of temperature, oxygenation, perfusion and fluid status is essential. Warm operating environments, appropriate vascular access and readiness with blood products are key.
- Postoperatively, nurses must monitor ventilation, circulation, glucose, urine output and wound/drain sites closely.

- Different surgical conditions have various associated risks and complications. Nurses caring for surgical neonates need to have an awareness of these, so as to be able to contribute with their expertise to the best possible outcome for each infant and family.
- Parents need clear communication, involvement in care and reassurance throughout the surgical journey. Their presence supports bonding and enhances recovery.

CASE STUDIES

CASE STUDY

Case study 1: The deteriorating preterm infant

Alex is now 1 week old following delivery at 28 weeks' gestation weighing 1.2kg. He is currently receiving full enteral feeds of expressed breastmilk at 180mL/kg/day. You notice on your shift that he is having frequent apnoeas and bradycardias associated with colour changes, and his mother expresses concerns that he is not himself.

On assessment Alex is lethargic, pale and vomits his recent feed, which is slightly green in colour.

Q.1. What are your immediate actions?

Alex's condition quickly deteriorates, and he needs to go to the operating room as he has a perforation near the terminal ileum.

Q.2. How can you optimise his condition in preparation for surgery?

It is now four weeks since Alex had his operation, during which he required partial bowel resection and formation of an ileostomy. He is receiving breastmilk feeds at 150mL/kg/day but is not gaining weight.

Q.3. What is your management strategy?
Q.4. What are the potential future risks?

Case study 2: The term infant with delayed passage of meconium

Fahim is admitted with a history of not having passed meconium since birth (30 hours ago). He also has a distended, tense abdomen.

Q.1. What do you do?
Q.2. What investigations will be required and at what stage will they take place?

CASE STUDY

Q.3. What could the diagnosis be?

Following rectal suction biopsy, Fahim is diagnosed with Hirschsprung's disease.

Q.4. What specific information and support do the parents need?

Case study 3: The term baby with bile-stained vomiting

Chen was born at term and has been admitted from the postnatal ward with a history of bile-stained vomiting.

Q.1. What do you do?
Q.2. Her mother is very anxious – what explanations would you give her, what can she expect to happen next?
Q.3. What information do you need?
Q.4. What investigations are required?
Q.5. Is this considered to be a surgical emergency? Why?

For suggested answer guides to the questions posed in these case studies, please refer to the web-based companion site specific to this chapter. See www.routledge.com/cw/petty

References

Ahmad, N., & Greenaway, S. (2018). Anaesthesia for inguinal hernia repair in the newborn or ex-premature infant. *BJA Education*, *18*(7), 211–217.

Alqahtany, L. Y., Alsharif, A., Alsharif, A., Alanazi, O., Altaf, M., Kaleemullah, A., Alsaedi, L., Wasaya, H. I., Alharbi, A. H., & Bawazir, O. (2025). Impact of surgical timing on outcomes in neonatal inguinal hernia repairs: A systematic review. *Pediatric Reports*, *17*(1), 12. https://doi.org/10.3390/pediatric17010012

Bischoff, A. (2016). The surgical treatment of cloaca. *Seminars in Pediatric Surgery*, *5*(2), 102–107.

British Association of Perinatal Medicine (BAPM). (2024). *Framework: Perioperative care of extremely premature babies at <28 weeks gestation: A framework for practice.* BAPM. https://www.bapm.org/resources/peri-operative-care-of-extremely-premature-babies

Bösenberg, A. T. (2024). Pediatric anesthesia in developing countries. In C. J. Coté, J. Lerman & B. J. Anderson (Eds.), *A practice of anesthesia for infants and children* (7th ed., pp. 1299–1313). Elsevier.

The Canadian Congenital Diaphragmatic Hernia Collaborative (TCCDH). (2018). Diagnosis and management of congenital diaphragmatic hernia: A clinical practice guideline. *Canadian Medical Association Journal*, *190*(4), E103–E112.

Chhabra, S., & Kenny, S. E. (2016). Hirschsprung's disease. *Surgery (Oxford)*, *34*(12), 628–632.

Chitale, R., Ferguson, K., Talej, M., Yang, W.-C., He, S., Edmond, K. M., & Smith, E. R. (2022). Early enteral feeding for preterm or low birth weight infants: A systematic review and meta-analysis. *Pediatrics*, *150*(Suppl. 1), e2022057092E. https://doi.org/10.1542/peds.2022-057092E

Department of Health. (2009). *Reference guide to consent for examination or treatment* (2nd ed.). Department of Health.

Duess, J. W., Sampah, M. E., Lopez, C. M., Tsuboi, K., Scheese, D. J., Sodhi, C. P., & Hackam, D. J. (2023). Necrotizing enterocolitis, gut microbes, and sepsis. *Gut Microbes*, *15*(1), 2221470. https://doi.org/10.1080/19490976.2023.2221470

Gallagher, M. E., Pacetti, A. S., Lovvorn, H. N., & Carter, B. S. (2020). Neonatal surgery. In S. L. Gardner, B. S. Carter, M. E. Hines & J. A. Hernandez (Eds.), *Merenstein & Gardner's handbook of neonatal intensive care: An interprofessional approach* (9th ed., pp 996–1038). Elsevier.

Gilliam, E. A., Vu, K., Rao, P., Krishnaswami, S., Hamilton, N., Azarow, K., Gingalewski, C., Jafri, M., Zigman, A., Butler, M., & Fialkowski, E. A. (2021). Minimizing variance in gastroschisis management leads to earlier full feeds in delayed closure. *Journal of Surgical Research*, *257*, 537–544. https://doi.org/10.1016/j.jss.2020.07.072

Golonka, N. R., & Hayashi, A. H. (2008). Early "sham" feeding of neonates promotes oral feeding after delayed primary repair of major congenital esophageal anomalies. *The American Journal of Surgery*, *195*(5), 659–662. https://doi.org/10.1016/j.amjsurg.2008.02.001

Hochart, V., Verpillat, P., Langlois, C., Garabedian, C., Bigot, J., Houfflin Debarge, V., Sfeir, R., & Avni, F. E. (2015). The contribution of fetal MR imaging to the assessment of oesophageal atresia. *European Radiology*, *25*(2), 306–314.

Hulscher, J., Irvine, W., Conforti, A., Di Cesare, A., Ichino, M., Sfeir, R., Madadi Sanjani, O., Strohm, J., Hukkinen, M., Moschino, L., Norsa, L., Kokešová, A., Bakx, R., Kooi, E., Obermann-Borst, S., Palleri, E., Vermeulen, M., Spruce, M., Rolle, U., . . . & Burgos, C. M. (2024). European reference network for inherited and congenital anomalies evidence-based guideline on surgical aspects of necrotizing enterocolitis in premature neonates. *Neonatology*, *122*(3), 376–384. https://doi.org/10.1159/000542540

Jevans, B., Cooper, F., Fatieieva, Y., Gogolou, A., Kang, Y.-N., Restuadi, R., Moulding, D., Vanden Berghe, P., Adameyko, I., Thapar, N., Andrews, P. W., De Coppi, P., Tsakiridis, A., & McCann, C. J. (2024). Human enteric nervous system progenitor transplantation improves functional responses in Hirschsprung disease patient-derived tissue. *Gut*, *73*(9), 1441–1453. https://doi.org/10.1136/gutjnl-2023-331532

Jyoti, J., James-Nunez, K., Spence, K., Parkinson, B., Thomas, G., & Trivedi, A. (2024). Evaluation of gastroschisis feeding protocol: A retrospective cohort study. *Journal of Paediatrics and Child Health*, *60*(11), 675–679. https://doi.org/10.1111/jpc.16657

Lau, P. E., Cruz, S., Cassady, C. I., Mehollin-Ray, A. R., Ruano, R., Keswani, S., Lee, T. C., Olutoye, O. O., & Cass, D. L. (2017). Prenatal diagnosis and outcome of fetal gastrointestinal obstruction. *Journal of Pediatric Surgery*, *52*(5), 722–725.

Laufer, M. R. (2024). Ovarian cysts in infants, children, and adolescents. In C. J. Lockwood & E. DeVore Berlan (Eds.), *UpToDate*. Retrieved September 17, 2025, from https://www.uptodate.com/contents/ovarian-cysts-in-infants-children-and-adolescents#H520749915

Lee, S., & Meeker, T. M. (2018). Basic knowledge of tracheoesophageal fistula and esophageal atresia. *Advances in Neonatal Care*, *18*(1), 14–21.

Lukish, J., Levitt, M., Burd, R. S., Kane, T., & Sandler, T. (2022). More evidence against appendectomy at the time of a Ladd procedure. *Journal of Pediatric Surgery*, *57*(11), 751.

Macrae, J., Ng, E., & Whyte, H. (2021). Anaesthesia for premature infants. *BJA Education*, *21*(9), 355–363.

Miyake, H., Chen, Y., Hock, A., Seo, S., Koike, Y., & Pierro, A. (2018). Are prophylactic anti-reflux medications effective after esophageal atresia repair? Systematic review and meta-analysis. *Pediatric Surgery International*, *34*(5), 491–497.

Ohliger, S., Cronin, J., & Deutsch, N. (2021). Induction, maintenance, and recovery. In P. J. Davis & F. P. Cladis (Eds.), *Smith's anesthesia for infants and children* (pp. 423–454). Elsevier.

Patel, R. M., Ferguson, J., McElroy, S. J., Khashu, M., & Caplan, M. S. (2020). Defining necrotizing enterocolitis: Current difficulties and future opportunities. *Pediatric Research*, *88*(S1), 10–15. https://doi.org/10.1038/s41390-020-1074-4

Pilkington, M., Nelson, G., Pentz, B., Marchand, T., Lloyd, E., Chiu, P. P. L., De Beer, D., De Silva, N., Else, S., Fecteau, A., Giuliani, S., Hannam, S., Howlett, A., Lee, K.-S., Levin, D., O'Rourke, L., Stephen, L., Wilson, L., & Brindle, M. E. (2024). Enhanced recovery after surgery (Eras) society recommendations for neonatal perioperative care. *JAMA Surgery*, *159*(9), 1071–1078.

Politis, M. D., Bermejo-Sánchez, E., Canfield, M. A., Contiero, P., Cragan, J. D., Dastgiri, S., De Walle, H. E. K., Feldkamp, M. L., Nance, A., Groisman, B., Gatt, M., Benavides-Lara, A., Hurtado-Villa, P., Kallén, K., Landau, D., Lelong, N., Lopez-Camelo, J., Martinez, L., Morgan, M., . . . & Nembhard, W. N. (2021). Prevalence and mortality in children with congenital diaphragmatic hernia: A multicountry study. *Annals of Epidemiology*, *56*, 61–69.e3.

Radmayr, C., Bogaert, G., Bujons, A., Burgu B., Castagnetti, M., 't Hoen, L. A., O'Kelly, F., Pakkasjärvi, N. A., Quaedackers, J., Rawashdeh, Y. F. H., Silay, M. S., Kennedy, U. K., Gnech, M., Skott, M., van Uitert, A., & Darraugh, J. A. (2025). *EAU guidelines on paediatric urology*. European Association of Urology. Retrieved September 17, 2025, from https://d56bochluxqnz.cloudfront.net/documents/full-guideline/EAU-Guidelines-on-Paediatric-Urology-2025.pdf

Riddle, S., Peiro, J. L., Lim, F.-Y., Habli, M., McKinney, D., & Kingma, P. (2023). Fetal tracheal occlusion for congenital diaphragmatic hernia. *NeoReviews*, *24*(4), e263–e269. https://doi.org/10.1542/neo.24-4-e263

Royal College of Anaesthetists. (2023). *Chapter 10: Guidelines for the provision of paediatric anaesthesia services 2025*. Royal College of Anaesthetists. Retrieved October 4, 2025, from https://rcoa.ac.uk/gpas/chapter-10#chapter-1

Spaeth, J. P., & Lam, J. E. (2024). The extremely premature infant (micropremie) and common neonatal emergencies. In C. J. Coté, J. Lerman & B. J. Anderson (Eds.), *A practice of anesthesia for infants and children* (7th ed., pp. 953–981). Elsevier.

Stafrace, S., Lobo, L., Augdal, T. A., Avni, F. E., Bruno, C., Damasio, M. B., Darge, K., Franchi-Abella, S., Herrmann, J., Ibe, D., Kljucevsek, D., Mentzel, H.-J., Napolitano, M., Ntoulia, A., Ording-Müller, L.-S., Perucca, G., Petit, P., Smets, A. M., Toso, S., . . . Riccabona, M. (2022). Imaging of anorectal malformations: Where are we now? Abdominal imaging task force of the European Society of Paediatric Radiology. *Pediatric Radiology*, *52*(9), 1802–1809. https://doi.org/10.1007/s00247-022-05395-7

Suen, H. C. (2018). Congenital H-type tracheoesophageal fistula in adults. *Journal of Thoracic Disease*, *10*(Suppl. 16), S1905.

Swanson, J. R., Hair, A., Clark, R. H., & Gordon, P. V. (2022). Spontaneous intestinal perforation (Sip) will soon become the most common form of surgical bowel disease in the extremely low birth weight (Elbw) infant. *Journal of Perinatology*, *42*(4), 423–429. https://doi.org/10.1038/s41372-022-01347-z

Tam, P. K. H., Wells, R. G., Tang, C. S. M., Lui, V. C. H., Hukkinen, M., Luque, C. D., De Coppi, P., Mack, C. L., Pakarinen, M., & Davenport, M. (2024). Biliary atresia. *Nature Reviews Disease Primers*, *10*, 47. https://doi.org/10.1038/s41572-024-00533-x

Troullioud Lucas, A. G., Barmani, S., Panda, S. J., & Mendez, M. D. (2023). Pediatric umbilical hernia. In *StatPearls*. StatPearls Publishing. Retrieved September 16, 2025, from https://www.ncbi.nlm.nih.gov/sites/books/NBK459294/

Varthaliti, A., Pergialiotis, V., Theodora, M., Lygizos, V., Daskalaki, M. A., Antsaklis, P., & Daskalakis, G. (2025). Advances in fetal surgery: A narrative review of therapeutic interventions and future directions. *Medicina (Kaunas)*, *61*(7), 1136. Retrieved August 13, 2025, from https://doi.org/10.3390/medicina61071136

Zhu, J., He, X., & Guo, M. (2025). Association of early hyperglycemia with morbidity and mortality in very low birth weight infants. *BMC Pediatrics*, *25*(1), 667. https://doi.org/10.1186/s12887-025-06035-3

23 NEONATAL DIAGNOSTIC PROCEDURES

Jenni Jones

CONTENTS

DOI: 10.4324/9781003591405-28

GUIDANCE ON HOW TO ENHANCE PERSONAL LEARNING FROM THIS CHAPTER

Key points covered in this chapter

- An overview of common neonatal diagnostic procedures, their background and normal and abnormal findings.
- Nursing considerations for neonatal blood sampling, lumbar puncture and radiographic, ultrasound and magnetic resonance image acquisition.
- Strategies to support babies and families during neonatal diagnostic procedures.

Reflection

Reading through the chapter, you are encouraged to engage with the key points and related literature in an enquiring way. Ask these questions:

- Which diagnostic procedures have you observed on the neonatal unit and what was the clinical question they were trying to answer?
- What is the nurse's role in individual diagnostic procedures?
- How can infants be prepared for and supported during some of the most common diagnostic procedures and how can parents be involved in this?

Implications for nursing care

- Finally, how will this chapter enable you to holistically plan and manage the care of infants and their families during diagnostic procedures? Consider the implications of what you learn for your nursing care relating to this area.

INTRODUCTION AND BACKGROUND

Diagnostic procedures are a vital tool in neonatal care, enabling the practitioner to assess the health status of infants, identify diseases and plan care accordingly. Due to major advances in technology and healthcare, a wide range of procedures is now available to facilitate the optimisation of care, improve survival and establish long-term prognosis of vulnerable and sick newborn infants. In this chapter, the most commonly used diagnostic procedures and the rationales for their employment on the neonatal unit will be discussed and related to relevant conditions and diseases. In addition, the nurse's role during individual procedures is considered and specific management strategies to support infants and their families during a range of investigative tests discussed.

BLOOD SAMPLING

Blood sampling is the most common diagnostic procedure on the neonatal unit (NNU). Premature and sick infants require close monitoring, and both point of care and laboratory testing of blood samples provides valuable information on health status and care requirement. Neonatal blood for analysis may be obtained via a number of routes, and both the infant's condition as well as the blood test required will dictate the most suitable method of collection.

Capillary sampling

This is the most frequently chosen method of blood sampling in the neonate, and the sample collected in this way is suitable for most blood tests. It is obtained from the capillaries located in the hypodermis after puncturing the skin with an automated lancet, and the sample yielded is composed of both venous and arterial blood. The only suitable site for capillary sampling is the **medial** or **lateral** plantar aspect of the infant's heel (Figure 23.1), as this avoids accidental injury to the **calcaneal** and **plantar nerves**, as well as the plantar arteries. Capillary

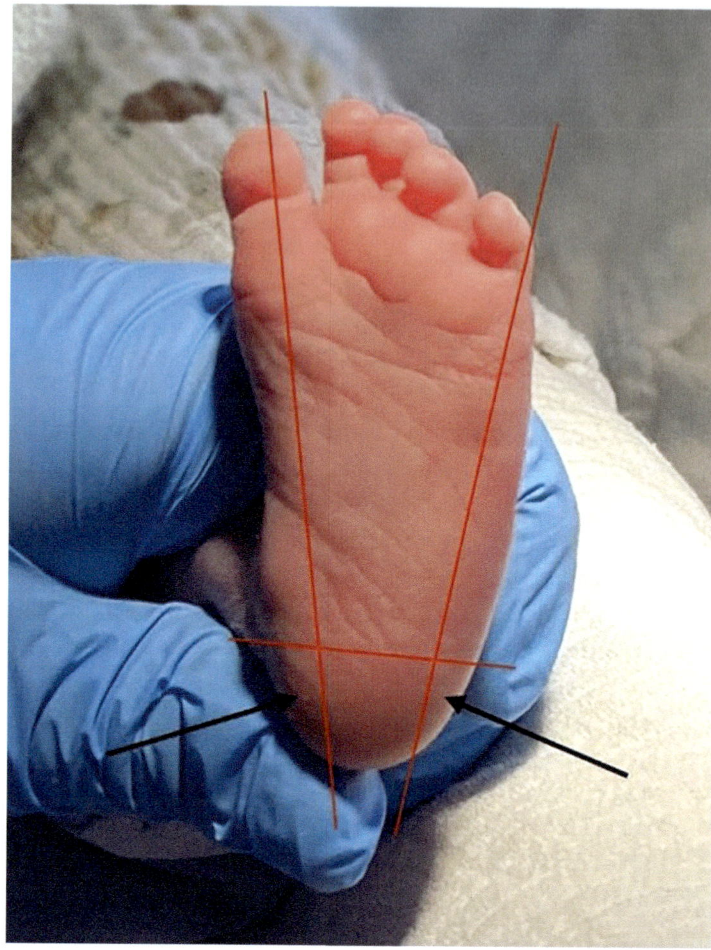

Figure 23.1 Suitable sites for capillary sampling: medial and lateral plantar aspect of the foot (Source: Jenni Jones)

sampling does not require specialist training and is frequently carried out by neonatal nursing staff following a competency assessment.

Venous sampling

This method of sampling, where blood is obtained via direct venepuncture, is the preferred method when larger volumes of blood are required than can practically be obtained from a capillary sample. In addition, samples for blood cultures should be obtained by venepuncture rather than capillary sampling, as this reduces the risk of accidental skin flora contamination and subsequent false positive results.

Arterial sampling

Arterial blood is most commonly collected for blood gas analysis. Although capillary samples can approximate many arterial blood gas values, they do not reliably reflect oxygen levels and therefore cannot be used to assess hypoxaemia. Arterial blood may be obtained by direct arterial puncture, but is more often collected via an umbilical artery catheter (UAC) or arterial percutaneously inserted central catheter (PICC). Where available, these lines should be accessed using a closed-circuit sampling system, primed with heparinised saline and connected immediately after line insertion. Closed-circuit systems significantly reduce infection risk associated with arterial puncture, but variations exist, so practitioners must be familiar with local systems and guidelines. Aseptic non-touch technique (ANTT) is essential when accessing the sampling port due to the high risk of pathogen transmission. This includes cleaning the port for 15 seconds with an appropriate disinfectant, allowing 30 seconds drying time and protecting all key parts. Arterial blood from closed systems is suitable for most tests, except coagulation studies due to heparin contamination. Heparinised syringes must be used for blood gases and non-heparinised syringes for other tests. After sampling, the line is flushed with heparinised saline. Throughout the procedure, infant limb perfusion must be monitored closely, and any signs of ischaemia require immediate cessation and urgent review.

Nursing considerations for skin-breaking procedures

Skin-breaking procedures are painful for infants and repeat exposure to pain and stress adversely affects physiological, neurological, psychosocial and behavioural development of infants (Williams & Lascelles, 2020). Measures must be taken to mitigate the stress response triggered by a skin-breaking procedure. A number of non-pharmacological methods can be utilised to comfort the infant during blood sampling. Most parents have a strong desire to actively participate in alleviating their infant's pain (Ullsten et al., 2021). Breastfeeding has been shown to be one of the most effective methods to alleviate procedural pain in neonates (Shah et al., 2023), and where possible, mothers should therefore be encouraged to breastfeed their infant during sampling. Furthermore, kangaroo care can be provided by either parent and has been shown to be beneficial in relieving pain during routine procedures (Sharma & Ruikar, 2022). Other beneficial methods of non-pharmacological pain relief include facilitated tucking, where the infant is placed in a midline position and the legs, arms, torso or head are gently cradled (Subedi et al., 2024), non-nutritive sucking (Pillai et al., 2023) and administration of breastmilk or 24% sucrose (Velumula et al., 2022). For more information on how to manage procedural pain, see Chapter 8.

Furthermore, blood sampling is a major cause of blood loss during the neonatal period, with research indicating that in preterm infants, it can account for as much as between one third and half of their total blood volume (Counsilman et al., 2019), leading to **iatrogenic** anaemia and an increased requirement of red blood cell transfusion. Therefore, blood samples should only be taken to answer a specific clinical question, and routine sampling must be avoided.

COMMON BLOOD TESTS AND CONSIDERATIONS FOR SAMPLE COLLECTION

Blood culture

Blood culture samples are collected in large bottles (Figure 23.2) containing nutrient-rich fluid to support microbial growth and an anticoagulant to prevent clotting. In adult practice, paired cultures, one aerobic and one anaerobic, are obtained to identify the widest range of pathogens (Gottschalk et al., 2024). However, the optimal 20–30 mL sample volume (Miller, 2018) is unsuitable for

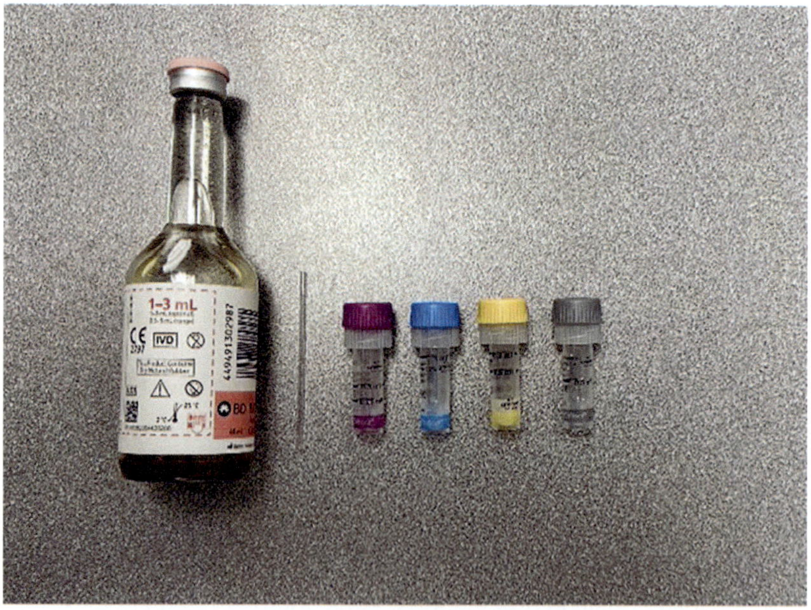

Figure 23.2 From left to right: Blood culture bottle, capillary sample tube for blood gas, EDTA bottle, coagulation sample bottle, SST bottle, whole blood biochemistry bottle (Source: Jenni Jones)

neonates. The Infectious Disease Society of America therefore recommends that when only limited blood volume is available, such as in neonates, a minimum of 1 mL should be collected and inoculated into a single aerobic bottle (Miller, 2018), as most bacteraemia is caused by aerobic organisms. Where possible, the sample should be taken before antibiotic therapy, as residual antibiotics may inhibit growth and lead to false negatives. Blood must be collected via direct venous access and obtained before all other samples to minimise contamination. Bottle tops must also be disinfected thoroughly before inoculation. Once received in the laboratory, a culture and sensitivity (C&S) test is performed: the sample is incubated for up to 10 days and monitored for growth, with preliminary results typically available at 36 hours. If positive, sensitivity testing identifies the most effective antimicrobial therapy.

Blood gas

Most commonly, blood gas analysis results are obtained via point of care testing, and samples are collected in either blood gas tubes during capillary sampling or dedicated syringes which allow sample collection by either direct arterial puncture or via closed-system sampling. Both are coated internally with a layer of heparin to prevent clotting, and following blood collection, the ends of the tube or syringe must be occluded and the sample agitated for 30 seconds to ensure adequate mixing with the anticoagulant.

In order to produce accurate results, capillary gas samples should be obtained first when multiple samples are collected, as during the sampling process, capillary blood becomes progressively venous. In addition, care must be taken to avoid air bubbles in the sample, as these lead to erroneous results and sample rejection. Following collection, blood gas samples should be analysed for various tests (Table 23.1) as soon as possible, as a delay may lead to clotting or falsely elevated carbon dioxide levels caused by continued cellular metabolism.

TABLE 23.1 COMMON ELEMENTS TESTED USING A BLOOD GAS ANALYSER

Acid-base balance and gases	To establish the blood pH and the partial pressures of tissue oxygen and carbon dioxide, along with an indication of the potential causes for acidosis or alkalosis. Blood gas values can be viewed in Chapter 14.
Blood glucose	To rapidly obtain a blood glucose value, in particular in hypoglycaemic neonates (Janjindamai et al., 2022).

TABLE 23.1 (Cont.)

Lactate	A byproduct of anaerobic metabolism, in which glucose is converted into the cellular energy source adenosine triphosphate (ATP). Elevated levels may indicate cardiovascular problems, hypoxia, sepsis, inborn errors of metabolism or organ dysfunction (Ganetzky & Cuddapah, 2017).
Ionised calcium	Whilst serum samples provide information on the total amount of calcium in the blood, ionised calcium describes the amount of calcium molecules not bound to proteins.
Bilirubin levels	Depending on the type of blood gas analyser and local policy, levels provided may be utilised to guide phototherapy treatment.
Other results	Some analysers provide additional values, including haemoglobin and electrolyte levels.

PRACTICE POINTS

Lactate levels are often erroneously elevated if there is excess squeezing of the foot during capillary sampling, or if sample analysis was delayed, and the potential causes for abnormal values must be considered before initiating treatment. In addition, Hb and electrolyte, results are usually less accurate than those provided by laboratory analysis and should therefore be interpreted with caution (Erturk et al., 2024).

Coagulation studies

Sample bottles for coagulation studies (Table 23.2) usually have a blue top and contain added sodium citrate, which binds to the calcium ions within the blood in order to render them inactive. Ionised calcium is required to activate a number of clotting factors during the coagulation cascade, and binding therefore prevents the sample from clotting prior to analysis. The process is reversible, allowing for calcium to become ionised again once received in the laboratory in order to conduct clotting time analysis. To ensure the correct ratio of blood to additive, sample bottles must be filled up to the specified level. In addition, blood for coagulation studies must be obtained via venous or arterial sampling, as capillary sampling may expedite clotting due to potential contamination with tissue factor (TF), the initiating substance of the clotting cascade.

TABLE 23.2 COMMON TESTS ANALYSED FROM COAGULATION STUDIES

Prothrombin time (PT)	The time in seconds it takes for the blood plasma sample to clot once the coagulation cascade begins. In neonates, the most common cause of prolonged PT is vitamin K deficiency.
Activated partial thromboplastin time (APTT)	This test investigates the intrinsic and common pathways of the clotting cascade, triggered when damage occurs to the vascular endothelium, by assessing the length of time in seconds until clot formation occurs once the reactive agent calcium chloride is added. A prolonged APTT may indicate coagulopathy, for example following a hypoxic event at birth.
Fibrinogen	A protein which, during the final step of the clotting cascade, is converted to fibrin, a crucial component for thrombus formation. Low fibrinogen, together with a prolonged PT and APTT can be an indicator of disseminated intravascular coagulopathy as discussed in Chapter 17.

PRACTICE POINT

In severely elevated PT and APTT, or when bleeding caused by coagulopathy is observed, a transfusion of fresh frozen plasma may be given, as it contains both clotting factors and fibrinogen and can therefore activate the clotting cascade.

Full blood count/complete blood count

Sample bottles usually have a purple top. They contain ethylenediaminetetraacetic acid (EDTA), an anticoagulant with a similar mode of action as sodium citrate, with the difference that the EDTA binding process is irreversible. Full blood count samples should be gently inverted several times to ensure thorough mixing with EDTA and prevent clotting. Table 23.3 outlines common tests carried out on a FBC. See Chapter 17 for more details on the diagnosis and management of common neonatal haematological problems.

Transfusion-related studies

Samples sent to the blood bank are usually collected in purple or pink topped bottles which, like FBC bottles, contain EDTA to prevent clotting. Care must be

TABLE 23.3 COMMON TESTS PERFORMED ON A FULL BLOOD COUNT

Haemoglobin (Hb)	The oxygen-binding component of red blood cells. A drop in Hb during the first weeks of life is usually due to normal physiological processes, or it may be pathological in origin. Pathological anaemia may be haemolytic (increased red blood cell destruction), haemorrhagic (loss of red blood cells) or caused by insufficient or inefficient erythropoiesis.
Haematocrit	The percentage of red blood cells, or ratio of red blood cells to total blood volume. Polycythemia is indicated by a venous hematocrit of >65%, caused by either excess red blood cell load or a decreased plasma volume. Hyperviscosity can impair end-organ perfusion and oxygen delivery.
Platelets	Thrombocytopenia is defined as a platelet count of < 150,000 per microlitre and severe thrombocytopenia at <50,000 per microlitre.
Reticulocytes	Immature, nuclei-lacking red blood cells, produced in the bone marrow and released into the circulatory system. On the FBC, the reticulocyte count is usually given as a total number per litre. In anaemia, it is useful to calculate the number of reticulocytes relative to total red blood cells in order to establish adequacy of the body's response to low Hb levels.
White blood cells	Neonatal reference values for white blood cell count vary considerably, depending on gestation at birth and postnatal age. See Chapter 20 for further details.
Blood film	Examines morphology, number and size of red blood cells, white blood cells and platelets to establish any abnormalities.

taken when preparing these samples prior to dispatch to the laboratory, as hospital guidelines often require labels to be hand-written at the cot-side immediately after blood collection, in order to reduce the risk of mislabelling and subsequent patient misidentification. Table 23.4 outlines the tests performed when a transfusion may be required.

Biochemistry studies

Most biochemistry studies (see Tables 23.5 and 23.6) are collected in a yellow or gold topped serum separating tube (SST), containing the agent silica, which initiates the clotting cascade and thereby causes aggregation of the whole blood cells, as well as a polymer gel, visible at the bottom of the tube. The latter forms a barrier between the clotted cells and the plasma following centrifugation in the

TABLE 23.4 COMMON STUDIES PERFORMED IN THE TRANSFUSION LABORATORY

Blood group and direct antiglobulin test (DAT)/ direct Coombs test (DCT)	Establishes blood group and tests for evidence of antibodies on the surface of the red blood cells, indicating haemolytic disease of the fetus and newborn caused by an incompatibility between maternal and infant blood groups. See Chapter 17 for more detail on feto-maternal blood incompatibilities.
Crossmatch	When the need for a blood-product transfusion arises, the blood group is established and the sample tested for antibodies, before matching it with the required donor blood product.

TABLE 23.5 COMMON BIOCHEMISTRY STUDIES

Urea and electrolyte profile (U&Es)	Urea is the end-product of protein metabolism, converted by liver enzymes from the highly toxic ammonia into this less-toxic, excretable compound. An elevated urea can be an early sign of acute kidney injury (AKI) or dehydration. U&Es include electrolytes sodium, potassium and chloride.
Creatinine	A byproduct of muscle metabolism, usually completely excreted via the kidneys. In the neonate, initial creatinine levels reflect maternal values, so are an unreliable marker of kidney function (Allegaert et al., 2020). However, during the first few days of life, levels should be gradually decreasing. Failure to do so, or an initial decrease followed by a subsequent rise in creatinine levels, is an indicator of AKI.
Liver function tests (LFTs)	LFTs measure alanine aminotransferase (ALT), aspartate aminotransferase (AST) and alkaline phosphatase (ALP). Elevated ALT and AST can suggest liver injury but both may also arise from non-hepatic causes. In preterm infants, raised ALP indicates metabolic bone disease, requiring further investigation to guide supplementation. LFTs also include serum bilirubin. In prolonged jaundice, a separate conjugated bilirubin level is useful, with values above 25 micromol/L suggesting liver disease. Albumin is also measured; low levels with severe unconjugated hyperbilirubinaemia may indicate the need for albumin transfusion.
Bone profile	A bone profile yields some values that are identical to those obtained as part of the LFTs, including ALP and albumin levels, as well as values for phosphate and calcium, which together with ALP are important for the diagnosis and management of metabolic bone disease.

TABLE 23.5 (Cont.)

C-reactive protein (CRP)	Produced in the liver as a response to inflammatory conditions, elevated CRP markers are suggestive of sepsis in the neonate, and serial testing can help establish success of antibiotic therapy.
Examples of other biochemistry studies	Gentamicin levels, magnesium, thyroid function tests, cortisol levels, paracetamol levels.

TABLE 23.6 WHOLE-BLOOD BIOCHEMISTRY STUDIES

Glucose	A laboratory glucose level must be obtained as part of the investigation panel for persistent hypoglycaemia, to enable interpretation of the insulin response and establish hyperinsulinaemia as a possible cause.
Lactate	This is usually tested using the blood gas analyser. If a sample is sent for laboratory analysis, the laboratory must be alerted in advance so the sample can be analysed immediately to ensure accuracy of the result. In addition, transportation in an ice-filled bag will further slow down the metabolic processes, thereby ensuring sample accuracy.

laboratory, facilitating extraction and analysis of the plasma. Vigorous shaking of the sample may cause haemolysis and subsequent release of the intracellular content into the serum, resulting in sample rejection due to inaccurate values. Once blood is obtained, the bottle should be gently inverted up to ten times to ensure thorough mixing of blood and additives.

Whole-blood biochemistry studies are also conducted in the biochemistry laboratory, but do not require separation of blood cells and plasma, as provided by the SST. Instead, whole-blood biochemistry studies are usually collected in a grey-topped bottle, containing an anticoagulant agent (usually potassium oxalate, but occasionally EDTA), as well as sodium fluoride, an agent inhibiting ongoing glucose metabolism.

RADIOGRAPHY

Since its discovery in 1895, X-ray technology has become one of the most frequently utilised diagnostic tools in medicine (Ou et al., 2021). X-rays are a form of electromagnetic radiation, obtained by producing a cloud of negatively charged electrons within an x-ray tube, through the production of heat, which are rapidly accelerated towards a positively charged electrode. This is followed by instant deceleration as the electrons collide with the x-ray tube. At the point of collision, the electrons release their energy in the form of x-ray beams, which have the ability to pass through matter (Behling, 2020). If the penetrated matter is composed of particles held together loosely, like water, the beams pass through easily, whereas denser structures absorb a proportion of the x-rays. Because the image becomes darker as more x-rays collide with the plate, solid structures such as bones, plastics or metals show up as white, or 'lucent' on the imaging plate, whereas air-filled structures such as the lungs are black, or 'radiopaque.' Whilst radiography is an invaluable tool in diagnostic medicine, x-rays are a form of ionising radiation, removing electrons from atoms and thereby producing free radicals (Chandimali et al., 2025). With repeated exposure, these compounds have the potential to damage DNA, resulting in mutations and increased growth of cancerous cells (Gunn et al., 2019). It is therefore imperative that x-ray procedures only be carried out after careful consideration and that efforts focus on limiting exposure and avoiding unnecessary repetition of the procedure.

THINK POINT

Think back to the last time you had to take a blood sample from a baby in your care. Did you have a good understanding of the why that particular sample was needed? Were you aware of the possible consequences of any abnormal results, and would you have been able to explain these to the parents?

Common radiographic images

- *Anterior-posterior (AP) view*: The baby is in a supine position with the imaging plate directly underneath their back, often in a pull-out compartment built into the incubator. An AP view of the chest is most commonly used to diagnose cardiac or pulmonary diseases and air leaks, to assess endotracheal tube or line positions, whereas an abdominal view allows for appreciation of bowel gas and bowel loop distribution as well as calibre. A combined AP view of both the chest and the abdomen is usually performed to confirm PICC tip placement if inserted via the lower limbs or positioning of umbilical lines.
- *Supine cross-table lateral view*: The baby is positioned supine with the x-ray plate along their side. This is a seldom used view of the chest, used primarily to confirm position of a chest drain tip or to establish the presence of an air leak.
- *Lateral decubitus view*: The infant is positioned on their side, either left side down (left lateral decubitus view) or right side down (right lateral decubitus

view), with the x-ray plate placed along their back. This view may be used to diagnose a pneumothorax or pleural effusion, in particular if an AP x-ray was inconclusive. The infant should be positioned with the affected side up for investigation of a pneumothorax and with the affected side down in a suspected pleural effusion. The left lateral decubitus view is the preferred view for the detection of free air within the peritoneal cavity, suggesting a bowel perforation: The free intra-abdominal air rises to the top and can be seen as a radiolucent area against the dense structure of the liver.

The following section addresses abnormal x-ray findings in brief. Further information about each condition can be found in Chapters 14, 15 and 22.

Abnormal findings on a chest x-ray

- *Ground glass appearance*: The diffuse granular appearance across both lung fields is a common finding indicating respiratory distress syndrome (RDS); see Figure 23.3.
- *Consolidation/collapse*: Dense, white, usually focal areas caused by alveoli filled with fluid or exudate.
- *Air bronchograms*: Bilateral dark, branching lines originating in the hilum and branching outwards, consisting of air-filled bronchi showing up against the lucency of the collapsed or consolidated alveoli.
- *Sunburst pattern*: Transient tachypnoea of the newborn (TTN) is caused by a delayed clearance of fluid from the lungs after birth. The lung fluid builds up in the blood vessels and lymphatic system and presents on the x-ray as streaks radiating out from the perihilar region. In addition, a fine line of fluid dissecting the superior and middle lobe of the right lung (horizontal fissure) is often clearly visible.
- *Air leaks*: These are caused by air escaping from ruptured alveoli and collecting in other spaces, such as the pleural cavity (pneumothorax), in the chest cavity between the lungs (pneumomediastinum) or within the sac enclosing the heart (pneumopericardium). As air is less dense than tissue, it shows up as a dark, radiolucent area on an x-ray. A less common type of air leak, pulmonary interstitial emphysema (PIE) develops due to overdistension and subsequent rupture of the alveoli or small conducting airways, followed by air trapping in the perivascular lung tissue. Chest radiography shows either small cystic or linear, non-branching lucencies.
- *Oesophageal atresia*: An incorrectly developed oesophagus, which instead of connecting with the stomach ends in a blind pouch. This is evident on a chest x-ray, where instead of extending into the stomach, a nasogastric or orogastric tube is seen to be coiling in the upper chest.

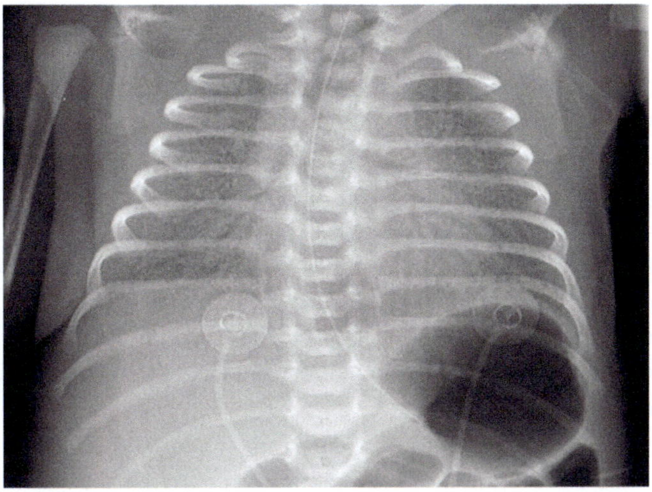

Figure 23.3 Classic presentation of RDS in a newborn infant a few hours old, born at 34 weeks of gestation: both lung fields show a diffuse, granular pattern that resembles ground glass (Source: Jenni Jones).

- *Diaphragmatic hernia*: A failure of the diaphragm to fully form during fetal development, allowing for herniation of intestine and/or liver into the thoracic cavity, visible on a chest x-ray.
- *Cardiac conditions*: X-rays alone are not a reliable tool to diagnose specific congenital heart defect (Chimoriya et al., 2024); however, an abnormal size or shape of the cardiac shadow can indicate a cardiac anomaly that should prompt further investigation. Some cardiac lesions have characteristic features on a chest x-ray. A boot-shaped heart, for instance indicates a Tetralogy of Fallot, whiles the appearance of an 'egg on a string' is consistent with a transposition of the great arteries.

Abnormal findings on an abdominal x-ray

- *Pneumoperitoneum*: Free air, which has escaped from the bowels into the peritoneal cavity. This usually presents as a linear area of lucency directly underneath the diaphragm. In addition, bowel loops may appear clearly defined, due to the presence of bowel gas both outside and inside of the bowels. In the advanced stages, an abdominal x-ray may show the 'football sign': the abdominal cavity is outlined in the oval shape of an American football, with the vertical stitching represented by a radiopaque falciform ligament.
- *Pneumatosis intestinalis*: Intramural gas, present within the bowel wall. On an abdominal x-ray, this may appear as 'tram tracks' along the bowel wall or alternatively present as 'soap bubbles.'

- *Pneumatosis portalis*: Air within the biliary tree, visible on the abdominal x-ray as radiolucent branches across the liver.
- *Thickening of bowel loops*: Visible separation of bowel loops, presenting as increased space between the loops on an abdominal x-ray. This may be a normal finding, caused by the presence of collapsed bowel loops between gaseous bowels, or it may indicate oedema caused by inflammation of the area.
- *Prominent bowel loops*: Referring to an abnormally large calibre of bowel loops. As an approximate guide, bowel loops can be classed as prominent if their diameter is more than twice the width of the sacral vertebrae. The finding may indicate inflammation, bowel stenosis or atresia, ileus or a mechanical obstruction.
- *Ascites*: Fluid in the peritoneal cavity causes structures within the area to appear more hazy and poorly defined on an abdominal x-ray.

For the x-ray guided assessment of endotracheal tube (ETT), umbilical line and PICC tip position, see online content. In addition, a description of x-ray presentation of common neonatal gastrointestinal tract conditions and example x-rays can be found online.

Contrast studies

These are performed to aid diagnosis of gastrointestinal (GI) problems in the neonate, including intestinal obstruction and necrotising enterocolitis. A radiopaque fluid or contrast agent is administered, either via the feeding tube or rectally, which coats the GI tract, thereby making it visible on an x-ray. The subsequently captured image can help identify mechanical or functional obstructions or evidence of perforation. Administering contrast agents rectally may have the added benefit of resolving obstructions caused by stool, such as a meconium plug or meconium ileus.

Fluoroscopy

Usually used in conjunction with a contrast study, neonatal fluoroscopy involves the technique of recording serial x-rays via a continuous x-ray beam in order to capture the image of the GI tract in motion. These can be useful when assessing upper or lower GI tract functioning.

Nursing considerations for neonatal radiography

When performing an x-ray on the NNU, the aim is to obtain the highest-quality image while minimising repeated exposure to ionising radiation. The infant's clinical condition must be considered, particularly if repositioning is required, as excessive handling may be poorly tolerated. Positioning should therefore balance minimal disruption with optimal image quality.

Before imaging, the infant's details must be checked carefully against the request to avoid identification errors. The infant is then positioned according to the required view. In incubators with built-in imaging drawers, the infant may need to be moved up or down to ensure all relevant anatomy is captured. If no drawer is available, a thin muslin sheet may be placed beneath the infant to improve comfort and reduce heat loss; however, folds or wrinkles must be avoided as they appear on the x-ray and can obscure interpretation. Gel pads or water-filled mattresses between the infant and the x-ray plate must be removed.

If a nasogastric or orogastric tube is required, it is helpful to insert it before imaging, as tube tip placement can be confirmed even without aspirates. Chest leads should be removed, but if continuous ECG monitoring is essential, stickers can be temporarily moved to the limbs or axillary line. Multiple lines, such as UVCs and UACs, should be untangled and positioned to either side of the infant to aid identification once the film is taken. For abdominal x-rays, the nappy should be folded down completely and any stool or meconium removed, as faeces can mimic the soap-bubble appearance of pneumatosis intestinalis. For AP chest x-rays, the head must be midline with no rotation and all nesting or boundaries removed to avoid obscuring key anatomy.

ACTIVITY

Next time one of the babies in your care has a radiography study, have a look and see if you can identify some of the features discussed here. Are you able to draw some conclusions about the baby's condition from what you can see on the images? Can you use these pictures to formulate a treatment plan?

Improper or rotated positioning is the most common reason infants are exposed to unnecessary radiation through repeated imaging (Su et al., 2022). To maintain optimal positioning and provide comfort, it is beneficial for a caregiver to remain at the bedside. A lead-lined apron must be worn, and depending on local availability, additional protective equipment such as thyroid collars or gloves may be used. In contrast, shielding radiosensitive infant areas, including the gonads, is no longer recommended (British Institute of Radiology, 2020). After the procedure, the x-ray should be reviewed immediately to confirm adequate quality. Once satisfactory, nesting, the nappy and any equipment can be replaced and the infant repositioned comfortably.

LUMBAR PUNCTURE

The most common indication for lumbar puncture (LP) is to obtain cerebrospinal fluid (CSF) to aid diagnosis of central nervous system (CNS) infections such as meningitis or encephalitis. It is an aseptic procedure involving insertion of a spinal needle into the subarachnoid space between L4 and L5. The National Institute for Health and Care Excellence (2021) recommends CSF sampling in the presence of strong suspicion of sepsis or clinical signs of meningitis, though thresholds vary by region and local guidelines. Less common indications include CSF drainage to relieve raised intracranial pressure, such as in acute progressive hydrocephalus or for investigation of inborn errors of metabolism.

For suspected CNS infection, 3–4 CSF specimens are typically collected for blood cell count, glucose measurement and gram staining. Accidental blood vessel damage or intracranial haemorrhage may introduce white and red cells into the CSF, but isolated white cells without erythrocytes may suggest infection. CSF glucose is compared with a serum glucose level ideally taken immediately beforehand; CSF glucose <80% of serum level may reflect bacterial **glycolysis** and strongly suggests bacterial meningitis. A dye is then added to stain bacteria, aiding identification. Although gram staining can help determine presence, size and morphology of organisms (Divya et al., 2023), some pathogens stain poorly, and a negative result does not rule out infection.

Depending on local policy, an additional CSF sample may be sent for polymerase chain reaction (PCR) testing. PCR testing may be more reliable than culture and sensitivity (C&S) testing because it detects a wider range of bacterial, viral and fungal pathogens (Kardjadj et al., 2025). Unlike C&S, PCR testing can identify pathogen DNA even after antibiotics have been started, and its specificity is higher. As LPs are often performed after initiation of antibiotics, PCR testing can detect organisms already killed by treatment. However, PCR testing does not provide antimicrobial susceptibility information and therefore cannot guide therapy in the way C&S can.

Nursing considerations during lumbar puncture

Before performing a LP, the infant's condition must be assessed. In the presence of cardiorespiratory instability, the procedure may worsen the baby's status and should be deferred until it is safe to proceed. LPs also carry increased bleeding risk in thrombocytopenic infants (Bauer et al., 2021), so many guidelines advise delaying the procedure until a platelet transfusion has been given when the platelet count is <50×10^9/L.

Effective pain management is essential. A recent Cochrane review reports that topical anaesthetics applied for up to 60 minutes may reduce procedural pain (Pessano, 2023b), but these agents are not licensed for infants <37 weeks gestation (Paediatric Formulary Committee, 2024). Therefore, initial analgesia should focus on sucrose or breastmilk and non-nutritive sucking.

Infants are usually positioned in the **lateral decubitus** position, although sometimes an upright, forward-flexed posture is preferred. Both allow maximal spinal flexion and widening of the intervertebral spaces. A Cochrane review found no significant difference in success between positions (Pessano et al., 2023a), but the lateral decubitus position allows easier cardiorespiratory monitoring and administration of oral comfort measures. Throughout the procedure, maximum spinal flexion and immobilisation are required to avoid injury and optimise success. One hand can be placed across the thighs and the other across the shoulders to flex the infant into a fetal posture, ensuring the spine, hips and shoulders remain aligned. Neck flexion should be avoided to maintain airway patency. A folded sheet across the shoulders and thighs may help maintain flexion, support self-soothing, conserve heat and improve immobilisation (Ramsay & Jackson, 2018).

To ensure one person can focus solely on positioning, a second assistant should provide comfort care and monitor the infant's physiological status, as desaturation events are common (Bedetti et al., 2021). Because the person performing the LP uses surgical ANTT and is scrubbed, a third assistant should pass the non-sterile collection tubes beneath the needle once CSF flow is confirmed. Clear communication among the team helps maintain sterility. To support thermoregulation, the LP should be performed in an incubator or under a radiant heater. Complications following neonatal LP are rare, and no additional monitoring is typically required (Bedetti et al., 2021). After the procedure, the infant should be observed for signs of pain and any discomfort managed accordingly.

POINT OF CARE ULTRASOUND SCAN

Bedside ultrasound imaging performed by a clinician other than a radiologist to support assessment or guide procedures is referred to as point of care ultrasound scanning (POCUS). In neonatology, it has traditionally been used for echocardiography and cranial ultrasound but is increasingly applied for broader clinical purposes (Recker et al., 2024). Its major advantages include rapid, real-time diagnosis and the absence of ionising radiation. Despite these benefits, POCUS remains underused due to the complexity of the skill and limited access to appropriate training opportunities (Carrera et al., 2022).

POCUS works by generating high-frequency soundwaves in the ultrasound transducer, which are directed at the area of interest. As waves encounter different tissues, they are reflected back to the probe at varying intensities; this returning energy is then converted into electrical signals to produce an image (Poggi & Palavecino, 2024). The brightness of structures depends on their echogenicity: hyperechogenic tissues appear bright, hypoechogenic tissues appear darker, and anechoic areas appear black. Increasingly, POCUS is used to investigate a wide range of neonatal conditions and to guide clinical decision-making. Some examples are given below.

Clinical application of point of care ultrasound scanning

CRANIAL ULTRASOUND SCAN

Preterm and extremely low birthweight infants are at an increased risk of intraventricular and germinal matrix haemorrhages and associated long-term neurodevelopmental complications. As a result, it is recommended that this patient group receives routine cranial ultrasound scans (CUSS) at regular intervals during the first few weeks of life (Hand et al., 2020). In addition, infants experiencing unexplained seizures and those requiring invasive respiratory support in the absence of an underlying clinical condition may undergo a CUSS for diagnostic purposes. Images are commonly obtained by applying the ultrasound probe to the anterior fontanelle, as sound waves do not transmit through the skull bone. Coronal views are obtained by directing the probe towards the anterior aspect of the head and moving it posteriorly, capturing images of relevant structures at regular intervals. The probe is then directed towards the left aspect of the head and swept towards the right, in order to obtain sagittal views. A CUSS can enable the identification and classification of any intraventricular haemorrhages or other intracranial bleeds and reveal calcifications or evidence of hydrocephalus.

ECHOCARDIOGRAPHY

POCUS can be utilised to assess the heart for structural abnormalities, as well as to assess the haemodynamic status of infants; however, there is a differentiation between POCUS and the more comprehensive targeted neonatal echography, with the former used to answer specific clinical, often time sensitive questions, whereas the latter is used to provide more comprehensive assessments, in particularly in the presence of complex pathologies such as patent ductus arteriosus (PDA), congenital heart disease or following hypoxia-ischaemia (McNamara et al., 2024). POCUS echocardiography on the other hand is a useful tool to investigate and guide treatment of haemodynamic instabilities and hypotension not related to structural heart disease or to guide treatment of conditions such as persistent pulmonary hypertension of the newborn or shock (Miller et al., 2019).

LUNG ULTRASOUND

It has been suggested that lung POCUS has a better sensitivity and specificity than x-ray studies to diagnose a number of neonatal pulmonary conditions and the technique has become increasingly popular in recent years (Liu et al., 2019). It can be utilised to diagnose a multitude of common neonatal conditions, including pneumothorax, pneumonia, meconium aspiration syndrome and TTN (Miller et al., 2019) In addition, information obtained through POCUS may aid clinical decision-making when considering clinical procedures such as surfactant administration or extubation (Liu et al., 2025).

ABDOMINAL ULTRASOUND

Application of abdominal POCUS is limited due to the high ultrasound beam attenuation by bowel gas. However, the modality can be helpful when assessing for signs of necrotising enterocolitis, in particular after a radiological examination has been inconclusive, as it can be more effective at revealing pneumatosis intestinalis, pneumatosis portalis and free intra-abdominal air than x-ray images (Singh et al., 2020). In addition, POCUS is utilised to assess severity of a number of gastro-intestinal tract conditions and thereby helps to assess the need for surgical intervention (Miller et al., 2019).

Procedural application of point of care ultrasound scanning

Most frequently, POCUS is utilised to guide peripheral and central catheter placement, as well as assessment of PICC tip positions. It can guide spinal needle placement during the LP procedure and facilitate endotracheal intubation by guiding ETT size selection and confirm correct placement (Pan et al., 2022). Altogether, the spectrum of clinical procedures that may be informed by the technique is wide, but very much depends on the skill of the practitioner.

Nursing considerations during point of care ultrasound scanning

This is a relatively non-invasive technique, and a skilled practitioner is able to conduct POCUS with minimal discomfort to the baby. However, infant handling may provoke a stress response, in particular in preterm infants, and a second practitioner should always be present to focus on providing comfort measures while the procedure is carried out. Non-nutritive sucking, provision of oral sucrose or breastmilk and containment holding are all suitable measures, and where possible, parents should be encouraged to take an active role in comforting their baby during the procedure.

While cares and procedures should normally be grouped together in order to ensure sufficient periods of rest for the infant, it may be prudent to defer POCUS until sometime after the infant has fed in order to avoid restlessness caused by hunger. Depending on the area to be investigated, some swaddling may provide additional comfort and help keep the baby still during the procedure. For the patient on continuous positive airway pressure (CPAP), it may be necessary to remove the hat and hold the interface in position manually during the CUSS procedure, as when left in place the equipment may make probe-placement difficult. In this case, it is helpful to have a third person assisting with comfort care, in order to allow the first helper to focus exclusively on airway management.

MAGNETIC RESONANCE IMAGING

Particularly useful to investigate disorders affecting the soft tissue, magnetic resonance imaging (MRI) is a non-invasive procedure designed to create a 2 or 3-dimensional image of internal body structures. Once inside, the MRI scanner produces a magnetic field around the body, causing the previously randomly spinning, positively charged proton particles within the hydrogen atoms of the body's water molecules to align, similar to the needles of a compass. The scanner then sends short bursts of a radio frequency pulse through the body, disturbing the proton particles' equilibrium and causing misalignment with the magnetic field. As soon as the radio waves stop, the protons re-align, releasing varying amounts of energy in the process, which is captured and transformed into a digital image. As MRI does not use the ionising radiation employed to create x-ray images, it is classed as a relatively risk-free procedure.

During the neonatal period, MRI is most frequently used to visualise the brain (Lollert et al., 2024), with less frequent indications including oncological investigations and evaluation of vascular or spinal malformations. Most commonly, a brain MRI is performed in order to determine the nature and extent of brain injury following a hypoxic-ischaemic insult (Thiim et al., 2022), with the aim to establish long-term prognosis and to predict future neurodevelopmental problems. In these infants, an MRI should be performed between day 4 and 14 of life (Austin et al., 2024; British Association of Perinatal Medicine, 2023), as earlier scanning may not reflect the extent of the injury.

MRI may also be conducted to investigate aetiology of seizures or to aid diagnosis and prognosis in infants with any other abnormal neurological signs. Further indications include perinatal stroke, metabolic disorders, meningitis or congenital malformation. When conducted to investigate ongoing symptoms, an MRI scan should be performed as soon as the infant is sufficiently stable, as early diagnosis can guide clinical management.

PRACTICE POINT

Consider the steps involved in performing a neonatal MRI study in your area. How would a baby be transported to the scanner? Do you know what equipment for respiratory support and ongoing infusions is available in your local MRI department? What is your local procedure to ensure a baby stays warm, comfortable and calm during an MRI scan?

As MRI scanners are usually located away from the NNU, the necessity to transport infants, in particular unstable ones in order to perform the procedure can present a major challenge, and benefits must be considered against the disruption caused, as well as the potential risks associated with transportation (Wong et al., 2021). Point of care MRI imaging at the bedside may be a feasible alternative (Singh et al., 2022), but whilst this is already practiced in some adult and paediatric intensive care settings, the application in neonatology is currently limited due to the requirement to adapt the technology for the neonatal brain (Cawley et al., 2023).

Nursing considerations during magnetic resonance imaging

Unless point-of-care MRI is available, transport to the scanner must be determined by the distance to the department and by the infant's gestational age and clinical stability. Infants requiring thermoregulation support, respiratory support, intravenous infusions or continuous monitoring must be transported in a neonatal transport incubator, while stable special-care infants may use alternatives such as a pram. Some hospitals have MRI-compatible transport incubators, which reduce heat loss and handling, but these are uncommon due to cost. Because MRI uses magnetic fields, the primary contraindication is the presence of metallic foreign bodies (Medicines and Healthcare Products Regulatory Agency, 2021). Devices used in neonatal surgery, such as PDA ligation clips, are generally non-ferromagnetic, but the accompanying practitioner must confirm compatibility before entering the MRI suite. A nurse typically remains in the MRI room to monitor and comfort the infant, so all metallic items, including jewellery and mobile phones, must be removed beforehand.

All accompanying equipment must also be non-ferromagnetic (Barkovich et al., 2021). Close liaison with radiology is essential to determine the availability of MRI-compatible ventilators, CPAP drivers and infusion pumps. Some centres require infants to be on minimal or no respiratory support if compatible devices are unavailable. Intravenous pumps may differ from those used routinely on the neonatal unit, requiring changes of syringes or infusion lines before transfer.

MRI-compatible monitoring equipment should be available in the radiology department and can replace standard neonatal leads just before entering the MRI room. To support thermoregulation, the infant's temperature should be optimised before transport, and heat loss during transfer must be avoided. Coordination with radiology to ensure an adequately warm scanning room can help. Additional methods include swaddling with warm blankets or using neonatal-appropriate self-warming blankets (Barkovich et al., 2021).

During scanning, infants must be protected from the significant noise produced by the MRI scanner. Neonatal ear-protectors, available on most NNUs or within radiology, should always be used. MRI image quality is highly sensitive to motion (King et al., 2023), creating difficulties when imaging newborns. Sedation is therefore frequently recommended to reduce movement, with chloral hydrate being the most common agent; however, it may cause respiratory depression and desaturations in neonates (Jung, 2020). A non-pharmacological alternative is the 'feed and wrap' technique, in which the infant is fed immediately before scanning and then tightly swaddled. This has been shown to produce images of comparable quality (Lollert et al., 2024), though effectiveness may decrease with advancing gestational age. Non-nutritive sucking can also be used to support comfort and minimise movement during the procedure.

Chapter takeaways

- Premature and sick infants undergo a multitude of diagnostic procedures during their stay on the NNU. Nurses play a crucial role in optimising diagnostic accuracy, ensuring asepsis, maintaining infant stability, supporting families, reducing procedural stress and interpreting the clinical significance of investigations.
- Blood sampling is central to neonatal diagnostics, with capillary, venous and arterial routes chosen according to clinical need; careful technique minimises contamination, iatrogenic anaemia and pain-related stress.
- Non-pharmacological pain relief is essential during skin-breaking procedures, with evidence supporting breastfeeding, kangaroo care, sucrose, facilitated tucking and involvement of parents to reduce physiological stress.
- Radiography remains a key diagnostic tool, requiring meticulous positioning, radiation-minimising practice and awareness of characteristic abnormal findings across chest and abdominal imaging.
- Lumbar puncture is vital for evaluating CNS infection, and safe performance depends on clinical stability, optimal positioning, skilled team support and effective pain-relieving strategies.

- Point-of-care ultrasound (POCUS) is increasingly integral, enabling rapid bedside assessment of cranial, cardiac, lung and abdominal pathology, while also guiding procedures such as line placement and intubation.
- MRI provides high-resolution imaging for neonatal neurological assessment, especially after HIE, but requires careful planning around transport, equipment compatibility, thermoregulation and noise protection.

CASE STUDIES

CASE STUDY

Case study 1: Admission of a term infant with signs of respiratory distress

Vincenzo is a 39+6-week baby who was born 2 hours ago via normal vaginal delivery. Vincenzo required no resuscitation at birth and was initially well, but over the past hour he has started persistent expiratory grunting. On examination his respiratory rate was 85 breaths per minute, the heart rate was 145 beats per minute, his axillary temperature was 36.8 degrees Celsius, his oxygen saturation was 92% and he had marked intercostal recession. He has been admitted to the NNU and commenced on CPAP therapy.

Q1. What initial blood tests would you expect to be ordered for Vincenzo and how do you think these should be collected?

Q2. How can you support Vincenzo during the blood sampling procedure?

Vincenzo is commenced on IV benzylpenicillin and gentamicin. Following this, a chest x-ray is ordered.

Q3. Vincenzo's parents are worried about the potentially harmful long-term effects of x-ray exposure. What could you say to reassure them?

Q4. How can you prepare both Vincenzo and his environment for the procedure?

Vincenzo's initial blood results show a raised white blood cell count and a CRP of 35mg/L.

Q5. What further investigations do you think Vincenzo might need now, and how can you support him while these are carried out?

Case study 2: The term infant requiring an MRI

Penelope is a 41+2 week baby born via emergency caesarean section following a pathological cardiotocography (CTG) reading in labour. She

CASE STUDY

required extensive resuscitation after delivery and was eventually admitted to the NNU spontaneously breathing and on CPAP therapy. Penelope underwent 72 hours of therapeutic hypothermia for her hypoxic-ischaemic insult, following by a period of rewarming. She is now 6 days old and remains on CPAP and a continuous infusion of parenteral nutrition and lipids. Penelope has been booked for an MRI scan. The department is on the other side of the hospital and your NNU does not have an MRI compatible transport incubator.

Q1. What do you need to consider prior to transporting Penelope to the MRI department? How will you prepare Penelope for the procedure?
Q2. Do you think Penelope should be sedated for the procedure? How would you justify your answer?
Q3. How can you support Penelope during the MRI scan?

For suggested answer guides to the questions posed in these case studies, please refer to the web-based companion site specific to this chapter. See www.routledge.com/cw/petty

References

Allegaert, K., Smits, A., van Donge, T., Van den Anker, J., Sarafidis, K., Levtchenko, E., & Mekahli, D. (2020). Renal precision medicine in neonates and acute kidney injury: How to convert a cloud of creatinine observations to support clinical decisions. *Frontiers in Pediatrics*, *8*(366), 1–10.

Austin, T., Connolly, D., Dinwiddy, K., Hart, A. R., Heep, A., Harigopal, S., Joy, H., Luyt, K., Malamateniou, C., Merchant, N., Rizava, C., Rutherford, M. A., Spike, K., Vollmer, B., & Boardman, J. P. (2024). Neonatal brain magnetic resonance imaging: Clinical indications, acquisition and reporting. *Archives of Disease in Childhood. Fetal and Neonatal Edition*, *109*(4), 348–361.

Barkovich, M. J., Williams, C., & Barkovich, A. J. (2021). Technical and practical tips for performing brain magnetic resonance imaging in premature neonates. *Seminars in Perinatology*, *45*(7), 1–6.

Bauer, M. E., Arendt, K., Beilin, Y., Gernsheimer, T., Perez Botero, J., James, A. H., Yaghmour, E., Toledano, R. D., Turrentine, M., Houle, T., MacEachern, M., Madden, H., Rajasekhar, A., Segal, S., Wu, C., Cooper, J. P., Landau, R., & Leffert, L. (2021). The Society for Obstetric Anesthesia and Perinatology interdisciplinary consensus statement on neuraxial procedures in obstetric patients with thrombocytopenia. *Anesthesia & Analgesia*, *132*(6), 1531–1544.

Bedetti, L., Lugli, L., Marrozzini, L., Baraldi, A., Leone, F., Baroni, L., Lucaccioni, L., Rossi, C., Roversi, M. F., D'Amico, R., Iughetti, L., & Berardi, A. (2021). Safety and success of lumbar puncture in young infants: A prospective observational study. *Frontiers in Pediatrics*, *9*(14), 1–6.

Behling, R. (2020). X-ray sources: 125 years of developments of this intriguing technology. *Physica Medica*, 162–187.

British Association of Perinatal Medicine. (2023). *Neonatal brain magnetic resonance imaging: Clinical indications, acquisition and reporting: A framework for practice*. British Association of Perinatal Medicine.

British Institute of Radiology. (2020). *Guidance on using shielding on patients for diagnostic radiology applications*. British Institute of Radiology.

Carrera, K. G., Hassen, G., Camacho-Leon, G. P., Rossitto, F., Martinez, F., & Debele, T. K. (2022). The benefits and barriers of using point-of-care ultrasound in primary healthcare in the United States. *Cureus*, *14*(8), 1–5.

Cawley, P., Padormo, F., Cromb, D., Almalbis, J., Marenzana, M., Teixeira, R., Uus, A., O'Muircheartaigh, J., Williams, S. C. R., Counsell, S. J., Arichi, T., Rutherford, M. A., Hajnal, J. V., Edwards, A. D., Deoni, S. C., Ljungberg, E., Bennallick, C., Kolind, S., Dean, D., & Pepper, M. S. (2023). Development of neonatal-specific sequences for portable ultralow field magnetic resonance brain imaging: A prospective, single-centre, cohort study. *EClinicalMedicine*, *65*, 1–17.

Chandimali, N., Bak, S. G., Park, E. H., Lim, H.-J., Won, Y.-S., Kim, E.-K., Park, S.-I., & Lee, S. J. (2025). Free radicals and their impact on health and antioxidant defenses: A review. *Cell Death Discovery*, *11*(1), 1–17.

Chimoriya, R., Kumar, G., Rana, K., Chimoriya, R., Anand, R., Dagar, K. S., & Awasthy, N. (2024). Role of chest radiographs and electrocardiograms in predicting the hemodynamics of congenital heart disease. *Exploration of Medicine*, *5*, 112–126.

Counsilman, C. E., Heeger, L. E., Tan, R., Bekker, V., Zwaginga, J. J., te Pas, A. B., & Lopriore, E. (2019). Iatrogenic blood loss in extreme preterm infants due to frequent laboratory tests and procedures. *The Journal of Maternal-Fetal & Neonatal Medicine*, *34*(16), 2660–2665.

Divya, B., Vijayakumar, T., Vasanthi, V., Narayan, M., Kumar, A., & Krishnan, R. (2023). Diagnostic utility of gram stain for oral smears – A review. *Journal of Microscopy and Ultrastructure*, *11*(3), 130–134.

Erturk, Z. K., Evrin, T., Ekici, B., Ertürk, B., Uzunget, S. C., & Çandar, T. (2024). Are blood gas analyzers reliable in electrolytes and other parameters? *Disaster and Emergency Medicine Journal*, *9*(2), 73–79.

Ganetzky, R. D., & Cuddapah, S. R. (2017). Neonatal lactic acidosis: A diagnostic and therapeutic approach. *NeoReviews*, *18*(4), 217–227.

Gottschalk, A., Coggins, S., Dhudasia, M. B., Flannery, D. D., Healy, T., Puopolo, K. M., Gerber, J., & Mukhopadhyay, S. (2024). Utility of anaerobic blood cultures in neonatal sepsis evaluation. *Journal of the Pediatric Infectious Diseases Society*, *13*(8), 406–412.

Gunn, C., O'Brien, K., Fosså, K., Tonkopi, E., Lanca, L., Martins, C. T., Muller, H., Friedrich-Nel, H., Abdolell, M., & Johansen, S. (2019). A multi-institutional comparison of imaging dose and technique protocols for neonatal chest radiography. *Radiography*, *26*(2), E66–E72.

Hand, I. L., Shellhaas, R. A., & Milla, S. S. (2020). Routine neuroimaging of the preterm brain. *Pediatrics*, *146*(5), 1–7.

Janjindamai, W., Tiwawatpakorn, N., Thatrimontrichai, A., Dissaneevate, S., Maneenil, G., & Phatigomet, M. (2022). Accuracy of neonatal venous blood glucose measurements using blood gas analyzer compared with central laboratory chemistry analyzer. *Journal of Clinical Neonatology*, *11*(1), 7–12.

Jung, S. M. (2020). Drug selection for sedation and general anesthesia in children undergoing ambulatory magnetic resonance imaging. *Yeungnam University Journal of Medicine*, *37*(3), 159–168.

Kardjadj, M., Chang, T. W., Chavez, R., Derrick, D., Spangler, F. L., Priestly, I. P., Park, L. Y., & Huard, T. K. (2025). The clinical validity and utility of PCR compared to conventional culture and sensitivity testing for the management of complicated urinary tract infections in adults: A secondary (ad hoc) analysis of pathogen detection, resistance profiles, and impact on clinical outcomes. *Microorganisms*, *13*(949), 1–22.

King, R., Low, S., Gee, N., Wood, R., Hadweh, B., Houghton, J., & Leijser, L. M. (2023). Practical stepwise approach to performing neonatal brain MR imaging in the research setting. *Children*, *10*(11), 1759–1759.

Liu, J., Inchingolo, R., Suryawanshi, P., Guo, B.-B., Kurepa, D., Cortés, R. G., Yan, W., Chi, J.-H., Acosta, C. M., Jagła, M., Sharma, D., Sorantin, E., Hsieh, K.-S., Graziani, G., Malta, B., Woods, P., Meng, Q., You, C.-M., Kruczek, P., & Kneyber, M. (2025). Guidelines for the use of lung ultrasound to optimise the management of neonatal respiratory distress: International expert consensus. *BMC Medicine*, *23*(1), 1–15.

Liu, J., Lovrenski, J., Ye Hlaing, A., & Kurepa, D. (2019). Neonatal lung diseases: Lung ultrasound or chest x-ray. *The Journal of Maternal-Fetal & Neonatal Medicine*, *34*(7), 1177–1182.

Lollert, A., Frey, K. S., Hoffmann, C., Herbst, M., König, J., Schmeh, I., Dette, F., & Staatz, G. (2024). "Feed-and-wrap" technique versus deep sedation for neonatal magnetic resonance imaging: A retrospective comparative study. *European Radiology*, *34*(11), 7104–7114.

McNamara, P. J., Jain, A., El-Khuffash, A., Giesinger, R., Weisz, D., Freud, L., Levy, P. T., Bhombal, S., de Boode, W., Leone, T., Richards, B., Singh, Y., Acevedo, J. M., Simpson, J., Noori, S., & Lai, W. W. (2024). Guidelines and recommendations for targeted neonatal echocardiography and cardiac point-of-care ultrasound in the neonatal intensive care unit: An update from the American Society of Echocardiography. *Journal of the American Society of Echocardiography*, *37*(2), 171–215.

Medicines and Healthcare Products Regulatory Agency. (2021). *Safety guidelines for magnetic resonance imaging equipment in clinical use.* HM Government.

Miller, J. M. (2018). A guide to utilization of the microbiology laboratory for diagnosis of infectious diseases: 2018 update by the Infectious Diseases Society of America and the American Society for Microbiologya. *Clinical Infectious Diseases*, *67*(6), e1–e94.

Miller, L. E., Stoller, J. Z., & Fraga, M. V. (2019). Point-of-care ultrasound in the neonatal ICU. *Current Opinion in Pediatrics*, *32*(2), 216–227.

National Institute for Health and Care Excellence. (2021). *Recommendations | Neonatal infection: Antibiotics for prevention and treatment. NICE clinical guideline 195.* NICE.

Ou, X., Chen, X., Xu, X., Xie, L., Chen, X., Hong, Z., Bai, H., Liu, X., Chen, Q., Li, L., & Yang, H. (2021). Recent development in x-ray imaging technology: Future and challenges. *Research*, 9892152, 1–18.

Paediatric Formulary Committee. (2024). *British national formulary for children 2024–2025.* BMJ Group and Pharmaceutical Press.

Pan, S., Lin, C., & Ban, T. C. H. (2022). Neonatal and paediatric point-of-care ultrasound review. *Australasian Journal of Ultrasound in Medicine*, *26*(1), 46–58.

Pessano, S., Bruschettini, M., Prescott, M. G., & Romantsik, O. (2023a). Positioning for lumbar puncture in newborn infants. *The Cochrane Library*, *10*(10), CD015592.

Pessano, S., Romantsik, O., Olsson, E., Hedayati, E., & Bruschettini, M. (2023b). Pharmacological interventions for the management of pain and discomfort during lumbar puncture in newborn infants. *The Cochrane Library*, *9*(9), CD015594.

Pillai, R. R., Bucsea, O., Shiff, I., Chow, C., Gennis, H. G., Badovinac, S., DiLorenzo-Klas, M., Racine, N. M., Kohut, S. A., Lisi, D., Turcotte, K., Stevens, B., & Uman, L. S. (2023). Non-pharmacological management of infant and young child procedural pain. *The Cochrane Library*, *6*(6), CD006275.

Poggi, C., & Palavecino, M. (2024). Ultrasound principles and instrumentation. *Surgery Open Science*, *18*, 123–128.

Ramsay, S., & Jackson, K. (2018). Improving practice using the wrapped tucked position for lumbar punctures. *Infant*, *14*(4), 135–136.

Recker, F., Kipfmueller, F., Wittek, A., Strizek, B., & Winter, L. (2024). Applications of point-of-care ultrasound in neonatology: A systematic review of the iterature. *Life*, *14*(6), 658–681.

Shah, P. S., Torgalkar, R., & Shah, V. (2023). Breastfeeding or breast milk for procedural pain in neonates. *The Cochrane Library*, *8*(8), CD004950.

Sharma, H., & Ruikar, M. (2022). Kangaroo mother care (KMC) for procedural pain in infants: A meta-analysis from the current evidence of randomized control trials and cross-over trials. *Journal of Family Medicine and Primary Care*, *11*(4), 1250–1256.

Singh, E., Thiim, K. R., Rostas, S., Cadogan, J., El-Dib, M., & Inder, T. E. (2022). Improving access to magnetic resonance imaging for the newborn. *Journal of Neonatal Nursing*, *29*(1), 199–202.

Singh, Y., Tissot, C., Fraga, M. V., Yousef, N., Cortes, R. G., Lopez, J., Sanchez-de-Toledo, J., Brierley, J., Colunga, J. M., Raffaj, D., Da Cruz, E., Durand, P., Kenderessy, P., Lang, H.-J., Nishisaki, A., Kneyber, M. C., Tissieres, P., Conlon, T. W., & De Luca, D. (2020). International evidence-based guidelines on Point of Care Ultrasound (POCUS) for critically ill neonates and children issued by the POCUS Working Group of the European Society of Paediatric and Neonatal Intensive Care (ESPNIC). *Critical Care*, *24*(1), 1–16.

Su, Y.-T., Chen, Y.-S., Yeh, L.-R., Chen, S.-W., Tsai, Y.-C., Wu, C.-Y., Yang, Y.-N., Tey, S.-L., & Lin, C.-H. (2022). Unnecessary radiation exposure during diagnostic radiography in infants in a neonatal intensive care unit: A retrospective cohort study. *European Journal of Pediatrics*, *182*(1), 343–352.

Subedi, R., Chaudhary, R., Karn, B. K., Yadav, U., Yadav, S. P., & Bhatta, M. (2024). Effectiveness of facilitated tucking on reducing pain during heelstick in neonates: A randomized controlled experimental study. *Annals of Medicine and Surgery*, *86*(9), 5211–5217.

Thiim, K. R., Singh, E., Mukundan, S., Grant, P. E., Yang, E., El-Dib, M., & Inder, T. E. (2022). Clinical experience with an in-NICU magnetic resonance imaging system. *Journal of Perinatology*, *42*(7), 873–879.

Ullsten, A., Andreasson, M., & Eriksson, M. (2021). State of the art in parent-delivered pain-relieving interventions in neonatal care: A scoping review. *Frontiers in Pediatrics*, *9*, 1–19.

Velumula, P. K., Elbakoush, F., Tabb, C., Farooqi, A., Lulic-Botica, M., Jani, S., Natarajan, G., & Bajaj, M. (2022). Breast milk vs 24% sucrose for procedural pain relief in preterm neonates: A non-inferiority randomized controlled trial. *Journal of Perinatology*, *42*(7), 914–919.

Williams, M. D., & Lascelles, B. D. X. (2020). Early neonatal pain – a review of clinical and experimental implications on painful conditions later in life. *Frontiers in Pediatrics*, *8*(30), 1–18.

Wong, J., Kalaniti, K., Castaldo, M., Whyte, H., Lee, K.-S., Schroff, M., & Campbell, D. M. (2021). Utilizing simulation to identify latent safety threats during neonatal magnetic resonance imaging procedure. *Simulation in Healthcare: Journal of the Society for Simulation in Healthcare*, *16*(3), 170–176.

24 NEONATAL TRANSPORT

Marina Loarce Montero, Patrick Turton, and Julia Petty

CONTENTS

DOI: 10.4324/9781003591405-29

GUIDANCE ON HOW TO ENHANCE PERSONAL LEARNING FROM THIS CHAPTER

Key points covered in this chapter

- An overview of the structure and function of the neonatal transport service and team.
- The different types of neonatal transport including clinical considerations relating to a range of different conditions.
- The safety and governance aspects surrounding transferring sick and high-risk neonates.

Reflection

Reading through the chapter, you are encouraged to engage with the key points and related literature in an enquiring way. Ask these questions:

- Which neonates in your care have had to be transferred, either out or in, and why?
- What considerations are required to ensure the neonate is as safe and risk-free as possible when stabilising them for transfer?
- How should the family be involved in the event of their baby needing transfer?

Implications for nursing care

- Finally: how will this chapter enable you to consider and understand the specific issues and challenges of neonatal transport for the high-risk neonate and their family? Consider the implications of what you learn for your nursing care relating to stabilisation and transfer of both neonates and parents.

INTRODUCTION AND BACKGROUND

Critically ill neonates are a highly vulnerable and unique population who require specialised teams for stabilisation and transport to achieve optimal outcomes (Aubertin et al., 2018; Meyer & Totapally, 2026). While *in utero* transfers are the preferred strategy (Watson et al., 2020), there are several reasons why a neonate may need to be transferred soon after birth; for example, if they require advanced respiratory care or surgery. Transfers require careful preparation and planning in order to minimise risks to the neonate and team involved. Having an awareness of the principles of safe neonatal transport will be helpful to those who are involved, including professionals who help to prepare the neonate and care for them after being transferred and who transfer neonates themselves. The logistic and clinical complexities of all transfers will vary, but due consideration should be given to common stages of the transport episode. These stages include:

- Referral or request for transfer
- Activation of the transferring team
- Handover of patient details
- Stabilisation and preparation for transfer
- Arrival at receiving location
- Handover of patient details
- Return of transferring team to base

This chapter aims to provide insight into preparing for and managing these stages safely and efficiently.

THE NEONATAL TRANSPORT SERVICE

In the UK, response times in the transfer of the sick and high-risk newborn improved significantly following the introduction of centralised transport services along with a shift in patterns of care leading on from the reorganisation of neonatal services in 2004, into managed clinical networks (British Association of Perinatal Medicine (BAPM), 2022; Heys et al., 2023; NHS England, 2023a). These networks were established to ensure collaborative working across Trusts, maintaining safe and equitable access to appropriate levels of neonatal care and facilitating transfers according to clinical need rather than geography alone. Neonatal transport teams are key to maintaining patient flow, coordinating the movement of critically ill neonates to units capable of providing required levels of care and repatriating them back to local units as soon as clinically appropriate (Adams, 2022).

This is recognised at a national level with policies such as the NHS neonatal transport service specification providing a structured framework for neonatal transport, defining service objectives (including time-critical response standards, transfer performance indicators and reporting requirements) and supporting high-quality, equitable care (National Health Service (NHS) England, 2024). Transfer reasons laid out within this framework are consistent with clinical practice: uplift (to higher-level care), resources/capacity (to manage unit pressures) and repatriation (back to local units when appropriate). More recent UK evidence also highlights ongoing challenges for neonatal transport services, including variable compliance with benchmark standards for response times and transfer coverage across networks, highlighting the importance of continued quality improvement and resourcing.

There are currently 14 neonatal transport services covering the UK, who carry out approximately 15,000 transfers per year (BAPM, 2025). The neonatal intensive care transport service specification identifies five key measures by which each transport service is benchmarked (Department of Health, 2015; NHS England, 2024). These are:

1 Dedicated neonatal transport services transfer at least 95% of patients requiring uplift within their defined catchment area on an annual basis.
2 For time-critical transfers, the transport team mobilises towards the patient within one hour from the start of the referral call (95% of transfers annually).
3 The transport team will arrive with the patient requiring uplift and intensive care transfers within 3.5 hours of the referring call on 80% of transfers.
4 Timely collection of data as requested by the NTG/BAPM dataset.
5 Publish an annual report.

Establishing a combined service requires time, hard work and support from the clinical and healthcare commissioning communities. Success depends on strong clinical leadership, a dedicated, highly skilled group of professionals who share a vision, financial support and a foundation based on quality and safety (Beccia et al., 2025). Given the high-risk nature of the activity, any new service needs to benchmark against recognised standards and key performance metrics to ensure the best care possible is provided to this vulnerable group of patients.

ACTIVITY

Comparing *in utero and ex utero* transfers

Read this paper on *in utero* transfers of neonates and note down why this approach is preferable, compared to an *ex utero* transfer.

- Watson, H., McLaren, J., Carlisle, N., Ratnavel, N., Watts, T., Zaima, A., Tribe, R. M., & Shennan, A. H. (2020). All the right moves: Why in utero transfer is both important for the baby and difficult to achieve and new strategies for change. *F1000Res*, *13*(9), F1000 979. https://pmc.ncbi.nlm.nih.gov/articles/PMC7429922/

Working on the transport team

Neonatal transport teams in the UK and indeed elsewhere globally, are multidisciplinary, combining experienced neonatal nurses, doctors (including advanced neonatal nurse practitioners (ANNPs) where available) and trained ambulance personnel to transfer critically ill or preterm neonates between hospitals safely. These teams provide 24 hourly clinical support, with consultant neonatologist advice available at all times. Team composition and training are guided by national specifications; however, they vary depending on the region and service model (NHS England, 2023; National Quality Board, 2023). The team may include a doctor and/or ANNP, a neonatal nurse and paramedic or a nurse-led team with medical support available. All teams are overseen by a neonatal consultant whilst undertaking a range of different transfers from acute uplifts to repatriations (Collier & Salgin, 2024).

Roles often overlap within the team due to the small size and its dynamics. Some activities such as equipment checks, monitoring, managing infusions, documentation and troubleshooting are normally shared; however, understanding individual skill levels within the team and clear protocols are essential to ensure safety and efficiency. Training therefore becomes key to enhance the multidisciplinary team skills focussing on human factors, clinical and technical skills, communication, advanced clinical assessment and decision-making (Murdoch et al., 2019).

Careful preparation of the transport team is key and can help to optimise performance regardless of the clinical complexity of the transfer. Challenges inherent to transport such as working in an unfamiliar or restricted environment as well as working under extreme pressure should not be underestimated. Regardless of the composition of the team, there are specific training and educational needs which address the challenges of working in the transport environment in line with the essential elements of team-working, outlined in Box 24.1.

BOX 24.1 ELEMENTS OF TEAM-WORKING FOR NEONATAL TRANSPORT

- Working effectively in small teams
- Working in restrictive and isolated environments

- Communicating in stressful situations
- Develop an enhanced level of clinical assessment and decision-making
- Independent working
- Team/peer support and debrief.

Neonatal transport episodes are often challenged by limitations such as confined spaces, continuous movement and fluctuating environmental conditions (Bekkevold et al., 2026). Careful preparation of the transport team can help to optimise their performance regardless of the clinical complexity of the transfer. The use of checklists, simulation and human factors training are key to building the skills of the team (Murdoch et al., 2019). The development of courses such as Neonatal, Adult and Paediatric Safe Transfer and Retrieval (NAPSTaR) by the Advanced Life Support Group provides a syllabus which aims to address the training needs of transport team staff. Learning from strategies and approaches adopted by high reliability organisations such as the aviation, construction and nuclear industries can add another dimension to safety in healthcare (Serou et al., 2021).

Equipment and vehicles for neonatal transport

Delivering a neonatal transport service requires the capability to provide mobile neonatal intensive care. For this, a transport incubator system (TIS) is needed, which includes an incubator mounted on a trolley with integrated monitoring, ventilation, infusion pumps and power supply systems (Figure 24.1). While TISs are broadly similar across services, individual configurations vary as they are often aligned with equipment already in use within the host organisation to maximise staff familiarity and patient safety (Lucas et al., 2021; NHS England, 2024)

Designing, procuring and maintaining a TIS is resource intensive and must comply with relevant UK and European safety and performance standards, including ambulance and medical device regulations. Service planning should take into consideration other costs such as servicing, equipment replacement and delivery of training and competency programmes to ensure staff can safely operate complex systems in the transport environment (British Standards Institution (BSI), 2020; NHS England, 2024). As a result, many services adopt a standardised TIS suitable for a wide range of transfers. Moreover, there are other utilised lighter, lower-dependency transport solutions, such as pod-and-trolley systems, that can be used

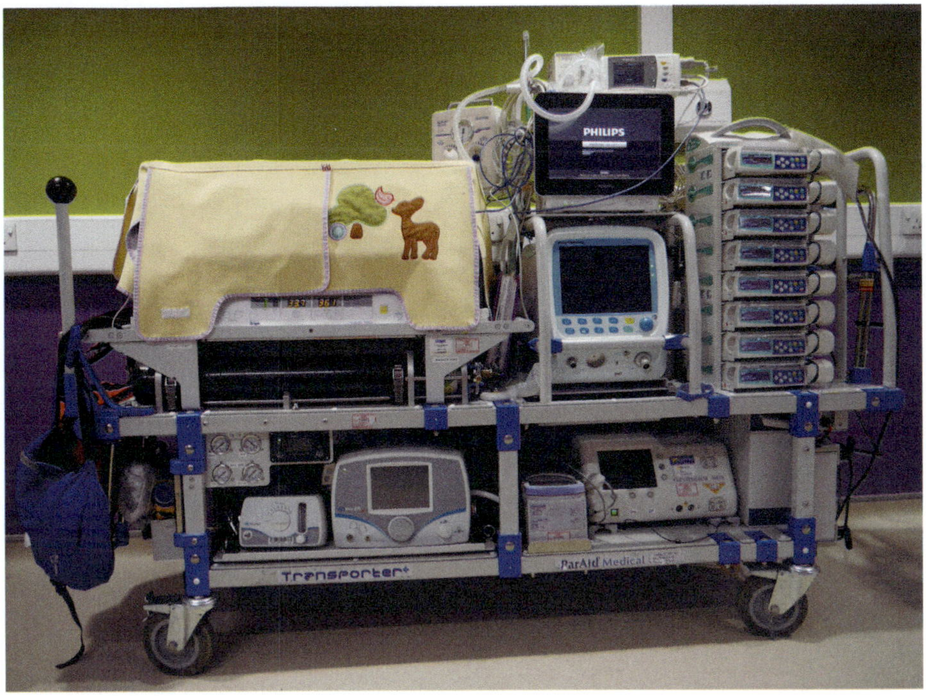

Figure 24.1 Neonatal transport incubator system (Source: Lisa Kaiser)

for appropriate transfers by some teams (BAPM, 2022). Regardless of system choice, secure fixation of equipment to the trolley and of the trolley to the ambulance is essential to ensure neonate and staff safety during transit (BSI, 2020).

Neonatal transport teams need to carry a comprehensive range of disposable emergency supplies to manage any incidents or interventions during transfer. Teams must balance minimising equipment load with ensuring readiness for clinical deterioration *en route*. Equipment is typically organised into portable transport bags (Figure 24.2) that allows safe transfer between ambulance and hospital environments. Equipment compatibility across regions will vary which means teams cannot always rely on local hospital equipment and must remain self-sufficient (BAPM, 2022).

The ambulance is an integral piece of equipment required for neonatal transport (Figure 24.3). Access to a dedicated neonatal ambulance allows teams to be familiar with vehicle layout, loading mechanisms and the provision of electrical and medical gas supplies. This familiarity supports efficient working, safe manual handling and effective troubleshooting during transfers, particularly in time-critical or high-acuity situations (Lucas et al., 2021; NHS England, 2024).

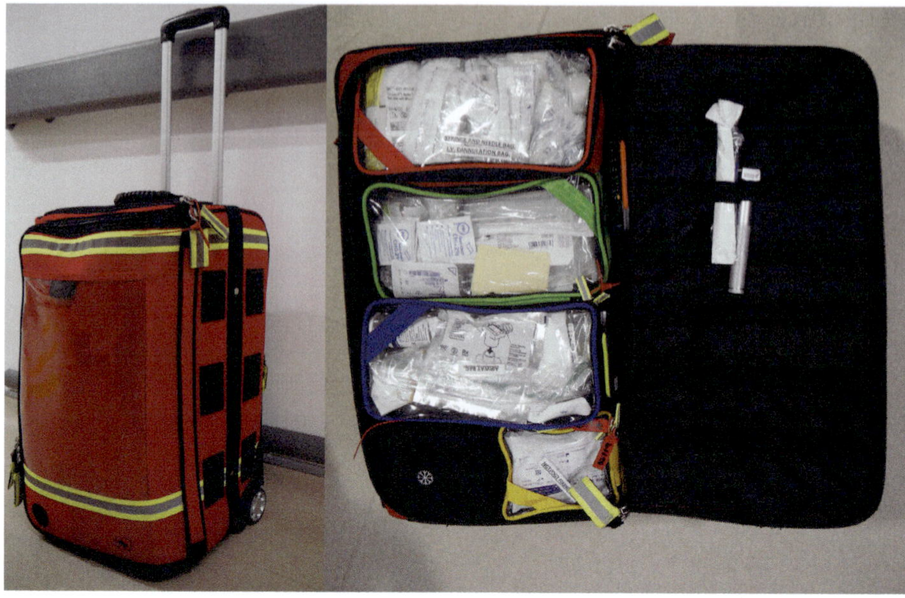

Figure 24.2 Neonatal transport pack/equipment (Source: Lisa Kaiser)

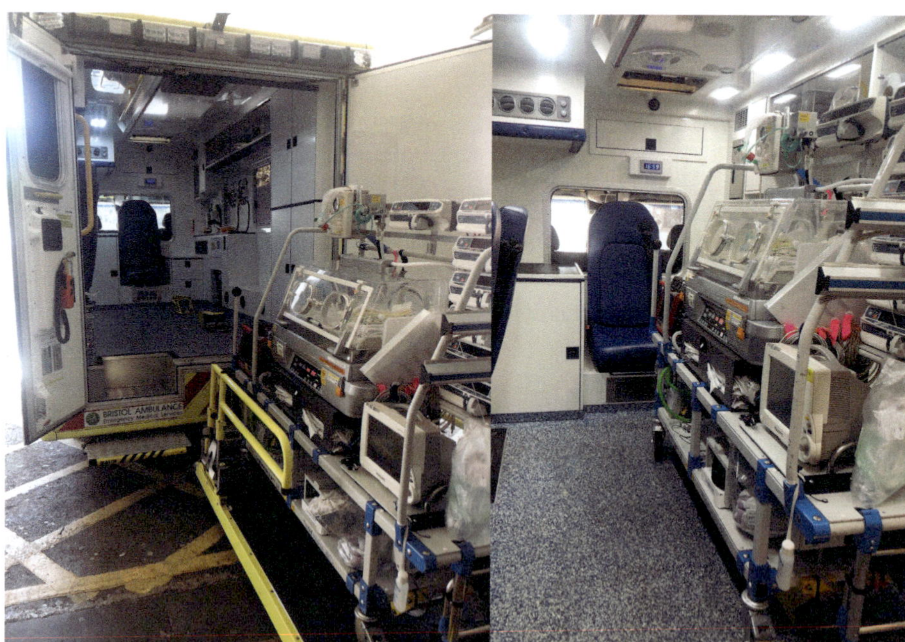

Figure 24.3 Neonatal transport ambulance (Source: Patrick Turton)

NEONATAL TRANSFERS NOT UNDERTAKEN BY THE TRANSPORT TEAM

There are occasions where a team other than a neonatal transport team might transfer a neonate. The likely alternatives are that the neonate is transferred by a paediatric critical care transport team, if they are moving into a paediatric intensive care unit or if the local team is required to transfer them. Examples of this are where any delay incurred waiting for the transport team to arrive will cause harm to the patient. There could also be certain surgical cases where the local team may be required to transfer the patient themselves.

There are other occasions where the referring team at the local hospital will need to undertake a transfer. This may be because the principal transport service for that area is committed to another transfer. In these cases, a careful discussion must take place between the referring, transport and specialist teams to consider the costs and benefits of waiting for the transport team to be available versus the local team moving the patient themselves. Key factors here are the underlying clinical problem, the clinical requirements of the infant at that time and a careful triage of the transport service's current workload. These transfers place significant burden on the local teams undertaking them. Access to the appropriate transport equipment is often difficult, and there are particular challenges with identifying an appropriately skilled team without critically depleting the staffing levels at base. Factors that can help reduce the stress and pressure that the transfers place on referring teams include:

- Early communication with relevant parties to aid in decision-making.
- Local guidance (developed with support from the regional transport team) to aid a prompt and safe dispatch.
- Checklists to assist in team and equipment preparation.

Simulation and scenario training for instigating a locally delivered transfer are excellent ways to identify issues pertinent to each centre. They give hospital teams the opportunity to rehearse the process and familiarise themselves with their transport equipment.

Intra-hospital transfers

Intra-hospital transfers are another example where neonates are not transferred by a specialist transport team. Even moving a neonate from the delivery suite to the intensive care department requires careful planning and transfers to operating theatre or for radiographical imaging can provide logistical and clinical challenges. Some hospitals have these departments in different buildings, necessitating a road transfer which may well be undertaken by practitioners who are not experienced in neonatal transport. Neonatal teams need to ensure that they have adequate equipment available and are appropriately practised in preparing for potential emergencies during the time off the neonatal unit (NNU).

AEROMEDICAL TRANSFERS

In the UK, the clear majority of neonatal transfers are undertaken by road, but at times air transport is needed depending on location and distance. Scotland has a well-established aeromedical capability, driven largely by factors such as geography and population spread as is the case in other larger countries, and it is increasingly accepted that helicopter (rotary wing) and aeroplane (fixed-wing) transfers have their place in UK neonatal transport provision (BAPM, 2021; Scottish Ambulance Service, 2026). Rotary-wing transfers may be considered when predicted road journey times exceed approximately two to three hours, while fixed-wing transfers are typically reserved for significantly longer distances. The use of fixed-wing aircraft is limited by airport availability and the need for additional secondary road transfers (NHS England, 2024). Subsequently, fixed-wing neonatal transfers are uncommon within the UK. As well as time related, decisions regarding aeromedical transfer must also consider clinical stability, availability of specialist teams, environmental factors and the risks associated with transfer physiology and handling (BAPM, 2021). It is not necessarily better to have shorter transport times, and this is often an assumption of air transport as a preferred method compared to road. There are a multitude of factors which will influence the decision-making regarding aeromedical transfers over and above the anticipated road transfer time (see Box 24.2).

BOX 24.2 FACTORS TO CONSIDER FOR DECIDING BETWEEN AIR AND ROAD TRANSFERS

- Patient stability and other clinical flight restrictions
- Requirement for/length of secondary transfer
- Weather
- Flight hours available
- Appropriately trained/competent team available
- Aircraft availability
- Equipment availability
- Requirement of family to travel with the neonate
- Funding arrangements

SAFETY DURING TRANSPORT

The neonatal transport environment is more restrictive and resource-limited than the hospital setting, with an increase on physical, cognitive and emotional demands on staff. Ensuring team safety is key and requires a systematic risk management process (NHS England, 2024). Transport teams must have access to appropriate personal protective equipment (PPE), including gloves, aprons, eye protection and hand hygiene products, alongside transport-specific items such as protective footwear and high-visibility clothing.

Manual handling presents a significant risk during neonatal transport; TISs may exceed 250–300 kg, increasing the risk of musculoskeletal and crush injuries. Staff should be trained in dynamic risk assessment and safe handling principles, to mitigate injury risk. Once loaded into the ambulance, safety considerations must continue. All equipment must be secured to approved mountings in line with ambulance safety standards, as loose items pose a serious risk during sudden braking or collisions (BSI, 2020). Team members must remain seated and restrained whenever possible. When clinical emergencies occur that require movement within the vehicle, clear communication with the driver is paramount and should be managed by stopping the vehicle where feasible (NHS England, 2024).

Environmental factors such as temperature, lighting, seating orientation can affect team performance and safety. They can contribute to fatigue, nausea and reduced situational awareness, particularly during prolonged journeys. Close communication between the clinical and driving teams is essential to determine an appropriate driving style that balances urgency with safety. Emergency driving has a role in neonatal transport, but its risks increase under adverse conditions; therefore its use should be discussed case by case.

Transport teams must also be prepared for safety challenges outside the vehicle, such as breakdowns or involvement in road traffic incidents. Training and guidance should support staff decision-making in these situations, recognising the complexity and emotional burden associated with balancing personal safety, professional duty and clinical responsibility (NHS England, 2024).

THINK POINTS

Think about the environment inside a fast-moving ambulance for a sick and/or premature baby. Consider the potential risks that are imposed on the neonate during such a journey from the start to the destination.

GOVERNANCE

Robust **governance** underpins the safety and quality of neonatal transport services in the UK. Transport services operate within the governance frameworks of their host NHS trust and broader neonatal operational delivery networks, with specific policies and procedures tailored to the unique risks of the transport environment (NHS England, 2024). Clear, locally ratified standard operating procedures (SOPs) guide practice and distinguish the transport setting from the hospital NNU.

Good documentation is crucial for safe and high-quality care. Transport teams maintain contemporaneous records of referrals, advice calls and transfer details for all transfers. These records support clinical accountability and are aligned with national quality and safety expectations (Nursing and Midwifery Council, 2018; NHS England, 2023b). Transport services are also required to have governance policies that define incident reporting, resolution pathways and mechanisms for multidisciplinary review.

Contemporary review of transport activity helps to identify emerging issues, such as equipment failures or unexpected clinical deterioration. The NTG plays a national role in promoting professional advice, benchmarking, adverse event reporting and data collection to support shared learning and improvement across UK services. Data submission and annual audit reports are part of quality assurance and enable comparative evaluation between services nationwide (BAPM, 2025).

Local governance mechanisms might vary, but many teams hold regular multidisciplinary meetings to examine transport outcomes, review policy adherence and support staff. Embedding these activities within formal local governance structures, ensure transport teams function effectively.

THE PATIENT JOURNEY

Each transport episode involves distinct phases that ensure continuity and safety, from referral through to return to base. The stages are agreed upon at a national level: referral and triage, team mobilisation, arrival and stabilisation at the referring unit, in-transit care, handover at the receiving unit and return back to base, all represented in Figure 24.4. It is worth considering that the transport episode should only be considered complete when the team and equipment are safely back at base.

Referral and triage

The journey begins with a referral, through a dedicated pathway between referring, transport and receiving clinicians. Structured referral improves early decision-making about urgency, team composition and equipment needs. Early

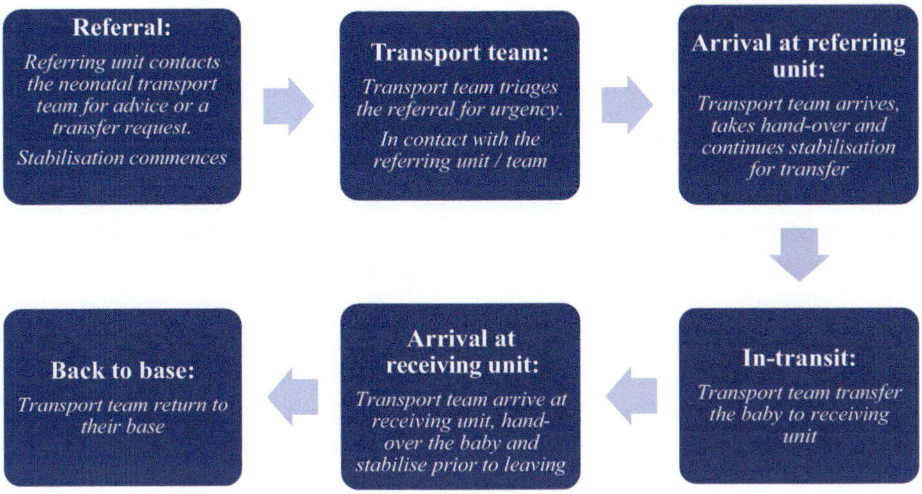

Figure 24.4 The neonatal transport journey

clinical advice can sometimes avoid an urgent transfer or reduce clinical risk before departure.

The patient journey starts with a referral call, which may be initially for clinical advice or a request for transfer. Many transport services offer a call conferencing facility which is an excellent way of sharing information and supporting clinical decision-making. The referring consultant, transport consultant, receiving consultant and specialty team, as well as other members of the transport service can be included in this call which supports the development of a shared mental model of the required actions. At this time, clinical advice for stabilisation can be given, which is sometimes all that is needed. On these calls, the transport team can arrange to make contact with the referring team in an agreed timescale in order to further assess the situation. On many occasions, it is clear that a transfer is required, and at this stage information is sought to help triage the transfer. This allows the transport team to agree the urgency of response required, the appropriate composition of the team and any additional specialist equipment required. At this stage the referring team still retains overall responsibility for the patient even though the process of transferring responsibility from referring team, to transport team and then on to the receiving team has started.

Arrival and stabilisation

On arrival at the referring unit, the transport team conducts a handover with the local staff, with all the clinical information required that allows stabilisation planning. This is a critical part of safe transfer and includes optimisation of respiratory and haemodynamic support, thermoregulation and other management (Jenkinson et al., 2025; Neonatal Network Southeast, 2025). The transport and referring teams should also introduce themselves to help improve team-working later in the transfer and identify who has been involved in the patient's care, making sure that there is opportunity to add information to the handover. Every effort should be made for a combined medical and nursing handover. This is a helpful way of ensuring a complete handover is provided and gives the referring team an opportunity to cross-check information provided. At this stage the transport team is starting to take overall responsibility for the patient.

Stabilisation is a vital component of the transport process. No matter how complex or sophisticated technological support becomes, adequate stabilisation of neonates will always be a critical determinant of a successful outcome (Wahab et al., 2019). Moreover, effective communication including handover and documentation is a very important issue. The information about the clinical condition, priorities and procedures must be reported in the same way in the files of the referring centre, the transport team and the receiving centre. Integral to the planning of this phase is preparing for an uneventful journey. Potential problems are identified and discussed and actions put in place so that they do not manifest in the ambulance, or, if they do occur, the team are primed to respond promptly and effectively (Collier & Salgin, 2024).

In-transit care

Once transfer begins, the specialised transport team is responsible for ongoing monitoring and interventions without immediate external support. Although evidence on specific clinical outcomes remains limited, specialist transport teams are associated with structured care in transit and better management of complex needs than *ad hoc* transfers by non-specialist professionals. Direct communication with the receiving unit during transit supports continuity of care (Fox et al., 2017).

Some of the potential clinical complications which teams might be faced with in transit include:

- Loss/blockage of airway
- Loss/blockage of IV access
- Snagging of monitoring lines/IV infusion lines/ventilator tubing
- Respiratory deterioration
- Cardiovascular deterioration
- Neurological deterioration.

Potential non-clinical complications include:

- Equipment failure
- Loss of power

- Gas supplies exhausted
- Team member becomes unwell
- Parent becomes unwell
- Deterioration in traffic/vehicle/road/weather conditions.

Handover at the receiving unit

Upon arrival at the receiving unit, a structured handover ensures that critical information, such as ventilation settings, vascular access, medication infusions and evolving physiological trends, is communicated clearly (Neonatal Networks Southeast, 2025). A clear transfer of responsibility at this stage minimises risks associated with incomplete handover. Minimising the risks to the neonate can be achieved by:

- Identifying a person who is leading this phase of the transfer
- Keeping the area as uncluttered as possible
- Ensuring a safety check of the receiving cot space has been carried out
- Allocating clear roles and responsibilities
- Planning the move and sharing this plan with the team
- Reassessment of the patient prior to and immediately following the move.

During this phase of the transfer, it is important to maintain attention in order to safely complete the task of transferring the care to the receiving team. Having arrived safely at the receiving location, the sense of relief mixed with fatigue from a long and potentially stressful transfer can contribute to errors occurring at this stage. Pre-briefing the transport team on arrival, ensuring the use of checklists and holding a team handover are all ways of minimising the chance of an error occurring.

Return to base

The journey is not complete until the transport team and equipment return to base, restock, clean equipment and document the transport episode. Debriefing at this stage is important, as it supports team learning and quality improvement.

CLINICAL CONSIDERATIONS IN NEONATAL TRANSPORT

Greater detail of the general management of specific clinical conditions can be found in the relevant sections of this book. However, there are times when the transport environment and process provide additional challenges to managing these conditions. While transport teams are well equipped, it is not feasible to carry every medication or piece of equipment for all eventualities. Sometimes additional subspecialty input or specialist equipment is required to refine a diagnosis and therefore assist in decisions about therapy or choice of receiving unit. An example of this could be trying to rule out a cardiac anomaly as a cause of hypoxia to ensure that the neonate is transferred to an appropriate centre. At other times, certain pieces of equipment are not available to all transport teams, such as a ventilator which can provide high frequency oscillatory ventilation.

Extreme prematurity

Neonates born at extremely low gestations are preferentially transferred *in utero* (Watson et al., 2020); however, *ex utero* transfer remains necessary in some circumstances. Extremely preterm neonates are particularly vulnerable to temperature instability, respiratory distress and haemodynamic instability during transfer.

TEMPERATURE CONTROL

Maintenance of normothermia is a core principle of neonatal care and strongly associated with improved outcomes (de Almeida et al., 2023). Transport incubators provide heating and humidification; however, environmental exposure during stabilisation and exposure to adverse conditions during loading into the ambulance increases the risk of hypothermia. UK frameworks emphasise pre-warming vehicles, minimising handling time, continuous temperature monitoring and use of adjuncts such as polyethylene wraps and warming mattresses (Neonatal Networks Southeast, 2025).

The transport team should give attention to:

- Taking care to pre-warm the ambulance
- Careful planning to minimise the time to transfer neonate from incubator to TIS
- Minimising the time the TIS is outside the vehicle
- Ensuring TIS batteries are fully charged and plugged in
- Close monitoring of the infant's temperature
- Use of thermal control adjuncts such as warming mattresses, hats, extra blankets.

SKIN INTEGRITY

Extremely preterm neonates have very fragile skin. As continuous ECG monitoring is usually essential during transfer, more UK teams utilise end-tidal or transcutaneous CO_2 monitoring to improve ventilation control, where probe placement needs careful consideration in order to maintain skin integrity (Jenkinson et al., 2025). Decisions regarding invasive monitoring and line placement must balance clinical benefit against risks of skin trauma.

VITAL SIGNS MONITORING

While an extremely preterm neonate may not routinely have electrocardiographic (ECG) monitoring in an NNU, continuous vital sign monitoring will most likely be necessary for the transport episode. These decisions should be made by the transport team caring for the neonate, considering all the clinical and logistic information available.

RESPIRATORY SUPPORT

Avoidance of ventilator-induced lung injury is paramount to modern neonatal practice. In order to achieve this, the early use of non-invasive ventilation such as CPAP is widely used across the UK and globally; however, during transport, many extremely preterm neonates are electively intubated to reduce the need for emergency intubation during transit (Jenkinson et al., 2025). Thoughtful consideration of sedation may facilitate safe ventilation while allowing early extubation at the receiving unit.

THE IMPACT OF VIBRATION AND NOISE

Physiologically unstable neonates may show exaggerated cardiovascular and neurological responses to acceleration and vibration. Earlier observational data suggested a possible association between transport and intraventricular haemorrhage, but recent UK evidence indicates the risk is more closely related to perinatal condition and early stabilisation rather than transport itself (Redpath et al., 2019). Ambulance journeys expose neonates to noise and vibration levels exceeding NNU standards, so smooth driving and careful route planning can help mitigate this stress.

Ambulance noise levels can reach 85–90 decibels (dB), far above the recommended NNU limit of 45 dB (Mayhew et al., 2022). Even standard NNU noise can cause short-term respiratory and cardiovascular effects, which are likely amplified in an ambulance. Hearing protection options for neonates are limited. Lower driving speeds and route selection can reduce noise and vibration, and extremely preterm neonates particularly benefit from a smooth, steady ride.

Acceleration, deceleration and cornering can further affect physiologically unstable neonates. Although these stimuli cannot be removed, driving style can reduce them, and teams can anticipate complications.

Surgical transfers

Concerning abdominal signs requiring surgical review are the reason for a significant number of neonatal transfers across the UK and globally. Necrotising enterocolitis (NEC) and congenital anomalies such as gastroschisis or oesophageal atresia (OA) are some of the conditions included in this category. National guidelines highlight the importance of collaborative decision-making between referring, transport and surgical teams in order to minimise any delay (BAPM, 2023). For all surgical transfers, decisions should be made by clinical collaboration between teams and, where appropriate, a swift transfer provided. Some examples are given now. Birthing in a hospital with on-site surgical facilities is considered preferable for neonates with surgical conditions. However, a recent systematic review concluded that transfer of neonates from the birth hospital to another facility for surgical intervention was not associated with increased risk of mortality or disability (Balasubramanian et al., 2025).

NECROTISING ENTEROCOLITIS

One such condition which can be managed medically but often requires surgical intervention is NEC. A particular concern for the transport team is that a tense and distended abdomen can have a negative impact on the respiratory status of the neonate. A significantly distended abdomen will reduce intrathoracic volume available for lung expansion and will be painful, so that the infant is at increased risk of apnoeas. The extra handling, vehicle vibrations and road surface issues are unfortunately likely to cause significant additional pain. Among other clinical considerations, these are two factors which may well support the decision to intubate, ventilate and sedate a neonate for transfer, who may otherwise have been stable enough to observe on a NNU. Adequate analgesia combined with sedation is vital.

GASTROSCHISIS

Most neonates with gastroschisis are delivered in regional neonatal intensive care units with surgical services, but transport teams must be prepared to stabilise and transfer these neonates within four hours of birth (Williamson et al., 2021). Many require substantial ongoing fluid resuscitation, which may continue during transfer, necessitating careful coordination with other aspects of care. Temperature control is also challenging, and maintaining normothermia requires close attention. A key objective is ensuring the neonate arrives with a pink, well-perfused gut. Reduced gut perfusion can have serious consequences (Rentea & Gupta, 2023). This is especially difficult to assess during transport because the bowel is not yet placed in a silo, and visibility is limited by lighting, seating and positioning. These constraints should be discussed in a team brief before departure, with plans to minimise risk. Close observation and documentation should occur before leaving the referring hospital, before setting off and at regular intervals during the journey. If concerns about perfusion arise, the surgical team at the receiving centre should be contacted for advice. They may arrange to meet the transport team immediately on arrival or prepare for direct transfer to theatre if required to protect bowel viability.

OESOPHAGEAL ATRESIA

Advances in antenatal ultrasonography allow early identification of surgical anomalies, enabling planned delivery at a surgical tertiary unit. However, some anomalies are missed or neonates must be born in non-surgical units. Postnatal detection may occur when nasogastric tube insertion fails, raising suspicion of OA, often associated with tracheo-oesophageal fistula (TOF). Isolated OA can be managed by placing a Replogle tube into the proximal pouch for continuous suction to prevent secretion accumulation, allowing safe transfer for surgical intervention (Puri & Zimmer, 2017). The main risk is aspiration of secretions or gastric contents via the fistula.

Primary management includes Replogle tube insertion with continuous suction and regular flushing. Some neonates may require respiratory support due to aspiration risk, but CPAP and invasive ventilation are contraindicated because positive pressure may pass through the fistula, causing gastric distension. Therefore, decisions about respiratory management during transfer of neonates with suspected TOF/OA must be made at a senior level.

PRACTICE POINTS

Specific considerations for transferring a neonate with an OA

Neonates with TOF/OA can be safely transferred breathing in air, with Replogle tube management. Continuous low flow suction is required, and the means to perform this will depend on the equipment available. Some portable suction units will permit low flow suction, though others may need an attenuating device to reduce the suction to an appropriate level.

CARDIAC ANOMALIES

Undiagnosed duct-dependent congenital heart disease can present with acute hypoxaemia or shock. When emergency transfer is required, pre-transport stabilisation and early prostaglandin infusion where indicated are critical and essential elements in order to reduce the risk of the transfer and for a favourable patient outcome. Antenatal diagnosis and pulse oximetry screening can facilitate early detection of this condition (Cloete et al., 2019).

Hypoxic-ischaemic encephalopathy and therapeutic hypothermia

Therapeutic hypothermia (TH) is the established standard of care for moderate-to-severe hypoxic-ischaemic encephalopathy (HIE) and should be delivered in tertiary centres. Many UK local neonatal units and some special care units now initiate active cooling prior to transport using servo-controlled systems, enabling neonates to reach and maintain the target temperature while awaiting transfer (BAPM, 2020). Many units also have access to cerebral function monitoring (CFM), which assists in identifying abnormal cerebral activity and detecting clinical or subclinical seizures. This information supports decision-making for TH and guides early management.

Portable cooling equipment supports safe temperature management during transit. However, portable CFM use during transport remains challenging due to vibration-related artefacts, which limit reliability and make seizure detection difficult. Nonetheless, having electrodes in situ allows CFM to be used when the vehicle is stationary if concerns arise.

Respiratory management is another key challenge. Neonates often hyperventilate in an attempt to correct acidosis, reducing $PaCO_2$. Even when intubated, they may breathe above the ventilator rate, risking hypocapnia, which is associated with poorer neurodevelopmental outcomes (Szakmar et al., 2022). Ventilation therefore requires cautious control during transfer (Redpath et al., 2022).

Palliative and end-of-life transfers

Transport for palliative care purposes, including transfer home or to hospice for redirection to comfort care, is recognised as part of family integrated care (FiCare). National perinatal palliative care frameworks emphasise advance planning, multidisciplinary communication and staff support (Wilkinson et al., 2025). The same principles apply in this special context: safe transfer planning, equipment preparation and team debriefing remain essential components of governance.

PARENTS AND NEONATAL TRANSPORT

It is vitally important to consider the experiences of parents whose child is being transferred (Lengauer & Grass, 2024). Parents are partners in the care that their baby receives in NNU the and this ethos should extend to the transport environment.

However, the opportunity to be involved in the actual care of the neonate may be limited due to many factors. These include the acute nature of many of these transfers, health of the mother, as well as the pastoral needs of the partner and related family. Professionals from the referring hospitals, transport teams and the receiving hospitals involved in these transfers can help to reduce the stress experienced by families and encourage them to feel as involved and supported as possible (Hodgson & Jackson, 2023). FiCare principles highlighted in Chapter 6 should continue at any point in a neonate's journey, including transport.

Communication

Parents often report that the lack of control experienced during childbirth is highly stressful, and transfer to referral neonatal intensive care units can further interrupt bonding (Yui & October, 2021). These experiences mirror those of parents on the NNU and are intensified when transfer to another hospital is required. Early, clear communication from the referring team about the possibility of transfer allows parents to ask questions and prepare. Neonatal professionals should prioritise effective communication, make use of video-calling platforms and support parental involvement in NNU and during transport whenever appropriate (Mason et al., 2024).

Communication between the transport team and parents is equally important. A clear introduction, explanation of the plan and brief outline of expected timelines help align expectations. Providing clinical updates and explaining responses to interventions can reduce anxiety. Where a neonate's prognosis is uncertain or poor, early communication helps prepare parents for what may lie ahead. Alongside clinical updates, parents should be informed of the risks of unexpected events during transfer and reassured that the team provide necessary expertise and equipment. They should also understand that transfer decisions are made carefully and are intended to benefit their baby.

Communication with the receiving team is another key element. Both the referring and transport teams play a role in ensuring a smooth transition. Parents who have been closely involved in their baby's care may feel they are losing control and can become anxious about meeting unfamiliar staff in a new environment. Involving parents in handover and ensuring proper introductions can help. Optimal communication about the transfer process alongside information about the receiving unit can lessen parental uncertainty (Chant et al., 2024).

Travelling in the ambulance

Over the past decade, neonatal transport services have increasingly supported parents travelling with their babies, and teams are encouraged to take parents on transfers when appropriate (Fraser & Harrison, 2025). However, parental travel is not always suitable, particularly soon after birth and caesarean section. Ambulance transport can be uncomfortable, making independent travel potentially preferable. Psychological factors are important; the ambulance environment can be overwhelming, and some anxious parents may cope better with support from family or friends. Pre-existing medical conditions may also prevent safe travel.

When parents travel with the team, careful preparation is essential. A safety brief should outline what to expect, driving style, estimated arrival times, emergency procedures and the need to wear a seatbelt and follow staff guidance. Space is limited, so luggage must be minimal and securely stowed. Whether a parent travels in the front or back depends on vehicle design, staffing needs and local SOPs, and teams must consider whether a parent's stress could distract clinicians or the driver. All team members should contribute to the decision. If a parent does not travel, they should receive clear information about the receiving hospital, including ward location, access, parking and the best contact number. All transfers can be stressful; capacity transfers move neonates away from support networks, while repatriation transfers, although generally lower risk and closer to home (BAPM, 2023) can still provoke anxiety due to transitions in staff, routines and memories of earlier illness.

PRACTICE POINT

Kangaroo care in neonatal transport

Recent evidence below advocates kangaroo care during transportation, where appropriate and if the neonate's condition allows. Read the paper below and consider this practice in terms of the feasibility, benefits and potential challenges.

Mason, L., Marufu, T. C., Warren, I., et al. (2024). Interventions for supporting parents of neonates requiring neonatal inter-hospital transport: A systematic review. *Nursing in Critical Care*, *29*(1), 164–177. https://onlinelibrary.wiley.com/doi/full/10.1111/nicc.12922

Chapter takeaways

- Neonatal transport requires specialised, highly trained multidisciplinary teams who can provide mobile intensive care, manage complex conditions and work effectively in restricted, high-pressure environments.
- Safe transfer depends on structured processes; namely, referral, stabilisation, equipment preparation, in-transit care and clear handovers, all

supported by national governance standards and robust risk-management systems.

- Environmental challenges such as noise, vibration, limited space and movement affect both neonates and staff, requiring mitigation through driving style, equipment security and anticipatory planning.
- Clinical needs vary by condition, with specific considerations for extremely preterm neonates, surgical cases, cardiac anomalies and neonates requiring therapeutic hypothermia.
- Parental communication and psychological support are essential, including clear explanations, involvement where possible, preparation for travel decisions and updates during and after transfer. Neonatal nurses need to be aware of the importance of their role in supporting parents through the distressing time of neonatal transport.
- Quality improvement and collaborative working across neonatal networks ensure equitable access to specialist care, efficient service delivery and consistent learning to enhance outcomes for neonates and families.

CASE STUDY

CASE STUDIES

These three case studies below present different neonates who all require transportation for further management of their conditions. For each case study, consider the following questions:

Q.1. Can you outline the nursing considerations when stabilising these neonates for transfer?
Q.2. Can you identify the potential risks relating to the actual transfer and how will these be minimised?
Q.3. What are the specific challenges for the families of these neonates?
Q.4. What specific care and information do the parents need?
Q.5. What information does the receiving unit need about these neonates?

Case study 1: Congenital cardiac lesion

Marcus is a term neonate born with a congenital heart defect, diagnosed following a collapse on the postnatal ward in the first day of life. He requires transfer to a specialist cardiac centre which is more than 40 miles away from the current NNU. He has a duct-dependent defect. Marcus' mother is single, and the father or partner is not present or contactable. She has her parents with her.

CASE STUDY

Case study 2: Surgical problem

Jeannie is a term neonate who after delivery was found to experience problems with feeding when she went blue and encountered coughing. A nasogastric tube was passed, but this coiled back up to the mouth and an oesophageal atresia is suspected. She is currently in a level 1 special care unit with no surgical care. Her parents have four other children.

Case study 3: Varying care levels in a set of twins

Aneesa and Jasmine are girl twins born at 27 weeks' gestation. There was a diagnosis of twin-to-twin transfusion during pregnancy. Aneesa is the receiving twin and, although she is experiencing some respiratory distress and a high packed cell volume, is being managed effectively and is stable. Jasmine, however, was born much smaller with a birthweight of 600g. She is very anaemic, hypovolaemic and is unstable with a high oxygen and ventilation requirement. She requires transfer to a level 3 neonatal intensive care unit for further management. The twins' mother Meera is currently unwell with high blood pressure and remains in the postnatal ward. Father Ali is present on the NNU. The extended family is caring for their other 2 older children at home.

For suggested answer guides to the questions posed in these case studies, please refer to the web-based companion site specific to this chapter. See www.routledge.com/cw/petty

References

Adams, E. (2022). *Neonatology GIRFT programme national specialty report.* https://gettingitrightfirsttime.co.uk/wp-content/uploads/2025/01/Neonatology-national-report-09-12i-FINAL.pdf

Aubertin, C. A., Speck, G., & Redpath, S. (2018). A dedicated neonatal transport unit pilot program: An innovative partnership. *Pediatrics*, *142*(1), 492.

Balasubramanian, H., Srinivas, A., Khedkar, P., Ananthan, A., Mohan, D., Kabra, N., & Patole, S. (2025). Association between transfer for surgery and mortality and disability among neonates in high income countries: A systematic review with meta-analysis. *PLoS ONE*, *20*(7), e0327971. https://doi.org/10.1371/journal.pone.0327971

Beccia, F., Gualano, M. R., Fevola, G., Capogna, E., Scarfagna, C., Bonacquisti, M., & Ricciardi, W. (2025). The impact of leadership interventions on neonatal care: A systematic review of current literature. *European Journal of Pediatrics*, *184*(2), 126. https://doi.org/10.1007/s00431-024-05968-8

Bekkevold, M., Solvik-Olsen, T., Lang, A. M., Heyerdahl, F., Hagemo, J. S., & Rehn, M. (2026). Data variables reported during neonatal transport: A systematic literature review. *Journal of Perinatology*, *46*(1), 6–11. https://doi.org/10.1038/s41372-025-02483-y

British Association of Perinatal Medicine. (2020). *Therapeutic hypothermia for neonatal encephalopathy: A framework for practice.* BAPM. https://www.bapm.org/resources/therapeutic-hypothermia-for-neonatal-encephalopathy

British Association of Perinatal Medicine. (2021). *Air transfer*. https://www.bapm.org/pages/air-transfer

British Association of Perinatal Medicine. (2022). *The British Association of Perinatal Medicine service and quality standards for provision of neonatal care in the UK*. https://www.bapm.org/resources/service-and-quality-standards-for-provision-of-neonatal-care-in-the-uk

British Association of Perinatal Medicine. (2023). *Safe and effective repatriation of neonates: A BAPM framework for practice*. https://www.bapm.org/resources/safe-and-effective-repatriation-of-neonates

British Association of Perinatal Medicine National Transport Group. (2025). *NTG annual transport data report: 2023/24*. https://www.bapm.org/pages/ntg-dataset

British Standards Institution. (2020). *BS EN 1789:2020: Medical vehicles and their equipment – Road ambulances*. BSI.

Chant, K., Ramesh, P., & Gallagher, K. (2024). Repatriation of babies between neonatal units: A parent survey. *Journal of Neonatal Nursing*, *30*(5), 456–460.

Cloete, E., Bloomfield, F. H., Cassells, S. A., Laat, M. W. M., Sadler, L., & Gentles, T. L. (2019). Newborn pulse oximetry screening in the context of a high antenatal detection rate of critical congenital heart disease. *Acta Paediatrica*, *109*(1), 93–99. https://doi.org/10.1111/apa.14946

Collier, L., & Salgin, B. (2024). The case for neonatal specialist transport teams. *Journal of Pediatrics: Clinical Practice*, *11*, 200105. https://doi.org/10.1016/j.jpedcp.2024.200105

de Almeida, M. F. B., Guinsburg, R., Sancho, G. A., Rosa, I. R. M., Lamy, Z. C., Martinez, F. E., & other collaborators. (2023). Neonatal thermoregulation: A cornerstone of care or forgotten principles? *Pediatric Research*, *93*, 1509–1516.

Department of Health. (2015). *Neonatal critical care retrieval (transport) service specification*. Department of Health.

Fox, G. F., Watts, T., & Hoque, N. (2017). Neonatal transport. In *Oxford handbook of neonatology* (2nd ed., 465–482). Oxford University Press.

Fraser, C., & Harrison, C. M. (2025). Parental experiences of the neonatal transfer process. *Pediatric Research*, 17. https://doi.org/10.1038/s41390-025-04402-5.

Heys, S., Yates, J., Main, C., Turton, P., & Kerslake, D. (2023). Exploring the pre-hospital setting for the emergency care and transfer of neonates: The role of UK ambulance and neonatal transport services. *Neonate*, *19*(6), 204–209.

Hodgson, H. S., & Jackson, A. (2023). Parental presence during neonatal transfers conducted by a national transport service. *Archives of Disease in Childhood – Fetal and Neonatal Edition*, *108*, 207–208.

Jenkinson, A., Dassios, T., Ratnavel, N., & Greenough, A. (2025). Respiratory support strategies in neonatal transport in the UK and Ireland. *European Journal of Pediatrics*, *184*(1). https://doi.org/10.1007/s00431-024-05947-z

Lengauer, C., & Grass, B. (2024). Neonatal transport: Parental needs and potential for improvement – a single-center cross-sectional study. *The Journal of Maternal-Fetal & Neonatal Medicine*, *37*(1). https://doi.org/10.1080/14767058.2024.2356036

Lucas, R. J., Boix, H., García, L. S., María, C. I., Couce, M. L., Losada, O. R., García, L. S., Giménez, T. E., Zafra, R. G., Ángel, M., Romero, M. C., Ángel, M., Simón, B. C., Rodríguez, N. M., Luengo, F. M., Rubio, J. D., Sánchez, M. S., Baena, L. P., & Ruiz, I. S. (2021). Recommendations on the skills profile and standards of the neonatal transport system in Spain. *Anales de Pediatría (English Edition)*, *94*(6), 420.e1–420.e11. https://doi.org/10.1016/j.anpede.2021.02.006

Mason, L., Marufu, T. C., Warren, I., Nelson, D., Cooke, S., Laparidou, D., & Manning, J. C. (2024). Interventions for supporting parents of neonates requiring neonatal inter-hospital transport: A systematic review. *Nursing in Critical Care*, *29*(1), 164–177.

Mayhew, K. J., Lawrence, S. L., Squires, J. E., & Harrison, D. (2022). Elevated sound levels in the neonatal intensive care unit: What is causing the problem? *Advances in Neonatal Care*, *22*(6), E207–E216. https://doi.org/10.1097/ANC.0000000000000996

Meyer, K., & Totapally, B. R. (2026). Neonatal and pediatric transport: A contemporary review. *Children (Basel)*, *13*(2), 175. https://doi.org/10.3390/children13020175

Murdoch, M., Kache, S., McNabb, L., Palmquist, A., Olson, M., & Sacks, L. (2019). A novel simulation based method for training pediatric & neonatal critical care transport teams. *Pediatrics*, *144*(2_MeetingAbstract), 875–875. https://doi.org/10.1542/peds.144.2ma9.875

National Quality Board/NHS England. (2023). *Safe staffing for neonatal services: Guidance*. NHS England.

Neonatal Network Southeast. (2025). *Prehospital management of preterm and term neonates: A framework for practice*. Neonatal Network Southeast. https://neonatalnetworkssoutheast.nhs.uk/professionals/guidelines/tvw-guidelines/prehospital-management/

NHS England. (2023a). *Neonatal critical care clinical network specification*. https://www.england.nhs.uk/wp-content/uploads/2024/05/PRN231107-neonatal-critical-care-network-specification-2023-.pdf

NHS England. (2023). *Towards a unified vision of nursing and midwifery documentation*. NHS England. https://www.england.nhs.uk/publication/towards-a-unified-vision-of-nursing-and-midwifery-documentation/

NHS England. (2024). *Service specification: Neonatal critical care*. https://www.england.nhs.uk/wp-content/uploads/2015/01/Neonatal-critical-care-service-specification-March-2024.pdf

Nursing and Midwifery Council (NMC). (2018). *The code: Professional standards of practice and behaviour for nurses, midwives and nursing associates*. NMC. https://www.nmc.org.uk/standards/code/

Puri, P., & Zimmer, J. (2017). Transport of the surgical neonate. In P. Puri (Ed.), *Newborn surgery* (4th ed.). Taylor and Francis.

Redpath, S., Moore, H., Sucha, E., Agarwal, A., Barrowman, N., Lemyre, B., & St Germain, L. (2022). Therapeutic hypothermia on transport: The quest for efficiency: Results of a quality improvement project. *Pediatric Quality & Safety*, *7*(3), e556. https://doi.org/10.1097/pq9.0000000000000556

Redpath, S., Shah, P. S., Moore, G. P., Yang, J., Toye, J., Perreault, T., & Lee, K. S. (2019). Do transport factors increase the risk of severe brain injury in outborn neonates <33 weeks gestational age? *Journal of Perinatology*, *40*(3), 385–393. https://doi.org/10.1038/s41372-019-0447-1

Rentea, R. M., & Gupta, V. (2023). Gastroschisis. In *StatPearls* [Internet]. StatPearls Publishing. https://www.ncbi.nlm.nih.gov/books/NBK557894/

Scottish Ambulance Service. (2026). *ScotSTAR: Scottish specialist transport and retrieval service*. https://www.neonataltransport.scot.nhs.uk/

Serou, N., Sahota, L. M., Husband, A. K., Forrest, S. P., Slight, R. D., & Slight, S. P. (2021). Learning from safety incidents in high-reliability organizations: A systematic review of learning tools that could be adapted and used in healthcare. *International Journal for Quality in Health Care*, *33*(1), mzab046. https://doi.org/10.1093/intqhc/mzab046

Szakmar, E., Munster, C., El-Shibiny, H., Jermendy, A., Inder, T., & El-Dib, M. (2022). Hypocapnia in early hours of life is associated with brain injury in moderate to severe neonatal encephalopathy. *Journal of Perinatology*, *42*(7), 892–897. https://doi.org/10.1038/s41372-022-01398-2

Wahab, M. G. A., Thomas, S., Murthy, P., & Chakkarapani, A. A. (2019). Factors affecting stabilization times in neonatal transport. *Air Medical Journal*, *38*(5), 334–337.

Watson, H., McLaren, J., Carlisle, N., Ratnavel, N., Watts, T., Zaima, A., Tribe, R. M., & Shennan, A. H. (2020). All the right moves: Why in utero transfer is both important for the baby and difficult to achieve and new strategies for change. *F1000Research*, *9*. https://doi.org/10.12688/f1000research.25923.1

Wilkinson, D., Bertaud, S., Mancini, A., & BAPM Working Group. (2025). Recognising uncertainty: An integrated framework for palliative care in perinatal medicine. *Archives of Disease in Childhood – Fetal and Neonatal Edition*, *110*, 236–244.

Williamson, S. L., Lawrence, L., Suren Arul, G., & Rasiah, S. V. (2021). Management and outcome for babies born with a gastroschisis. *Neonate Journal*, *17*(1), 9–12.

Yui, Y., & October, T. W. (2021). Parental perspectives on the postpartum bonding experience after neonatal intensive care unit transfer to a referral hospital. *American Journal of Perinatology*, *38*(13), 1358–1365.

25 FINAL COMMENTS: THE IMPORTANCE OF EVIDENCE-BASED NEONATAL PRACTICE

Julia Petty

CONTENTS

DOI: 10.4324/9781003591405-30

GUIDANCE ON HOW TO ENHANCE PERSONAL LEARNING FROM THIS CHAPTER

Key points covered in this chapter

- What is evidence-based practice applied to neonatal care?
- What are the forms of knowledge applicable to neonatal nursing practice?
- The importance and value of an evidence-based approach to neonatal care.

Reflection

Reading through the chapter, you are encouraged to engage with the key points and related literature in an enquiring way. Ask these questions:

- How has research generated new knowledge in neonatal care?
- How has new knowledge and evidence influenced your own practice?
- Can you think of any specific examples of research that has had a positive impact on infants and their families?

Implications for nursing care

- Finally: how will this chapter enable you to consider and understand the importance of research and evidence-based practice in neonatal care? Consider the implications of what you learn as relevant to current and future practice development.

INTRODUCTION AND BACKGROUND

This final chapter builds upon the foundational knowledge explored in previous sections, focusing on the integration of **evidence-based** practice (EBP) within neonatal care. It highlights the significance, relevance and practical application of EBP in neonatal settings, emphasising the need for neonatal nurses and allied health professionals to critically engage with diverse forms of knowledge. The chapter also explores the resources available to support clinical decision-making and highlights a balanced, pragmatic approach when addressing the complex needs of neonates and their families. Again, while the UK perspective is drawn upon, reference will be made to the global picture in the name of the importance of shared learning and networking across international boundaries (Petty et al., 2022; Council of International Neonatal Nurses (COINN), 2021, 2025)

NEONATAL KNOWLEDGE AND EVIDENCE-BASED PRACTICE

To effectively implement EBP, the neonatal healthcare team must understand the various forms of evidence and how they can be integrated into clinical care. The source of evidence used to acquire knowledge is depicted in Figure 25.1. This includes not only research-based knowledge but also clinical expertise, patient preferences and contextual factors.

Knowledge derived from research

Historically, neonatal care relied heavily on textbooks and peer-reviewed journals, which, while valuable, were limited by publication delays and accessibility. The digital era has transformed this landscape, enabling rapid access to a vast array of research through online databases. This shift has coincided with a surge in neonatal research output, driven by both technological innovation and a growing emphasis on family integrated care. A widely accepted model for evaluating research quality is the hierarchy of evidence (Wallace et al., 2022), which ranks sources based on methodological rigor (Figure 25.2). At the top are systematic reviews, meta-analyses and national clinical guidelines, which according to advocates of this model, provide the most reliable evidence for practice. Randomised controlled trials (RCTs) and cohort studies follow, while case reports, expert opinions and patient experiences are considered lower-tier evidence.

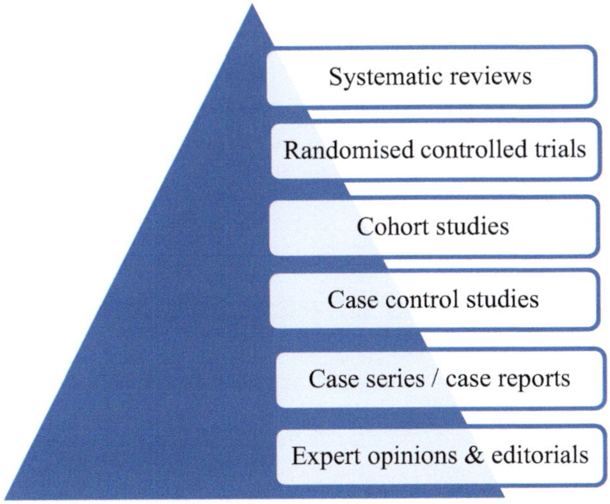

Figure 25.1 Sources of knowledge for evidence-based nursing practice

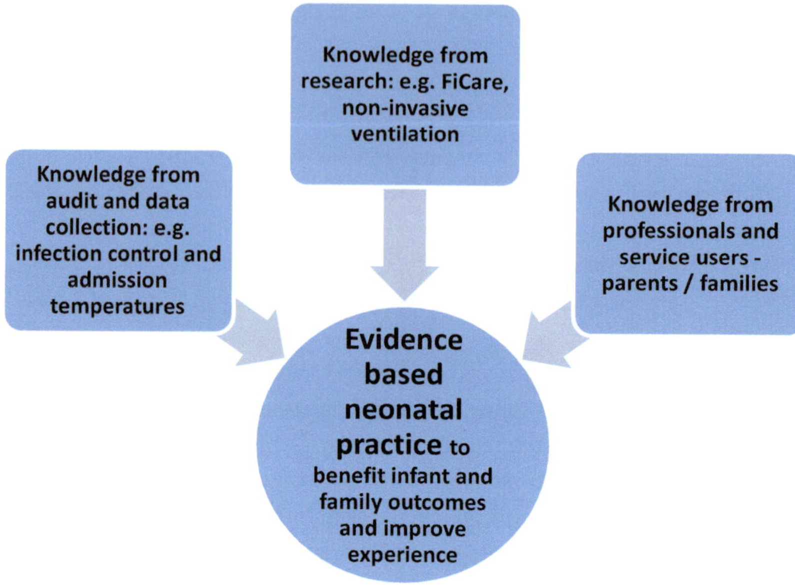

Figure 25.2 The hierarchy of evidence

However, the value and application of qualitative, interpretive and/or narrative-based research to explore the human experience and the humanistic elements of healthcare, that cannot be measured quantifiably, should not be underestimated. This is especially so within the context of nursing care and research where such methodologies are well-suited and highly valuable for us to understand our patients. Qualitative research is invaluable in facilitating knowledge and insights into the patient or parent experience in order to learn and improve practice (Petty et al., 2025), raising a critical question about the appropriateness of an evidence hierarchy. Most importantly, whatever type of research is undertaken, it should positively impact on infants and families in our care. A summary of EBP that has been shown to influence outcomes of infants and/or families is outlined in Box 25.1.

BOX 25.1 EXAMPLES OF RESEARCH WHICH HAVE IMPACTED NEONATAL PRACTICE

- Family integrated care
- Developmental care/individualised developmental care programmes
- Parents' experiences
- Skin-to-skin care

- Pain assessment and management
- The first hour of care (golden hour)
- Optimised cord management at birth
- Newborn resuscitation and stabilisation
- Feeding regimes and the value of breastmilk
- Thermal care (e.g. polyethylene bags/wraps for preterm infants)
- Non-invasive ventilation
- Surfactant therapy
- Antenatal corticosteroid and magnesium sulphate administration for preterm birth
- Therapeutic hypothermia for hypoxic-ischaemic encephalopathy.

Knowledge from critical appraisal and practical application

One vital skill in nursing and healthcare, in order to provide best practice for neonates and families, is accessing appropriate, recent and quality research-based evidence and to approach this in a critical way to ensure it is robust and relevant. Given the ethical and logistical challenges of conducting RCTs in neonatal populations, much of the available research may be observational and/or interpretive. While valuable, such studies must be critically appraised for validity, bias and clinical relevance. Importantly, statistically significant findings do not always equate to meaningful clinical outcomes. Several key literature databases are prominent in the healthcare field, offering access to a vast collection of research and evidence. PubMed, CINAHL, Embase and the Cochrane library are frequently cited as essential resources for healthcare professionals and researchers. Peer-reviewed journals such as the *Journal of Neonatal Nursing, Archives of Disease in Childhood – Fetal and Neonatal Edition* and *Journal of Perinatal & Neonatal Nursing* continue to expand the body of neonatal-specific literature. The accessibility of online and open access platforms has further accelerated the translation of research into practice, such as PubMed Central (PMC), a free full-text archive of health, biomedical and life sciences journal literature at the U.S. National Institutes of Health's National Library of Medicine (NIH/NLM). The International Society for Evidence-Based Neonatology (EBNEO) was founded in 2015 with a vision that neonatal care should be firmly based on the best available evidence. This vision includes a short passage from research-based knowledge to implementation in neonatal care (translation), thereby improving survival, decreasing morbidities and promoting long-lasting health for newborn infants.

Knowledge from national and international data resources

Several key national and international data resources are currently used in neonatal healthcare to improve patient care and outcomes. The National Neonatal Research Database (NNRD) in the UK is a comprehensive, longitudinal dataset containing information on all admissions to NHS neonatal units (NNUs). This supports initiatives such as the National Neonatal Audit Programme (NNAP), which aims to standardise care and improve outcomes. As an example of data usage and benchmarking, the UK Neonatal Transport Group (UK NTG) collects annual national data, allowing quality comparisons across teams (British Association of Perinatal Medicine (BAPM), 2025). This approach helps optimise transport protocols and improves patient outcomes. Internationally, the Vermont Oxford Network (VON) provides a global neonatal database with quality improvement and educational resources. These resources facilitate research, audit, benchmarking and quality improvement initiatives in neonatal care. To enhance transparency and reduce research duplication, clinical trial registries have become essential. Platforms such as ClinicalTrials.gov and the UK's National Perinatal Epidemiology Unit (NPEU) allow neonatal healthcare professionals to track ongoing studies and anticipate future evidence that may influence practice.

Knowledge from national and global clinical guidance and standards

National and global guidelines along with position statements provide evidence-based, current standards of care to ensure consistent knowledge to apply to practice. UK-based examples are provided by the Neonatal Nurses Association (NNA), the National Institute for Health and Care Excellence (NICE) and Getting It Right First Time (2022). Overseas, the European Standards of Care for Newborn Health, the Global Foundation for the Care of Newborn Infants (GFCNI), the Jessica Briggs Institute (JBI) and the World Health Organization (WHO), all provide open-access, accessible web-based resources on their online platforms.

It is also imperative that the various guidelines align with each other. A good example of this was demonstrated in 2024, when two significant guidelines were released emphasising the need for inclusive clinical practice and education in neonatal care. BAPM introduced a new framework for practice, recommending routine pulse oximetry testing for all asymptomatic newborns of 34 weeks and above. Additionally, in November 2024, NHS England (NHSE) published National standards for neonatal Qualified in Specialty (QIS) education. Both guidelines incorporate recommendations from the NHS Race and Health Observatory's (NHS RHO, 2023) review of neonatal assessment and practice report.

Knowledge from clinical audit and data collection

Clinical audit remains a cornerstone of quality improvement in neonatal care. It involves evaluating clinical performance against evidence-based standards to identify areas for improvement (Foy et al., 2020). The NHS's original quality framework emphasised audit as a key component of clinical effectiveness. More recently, audit and feedback have been shown to improve patient care when implemented thoughtfully, especially when combined with educational strategies and tailored interventions (Fontaine et al., 2024). The NNAP continues to be a vital tool in the UK, measuring key indicators such as admission temperature, antenatal steroid use and breastmilk feeding at discharge. These metrics help NNUs benchmark performance and drive improvements in care quality. The Neonatal Data Analysis Unit (NDAU) supports this by analysing data from BadgerNet, a digital platform used primarily in the UK that replaced traditional paper records with a secure, electronic system. This type of system ensures that audit findings are actionable and relevant to frontline practice.

Knowledge from professionals and service users

Research evidence from RCTs is not always feasible in neonatal settings. In such cases, qualitative research provides valuable insights into the experiences of both families and healthcare professionals. Recent studies continue to support its use in exploring sensitive topics such as bereavement care and parental involvement in NNUs. However, as well as national data on parent experience, it is important that local experience is also demonstrated and shared. This can be done through several approaches, including questionnaires such as local unit surveys of parental experiences, thematic review of complaints and correspondence from parents and families along with face-to-face discussion. Integrated workshops with both service users and neonatal staff also provide valuable knowledge about the local service. The lived experience of the babies in neonatal care and their families is a valuable, enlightening and important source of evidence that neonatal nurses and AHPs should synthesise into their EBP.

The code of practice of the UK professional regulator requires nurses to work in partnership with patients to ensure care is delivered effectively, so that patients are empowered to share clinical decisions (Nursing and Midwifery Council (NMC), 2018). Figure 25.2 outlines the different sources of knowledge. Tacit knowledge, gained through experience rather than formal study, remains essential in neonatal nursing in particular. It includes intuitive skills which develop over time and contribute to expert clinical judgment. This aligns with Benner's 'novice to expert' model and is reinforced through mentorship, preceptorship and peer learning.

Knowledge from professional organisations

Professional organisations provide a rich and valuable source of information, resources and support. These include the aforementioned NNA in the UK, and other professional organisations such as the Royal College of Nursing (RCN), BAPM and the Royal College of Paediatrics and Child Health (RCPCH). The UK NNA (2026) provides a comprehensive interactive careers framework to guide nurses through their professional progression from pre-registration student up to advanced practice. Global organisations also serve to provide support, guidance, benchmarking and tailored information such as the COINN, GFCNI, WHO and UNICEF.

Charities provide resources for both professionals and, importantly, for parents who are a key resource for qualitative evidence regarding neonatal care. Charities also publish and disseminate key reports and data from both research and national audits. Bliss, Tommy's and TinyLife, as UK examples, are service user advocate organisations utilising parental experiences to promote optimal baby-centred care for those neonates nursed in NNUs. Bliss undertakes surveys of parental experiences and generates reports that inform policy and national guidance for neonatal care. Members work alongside the government, commissioners and with local stakeholders to provide a user perspective for necessary resources, unit guidelines and support for families in the NNUs.

EDUCATION AND APPLICATION OF KNOWLEDGE TO PRACTICE

EBP is a foundational element of both undergraduate and post-registration healthcare education. Recent curriculum guidelines, for example, from NHS England (2024), the National Association of Neonatal Nurse Practitioners (NANNP) in the United States and COINN (2021) emphasise the integration of EBP competencies into neonatal nurse training, ensuring that nurses are equipped to apply research in clinical settings. Despite this, translating EBP from theory to practice remains challenging. Literature suggests that while student nurses value EBP, they often struggle to apply it during placements due to limited support and time constraints (Dabkowski et al., 2026). Preceptors may also lack the skills to mentor students effectively in EBP, highlighting a need for ongoing professional development.

Protected time, access to digital resources and librarian support are essential to help neonatal nurses develop critical appraisal skills and stay current with research. Digital platforms are increasingly used to share innovations, such as the Red Hat Project linked to the ATAIN initiative, which gained traction through social media engagement. Conferences (e.g. NNA, RCN, COINN, REaSoN,

SIGNEC UK) and special interest groups like NNA LEARN and the Improvement Science Research Network (ISRN) also provide valuable opportunities for knowledge exchange and professional networking. Finally, participation in national research initiatives, such as those led by the NPEU, allows neonatal healthcare professionals to engage directly with clinical research, enhancing their understanding and application of EBP in practice.

THINK POINTS

- How will you apply the learning from this chapter to your practice? On your next shift? Next month? Next year?
- Are your literature searching skills up to date?
- Does your organisation provide training to improve evidence-based practice skills?
- Could you set up a journal club in your unit? Or could you support one that already exists?

Activities

Can you identify any areas of care that require change or that need to be introduced into the clinical area to improve care of neonates and families? What further research and enquiry is required? Is it possible to address the gaps or areas of improvement by a quality-improvement (QI) project?

Consider how we learn from both national and global standards and guidelines. What is universally applicable across global boundaries to apply to the care of neonates and families born anywhere in the world?

Practice points

Think about an area of practice that you take part in when caring for a neonate/family on the NNU or in the community setting.

What forms of evidence did you use to guide your clinical practice?

How did you know these sources were up to date and reliable?

Was your practice evidence-based?

Were there any areas of care that are not supported by evidence or research or that require an update in knowledge?

Chapter takeaways

- Evidence-based practice in neonatal nursing and healthcare practice is dynamic and multifaceted.

- By critically engaging with high-quality evidence, leveraging national data resources and staying informed through service-user/family engagement, professional organisations, journals and registries, neonatal nurses and the team of allied healthcare professionals can ensure their practice remains current, compassionate and clinically effective.
- This book endeavours to contribute to the body of knowledge from the above sources, aiming to impart key information for neonatal healthcare professionals to learn from and apply to best practice of the neonate and family, wherever they work in the world.

CASE STUDY

CASE STUDIES

Case study 1: Producing an evidence-based guideline

You work on a NNU where parents can visit any time, but extended family can only visit at set times which are limited to 1-hour periods. You are aware that a family were upset that the grandparents weren't allowed free access to their first grandchild. Professionals have also expressed that it can be difficult with lots of visitors in the unit, especially when babies are very sick. You are asked to update the unit visiting guideline.

Q.1. Which sources would you use in order to provide the most evidence-based guidance?
Q.2. What are you expecting each source to add to the process?
Q.3. What obstacles do you envision occurring?
Q.4. How will you overcome these obstacles?

Case study 2: The expert vs. the novice approach

Jane is a midwifery student on her NNU placement. Her mentor is an experienced neonatal nurse. They are caring for an extremely preterm infant who has redirection of care and dies shortly afterwards.

Q.1. What forms of knowledge will Jane use to provide care for the family at this time?
Q.2. What forms of knowledge will her mentor use to support the family?
Q.3. What forms of knowledge will her mentor use to support Jane?
Q.4. How will Jane use this experience in future practice?

For suggested answer guides to the questions posed in these case studies, please refer to the web-based companion site specific to this chapter. See www.routledge.com/cw/petty

References

British Association of Perinatal Medicine. (2025). *Neonatal transport group dataset*. https://www.bapm.org/pages/ntg-dataset

Council of International Neonatal Nurses. (2021). *COINN core competencies*. https://www.coinnurses.org/competencies

Council of International Neonatal Nurses. (2025). *Unifying neonatal nurses globally*. https://www.coinnurses.org/about-us

Dabkowski, E., Winchester, T., & Barbagallo, M. (2026). Exploring student nurses' perspectives of research and evidence-based practice: A pre-and postintervention study using authentic assessment. *Teaching and Learning in Nursing*. https://doi.org/10.1016/j.teln.2025.12.027

Fontaine, G., Vinette, B., Weight, C., Maheu-Cadotte, M.-A., Lavallée, A., Deschênes, M.-F., Lapierre, A., Castiglione, S. A., Chicoine, G., Rouleau, G., Argiropoulos, N., Konnyu, K., Mooney, M., Cassidy, C. E., Mailhot, T., Lavoie, P., Pépin, C., Cossette, S., Gagnon, M.-P., . . . Middleton, S. (2024). Effects of implementation strategies on nursing practice and patient outcomes: A comprehensive systematic review and meta-analysis. *Implementation Science*, *19*, 68. https://doi.org/10.1186/s13012-024-01398-0

Foy, R., Skrypak, M., Alderson, S., Ivers, N. M., McInerney, B., Stoddart, J., Ingham, J., & Keenan, D. (2020). Revitalising audit and feedback to improve patient care. *British Medical Journal*, *368*. https://doi.org/10.1136/bmj.m213

Getting It Right First Time. (2022). *Neonatology – workforce*. GIRFT Programme National Specialty Report. https://gettingitrightfirsttime.co.uk/wp-content/uploads/2025/01/Neonatology-workforce-report-09-12f-FINAL.pdf

Neonatal Nurses Association. (2026). *Neonatal careers framework*. https://nna.org.uk/neonatal-nurse-career-framework/

NHS England. (2024). *National standards for neonatal qualified in specialty (QIS) education*. https://www.england.nhs.uk/long-read/national-standards-for-neonatal-qualified-in-specialty-qis-education/

NHS Race and Health Observatory. (2023). *Review of neonatal assessment and practice in Black, Asian, and minority ethnic newborns*. https://nhsrho.org/wp-content/uploads/2023/08/RHO-Neonatal-Assessment-Report.pdf

Nursing and Midwifery Council (NMC). (2018). *The code: professional standards of practice and behaviour for nurses, midwives and nursing associates*. NMC. https://www.nmc.org.uk/standards/code/

Petty, J., Harding, C., & Whiting, L. (2025). Investigating parental perspectives of the enablers and barriers to communication with their preterm infants: A narrative study. *Journal of Child Health Care*, *26*, 13674935241302437. https://doi.org/10.1177/13674935241302437

Petty, J., Jones, T., van den Hoogen, A., Walker, K., & Kenner, C. (Eds.). (2022). *Neonatal nursing: A global perspective*. Springer Publishing.

Wallace, S. S., Barak, G., Truong, G., & Parker, M. W. (2022). Hierarchy of evidence within the medical literature. *Hospital Pediatrics*, *12*(8), 745–750. https://doi.org/10.1542/hpeds.2022-006690

INDEX

Note: page numbers in *italics* indicate a figure, page numbers in **bold** indicate a table, and page numbers in ***bold italics*** indicate a box on the corresponding page.

For Product Safety Concerns and Information please contact our
EU representative GPSR@taylorandfrancis.com Taylor & Francis
Verlag GmbH, Kaufingerstraße 24, 80331 München, Germany